Spiritual Care in Palliative Care

Megan C. Best
Editor

Spiritual Care in Palliative Care

What it is and Why it Matters

Springer

Editor
Megan C. Best
Institute for Ethics and Society
University of Notre Dame
Sydney, NSW, Australia

ISBN 978-3-031-50863-9 ISBN 978-3-031-50864-6 (eBook)
https://doi.org/10.1007/978-3-031-50864-6

This Springer imprint is published by the registered company Springer Nature Switzerland AG
The registered company address is: Gewerbestrasse 11, 6330 Cham, Switzerland

Foreword

Spirituality is an essential element of whole person care. For centuries, healers from different cultures and religions were integrated into the holistic care of people. Scientific advances in the twentieth century shifted the emphasis of care to the physical aspect of care. However, leaders such as Dr. Paul Tournier in the 1950s and Dr. Cicely Saunders, the founder of Hospice and Palliative Care in London in the 1960s, resurfaced the importance of attending to the whole person. I was privileged to build on this work by establishing consensus models with a focus on addressing spiritual health and attending to spiritual distress. These models and the resurgence of research in spiritual care practice by clinicians and spiritual care specialists have helped to advance this important clinical area of care, particularly for patients with serious illness. It also impacted the inclusion of spiritual care in the World Health Assembly Resolution on Palliative Care.

This book, *Spiritual Care in Palliative Care: What It Is and Why It Matters*, is an excellent compilation of scholarly work from an international panel of authors offering guidance for adapting to cultural and religious diversity for a range of patient cohorts, as well as considering the differing roles in the multidisciplinary team. I strongly recommend this resource for all those interested in addressing the critical need for spiritual care in those with complex, serious, and life-limiting illness.

GW Institute for Spirituality and Health
George Washington University,
Washington, DC, USA

Christina Puchalski

Foreword

Preface

I once heard the founder of the modern palliative care movement, Cicely Saunders, talk about how she would sit at the end of her patients' beds and record their stories. As she listened, she became aware of the multifaceted nature of their suffering, resulting from the many losses inherent within the end of life trajectory. Sources of distress were identified across all dimensions of the human experience—including not only the physical but also domains such as the psychological, emotional, social, financial, and of course, spiritual. This led to her conceptualisation of 'total pain', which is a key to understanding the need for spiritual care in palliative care. The World Health Organization has embraced this perspective in defining palliative care as healthcare that relieves 'serious health-related suffering, be it physical, psychological, social, or spiritual'. All dimensions of the person need attention if we are to provide the best possible care.

But spiritual care is not 'one size fits all'. As there are many sources of suffering, so are there a range of spiritual needs and ways to find spiritual strength. This book is an attempt to provide instruction on how to best support patients across a breadth of contexts, whatever your professional perspective. It combines the findings of empirical research with clinical wisdom from international leaders in the field to provide guidance for our quest to support our patients and their families through some of the most difficult experiences they will ever face. Patient case histories are provided throughout this book to assist in practical application of spiritual care principles. Patient details have been altered to ensure confidentiality.

We begin with a reminder of the spiritual nature of the end of life journey through hearing palliative care patients recount their experience of dreams and visions. We then explore the nature of spirituality in the context of healthcare and how our terminology developed, before considering spiritual needs for patients approaching the end of life, including challenges for their measurement.

Diversity exists within spiritual experience. Religion is one way of experiencing spirituality and at times will lead to distinctively religious needs which require familiarity with that religion's tenets if those needs are to be met. We therefore include a focus on religious care in the second section, addressing indigenous and major world faiths, and compare it to a non-religious approach.

One justification for spiritual care provision is the positive impact it can have. This is examined in the third section of this book. We examine some of the main areas where spirituality can impact patient outcomes, with a special focus on areas of particular interest in the palliative care setting, namely the interaction between spirituality and pain management, and mental health.

The fourth section focuses on the practice of spiritual care. We start by considering the nature of compassion as an essential component of care provision, before exploring a range of approaches to care. Barriers to care provision and ways to overcome them are also addressed.

Diagnosis of a life-limiting illness challenges the world view of the patient, and spiritual resources are required to cope with the threat to mortality. If existential questions remain unanswered, suffering can ensure. And so, in the fifth section of this book, we focus on the experience of spiritual suffering and existential distress—how it manifests, and ways it can be addressed.

Training in spiritual care is the strongest predictor of its provision, so in the sixth section we look at aspects of spiritual care training across the multidisciplinary team. We begin by considering some extant examples of interprofessional training and the need for practices to be both culturally safe for our patients and promoting well-being for ourselves. The distinctive nature of spiritual care for the doctor, nurse, chaplain, and social worker is described in detail.

Our spiritual journey across the lifespan and in different settings is not consistent, and so we then explore the variations in spiritual care that may at times be required. We traverse the spectrum of patients we may encounter in our work and illustrate how to care for the family members who accompany them.

We end by looking at policy issues, including the ethics that should guide our practice, and the difference that leadership at the institutional level can make in ensuring spiritual care provision for all who need it.

I am delighted that we have been able to include such a wide range of approaches to spiritual care and give some insight into the exciting areas of research that are advancing this field of knowledge. I hope it will spark new cross-disciplinary paths of inquiry. Our patients can only benefit from these initiatives.

I am greatly indebted to the authors who have generously contributed to this work and thank them for their involvement in this project. I can see that many of them have also sat with their patients and learned from their stories. I have learnt a lot from this book and hope that you will also.

Sydney, Australia
December 2023

Megan C. Best

Contents

Part I
Introduction

Dreams and Visions at the End of Life

Christopher Kerr and Carine Mardorossian

Abstract Pre-death dreams and visions (end-of-life experiences) have been documented throughout history and across cultures. Yet, despite their universality and clinical significance, they have rarely been explained in a care-giving framework or presented as being clinically relevant. This chapter will explore this topic from the perspective of the dying rather than the observer. It is based on published, quantified data that draw on the dying experiences of over 1200 patients and their families. The objective is to explain, often in the patients' own words, why pre-death dreams and visions are extraordinary occurrences that bring comfort and exemplify human resilience. These are not regular dreams and distinct from states of confusion or delirium. They are momentous occurrences in patients' experience of dying, which they describe as 'more real than real' and that often marks a transition from distress to acceptance. These end-of-life experiences help patients restore meaning, make sense of the dying process and assist in reclaiming it as an experience in which the dying have say.

Keywords End-of-life experiences · Pre-death dreams and visions · Delirium Hospice · Palliative care · Dying process · Spiritual care

C. Kerr (✉)
Hospice & Palliative Care Buffalo, Cheektowaga, NY, USA
e-mail: ckerr@palliativecare.org

C. Mardorossian
University of Buffalo, Buffalo, NY, USA
e-mail: cmardoro@buffalo.edu

M. C. Best (ed.), *Spiritual Care in Palliative Care*,
https://doi.org/10.1007/978-3-031-50864-6_1

1 Introduction

I am a doctor, and all of my patients die.

What we know of dying we know as witnesses: scenes of grim physical decline and feelings of profound loss. Yet, as a Hospice doctor, I have been at the bedside of thousands of patients who, in the face of death, often speak of love, meaning, and grace. They reveal that there is often hope beyond cure as patients transition from a focus on cure to notions of personal meaning. As illness advances, 'grace and grit' collide and often bring new insight to the dying, insight that is often paradoxically life-affirming. These end-of-life experiences include pre-death dreams and visions that are manifestations of a time of integration and coming into oneself. So yes, all my patients die, but not before they find a path to affirming the love they felt, the relationships they cherished, and the life they led.

My own understanding of this process first came into focus after caring for a young man named Tom. Tom was only 40 when he arrived at hospice with end-stage HIV. Unlike most of my patients, he was not surrounded by loved ones. Not a soul came to visit. Ever. He was rather stoic, so I wondered if the absence of visitors was his choice rather than a symptom of his loneliness. Maybe that was his way of refusing to give death an audience.

I was puzzled but, wanting to respect his privacy, did not inquire. Despite a gaunt and haggard appearance, Tom's emaciated body showed traces of once chiselled muscles. He had kept fit and was still quite young, which immediately gave me hope. In light of his age and physical conditioning, I thought that his body would be more likely to respond positively to life-prolonging treatment. Not long after he was admitted, I went to the nurses' station and decreed that 'I think we can buy Tom some time. IV antibiotics and fluids should do it'.

The charge nurse, Nancy, had been at hospice for much longer than I had. She knew her job, and everyone looked up to her. She was also not one to mince her words. Still, her response took me by surprise: 'Too late. He's dying'.

I said, 'Oh really?'

She said, 'Yep. He's been dreaming about his dead mother'.

I chuckled awkwardly—equal parts disbelief and defensiveness.

'I don't remember that class from medical school', I said.

Nancy did not miss a beat, 'Son, you must have missed a lot of classes'.

I was a 30-year-old cardiology fellow, working weekends at Hospice to pay the bills while I was finishing my specialty training. Nancy was an exceptional veteran nurse who had little patience for young idealistic doctors. She did what she always did when someone was out of their depth, she rolled her eyes.

I went about my business, mentally running through all that modern medicine could bring to bear to give Tom another few weeks or even months. Knowing that Tom could not be 'saved', I was still determined to do everything possible to give him more time and make him less miserable. He was riddled with infections, so we administered antibiotics. Since he was also severely dehydrated, I asked for a saline drip. I did all I could do as a doctor to prolong his life, and within 48 hours, Tom was dead.

Nancy had been right in her estimation of where he was on the downwards slope. But how could she have known? Was it just pessimism—the numbing effect of having watched so many people die? Was she truly using a patient's dream as predictor of life span? Nancy had worked in hospice a long time. She was tuned into aspects of dying I knew nothing about—the subjective dimensions of dying which were exactly what my training and expertise as a doctor had taught me to ignore.

Like many physicians, I'd never even considered that there's more to death than an enemy to be fought. I knew about blind intervention—doing everything possible to keep people conscious and breathing—but had little regard for how any given individual might wish to die, or for the fact that, ultimately, death is inevitable. Since it had not been part of my medical education, I failed to see how the subjective experience of dying could be relevant to my role as a doctor.

It was ultimately the remarkable recurrence of pre-death dreams and visions among dying patients that made me realise how profound and widespread a phenomenon this was. These were powerful and stirring experiences that occurred in the last days or hours of life, moments of genuine insight or vivid re-centring that often brought them a sense of wholeness and tranquillity. These are not regular dreams. They are momentous occurrences in patients' experience of dying, which they describe as 'more real than real' and that often mark their transition from distress to acceptance. They are unique to every individual and their needs, and give insight into the life that was led, lessen the fear of impending death, and establish connectivity between and across lives, both living and dead. They are centred on self-understanding, concrete relationships, personal histories, and singular events, not abstract preoccupations with the great beyond. They are made of images and tapestries that are rooted in each person's unique life experiences. They are about a walk in the woods relived alongside a loving parent, car rides or fishing trips taken with close family members, or seemingly insignificant details like the colour of a loved one's dress, the touch of a horse's velvety muzzle, or the rustling sound of a cottonwood's shimmering leaves in the backyard of one's childhood home. Long-lost loved ones come back to reassure; past wounds are healed; loose ends are tied; lifelong conflicts are revisited; forgiveness is achieved. These are the intimate, ordinary but meaningful elements that populate my patients' inner world before death, and amazingly, it is precisely in these seemingly unremarkable occurrences that the dying often find the most profound resolution to lifelong regrets and conflicts.

In restoring meaning, end-of-life dreams and visions help us by making sense of our final process and assist in reclaiming it as an experience in which we have a say. Dreams and visions at the end of life also benefit those left behind, the bereaved, who get relief from seeing their loved ones pass with a sense of calm closure. These subjective experiences are powerful reminders that beauty and love in human existence often manifest themselves when we least expect it. The patients who summon up comforting processes at life's end are beset by symptoms of a failing body over which they have limited control. They are at their most frail and vulnerable, existing within suffering states of aching bones and air hunger. Catheters, IV's, and pills may now be part of their everyday, sometimes literally functioning as extensions of their bodies under the daily medical management that is their new and irreversible lot.

They may experience various degrees of cognitive, psychological, and spiritual dissonance. Yet even as the inexorable march of time is taking its toll on their bodies and minds, many also have pre-death dreams and visions in the context of which they display remarkable awareness and mental sharpness. Herein lies the paradox of dying: patients are often emotionally and spiritually alive, even enlightened, despite their precipitous physical deterioration. Doing justice to their end-of-life experiences means accounting for this paradox, one in which death and dying are about physical decline and sadness, but also about spiritual awakening, beauty, and grace. It also means recognising the degree to which the self-soothing power of people's end-of-life experiences may be compromised by the medicalisation of the dying process.

Interestingly, the richest, most thoughtful and resonant discussions on the subject have come from the humanities: from writers, poets, and philosophers, rather than from the work of psychoanalysts, scientists, sociologists, or medical professionals. These latter disciplines aim to describe and prove hypotheses in a more or less objective fashion. By contrast, it is the role of the humanities to bear witness to the irreducible complexity of humanity's subjective experiences. There is no doubt a place for both of these perspectives in our approach to dying, but this difference is crucial when trying to redress the overmedicalisation of mortality in our contemporary lives. It explains why patients themselves, as well as their caretakers, are more drawn to the imaginative and creative arts to make sense of their end-of-life journey. The acceleration of the science of medicine has tended to obscure its art. Medicine, always less comfortable with the subjective, is more concerned with disproving the unseen rather than revering its meaning. Yet, it is through the humanities that we can touch human emotions that are inaccessible to science alone.

In the West, end-of-life dreams and visions have more recently been discussed as evidence of phenomena ranging from the neuronal workings of a dying brain to the consequences of oxygen deprivation, an approach that did not account for the view from the bed any more than previous ones. We have lost our way with dying, and with death. It has become easier to live longer, but harder to die well. Most Americans want to die at home in the care of loved ones, yet most die in institutions, often alone or in the care of strangers. The death people wish for often becomes the one they fear, a sanitised and undignified one. Amidst the current madness of medical excess, there is a need for spiritual renewal that medicine alone cannot address. By exploring the non-physical experience of dying, there is an opportunity to reframe and humanise dying from an irredeemably grim reality to an experience that can contain richness of meaning for patients and loved ones alike.

To this end, our research team conducted studies that used structured interviews aimed at defining a patient-centred perspective. We produced quantifiable data that drew on interviews of patients and their families, videotaped testimonies and written records of over 1200 discrete pre-death dreams and visions to explain, often in the patients' own words, how these extraordinary occurrences brought them comfort and exemplified human resilience at life's end.

We set out to make the collected data quantifiable rather than anecdotal. We made sure it came directly from the patients, not the observers. This was the gap that needed to be filled. But to be able to do so, we first had to rule out the possibility that these experiences were just manifestations of confusional states such as delirium. Even a quick online scan of the literature on the topic will reveal how often end-of-life experiences get confused with altered mental states. Clinicians unfamiliar with end-of-life experiences routinely discount them as hallucinations caused by medications, fever, or confusional states like delirium. In doing so, they insinuate that these experiences hold little intrinsic value. Yet the distinction between the two is critical. Patients with delirium, by definition, exhibit disorganised thinking, loss of connectivity, and an inability to interpret their surroundings that often results in agitation, restlessness, and fear [1]. The experience of delirium is typically very distressing not only for the patients but also for the families and caregivers, while end-of-life experiences typically occur in patients who have clear consciousness, heightened acuity, and awareness of their surroundings. They are recalled with clarity and are memorable. They differ most from hallucinations or delirium by the nature of the responses they evoke, including inner peace, acceptance, subjective meaning, and a sense of one's impending death [2–5]. The distinction is crucial since end-of-life experiences, when mistaken for delirium, result in the patient being medicated, which robs the dying patient of the opportunity to have the comforting experience inherent in the dying process [4, 5]. An inappropriate medical intervention may further the isolation experienced by the dying and impair the person's ability to experience and communicate meaning at the end of life.

Neuroscientists and physicians too often interpret end-of-life processes as restricted to the last few minutes or hours in a patient's life, which is when delirious states are likely to happen. These are moments when the brain is compromised by diminished oxygen and alterations in neurochemistry. But these episodes of altered brain function, mostly restricted to the last hours to moments of life, are not representative of the sum total of each patient's end-of-life experiences. The point of reference is what counts. Dying is a process that cannot be judged solely on the last chapter of what is a protracted journey. Some patients live with a terminal illness for months or years before passing and begin experiencing pre-death dreams and visions when their minds are fully functional. They are able to do their taxes, drive, read, walk, and entertain company. A fair amount of the literature that confuses end-of-life experiences with hallucinations does so because it is referring to the hours or minutes before death when patients drift in and out of consciousness and may indeed have delirious moments. Just like we know better than to judge books by their cover, we may do well to remember not to judge end of life, or life itself for that matter, by its last lines or moments.

In the first of what would become a series of studies, we proceeded to gather over 400 interviews with 66 study patients, some of whom were enrolled for as long as three months [6]. Patients were interviewed near daily until their passing. This was significant as previous researchers had collected data either during random moments or very near death and failed to capture dying as a process that lasts from days to months. The first part of our study, the questionnaire, included unambiguous questions related to the presence or absence of end-of-life dreams and visions: whether these experiences occurred during sleep or wakefulness, whether they were comforting or discomforting and what imagery they included. We asked every participant the same questions about dream/vision content, frequency, and degree of realism. We used a numbered scale so answers could be quantified and compared.

The near universal response we received about end-of-life experiences was that they are categorically 'distinct' from 'normal dreams'. One of the most common statements we recorded was 'I don't normally remember my dreams, but these were different', 'they felt more real than real', and it was 'as though it actually happened'. Patients emphatically maintained that their dreams were not just lifelike, they were lived. When asked to rate the degree of realism of these episodes, most patients rated their end-of-life experiences as the maximum 10 out of 10. And that was the case whether they were asleep or awake, or both, during these events. What we would refer to as 'dreams' because they happened during sleep, patients themselves would call 'visions', as insistently as those who claimed to have seen dead people with their eyes open. In fact, in our survey of patients, 45% of pre-death experiences had occurred during sleep, while 16% took place in wakefulness and more than 39% in both states. Certainly, these statistics reflect the shifting levels of alertness that define the dying process, the bouts of realistic lucid dreaming when patients are aware that they are dreaming, as well as sleep punctuated by a degree of dream intensity that carries over into wakefulness. But in all these cases, our patients talked about their end-of-life experiences as the most awake, alert, and present they had ever felt. While this may make it more difficult for researchers to define wakefulness at end of life, the ambiguity is completely irrelevant to the dying patient, for whom the experience is as vivid, palpable, and impactful as if it had been experienced when awake, if not more so.

We also asked patients to score the degree of comfort or discomfort of their end-of-life experiences, and those dreams or visions that involved deceased relatives and friends were shown to provide the highest comfort rating. This may be a startling reversal of our cultural association of death with grief, sadness, and struggle, but the numbers speak for themselves: patients rated the comfort level of seeing the dead as 4.08 out of 5 (with 5 being the highest comfort) as opposed to an average of 2.86 out of 5 when seeing the living. And the end-of-life experiences that they most frequently reported as soothing included the presence of dead friends and relatives (72%) followed, in order, by living friends and relatives, dead pets or other animals, past meaningful experiences, and only last, religious figures. Taken together, the data suggest that the dying process includes a built-in mechanism which soothes our fears as our inner world becomes ever more populated by those we have loved and lost. Remarkably, the greatest comfort comes from our most basic and foundational needs and relationships, and from moments that capture the beautiful simplicity of everyday life.

When 91-year-old Anne was admitted to our inpatient facility with congestive heart failure, she was having such vivid visions of her long-deceased sister, that, upon waking one day, she looked around and asked 'where is Emily?' Emily had passed away 16 years ago, but to Anne, her presence and appearances were as real as her doctor's. Anne was subsequently admitted to our inpatient unit in acute respiratory distress, where she woke up, stared up at the ceiling, and acted like she was seeing things that were not there. At one point, she sat up straight in bed and stretched her arms out to the ceiling as if to embrace someone. She asked her family, 'Am I going to die now?' When her condition improved, she awoke, looked around and asked again for her dead sister, explaining that Emily had been there all along, sitting beside her on the bed. Anne also reported having frequent dreams of a more youthful Emily, going about 'doing the usual things' around the house. She could describe her sister's appearance in detail: the strong, jutting chin, the dark blond hair pulled in a high, loose bun, the sagging pea green cotton jersey dress whose sleeves were rolled carelessly at the elbows. Sometimes, Emily put her hand over her mouth and laughed, before moving on to the next task at hand. Few words were uttered but the dreams were heart-warming and invigorating, with Anne often envisioning herself as a much younger self going for walks with her sister. She had been one of five siblings, but she was closest to Emily, who 'had raised' her: 'I am not going alone—Emily will be with me', she insisted.

Despite my inability to share in her perception, I was nonetheless grateful that Anne was not alone, that she was comforted by Emily. The next day, Anne continued to have dreams of her sister, and two days later, after she had stabilised clinically and resumed sleeping, she was discharged home. Like most patients, the stalling of her physical decline towards death coincided with a cessation of her pre-death experiences, and like Ryan, she regretted not having visions anymore. Anne died peacefully at home about a month later, and although I was not at her bedside when she made the transition, I doubt that she went alone.

Another striking feature of end-of-life experiences is their ability to reconstruct or edit memories. Significant moments, often derived from childhood, are condensed, modified, and restructured, so patients' most pressing needs can be addressed and redressed. Tim, a 73-year-old lifelong labourer with end stage colon cancer, had end-of-life experiences that both evoked and restructured his childhood memories so he could relive them free from the pain of poverty with which he had grown up. He first began seeing his parents, grandparents, and old friends, who kept 'telling me I will be okay'. Then, four days before passing on, his dreams placed him back in the formative years of his early teens. He had grown up amidst the tragedies of the Great Depression, in a blue-collar neighbourhood of South Buffalo in the United States of America (USA) where he had helplessly watched lives get broken and displaced. His own father had fought to support his family with low-paying and sporadic work. Like many who lived through those hard times, the single most important fear that overshadowed their happiness was about the family's collective struggle to make ends meet and find hope and purpose among the despair.

Tim's end-of-life dreams helped ease the burden of insecurity that this pivotal period in his life had occasioned. He reimagined himself as a young boy walking through and out of his house, a metaphor for his childhood journey. First, he passed the kitchen where, from the corner of his eye, he could see his mother kneeling in prayer. The meaning was clear: Tim had described his mother's devotion to God as his family's source of strength. He then saw himself walking out of the house, only to be overtaken by his best friend who lived next door. The boy was holding a baseball bat and a ball and summoning him to come and play. Significantly, this friend would remain his lifelong best friend and 1 day even become his brother-in-law. Finally, he sees his father pushing a wheelbarrow, a sign of employment and a sense of worth restored. Tim's old psychic wounds were healed; his world was now safe, sustaining, and complete.

As Tim recounted his dream, I was no longer looking at a frail dying man but at the sparkling eyes of a child who had rediscovered the early love that had nurtured and warmed his life. What had first looked like the separate acts of a three-act play, his mom in prayer, his friend playing ball, and his dad walking off to work, provided instead visions of the most important forces at play in his early life, variants on the same theme of love. These were rich and connective enactments of the layered relationships that had mattered to him most growing up and that made him who he was. Far from containing a singular content or meaning, they offered a multi-faceted and meaningful version of an imagined but essential reality in response to his most deep-seated fears and needs. Tim himself interpreted his dream as an archetypal resolution that brought him back to a sense of wholeness and peace. He felt a profound sense of connection that, as for many other patients, ironically bypassed words and language. In end-of-life experiences, little may be said but much is understood.

In Tim's dreams, meaningful past events were condensed, reordered, and repackaged to put him back in touch with the most sustaining and uplifting aspects of his past life. For others, this reality makeover entailed a much more radical editing process that excluded as much as it selected and abbreviated.

One of the most touching realisations we had early on in our study was that it was not the fear of death that end-of-life experiences confront. We uncovered instead a remarkably expansive ability to address the injuries people acquire from having lived, those they don't speak of, the ones that haunt and send them to therapy and the traumas that could not be cured. We had designed the study thinking that the therapeutic value of end-of-life experiences resided in easing the dying process. We had no idea that their potency extended to injuries whose genesis could be traced back to childhood. End-of-life experiences are not just about life's final transition; they address life in its entirety. Sometimes, they do so by cutting out the injurious past or by offering an alternate ending. The means is as varied as the goal is consistent, namely the resolution of what was once a crippling affliction into healing and redress.

The story of John, a decorated war veteran, was a case in point. John was admitted to our facility due to persistent insomnia. When I walked into his room, I was struck by this broad-shouldered man who wore the distraught and exhausted face of someone who had seen too much. John had participated in the battle that General Eisenhower had named the 'Great Crusade' of World War II, the Battle of Normandy, and when I asked him about his condition, he summed it up with three words: 'A war problem'. He then let his family members elaborate.

John's family explained that although he had never so much as mentioned his war experiences until the last few weeks, he was now unable to close his eyes without reliving the unimaginable carnage of D-Day. He had recurring nightmares from which he woke up drenched in sweat. It took his end-of-life experiences for John to come to terms with the haunting memories of his war experiences. He went on to share with me details of the past he had kept only to himself. Maybe he had wanted to spare his loved ones the knowledge of the agony and nightmares that had defined his troubled sleep after the war or perhaps he could not find words to describe his horror.

John was only 20 when he enrolled as a gunner on the SS James L. Ackerson which entered Normandy beside the USS Texas. He was and would always remain a proud Texan who took his duty as a soldier to heart and believed in the ideals of his country. On June 7, 1944, he was part of the Infantry Division that was sent ashore to Omaha, the bloodiest of the D-Day beaches. Their assignment was to retrieve the soldiers who had been isolated from the rest of the forces ashore. The mission was successful, and the landing craft came back with the wounded Rangers they had been sent to rescue. Still, John would never be able to wipe away the vision of the bloodied beach strewn with the mutilated bodies and floating limbs he saw upon landing. This was the experience in the war that was going to haunt him for the rest of his life.

As he lay dying in the Hospice, John was assailed by nightmares about the fallen American soldiers he could not save: 'There is nothing but death, dead soldiers all around me'. I had witnessed people in a state of fear before, but John was not just frightened. He was terrified. His terror was palpable. I had never been able to adjust to the idea of a young man facing the horrors of war, the possibility of death at life's beginning, but watching John return to that site of terror a second time as an old man defied words. He described his nightmares as so intensely real that they felt lived. He could not overcome his pain, and his dreams reflected it.

This is why the complete transformation he underwent a few days later was all the more remarkable. I came to see him, and he was visibly comfortable, even at peace; he could sleep, he said smiling. He credited two of his more recent dreams for this welcome development. In a first joyful dream, he had relived the day he had finally gotten his discharge papers from the military. His second dream sounded more like a nightmare, but to him it was anything but. He dreamt he was approached by a soldier who had been killed on Omaha Beach and had come back to tell him: 'Soon, they are going to come and get you'. John instinctively knew that 'they' referred to his fellow soldiers, and that the dream was about reuniting with his comrades, not judgement. He finally had closure. He could close his eyes and rest.

John's end-of-life experience did not deny his reality, or his war, but it did recast these in such a way as to grant him his hard-earned peace. The soul within that courageous 20-year-old boy had fought the war's ghosts for 67 years was finally released from his enormous obligation and from its injustice.

John's story exemplifies the process through which even the most difficult dreams can provide substantial psychological or spiritual benefits to the dying patient. For him, the tortured memory of the deadliest of the D-Day assaults morphed into the site of the very military camaraderie he thought he had betrayed. He needed to be released from the obligation he had been unable to fulfil and from the overwhelming shame he could not escape. Most importantly, he needed to forgive himself for his inability to save his brothers in arms. Thankfully, his end-of-life experiences allowed him to do just that.

In another study, we identified distinct thematic categories in the wide variety of end-of-life experiences we were surveying [7]. For instance, a large group of patients described dead friends and relatives in their dreams as 'waiting for them' while standing 'just there', in a quiet presence that felt like the tightest embrace. This watchful silence involved no judgement, just pure love and guidance. Bridget had no doubt about the supportive nature of her vision when her two dead aunts appeared to her, simply standing and watching silently over her in her sleep. She needed no explanation to decipher the meaning of their presence or to take in the ubiquity of their love.

After demonstrating the soothing role of end-of-life experiences, we soon discovered that the dying patient is often graced with more than a feeling of comfort. One of our more recent studies confirmed the role that pre-death dreams and visions play in post-traumatic growth as well, the growth an individual experiences after encountering stressful life events such as dying [8]. In other words, there is meaningful adaption, substantive, spiritual yet cognitively meaningful, a mechanism through which the patient can emerge from the dying process with a positive psychological change. After comparing dreamers to non-dreamers, we found that patients who reported end-of-life experiences had higher scores in positive growth in multiple areas, whether it was in terms of personal strength or spiritual development. Interestingly, although research shows a lack of religion in dream content, spiritual growth is by far the largest change we see in our dreamers.

In light of the inseparable nature of the spiritual to the physical aspects of dying, it is somewhat paradoxical that patients rarely report religious content in their end-of-life experiences. Although our studies have documented several accounts of patients dreaming of religious themes, this trend is disproportionate when compared to the totality of our data. Other investigators have similarly shown a near absence of religious references in the dreams and visions of the dying. Still, while this paradox is certainly remarkable, it is also hardly the point. Family is our first church, and the tenets of faith are love and forgiveness, the very themes of pre-death dreams and visions.

This is an insight that is exemplified in the writings of Kerry Egan, a hospice chaplain in Massachusetts, USA. In her short but powerful piece 'My Faith: What people talk about before they die', Egan explains that she is routinely called to the bedside of dying patients who want to talk, not about God or any big spiritual questions, but about their families and 'the love they felt, and the love they gave [or] did not receive, or the love they did not know how to offer, the love they withheld, or maybe never felt for the ones they should have loved unconditionally…. people talk to the chaplain about their families because that is *how* we talk about God. That is *how* we talk about the meaning of our lives…. We live our lives in our families: the families we are born into, the families we create, the families we make through the people we choose as friends' [9]. In a world where people's success is often measured by the number of relationships they sacrifice along the way, the dreams of the dying help us visualise a world where human relationships define our purpose and our true accomplishment.

To Egan, not mentioning God directly does not create conflict with her own religious faith or role as chaplain because it is in the love felt by family members for each other that she recognises God and the teachings of her religion: 'If God is love, and we believe that to be true, then we learn about God when we learn about love. The first, and usually the last classroom of love is the family'. At the bedside, I have witnessed again and again a quiet process of peaceful surrender and well-being, a version of grace and beauty that can indeed only be described as spiritual. But if end-of-life dreams are spiritual, they are not so in content so much as in experience. They are spiritual in the manner in which they alter perception and the sense of well-being they provide. They are spiritual because of the deeply personal process of renewal they trigger in the most secret corners of the self. They are spiritual insofar as they free us from fear and pain and connect us to each other. At the hour of our death, spiritual transformation is no longer external to the self. It happens in the innermost recesses of our being. As we progress towards acceptance, illness and death place us on a spiritual path that ultimately affirms who we are and how to love and forgive. In chaplain Egan's words, 'We don't have to use words of theology to talk about God; people who are close to death almost never do. We should learn from those who are dying that the best way to teach our children about God is by loving each other wholly and forgiving each other fully—just as each of us longs to be loved and forgiven by our mothers and fathers, sons and daughters'.

End-of-life experiences are also rarely of a deep philosophical nature. They don't involve punch lines, big existential questions, exuberant pronouncements, epiphanies, or reckonings. They often simply consist of dreams or visions about family, everyday events, or even pets. It is through these reconstituted relationships that the dying often put themselves back together and recover a sense of self. It is exactly this act of connecting, reconnecting, and connectedness that patient after patient testifies to experiencing when they describe the effects of their dreams and visions at life's end. Our patients' pre-death dreams and visions help the dying reunite with a more authentic sense of self, with the people they have loved and lost, those who have secured them, who have brought them forgiveness and peace. Their needs are addressed, whether it is to be guided, reassured, forgiven, or simply loved.

All of us get injured or injure for having lived, yet end-of-life experiences appear to make us whole again, through forgiveness, love, and the return of those we lost. Old wounds heal as time and distance fade and the span of one's life narrows to what matters. There appears to be some of final justice as end-of-life experiences exclude those who have caused us harm and embrace those who have nurtured and loved best. It's fitting, perhaps, that the circle that gets completed is one of restoration, and we return to the best parts of having lived. End-of-life experiences deserve to be recognised as evidence of the life-affirming and inspiring resilience of the human spirit that drives them. They are proof of humanity's built-in, natural, and profoundly spiritual capacity for self-sustenance and self-healing, grace and hope.

From a clinical perspective, I believe presence is more important than intervention. Presence brings acceptance, creates space for reflection and allows times for expression and therefore dignity. In fact, I have rarely encountered a patient who requested interpretation of their end-of-life experiences. The journey is over; we are behind the curtain. Perhaps, it is even worth asking whether the analysis of dreams serves the needs of the clinician as opposed to the patient. End-of-life experiences provide answers to questions that no longer need answering. They represent a culmination point rather than a doorway. These experiences are not about thinking so much as about remembering, feeling, sensing, breathing, and smiling.

Despite their significance, end-of-life experiences are rarely validated or placed within any clinical context, particularly within a pure medical model. A humanising approach to care at the end of life must recognise that dying is a unique vantage point that brings distinct perceptions and perspectives, such as end-of-life experiences. The isolation and loneliness of dying are made worse when the patient's inner experiences are ignored, denied, or refuted. In fact, patients' end-of-life experiences may be 'medicalised' and mistaken for delirium. Such patients may even receive medication to treat delirium and thereby sterilise the patient from their own meaningful inner end-of-life processes.

The role of any palliative or spiritual care provider is to address the totality of suffering which includes existential or spiritual distress as well as create space or permission for the patient to acknowledge end-of-life experiences. There is even some data which suggest that patients are reluctant to share end-of-life experiences for fear of being ridiculed. It is often helpful to introduce the topic of end-of-life experiences with patients by stating that it is common for dying patients to report vivid dreams that feel real to the point of feeling virtual. Moreover, the dying process is typically defined by progressive sleep that alters normal sleep architecture such that realities blur between dreams and wakefulness. Once defined and explained, patients will often freely acknowledge their end-of-life experiences. Again, the emphasis is on validation and providing space for acceptance as well as reflection.

When caring for the dying patient, we are caring for them in the context of their lives, which includes those they love. Sadly, we often see families and friends unsettled by a patient's end-of-life experiences and references to unshared realities. We hear uninformed families attribute end-of-life experiences to the effects of medication, a brain metastasis or even fear of death. For example, I once saw a patient's daughter sitting in the corner of the room, hands on lap and staring out the window—avoiding looking at the direction of her mother in the bed. The patient was speaking in her native Polish language and making frequent references to her inner experiences. We explained to the daughter that end-of-life experiences are common and overwhelmingly comforting for the patient. The next day, the daughter was sitting beside her mother's bed, taking notes and documenting aspects of her mother's childhood that were previously unknown—vivid descriptions of her childhood friends and experiences that had drifted over time and distance. This is an example of one of the critical roles of the team, which is to help interpret the patient experience and thereby narrow the space between the person in the bed and those at the bed side. We have looked at the impact of end-of-life experiences on the bereaved and published several papers [10, 11]. Simply put, what is good for the patient is good for those left behind. Families commonly witness their dying loved one's experiences of pre-death dreams, and they are reported as overwhelmingly positive. The effect on grief was quantifiable using validated measures—family members felt that witnessing these experiences helped with their overall grief, accepting their loss, working through the pain of grief and continuing the bond with their loved one.

Dying is so much more than a physical event. Where medicine fails, dying becomes what it has always been, a human event—the closing of a life. And dying with dignity, just as living with dignity, is so much more a spiritual event than a biomedical process. There is nothing new in this observation. The German poet Rainer Maria Rilke best captured the importance of each individual's spiritual expression of meaning in life's final moments when he stated 'I don't want the doctor's death. I want my own freedom'.

References

1. American Psychiatric Association. Diagnostic and statistical manual of mental disorders. 4th ed., text revision. Washington, DC: American Psychiatric Association; 2000. ISBN 978-0890420256.
2. Brayne S, Lovelace H, Fenwick P. End-of-life experiences and the dying process in a Gloucestershire nursing home as reported by nurses and care assistants. Am J Hosp Palliat Care. 2008;25:195–206.
3. Houran J, Lange R. Hallucinations that comfort: contextual mediation of deathbed visions. Percept Mot Skills. 1997;84:1491–504.
4. Mazzarino-Willett A. Deathbed phenomena: its role in peaceful death and terminal restlessness. Am J Hosp Palliat Care. 2010;27:127–33.
5. Fenwick P, Brayne S. End-of-life experiences: reaching out for compassion, communication, and connection-meaning of deathbed visions and coincidences. Am J Hosp Palliat Care. 2011;28:7–15.
6. Kerr CW, Donnelly JP, Wright ST, Kuszczak S, Banas A, Grant P, Luczkiewicz D. End-of-life dreams and visions: a longitudinal study of hospice patients' experiences. J Palliat Care. 2014;17(3):296–303.
7. Nosek CL, Kerr CW, Woodworth J, et al. End-of-life dreams and visions: a qualitative perspective from hospice patients. Am J Hosp Palliat Med. 2015;32(3):269–74.
8. Levy K, Grant PC, Depner RM, Byrwa DJ, Luczkiewicz DL, Kerr CW. End-of-life dreams and visions and posttraumatic growth: a comparison study. J Palliat Med. 2020;23(3):319–24.
9. Egan K. What people talk about before they die. https://www.cnn.com/2016/12/20/health/...people-talk-about...kerry-egan/index.html
10. Grant PC, Levy K, Lattimer TA, Depner RM, Kerr CW. Attitudes and perceptions of end-of-life dreams and visions and their implication to the bereaved family caregiver experience. Am J Hosp Palliat Med. 2021;38(7):778–84.
11. Grant PC, Depner RM, Levy K, LaFever SM, Tenzek KE, Wright ST, Kerr CW. Family caregiver perspectives on end-of-life dreams and visions during bereavement: a mixed methods approach. J Palliat Med. 2019;38(7):778–84.

Health-Related Spirituality: Empirical, Historical, and Conceptual Clarifications

Simon Peng-Keller

Abstract To clarify the term of 'health-related spirituality', this chapter takes three approaches: historical research on the genealogy of this term, empirical research on current forms of spirituality, and conceptual analysis. An improved understanding of the many pasts of 'spirituality', of its distinct current usages, and of its multidimensionality, contributes to a better perception and understanding of the fluid, emergent and sometimes contradictory phenomena related to this term. It is argued that in the diversity of contemporary popular and academic usages of the term 'spirituality', distinguishable strands of a long conceptual history converge. This term's success is that it transcends a duality constitutive of (Euro-American) modernity: the distinction between religious and secular. However, the integration of spiritual aspects responds not only to a societal change but also to a functional differentiation and reintegration in healthcare. Using the example of the World Health Organisation (WHO) discussion on the 'spiritual dimension' of health, it is pointed out that health-related spirituality is inevitably imbued with values and connected with healthcare politics and law.

Keywords Health-related spirituality · Spiritual beliefs · Spiritual practices
Spiritual experiences · Spiritual attitudes · Spiritual distress · Spiritual needs
Spiritual resources · World Health Organisation · Spiritual care · Palliative care

More than a decade ago, Swedish psychologist Pär Salander criticised the tendency to broaden the concept of spirituality. His thesis was: 'Outside of the religious context, "spirituality" lacks a theoretical foundation and a systematic meaning' [1]. If the vertical-religious dimension is removed from the term, as is often the case in

S. Peng-Keller (✉)
Department of Theology, University of Zürich, Zürich, Switzerland
e-mail: simon.peng-keller@uzh.ch

M. C. Best (ed.), *Spiritual Care in Palliative Care*,
https://doi.org/10.1007/978-3-031-50864-6_2

health-related discourses, it arguably loses its specificity and is therefore not suitable for describing a professional activity. To the extent that spiritual care is guided by such a vague understanding of spirituality, it adapts like a chameleon to the tasks of psychological counselling and psychosocial support. Salander's criticism points to the need for conceptual clarification. To this end, this article, drawing on previous studies [2–4], choses three approaches to this topic: the empirical research on current spiritualities is deepened by a genealogy of this term and leads to a conceptual analysis. The aim is to show that in the diversity of contemporary popular and academic discourses on spirituality, distinguishable strands of a long conceptual history converge.

I proceed in four steps: First, I overview the empirical knowledge about contemporary usages of the term 'spirituality', before I turn to their complex genealogy in the second part. With regard to the topic of this book, the third section summarises a remarkable discussion on the 'spiritual dimension' of health taking place within the World Health Assembly at the beginning of the 1980s. Against this background, in the final section I outline some perspectives for a conceptual clarification of 'health-related spirituality'.

1 Plural and Hybrid Spiritualities

The usage of the term 'spirituality' has expanded greatly over the course of the twentieth century, and with it the range of ways in which one can understand oneself as 'spiritual'. To describe oneself or others as spiritual is often to relativise the modern contrast between religious and secular beliefs. Those who use the term 'spiritual' as a self-designation today are not necessarily saying anything about their relationship to religious institutions and traditions. The concept of spirituality owes its current popularity not least to the increasing restriction of the concept of religion to its institutional forms. As will be shown in the next section, what is currently described as religious and spiritual diversity, spiritual hybridisation, 'fluid religion' [5], or multiple belonging, is anything but new. What is new, however, is the wider establishment of these trends, which can be seen in the increasing popularity of describing oneself as 'spiritual, but not religious' [6]. This development bespeaks a form of globalisation marked by the worldwide circulation of spiritual and religious ideas and practices [7]. While modernity appears to be characterised by the need to decide between a religious and a secular orientation, there is now, within the space of (post-)secular society, a burgeoning spectrum of options which often do not belong exclusively to one tradition but draw on many. These, in turn, extend into the sphere of traditional religiosity, such that the boundaries between religious and secular spheres are blurred. According to John Cottingham, the term 'spirituality' is perfectly suited for our collective situation:

> The concept of spirituality is an interesting one, in so far as it does not seem to provoke, straight off, the kind of immediately polarised reaction one finds in the case of religion. This may be partly to do with the vagueness of the term [...] Yet at the richer end of the spectrum,

> we find the term used in connection with activities and attitudes which command widespread appeal, irrespective of metaphysical commitment or doctrinal allegiance. [...] In general, the label 'spiritual' seems to be used to refer to activities which aim to fill the creative and meditative space left over when science and technology have satisfied our material needs. So construed, both supporters and opponents of religion might agree that the loss of the spiritual dimension would leave our human existence radically impoverished. [...] Spirituality has long been understood to be a concept that is concerned in the first instance with activities rather than theories, with ways of living rather than doctrines subscribed to, with praxis rather than belief. [8]

Despite all the individualisation and hybridisation, spiritual pluralisation is not haphazard. Rather, a limited number of basic types of contemporary spirituality are emerging. Nancy Ammerman distinguishes three of these [9]. She assigns to the first type all those forms that are defined by an explicit reference to God. The second group consists of those forms that deny any reference to God but affirm a belief in something 'higher'. The third type is characterised by a belief in 'horizontal transcendence', where this may be construed in humanistic or cosmologic terms.

Ammerman's typology can be further differentiated. On the basis of extensive empirical data, Heinz Streib, Ralph W. Hood and colleagues [10] distinguish the basic forms of contemporary spirituality with regard to their ideas of transcendence (*theistic* vs. *non-theistic*), their relationship to institutional forms of religion (*close to religion* vs. *distant from religion*) and their primary form of self-transcendence (*mystical* vs. *humanistic*). If one applies these distinctions to the statement above, it represents a spirituality that is non-theistic and distant from religion, and which exhibits a clearly mystical character. If the three types described by Ammerman are transposed into Streib and Hood's coordinate system, the following dimensions emerge (see Fig. 1):

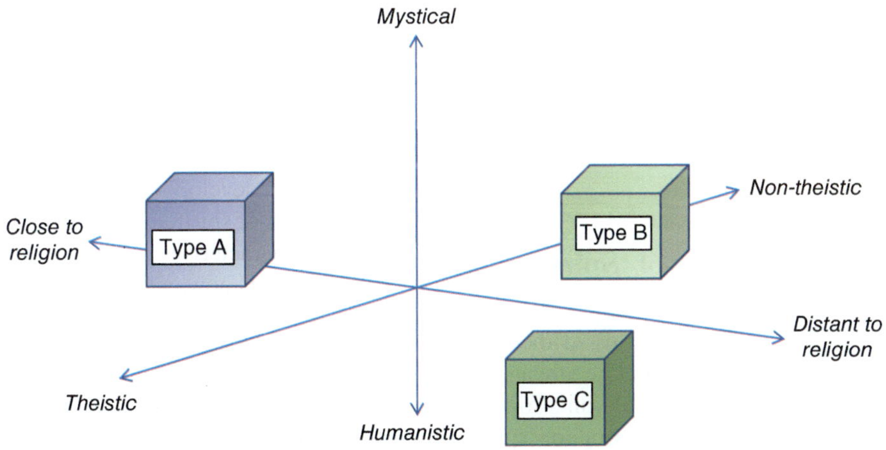

Fig. 1 Types of contemporary spirituality. According to H. Streib and R. W. Hood, these appear in forms that are more or less religious, theistic or non-theistic, and more mystical or more humanistic [2]

As helpful as such typologies may be for providing an initial orientation in the sometimes confusing field of religious and spiritual convictions and practices, they should nevertheless be treated with caution. Typological approaches tend to underplay ambivalences and ossify exploratory movements into fixed positions. Neither the developmental dynamics nor the inner tensions of actual spiritual experience are adequately represented in such cartographies.

Trajectories of spiritual exploration and transformation can be found today in both religious and secular variants. They are often sparked by an encounter with serious illness or death and move the individual beyond previously unquestioned ideas and practices. The Czech theologian Tomáš Halík, who has studied these experiences with particular care, notes that 'seekers among believers (those for whom faith is not a legacy, but a way) and among non-believers, who reject the religious notions put forward to them by those around them nevertheless have a yearning for something to satisfy their thirst for meaning' [11]. The function of this appeal to the vocabulary of the spiritual is often precisely to 'describe experiences and denote positions and aspirations that are "more than" or "move beyond" either secularity or religion' [12]. In this sense, 'spiritual' points towards a sphere that both presupposes and transcends the religious/secular dichotomy typical for Modernity.

There are some paradoxical aspects of contemporary 'spiritualities of life' [13]. For example, the simultaneous emphasis on intense relationship to the sensual world and a trans-sensory inner orientation: 'Rather than being flatly individualistic or purely 'internal' in nature, spirituality appears today to designate an ensemble of (often disparate) technologies—linguistic, ritual, praxiological, associative, etc.—through which inner and outer worlds are connected' [10].

This diversification of the religious-spiritual field is most noticeable at the micro level of everyday spiritual care. As Wendy Cadge and Emily Sigalow have observed, healthcare chaplains navigate the pluralised life-worlds of their patients with the aid of two different communication strategies: on the one hand, by using religiously neutral language; and on the other hand, by moving back and forth between different forms of language, a kind of 'code-switching' [14]. These communicative strategies reflect a specific challenge that spiritual care faces in pluralistic contexts: the task of dealing with indeterminacies and ambiguities in a relationship.

2 Genealogies of 'Spirituality'

This first section responds to the critique that current discussions of spirituality, especially in the realm of healthcare, lack a sense of its historical and cultural background [15]. Mikhail Bakhtin's formula 'every meaning will have its homecoming festival' [16] is certainly true for 'spirituality' and its metaphorical background. The older meanings survive while new amalgamations arise in highly complex interactions. What is often decried as the 'fuzziness' of the term might be better described as the co-presence of diverging usages. As already indicated, the career of this 'travelling term' [17] in the twentieth century is closely linked to that of 'religion'. A closer look at the complex history of this term helps to better understand how it came about.

Firstly, note that what follows is not just a history of 'spirituality' as a concept, but also a history of its fluid metaphorical matrix. The semantic richness to the Latin word *spiritus* is due to its metaphorical quality and its oscillation between anthropological, cosmological, and theological meanings typical to classical Roman literature as well as biblical writings. The biblical Old Testament term *ruah*, which was consistently translated into Latin as *spiritus*, was used for the human spirit as well as for the spirit of God. In St Paul's letters in the New Testament of the Bible, *pneumatikos* is to be understood exclusively in the theological sense of 'inspired by the Holy Spirit', while the noun *pneuma* is also used in an anthropological sense (e.g. in 1 Thessalonians 5:23 where 'spirit', 'soul', and 'body' constitute the totality of human being). Regarding the complex reception of this broad metaphorical fund, the history of spirituality can be considered as numerous parallel attempts to conceptualise metaphorical language in theological, philosophical, legal, or scientific discourses.

The tension between metaphorical density and conceptual disambiguation is a constant in this history to this day. With the emergence of the abstract noun *spiritualitas* in the fifth century, the threshold between metaphorical and conceptual language was crossed at an identifiable historical point. This abstract noun partly preserves the pneumatological meaning of the biblical term *pneumatikos* (*'spirit[u]alis'*). Nonetheless, it already foreshadows the more ontological denotations which became dominant no later than in the twelfth century. In the context of the emerging scholasticism, *spiritualitas* was increasingly used in contrast to the term *corporalitas* and served as an umbrella term for all things and practices that did not belong to the realm of worldly affairs but to an ontologically higher sphere of things with immaterial value. Even more important for the later development is the circumstance that the contrast between the spiritual (eternal) and the secular (temporal) realm, between the spiritual care of the priesthood and the bodily care of the physicians, was politically shaped by the Gregorian Reform (eleventh–twelfth century) and is consequently reflected in canon law. The jurisdiction of the Church, in distinction to the worldly law, is bound to the spiritual realm. Whoever and whatever belonged to it was to be called *spiritual.* With this legal denotation, the Latin term was later translated into the vernacular.

With the *longue durée* of the canon law, the legal distinction between spiritual and secular influenced terminological usage until the twentieth century. To quote only one remarkable example: Article 37 of the Geneva Convention for the Amelioration of the Condition of the Wounded and Sick in Armed Forces in the Field, ratified in 1949, reads as follows: 'The religious, medical and hospital personnel assigned to the medical or spiritual care [...] shall, if they fall into the hands of the enemy, be respected and protected' [18]. Although the Geneva Convention abstains from any ontological commitment, in discriminating between spiritual and medical care it harks back to a distinction formed by medieval theology and politics.

While the ontological and legal reframing of *spiritualitas* was the work of scholastic theology and as such a product of the defining culture of those times, the later history of the term 'spirituality' was equally influenced by heterodox spiritual movements as it was by mainstream theology. In addition to the radical Franciscan followers of Joachim of Fiore who preached the new age of the Holy Spirit, the late Medieval period knew many and various 'free spirits'. A common trait of the heterogeneous people and groups which were subsumed under this heresiological term was the claim of having found direct access to the Holy Spirit. Regularly quoting Paul's '*ubi spiritus, ibi libertas*' (2 Cor 3:17) they understood themselves as Christians who were freed by the Holy Spirit. In contrast, official theology tended to regard them as wayward spirits and as such a danger to the Church and society.

The dissemination of the term 'spirituality' in the modern vernacular started with the mystical current in seventeenth-century France, which was seen by its opponents as a descendant of medieval and protestant spiritualism. The label 'nouvelle spiritualité', which emerged at the same time as the noun '*mystique*' and was used to characterise this current, might initially have had a derogative meaning. The approbatory one is documented, a century later, in d'Alembert and Diderot's *Encyclopaedia*. In its short article on 'spiritualité', published in 1751, two meanings of the term are registered. First, the 'spirituality of the soul that is used to signify its quality which is unknown to us and is essentially distinct from matter'; second, 'the same term is also used for an honest and special piety, which is devoted to meditation on the most subtle and detached aspects of religion' [19].

The mystical imprint, which characterises the French coining of 'spiritualité', will remain typical up to and throughout the modern era. It is likely that the English term 'spirituality' was derived from the French 'spiritualité'. The passage from French mysticism to American Protestantism foreshadows the future journey of the term. One of the writers who might have introduced its mystical flavour into modern English was John Fletcher, born at Lake Geneva in 1729 as Jean Guillaume de la Fléchère. Of Huguenot ancestry, de la Fléchère studied in Geneva and read the works of seventeenth-century French mystics in the original. During a stay in London, he met Charles Wesley and became one of the most fervent supporters of the Methodist's evangelical mysticism. Fletcher may not have been the first to use the newly coined term in this way. Twenty years earlier, the Anglican Thomas Hartlex, who also belonged to the evangelical revival, had already used the term in his *Short Defense of the Mystical Writers*. For Hartlex, the mystics were the guardians of the 'spirituality of true religion' [20].

On the threshold of the eighteenth century, a new factor emerged out of Mesmerism and related currents, one which would have a strong impact on the subsequent history of spirituality and its relationship with medicine. Physician Anton Mesmer's 'animal magnetism' melded the scientific understanding of his time with occultist traditions, and attempted to create a theoretical framework for therapeutic experiments [21]. The enormous success of Mesmerism, spreading from Vienna to France, Scotland, and the United States, was due to its combination of modern medical science and energetic healing. In the mesmeric crucible, spirituality was enriched with new connotations. In mesmerist writings, the term spirituality was connected to the cosmic flow of healing energies. What differentiated Mesmerist concepts from medieval theology or ontology was the mesmerist's distance from religious beliefs and the emphasis on scientific justifications.

Although Mesmerism was on the wane by the middle of the nineteenth century, it formed an influential and enduring model of a scientifically based spirituality which was linked to modernity and innovation, as well as to therapeutic practices. Among the heirs of this model, the American Transcendentalists were probably among the most seminal. Leading figures like Amos Bronson Alcott, who was also acquainted with seventeenth-century French mysticism [20], strove for a spirituality which would transcend all religious and political divisions of the past. A remarkable instance of the new, refashioned term is to be found in Walt Whitman's *Democratic Vistas*, published in 1871 following the American Civil War. For Whitman [22], spirituality is to be considered the highest form of religion, which cannot be reached by dint of church piety but rather in lonely meditation and aesthetic ecstasy. Despite his emphasis on self-reliance, the final goal Whitman pleaded for was not the perfection of the individual but of a democratic community. The lasting success of American transcendentalism can be found in its ability to meld divergent traditions in creative ways. Along with the French mystics and the Mesmerists, the Unitarians, Romantic poetics and the writings of Swedenborg also contributed to this spiritual crucible [6].

Among these influences, romantic orientalism deserves special consideration. The first German and English translations of Sanskrit texts were widely read in Mesmerist and transcendentalist circles, nourishing an orientalist vision of the 'spiritual wisdom of the East' [23–25]. Mediated by theosophical movements, this vision was ultimately rooted in colonial India, whence it spread to North America and Europe in the following decades. The most important figure for the circulation of ideas might be Swami Vivekananda, who imbued the term 'spirituality' with connotations that remain in currency today. Between 1893 and 1896, during Vivekananda's first lecture tour of Europe and the United States, spirituality became the watchword of his Neo-Hindu message. He criticised the materialism of the West as well as the intolerance of the monotheistic faiths while praising India as 'the treasure-house of religion and spirituality' (1970, 148) and as a 'glorious land of religious toleration' (1970, 187).

This discourse is congruent with Vivekananda's anti-colonial reform programme, which contrasted the spiritual poverty of the secular West with India's religious wealth. Swami Vivekananda's concept of spirituality was shaped not only by the contrast between East and West, but even more by the binary distinction between ritualistic forms of religion and more interior ones. Like the way in which Transcendentalists praised Christian mysticism while criticising church ceremonies and institutions, Vivekananda distinguished between the ceremonial and the spiritual aspects of Hinduism. In his version, Hindu spirituality encompasses a certain philosophy and meditative practice, but not ritual practices and popular beliefs.

The trajectory of the term 'spirituality' in the twentieth century is due not least to the increasing restriction of the concept of religion to the institutional. In his book *The Varieties of Religious Experience* published in 1902, William James used the term 'personal religion' in a way that corresponds to today's understanding of spirituality: as opposed to the institutional and theological aspects of religion. He was concerned with 'the inner dispositions of man himself which form the centre of interest, his conscience, his deserts, his helplessness, his incompleteness' and thus, ultimately, with 'human nature', as the subtitle of his book indicates (*A Study in Human Nature*) [26]. The American transcendentalists, Ralph Waldo Emerson, and Walt Whitman in particular, played an important role for James, as did the Mind Cure or New Thought movement, which he treated in detail in two of his lectures—a movement that anticipated many aspects of contemporary mindfulness movement.

Outside organised religion, the heirs of the Mesmerists and the Transcendentalists refined and disseminated their concepts of 'unchurched spirituality' [6, 21, 27], while ambassadors of the 'spiritual East' found their way to Europe and America. As in the case of Vivekananda, the interchange between Western concepts of spirituality and the message of Eastern masters like Inayat Khan (1882–1927), D. T. Suzuki (1870–1966), and Maharishi Mahesh Yogi (1918–2008) resulted in a 'whirlpool effect'. In highly complex cross-fertilisations, practices like *hatha yoga*, Sufi contemplative practice, or Japanese *zazen* were extracted from their interpretative contexts and labelled 'spiritual'. This 'healthification' of Hindu and Buddhist practices [28] was embedded in a broad range of twentieth-century movements which aimed to foster physical and mental health through bodily and spiritual exercise. While some of them were explicitly secular or trans-religious, such as the New Thought movement, others were firmly Christian, like the Young Men's Christian Association (YMCA) [27, 29], or had a Christian background, as for instance Alcoholics Anonymous [30, 31]. Maybe one of the most significant examples of the 'healthification' of spirituality in the twentieth century, however, is probably the WHO's debate on the 'spiritual dimension of health', to which I turn in the following section.

3 The Debate in the World Health Organisation on the 'Spiritual Dimension' of Health

Contrary to the widespread perception that the 'spiritual dimension' has emerged relatively recently within the WHO, its history is considerably longer and more complex. As will be shown in this section, the discussion about the spiritual dimension of health in WHO discourse was connected to aspirations for universal primary healthcare, attempts to deliver a more holistic form of healthcare, and the search for a shared ethical framework to unify the disparate national interests represented in the organisation.

At the 61st session of the WHO's Executive Board, held in 1978, a Libyan physician named A. M. Abdulhadi criticised a report on adolescents' health needs because it 'made no reference to spiritual values and their impact on adolescent development' [32]. At the same session of the Executive Board, only few days later, the

Indian health official Desh Bandhu Bisht argued: ‘If the ultimate aim of health was peace and happiness for mankind, then the spiritual parameter should be added to those already included, namely, physical, mental and social health’ [32]. In the same year, at the International Conference on Primary Health in Alma-Ata (now Almaty, Kazakhstan), the Alma-Ata Declaration made the provision of primary healthcare the flagship strategy of the WHO.

One of the main architects of the primary healthcare concept adopted with the Declaration of Alma-Ata at the WHO was Halfdan Mahler (1923–2016), who served as Director-General of the WHO between 1973 and 1988. The son of a Danish Baptist preacher, Mahler ‘developed the need to dedicate his life to a useful mission. His asceticism and Protestant work ethics were to fuel his entire career’ [33]. For Mahler, the WHO’s definition of health was a statement of ‘transcendental beauty and significance’ which generated a ‘complete light’ that would guide the organisation on its path towards primary healthcare reform [34]. In his experience, the Alma-Ata conference was a ‘sacred moment’ which united the pantheon of nations behind the ‘gospel of health for all’ [35]. Under Mahler, the World Health Assembly (WHA) in 1979 launched the *Health for All*-initiative, a programme infused as much by the new primary healthcare paradigm as by a humanistic ethos. It formed a major reference point for subsequent discussion, which will be examined more closely below. It was initiated by the representative of a small African country with a colonial past: Samuel Hynd (1924–2016), the Health Minister of Swaziland. Hynd was a committed member of the Church of the Nazarene [36], and his father had worked as a medical missionary to build Swaziland’s healthcare system on European models. In his address to the plenary meeting on 4th May 1983, Hynd made the following statement:

> At the risk of being misunderstood, but in order to identify an area to give further impetus to our unquestionably noble efforts, I find the definition of health in our Constitution is wanting. […] there is a dimension to a man or a woman that goes beyond and above his physical, mental and social wellbeing. There is something within a person – […] what one could call attitude, motivation, driving force, or by whatever name you wish to call it or define it, but which I prefer to call spirit. [37]

With this, Hynd put the ‘spiritual dimension’ into the spotlight of the WHA. He continued by linking it directly to the organisation’s efforts for more effective and equitable healthcare systems:

> Our founding fathers may have been afraid of this word for various reasons, but let us face it, the programmes in health that are proving successful in our countries are those led by people whose healthy spirit makes it a success. A programme can have all the ingredients of being good and successful, but it comes out dry and lacking the spiritual quality it needs. I may be accused of introducing some religious concept into WHO but let me say that whether you are a priest or a mullah or a commissar, you are a success or otherwise by virtue of the spirit in which you conduct your programme and of your inner spiritual being. What I am really saying is, that if we want a healthy WHO and a healthy health for all, I want to see health in our Constitution this way: ‘Health is a state of complete physical, mental, social and spiritual wellbeing’. [38]

Various elements of the resolution text ultimately adopted can already be found in Hynd's speech: the link to the Health for All-initiative; the reference to the WHO's constitutional definition of health; the identification of a 'spiritual dimension' as a motivating factor in the promotion of healthcare; and the interreligious understanding of this dimension. Hynd's plan was supported by several African countries, but most enthusiastically by delegates from Arab nations. The most prominent among them was Abdul Rahman Al-Awadi, Kuwaiti Minister of Health and a former member of the WHO's Executive Board. Al-Awadi took up the cause while adding elements of his own, including criticism of the prevailing, U.S.-dominated geopolitical and cultural world order. The anxiety and insecurity characterising our age, he said, was due to a spiritual 'vacuum'.

However, there was also clear opposition voiced against the proposal. The spokesman of the opposing side was M. N. Savel'ev, representative of the USSR. Several speakers highlighted uncertainty regarding the precise meaning of the 'spiritual dimension' in the draft resolution. The most forceful input in this respect came from the representative of West Germany, who admitted that his delegation was 'in the awkward position of no longer knowing what was really being talked about. The text of the draft resolution mentioned a spiritual dimension, but other delegations had spoken of a religious dimension; perhaps it was even the mental dimension that was meant. For that reason, his delegation would greatly appreciate any clarification of what was understood by "spiritual dimension"' [37]. The plenary meeting finally approved the proposal to instruct the Executive Board to further clarify matters.

As a basis for further discussions, Halfdan Mahler drafted an extensive report, which was approved by the Executive Board without reservation. A number of Mahler's formulations were later integrated into the resolution text. To narrow down the range of possible interpretations, the report began with terminological considerations. The adjective 'spiritual', said the report, indicates 'a phenomenon that is not material in nature but belongs to the realm of ideas that have arisen in the minds of human beings, particularly ennobling ideas' [39]. Thus, the 'spiritual dimension' was differentiated in two ways: by qualifying it ontologically (spiritual vs. material), and by linking it to a realm of higher values ('ennobling ideas').

For diplomatic reasons, Mahler's position oscillated between conceptual 'thinning' and 'thickening' [40]. He avoided turning 'spirituality' into a non-committal residual category by linking it to a humanistic ethos that informed efforts to build more equitable healthcare systems. Therefore, the concept of 'ennobling ideas', in the form of universal ethical principles and attitudes, formed the criterion for what was to be understood by the 'spiritual dimension'. Mahler's report paved the way for the resolution A37.13 adopted by the 37th World Health Assembly in 1984. It affirmed 'that ennobling ideas have not only stimulated worldwide action for health but have also given to health, as defined in WHO's Constitution, an added spiritual dimension', and invites 'Member States to consider including in their strategies for health for all a spiritual dimension as defined in this resolution in accordance with their social and cultural patterns' [41].

Irrespective of how the process and its result are to be interpreted: The discussions around resolution WHA37.13 represent a milestone for the WHO's approach to the 'spiritual dimension'. It was the first and, so far, the only time in the history of the WHO that the WHA discussed this topic explicitly and in some detail. The process that culminated in the adoption of resolution WHA37.13 can be described in a threefold way: First, as a quest for a health policy compromise, in which the term 'spiritual dimension' with its wide range of possible meanings served the purpose of bridging the divide between opposing world views. From this perspective, the course of the discussion described represents a process of conceptual 'thinning', in which the primarily religiously connoted term 'spiritual' was translated into a secular and abstract language. Second, from the perspective of the principal actors in the process, it might be more appropriate to speak of an unfolding process, during which an aspect that was already implicitly present in the WHO's definition of health was made explicit and henceforth impossible to ignore. Finally, the discussion described can also be viewed as a creative process of 'value generalisation' [42] or 'norm construction' [40], in which the commitment to better and fairer global healthcare was reinforced by framing it with a spiritual and cosmopolitan 'order of worth' [40, 43].

More lasting than the resolution WHA37.13, which soon fell into institutional oblivion, were the WHO's efforts to promote palliative care and to anchor spiritual care within this framework. The idea of palliative care challenged the WHO's focus on prevention, the fight against infectious diseases, and drug control. In a report written by an expert committee and published in 1989, palliative care is defined as 'the active total care of patients whose disease is not responsive to curative treatment. Control of pain, of other symptoms, and of psychological, social and spiritual problems is paramount' [44]. In a separate section on 'spiritual aspects', this report emphasised that 'all programmes of palliative care should respect and incorporate the basic values of spiritual and religious diversity that are enshrined in the United Nations' 1981 Declaration on the elimination of all forms of intolerance and of discrimination based on religion and belief'. According to that declaration, everyone shall have the right to 'freedom of thought, conscience, religion and belief' [44]. The report attempted to differentiate between 'spiritual' and 'religious': The notion 'spiritual' referred 'to those aspects of human life relating to experiences that transcend sensory phenomena. This is not the same as 'religious', though for many people the spiritual dimension of their lives includes a religious component'. Furthermore, 'spiritual' was characterised as 'an integrating component, holding together the physical, psychological and social components'; as 'being concerned with meaning and purpose'; as 'associated with a need for forgiveness, reconciliation and affirmation of worth' as well as with 'inner healing' [44].

In the following section, I discuss the WHO's approaches towards the 'spiritual dimension' of health in the wider context of current discussions on health-related spirituality.

4 Conceptual Conclusion

Against the background of the discussions just outlined and in the context of empirical spirituality research, the concept of 'health-related spirituality' can be understood in two ways: According to the first understanding, spiritual beliefs, practices, experiences, and attitudes are considered (external) determinants of physical or mental health. According to the second understanding, health, understood as comprehensive wellbeing, includes a spiritual dimension, namely 'spiritual wellbeing'. In both ways, 'health-related spirituality' is a value-laden term. Where people today claim being spiritual for themselves or attribute it to others, they usually use it in an evaluative way. Anyone who says that they are (not) spiritual is not only describing something, but also evaluating it with regard to a certain way of being. This applies in particular to *health-related* spirituality: It is inevitably imbued with value and connected to healthcare politics and law [45]. For stakeholders in healthcare and health-related research, spirituality is important *insofar* as it fosters health and dignity, and helps people cope with illness and death—*or insofar* it poses a problem to this.

Empirical constructs like 'spiritual wellbeing' and 'spiritual distress' are located in the realm of the value-laden and contested concepts of health, illness, and mental disorder. Therefore, research in the field of health-related spirituality must free itself from the illusion of universally valid concepts with stable meanings. Or to put it positively: the indeterminations and the overdeterminacy of these terms are part of the object to be studied. An improved understanding of the many pasts of 'spirituality' and of its distinct current usages contributes to a better perception and understanding of the fluid, emergent and sometimes contradictory phenomena related to this term. To avoid a narrow view of the complexity of lived spirituality, its various dimensions—beliefs, experiences, practices, and attitudes—should be studied separately and examined in their interdependence.

If a spiritual dimension of health is assumed, then the question arises as to how it can be distinguished from the mental dimension. Again, there are two options for understanding: The spiritual dimension may either consist in a *linear extension* where it is attached to physical, mental, and social dimensions, or it may be conceived as orthogonal to these dimensions, as their *depth dimension*. In the first case, 'spiritual' refers to an additional realm, in the second case, to something that can be found in all dimensions of human life. The distinction between mental and spiritual wellbeing becomes manifest when the latter occurs in the midst of mental distress. As the WHO's 2004 report *Promoting Mental Health* highlighted, 'Spirituality can enable people to step outside or beyond the mental distress and experience comfort and calm. Especially in the midst of crisis, particular kinds of spirituality can prove to be a powerful resource which can be a real buffer against excessive mental distress and despair' [46].

The integration of a 'spiritual dimension' into healthcare responds not only to a societal change, but also to the functional differentiation and professional specialisation of medicine. A professional inclusion of spiritual aspects into healthcare requires specialists (chaplains) and generalists (nurses, physicians, psychotherapists, etc.). This affects professional identities, boundaries, and cooperation: While chaplains face the challenge of integrating themselves into interprofessional teams, doctors, nurses, and therapists of all kinds are faced with the task of understanding attention to spiritual aspects as part of their professional role and acquiring the corresponding skills. Insofar as a 'spiritual dimension' of health refers to something which encompasses and permeates all other dimensions (and does not stand solely for a further particular aspect of human life), spiritual caregivers are, paradoxically, specialists for the whole (patient).

Acknowledgements I would like to thank Dr. Fabian Winiger for reviewing and correcting a first version of this article and for his helpful feedback.

References

1. Salander P. The Emperor's new clothes: spirituality. A concept based on questionable ontology and circular findings. Arch Psychol Relig. 2012;34(1):17–32.
2. Peng-Keller S. Healthcare chaplaincy as specialised spiritual care – the Christian call for healing in a global health context. Göttingen: Vandenhoeck & Ruprecht; 2024.
3. Peng-Keller S, Winiger F, Rauch R. The spirit of global health: the World Health Organization and the 'spiritual dimension' of health, 1946–2021. Oxford/New York: Oxford University Press; 2022. 256 p.
4. Peng-Keller S. Genealogies of 'spirituality' – an historical analysis of a travelling term. J Study Spiritual. 2019;9(2):86–98.
5. Lüddeckens D, Walthert R, editors. Fluide Religion: neue religiöse Bewegungen im Wandel; theoretische und empirische Systematisierungen. Bielefeld: Transcript; 2010. 270 p. (Sozialtheorie).
6. Fuller RC. Spiritual, but not religious: understanding unchurched America. Oxford: Oxford University Press; 2001. 238 p.
7. Borup J. Pizza, Curry, Skyr and Whirlpool effects – religious circulations between east and west. In: Borup J, Fibiger MQ, editors. Eastspirit: transnational spirituality and religious circulation in East and West [Internet]. Leiden: Brill; 2017 [cited 2021 June 30]. p. 11–35. https://brill.com/view/book/edcoll/9789004350717/B9789004350717_003.xml
8. Cottingham J. The spiritual dimension: religion, philosophy and human value. Cambridge, UK/New York: Cambridge University Press; 2005. 200 p.
9. Ammerman NT. Spiritual but not religious? Beyond binary choices in the study of religion. J Sci Study Relig. 2013;52(2):258–78.
10. Streib H, Hood R, editors. Semantics and psychology of spirituality: a cross-cultural analysis [Internet]. Cham: Springer International Publishing; 2016 [cited 2021 June 30]. https://www.springer.com/gp/book/9783319212449
11. Halík T. Christianity in a time of sickness. America Magazine [Internet]. 2020 Apr 03 [cited 2024 Jan 17]; (April 30, 2020). https://www.americamagazine.org/faith/2020/04/03/christianity-time-sickness
12. Bender C, Taves A. Introduction: things of value. In: Bender C, Taves A, editors. What matters?: ethnographies of value in a not so secular age. New York: Columbia University Press; 2012. p. 1–33.
13. Heelas P. Spiritualities of life: new age romanticism and consumptive capitalism. Malden: Blackwell Publishing; 2008. (Religion and spirituality in the modern world).

14. Cadge W, Sigalow E. Negotiating religious differences: the strategies of interfaith chaplains in healthcare. J Sci Study Relig. 2013;52(1):146–58.
15. Inbadas H. History, culture and traditions: the silent spaces in the study of spirituality at the end of life. Religions. 2016;7(5):53.
16. Bakhtin MM. Speech genres and other late essays. In: Speech genres and other late essays [Internet]. University of Texas Press; [cited 2024 Jan 17]. https://www.degruyter.com/document/isbn/9780292792562/html?lang=en
17. Bal M. Travelling concepts in the humanities: a rough guide. Toronto/Buffalo/London: University of Toronto Press; 2002.
18. Amelioration of the condition of wounded, sick and shipwrecked members of armed forces at sea. Geneva, 12 August 1949. Oct 21, 1950.
19. Diderot D, d'Alembert JLR. Spiritualité. In: L'Encyclopédie. 1st ed. Paris; 1751.
20. Schmidt LE. Restless souls: the making of American spirituality, with a new preface. 2nd ed. Berkeley: University of California Press; 2012. 360 p.
21. Baier K. Meditation und Moderne: Zur Genese eines Kernbereichs moderner Spiritualität in der Wechselwirkung zwischen Westeuropa, Nordamerika und Asien. Würzburg: Königshausen u. Neumann; 2009. 980 p.
22. Whitman W. Democratic vistas: the original edition in facsimile. 1st ed. Folsom E, editor. Iowa City: University of Iowa Press; 2009. 214 p.
23. Halbfass W. India and Europe: an essay in understanding. New York: State University of New York Press; 1988.
24. King R. Orientalism and religion: postcolonial theory, India and 'the mystic East'. London/New York: Routledge; 1999. 283 p.
25. App U. The birth of orientalism. Philadelphia: University of Pennsylvania Press; 2011. 570 p.
26. James W. The varieties of religious experience – a study in human nature. London/Bombay: Longmans, Green, and Co; 1902.
27. White CG. Unsettled minds: psychology and the American search for spiritual assurance, 1830–1940. Berkeley/Los Angeles: University of California Press; 2008. 278 p.
28. Borup J, Fibiger MQ, Borup J, Fibiger MQ, Borup J, Fibiger MQ, editors. Eastspirit: transnational spirituality and religious circulation in East and West [Internet]. Brill; 2017 [cited 2021 Dec 14]. https://brill.com/view/title/34500
29. Putney C. Muscular Christianity: manhood and sports in protestant America, 1880–1920. Repr. Cambridge, MA: Harvard University Press; 2011. 300 p.
30. Kaskutas LA, Galanter M, editors. Recent developments in alcoholism: research on alcoholics anonymous and spirituality in addiction recovery [Internet]. New York: Springer; 2008 [cited 2024 Jan 22]. (Recent Developments in Alcoholism; vol. 18). http://link.springer.com/10.1007/978-0-387-77725-2
31. Taves A. Revelatory events: three case studies of the emergence of new spiritual paths. Princeton: Princeton University Press; 2016. 384 p.
32. World Health Organization. Sixty-first session of the executive board, Geneva, 11–26 January 1978: part III: summary records [Internet]. World Health Organization; 1978 [cited 2019 Nov 7]. https://apps.who.int/iris/handle/10665/86042
33. Hanrieder T. Mahler, Halfdan Theodor. In: Reinalda B, Kille KJ, Eisenberg J, editors. IO BIO, biographical dictionary of secretaries general of international organizations [Internet]. http://www.ru.nl/fm/iobio
34. Mahler H. WHO media centre. 2008 [cited 2019 Nov 1]. Address to the 61st World Health Assembly. https://www.who.int/mediacentre/events/2008/wha61/hafdan_mahler_speech/en/
35. Primary health care comes full circle. An interview with Dr Halfdan Mahler. Bull World Health Organ. 2008;86(10):737–816.
36. Ellis G, Hynd E. Footprints on African hearts and lands: the life and work of Dr. Samuel W. Hynd. Nashville: Seaside Creative Services; 2014. 268 p.

37. World Health Organization. Thirty-sixth World Health Assembly, Geneva, 2–16 May 1983: summary records of committees [Internet]. Geneva: World Health Organization; 1983 [cited 2019 Nov 7]. https://apps.who.int/iris/handle/10665/159888
38. World Health Organization. Thirty-sixth World Health Assembly, Geneva, 2–16 May 1983: verbatim records of plenary meetings, reports of committees [Internet]. WHO; 1983 [cited 2019 Nov 4]. https://apps.who.int/iris/handle/10665/159887
39. World Health Organization. Seventy-third session of the executive board, Geneva, 11–20 January 1984: resolutions and decisions annexes. Geneva: World Health Organization; 1984.
40. Hanrieder T. The public valuation of religion in global health governance: spiritual health and the faith factor. Contemp Polit. 2017;23(1):81–99.
41. World Health Organization. Thirty-seventh World Health Assembly, Geneva, 7–17 May 1984: summary records of committees [Internet]. Geneva: World Health Organization; 1984 [cited 2019 Mar 5]. https://apps.who.int/iris/handle/10665/160776
42. Joas H. The genesis of values. 1st ed. Chicago: University of Chicago Press; 2001. p. 256.
43. Hanrieder T. Orders of worth and the moral conceptions of health in global politics. Int Theory. 2016;8(3):390–421.
44. World Health Organization, Expert Committee on Cancer Pain Relief and Active Supportive Care. Cancer pain relief and palliative care: report of a WHO expert committee – meeting held in Geneva from 3 to 10 July 1989 [İnternet]. Geneva: World Health Organization; 1990 [cited 2019 Dec 18]. https://apps.who.int/iris/handle/10665/39524
45. Sullivan WF. A ministry of presence – chaplaincy, spiritual care, and the law. Chicago: University of Chicago Press; 2014.
46. World Health Organization. Promoting mental health: concepts, emerging evidence, practice – a report of the World Health Organization, Department of Mental Health and Substance Abuse in collaboration with the Victorian Health Promotion Foundation and the University of Melbourne [Internet]. Geneva: World Health Organization; 2005 [cited 2019 Apr 23]. https://apps.who.int/iris/handle/10665/43286

Spiritual Needs and Spiritual Wellbeing of Palliative Care Patients

Arndt Büssing

Abstract Patients with chronic or life-threatening diseases but also stressed or old people have specific existential/spiritual needs which are in most cases not known by healthcare professionals. These needs can be assessed in a standardised manner for example with the Spiritual Needs Questionnaire (SpNQ-20). The intensity of spiritual needs is influenced by cultural and religious issues, personality, mood states, course of disease, life situation and thus place of treatment. However, spiritual wellbeing and spiritual needs are only marginally related; both are more or less independent dimensions with differentiated meanings as potential resources. Healthcare professionals may be the first to perceive such unmet needs and specifically support patients. For that purpose, the development of spiritual care competencies is necessary.

Keywords Spiritual Care · Spiritual needs · Spiritual wellbeing · Quality of life Patients · Palliative care

1 Introduction

Spiritual care means to support existential and spiritual needs and to care for the related fears and worries of sick, old and stressed people as a 'whole person' [1–3]. It is not a synonym for pastoral care; instead, pastoral care can be seen as a specialised aspect of spiritual care [4]. In the context of palliative care, the World Health Organisation stated that 'relieving serious health-related suffering, be it physical, psychological, social, or spiritual, is a global ethical responsibility' [5]. This requires

A. Büssing (✉)
Department of Health, Witten/Herdecke University, Herdecke, Germany
e-mail: Arndt.Buessing@uni-wh.de

M. C. Best (ed.), *Spiritual Care in Palliative Care*,
https://doi.org/10.1007/978-3-031-50864-6_3

being able to perceive these needs and support them adequately. Yet, with the exception of palliative care units and hospices, this is more often an ideal than practice.

Findings among patients with advanced cancer showed that 72% felt their spiritual needs were not or only minimally supported by the medical system; and further, 47% did not feel supported by representatives of a religious community [6]. These findings underlined that many of these patients had specific spiritual needs that remained unrecognised - and they had no one to talk to about these needs. Meanwhile, empirical data from various countries showed that spiritual needs, which are often regarded as outside of the expertise of healthcare professionals, are prevalent in various groups of people [7]. A narrative review by Mercier et al. clearly underlined that 'many adult patients with cancer report spiritual needs and a desire for the treatment team to address their spiritual needs' [8].

To assess such needs, there are a few standardised instruments available. In their literature reviews of spiritual care instruments, the *Spiritual Needs Questionnaire* was highlighted both by Seddigh et al. and by Nissen et al. [9, 10]. The *Spiritual Needs Questionnaire* (SpNQ) with 20 (+7) items and three free text fields was developed in 2009 and is currently available in 16 languages [1, 7, 11]. Its easy handling allows a structured assessment of the intensity ('importance') of spiritual needs in different groups of people [7]. The SpNQ differentiates four main dimensions: religious needs, existential needs, inner peace needs, and generativity needs [7, 11, 12]. Family support needs is an optional factor that is more a psychosocial than a spiritual need category.

The intensity of needs varies, depending on people's cultural and religious background, underlying disease and prognosis, interpretation of disease, mental health status, and various other variables [13]. Patients with cancer report higher spiritual needs than patients with chronic pain diseases [14], while residents in retirement/nursing homes have much lower needs scores [15]. These differences could be explained by differences in hope, treatment options, and expectations of life. Patients in palliative care units (PCU) and hospices may struggle more with their underlying disease and life situation, and thus, the intensity of their needs would differ from those of residents in retirement/nursing homes. It seems that many of the respondents from retirement/nursing homes have downregulated their needs because they assume they have to be satisfied with the situation as it is, and thus, they may not expect too much from their lives anymore [12].

In the following study, the aim was thus to analyse whether patients´ spiritual needs and wellbeing differ concerning the place of treatment or where they live and stay. For that purpose, participants' data from two surveys were combined and evaluated with respect to the intensity of their spiritual needs (SpNQ) [16] and spiritual wellbeing (measured by the 12-item *Functional Assessment of Chronic Illness Therapy-Spiritual Wellbeing*—FACIT-Sp) [17]. Of further interest was how these relate to the perception of health or impairment (measured by numeric rating scales-NRS) and psychological wellbeing (measured by the 5-item *World Health Organization Well-Being Index*—WHO-5) [18] as well as their satisfaction with the support they receive from family, friends, treatment staff, and pastoral workers (measured by the 10-item *Brief Multidimensional Life Satisfaction Scale*—BMLSS Support) [19].

2 Findings

The place where recruited participants (n = 899; 72% women, 28% men; 82% Christians, 2% other and 16% no religious affiliations) were living or were treated (49% Senior care facilities/Nursing homes [SCNH], 14% Geriatrics/Hospitals, 26% PCU, 12% Hospice) significantly depends on their age (mean age 78 ± 13 [29–102] years) and underlying diagnoses (43% cancer, 16% cardiovascular diseases, 4% old age/mild dementia, 37% other), and thus their health situation and perceived impairment. In PCU, 94% of patients had cancer, while in hospice 86% had cancer, 6% cardiovascular diseases, and 8% other diagnoses. In contrast, in geriatric wards and hospitals, 47% were treated for various other reasons (including stroke, Parkinson's disease, age-related fractures/falls, etc.), 28% had cancer, 23% had cardiovascular diseases, and 2% were of very old age (frailty) and had mild dementia. Also, in SCNH, residents had various other diseases (58%), 25% cardiovascular diseases, 8% old age/mild dementia, and 9% cancer. The distribution of diagnoses clusters differs significantly ($p < 0.001$; Pearson Chi^2). Within this sample, there are further significant age-related differences with a strong effect size (Table 1); the oldest people were found in SCNH, while patients in PCU were younger ($Eta^2 = 0.270$).

Table 1 Spiritual needs and treatment places

		Religious needs	Existential needs	Inner peace needs	Generativity needs	SpNQ-20 mean score	SpNQ-10 sum score (Screener)
All participants (n = 899)	Mean	1.20	0.86	1.72	1.71	1.30	13.56
	SD	0.94	0.76	0.79	0.78	0.63	6.72
Treatment places							
Senior care facilities/ Nursing homes (n = 438)	Mean	1.38	0.78	1.64	1.72	1.32	14.04
	SD	0.92	0.71	0.73	0.76	0.61	6.46
Geriatrics/ Hospital (n = 127)	Mean	1.00	0.90	1.80	1.69	1.27	13.45
	SD	0.93	0.76	0.79	0.68	0.62	6.82
Palliative care units (n = 231)	Mean	0.98	0.91	1.71	1.63	1.23	12.10
	SD	0.93	0.83	0.87	0.86	0.68	7.12
Hospice (n = 103)	Mean	1.12	1.01	2.04	1.89	1.42	14.94
	SD	0.92	0.78	0.74	0.77	0.59	6.27
p value		**<0.001**	0.019	**<0.001**	0.050	0.046	**<0.001**
Eta^2 value		0.040	0.011	0.026	0.009	0.009	0.019

Effect sizes $Eta^2 < 0.06$ are regarded as small, between 0.06 and 0.14 as moderate, and >0.14 as strong. Significance levels <0.001 are highlighted (bold)

2.1 Spiritual Needs

The spiritual needs of participants were differentiated into religious, existential, inner peace, and generativity needs [7]. To make data comparable, additionally, the SpNQ-20 scores (which are mean scores of these four factors) and the SpNQ-10 Screener scores (which are a sum score of three reduced factors) were depicted (Table 1). Usually, needs for inner peace and generativity scored higher than existential and religious needs.

With regard to the care facilities, there are significant differences for religious needs, existential needs, and inner peace needs ($Eta^2 = 0.034$; $p = 0.006$), but not for generativity needs (Table 1). In SCNH, existential needs and inner peace needs are lower when compared to the respective needs of patients from other treatment places, while their religious needs are stronger. Particularly in hospice, inner peace needs, and generativity needs were higher than in the other patients. However, these differences are small only.

Compared to women, men have significantly lower religious needs ($Eta^2 = 0.049$; $p < 0.001$) and in trend also generativity needs ($Eta^2 = 0.011$; $p = 0.032$), although these differences are only weak, while there were no significant gender-related differences for existential needs ($Eta^2 = 0.001$) and inner peace needs ($Eta^2 = 0.006$) (data not shown).

2.2 Spiritual Wellbeing

Spiritual wellbeing is differentiated into Meaning, Peace, and Faith sub-scales [17]. The Faith scale is contextual and refers to the experience of illness, while Meaning and Peace are generic scales. The scale may be regarded as an indicator of psychological wellbeing and mental health rather than spirituality as a generic dimension. As shown in Table 3, the level of spiritual wellbeing is high for Meaning, moderate for Peace, and rather low for Faith (Table 2).

For the care facilities, there were significant differences in the dimension of Peace and Faith, with this being highest in residents from SCNH as compared to patients from other treatment places. However, the effect sizes are only small (Table 2). For meaning, there were no significant differences.

For men, all spiritual wellbeing dimensions (Meaning: $Eta^2 = 0.016$, $p = 0.016$; Peace: $Eta^2 = 0.029$, $p < 0.001$; Faith: $Eta^2 = 0.054$, $p < 0.001$) were lower compared to women; however, effect sizes were small (data not shown).

Table 2 Spiritual wellbeing and treatment places

		Meaning	Peace	Faith	Spiritual wellbeing mean score (FACIT-Sp)
All participants (n = 899)	Mean	3.14	2.59	2.15	2.63
	SD	0.76	0.91	1.25	0.76
Treatment places					
Senior care facilities/nursing homes (n = 438)	Mean	3.13	2.74	2.36	2.74
	SD	0.75	0.86	1.22	0.74
Geriatrics/Hospital (n = 127)	Mean	3.22	2.43	1.96	2.53
	SD	0.68	0.91	1.23	0.71
Palliative care units (n = 231)	Mean	3.16	2.44	1.93	2.51
	SD	0.76	0.90	1.30	0.76
Hospice (n = 103)	Mean	3.05	2.47	2.00	2.50
	SD	0.86	1.01	1.20	0.80
p value		0.389	**<0.001**	**<0.001**	**<0.001**
Eta^2 value		0.003	0.026	0.026	0.022

Effect sizes $Eta^2 < 0.06$ are regarded as small, between 0.06 and 0.14 as moderate, and >0.14 as strong. Significance levels <0.001 are highlighted (bold)

Table 3 Quality-of-life indicators and treatment places

		Mean age (Years)	Psychological wellbeing (WHO-5)	Perceived health situation (NRS)	Perceived impairment (NRS)	Support satisfaction (BMLSS-Support)
All participants (n = 899)	Mean	77.84	12.18	45.11	56.08	76.26
	SD	12.64	6.15	21.46	23.66	17.49
Treatment places						
Senior care facilities/ Nursing homes (n = 438)	Mean	83.53	13.66	52.75	48.84	72.58
	SD	9.86	5.81	19.56	22.97	16.93
Geriatrics/ Hospital (n = 127)	Mean	78.58	11.11	44.50	60.24	72.79
	SD	9.76	6.54	20.41	22.99	17.63
Palliative care units (n = 231)	Mean	67.67	9.20	34.59	67.61	82.20
	SD	12.35	5.49	19.05	21.47	17.13
Hospice (n = 103)	Mean	75.42	10.30	36.92	70.00	82.98
	SD	12.22	5.93	22.59	16.54	14.85
p value		**<0.001**	**<0.001**	**<0.001**	**<0.001**	**<0.001**
Eta^2 value		0.270	0.082	0.141	0.137	0.074

Effect sizes $Eta^2 < 0.06$ are regarded as small, between 0.06 and 0.14 as moderate, and >0.14 as strong. Significance levels <0.001 are highlighted (bold)

2.3 Indicators of Quality of Life

The participants assessed their health situation as 'moderate' and regarded their health impairment as 'moderate' to 'severe'; their psychological wellbeing was in the 'moderate' range (Table 3). However, they felt well-supported by their family, friends/acquaintances, therapeutic team (nurses, physicians, psychologists, etc.), and pastoral care providers.

Concerning the care facilities, there are significant differences for all four indicators with moderate effect sizes (Table 3). Psychological wellbeing and the perceived health situation were lowest and perceived impairment highest in PCU; nevertheless, PCU patients felt best supported. In contrast, residents from SCNH had the highest wellbeing and perceived health situation and the lowest perceived impairment. However, support satisfaction was lowest in SCNH and Geriatrics/Hospitals (Table 3).

There were further weak differences based on gender for perceived impairment ($Eta^2 = 0.012$; $p = 0.024$), perceived health situation ($Eta^2 = 0.012$; $p = 0.024$), and support satisfaction ($Eta^2 = 0.011$; $p = 0.031$) but no for psychological wellbeing ($Eta^2 = 0.005$) (data not shown). These differences should be regarded as trends only.

2.4 Correlations Between Spiritual Needs, Spiritual Wellbeing, and Quality-of-Life Indicators

The spiritual needs dimensions were moderately interrelated, and particularly existential and inner peace needs were strongly correlated (Table 4). However, the putatively similar topics of existential needs and meaning wellbeing are not significantly related, and inner peace needs and peace wellbeing are marginally to weakly associated, while religious needs and faith wellbeing are strongly related (Table 4). Therefore, both the SpNQ-20 mean scores and SpNQ-10 sum scores of the Screener version are only weakly related to the FACIT-Sp mean scores. Spiritual needs and spiritual wellbeing are thus more or less independent dimensions with their meaning and justification as unmet resources [13].

Table 4 Correlations between spiritual needs and spiritual wellbeing

	Religious needs	Existential needs	Inner peace needs	Generativity needs	SpNQ-20 mean score	SpNQ-10 sum score (screener)
Spiritual needs						
Religious needs	1.000					
Existential needs	0.397*	1.000				
Inner peace needs	.0334*	0.563*	1.000			
Generativity needs	0.380*	0.490*	0.459*	1.000		
SpNQ-20 mean score	0.770*	0.795*	0.717*	0.710*	1.000	
SpNQ-10 sum score	0.755*	0.738*	0.778*	0.551*	0.943*	1.000
Spiritual wellbeing						
Meaning	0.111*	–0.048	0.008	0.188*	0.084	0.046
Peace	0.083	–0.219*	–0.156*	0.034	–0.069	–0.072
Faith	0.637*	0.144*	0.110*	0.203*	0.411*	0.408*
FACIT-Sp mean score	0.430*	–0.019	0.003	0.189*	0.234*	0.217*

*$p < 0.0001$ (Spearman rho); moderate and strong correlations are highlighted (yellow or orange)

Are spiritual needs and spiritual wellbeing related to perceived health impairments and low quality of life? For obvious reasons, psychological and spiritual wellbeing are moderately related (here it is the Peace dimension that is strongly related to psychological wellbeing) (Table 5). Perceived impairment, perceived health situation, and support satisfaction (i.e. patient perceptions) are weakly related to spiritual wellbeing. In contrast, participants' spiritual needs are not triggered by reduced quality of life alone (Table 5). Perceived impairment and psychological wellbeing are weakly related to existential and inner peace needs, but not to religious needs.

Table 5 Correlations between quality-of-life indicators and spiritual needs and spiritual wellbeing

	Psychological wellbeing (WHO-5)	Perceived health situation (NRS)	Perceived impairment (NRS)	Support satisfaction (BMLSS-Support)
Quality of life indicators				
Psychological wellbeing	1.000			
Perceived health situation	0.446*	1.000		
Perceived impairment	−0.399*	−0.516*	1.000	
Support	0.161*	−0.041	0.016	1.000
Spiritual needs				
Religious needs	0.077	0.086	−0.030	0.065
Existential needs	−0.208*	−0.076	0.217*	−0.023
Inner Peace needs	−0.196*	−0.075	0.216*	0.065
Generativity needs	0.018	0.030	0.100*	0.091*
SpNQ-20 mean score	−0.090	0.005	0.146*	0.063
SpNQ-10 sum score	−0.096*	0.023	0.135*	0.042
Spiritual wellbeing				
Meaning	0.310*	0.162*	−0.135*	0.272*
Peace	0.527*	0.267*	−0.270*	0.167*
Faith	0.279*	0.185*	−0.151*	0.184*
FACIT-Sp mean score	0.470*	0.254*	−0.230*	00.256*

*$p < 0.0001$ (Spearman rho); moderate and strong correlations are highlighted (yellow or orange)

3 Discussion

The basic pattern of spiritual needs as well as the spiritual and psychological wellbeing of people from different care areas in this study is similar to that of other palliative care patients from South-West Germany [20]. For the latter, these variables hardly changed over the course of their 2–3 weeks stay at the PCU; their satisfaction with the support from the therapeutic team was nevertheless very high [20]. This means, that even at the end of their PCU stay, patients still had spiritual needs, but they also saw that the therapeutic team cared for them and supported them as well as possible.

While it is important to assess patients' psychosocial, existential, and spiritual needs, particularly at the end of their lives, patients in the early stages of the disease have the same pattern and intensity of unmet spiritual needs. Comparing the findings of the spiritual needs of cancer patients receiving palliative care [20, 21] with those in earlier stages of the disease [14, 22] clearly indicates that they have the same intensity [3]. Thus, not only patients at the end of life require support but already at the time of diagnosis, and also when people have to live in nursing homes and may have lost their independence and courage to live.

Patients' basic stress caused by their life situation (as a sick or dying person) is only marginally related to the intensity of spiritual needs. In fact, spiritual needs arise from many reasons and causes, not just from the lack of something [13]. Spiritual needs may rather be an expression of patients' longing for life in abundance—which always remains, even in PCU and hospices.

Both dimensions, spiritual needs and spiritual wellbeing, have to be assessed in spiritual care processes: the burden experienced by the patient (indicated for example by the absence of spiritual wellbeing) and the resources that might be available to them (indicated by the spiritual needs). The resulting conversations with healthcare professionals and pastoral workers may help patients to cope with their fears and worries; talking with someone may provide hope and comfort, it helps them to reconcile with life and to reconnect with the specifically Sacred—and thereby restoring dignity and finding peace and acceptance.

Even if these spiritual needs are still prevalent until the end of life and cannot be 'resolved' at all (as they may express basic longings for salvation, meaning, purpose, and finally inner peace that cannot be satisfied), patients were mostly satisfied with the support from their family (4.9 ± 1.5) and the therapeutic staff (4.8 ± 1.1). They were also satisfied with the support from friends and acquaintances (4.3 ± 1.7) but less satisfied with pastoral care (3.9 ± 1.6). A relevant finding is that the pastoral care support was much higher in PCU as compared to SCNH (4.4 ± 1.6 vs. 3.6 ± 1.6; $Eta^2 = 0.051$, $p < 0.011$). It could be that pastoral care providers are less often available in SCNH, despite the residents expressing unmet spiritual needs, and they may, as a result, have felt lonely and isolated.

Person-centred care at the end of life means taking patients' needs and burdens seriously [23]. Mercier et al. suggested that 'addressing spiritual needs helps patients maintain hope, assists clinicians in sustaining cultural humility during times of medical decision-making, and promotes well-being among survivors' [8]. The fact that nurses, in particular, have special importance in perceiving and supporting the spirituality of residents in SCNH and patients in PCU has been described and discussed many times [24–28]. This requires the development of spiritual care competencies not only as an individual but as a multi-professional team [29–31]. Everyone in the team contributes specific skills based on their own professional qualifications, and these should be supplemented by spiritual competencies to best support patients.

4 Conclusion

Spiritual care is a multi-professional approach where healthcare professionals may be the first to perceive patients' unmet needs and their fears and worries. It is important to address psychosocial, existential, and spiritual needs, particularly at the end of their lives [32]. These needs can be assessed in a standardised way either with the extended version of the *Spiritual Needs Questionnaire* (SpNQ-20) or with its 10-item Screening version. There are significant differences in the intensity of spiritual needs depending on cultural and religious issues, personality, mood states, the course of disease and how they perceive their life situation, and thus place of treatment, which should be considered in Spiritual Care approaches.

Acknowledgement Many thanks to all cooperation partners who contributed to the Spiritual Needs project, and to all participants for filling out the anonymous questionnaires.

References

1. Frick E, Roser T. Spiritualität und Medizin. Gemeinsame Sorge um den kranken Menschen. Stuttgart: Kohlhammer; 2011.
2. Gijsberts M-JHE. Spiritual care in palliative care: a physician's perspective. Religions. 2022;13(4):323. https://doi.org/10.3390/rel13040323.
3. Büssing A. Spirituellen Bedürfnissen begegnen: Welche Relevanz hat es für Krebspatient*innen? Die Onkologie. 2024;30 (Suppl. 1):S19–S24
4. Peng-Keller S. Klinikseelsorge als spezialisierte Spiritual Care. Der christliche Heilungsauftrag im Horizont globaler Gesundheit. Göttingen: Vandenhoeck & Ruprecht; 2021.
5. WHO. Palliative care. 2023. Available at: https://www.who.int/health-topics/palliative-care. Last accessed on 6 Nov 2023.
6. Balboni TA, Vanderwerker LC, Block SD, Paulk ME, Lathan CS, Peteet JR, Prigerson HG. Religiousness and spiritual support among advanced cancer patients and associations with end-of-life treatment preferences and quality of life. J Clin Oncol. 2007;25:555–60. https://doi.org/10.1200/JCO.2006.07.9046.
7. Büssing A. Spiritual needs in research and practice. The spiritual needs questionnaire as a global resource for health and social care. Cham: Palgrave Macmillan; 2021.
8. Mercier M, Maglio J, Almhanna K, Guyer D. Spiritual care for adult patients with cancer: from maintaining hope and respecting cultures to supporting survivors—a narrative review. Ann Palliat Med. 2023;12(5):1047–58. https://doi.org/10.21037/apm-22-1274.
9. Seddigh R, Keshavarz-Akhlaghi AA, Azarnik S. Questionnaires measuring patients' spiritual needs: a narrative literature review. Iran J Psychiatry Behav Sci. 2016;10:e4011. https://doi.org/10.17795/ijpbs-4011.
10. Nissen RD, Falkø E, Toudal DV, Assing-Hvidt E, Büssing A, Søndergaard J, Walin JA, Hvidt NC. The catalogue of spiritual care instruments: a scoping review. Religions. 2020;11:252. https://doi.org/10.3390/rel11050252.
11. Büssing A, Recchia DR, Koenig H, Baumann K, Frick E. Factor structure of the spiritual needs questionnaire (SpNQ) in persons with chronic diseases, elderly and healthy individuals. Religions. 2018;9:13. https://doi.org/10.3390/rel9010013.

12. Büssing A, Koenig HG. Spiritual needs of patients with chronic diseases. Religions. 2010;1:18–27. https://doi.org/10.3390/rel1010018.
13. Büssing A. The spiritual needs questionnaire in research and clinical application: a summary of findings. J Relig Health. 2021b;60:3732–48. https://doi.org/10.1007/s10943-021-01421-4.
14. Büssing A, Janko A, Baumann K, Hvidt NC, Kopf A. Spiritual needs among patients with chronic pain diseases and cancer living in a secular society. Pain Med. 2013;14:1362–73. https://doi.org/10.1111/pme.12198.
15. Erichsen NB, Büssing A. Spiritual needs of elderly living in residential/nursing homes. Evid Based Complement Alternat Med. 2013;2013:913247. https://doi.org/10.1155/2013/913247.
16. Büssing A, Balzat HJ, Heusser P. Spiritual needs of patients with chronic pain diseases and cancer – validation of the spiritual needs questionnaire. Eur J Med Res. 2010;15:266–73. https://doi.org/10.1186/2047-783X-15-6-266.
17. Bredle JM, Salsman JM, Debb SM, Arnold BJ, Cella D. Spiritual well-being as a component of health-related quality of life: the functional assessment of chronic illness therapy – spiritual well-being scale (FACIT-Sp). Religions. 2011;2:77–94. https://doi.org/10.3390/rel2010077.
18. Bech P, Olsen LR, Kjoller M, Rasmussen NK. Measuring well-being rather than the absence of distress symptoms: a comparison of the SF-36 mental health subscale and the WHO-Five well-being scale. Int J Methods Psychiatr Res. 2013;12:85–91.
19. Büssing A, Fischer J, Haller A, Heusser P, Ostermann T, Matthiessen PF. Validation of the brief multidimensional life satisfaction scale in patients with chronic diseases. Eur J Med Res. 2009;14:171–7.
20. Büssing A, Baumann K, Rentschler J, Becker G. Spirituelle Bedürfnisse von Tumorpatien-ten verändern sich während der palliativmedizinischen Betreuung kaum. Deutsche Zeitschrift für Onkologie. 2020;52:111–6. https://doi.org/10.1055/a-1135-3566.
21. Büssing A, Scheer K, Tewes M, Niesert W, Büntzel J, Rentschler. Erfassung existenzieller und spiritueller Bedürfnisse in der palliativen Betreuung – Erste Erkenntnisse zur Implementierung des Spiritual Needs Screeners. Spirit Care. 2022;11:278–81. https://doi.org/10.1515/spircare-2022-0045.
22. Höcker A, Krüll A, Koch U, Mehnert A. Exploring spiritual needs and their associated factors in an urban sample of early and advanced cancer patients. Eur J Cancer Care. 2014;23:786–94. https://doi.org/10.1111/ecc.12200.
23. Stevenson-Baker S. Promoting person-centred care at the end of life. Nurs Stand. 2023;38(11):76–82. https://doi.org/10.7748/ns.2023.e12171.
24. Baldacchino DR. Nursing competencies for spiritual care. J Clin Nurs. 2006;15(7):885–96. https://doi.org/10.1111/j.1365-2702.2006.01643.x.
25. McSherry W. The principal components model: a model for advancing spirituality and spiritual care within nursing and health care practice. J Clin Nurs. 2006;15(7):905–17. https://doi.org/10.1111/j.1365-2702.2006.01648.x.
26. Wallace M, O'Shea E. Perceptions of spirituality and spiritual care among older nursing home residents at the end of life. Holist Nurs Pract. 2007;21(6):285–9. https://doi.org/10.1097/01.HNP.0000298611.02352.46.
27. Edwards A, Pang N, Shiu V, Chan C. Review: the understanding of spirituality and the potential role of spiritual care in end-of-life and palliative care: a meta-study of qualitative research. Palliat Med. 2010;24(8):753–70. https://doi.org/10.1177/0269216310375860.
28. Gijsberts MHE, Liefbroer AI, Otten R, Olsman E. Spiritual care in palliative care: a systematic review of the recent european literature. Med Sci. 2019;7(2):25. https://doi.org/10.3390/medsci7020025.
29. Ross L, McSherry W, Giske T, van Leeuwen R, Schep-Akkerman A, Koslander T, Hall J, Steenfeldt VØ, Jarvis P. Nursing and midwifery students' perceptions of spirituality, spiritual care, and spiritual care competency: a prospective, longitudinal, correlational European study. Nurse Educ Today. 2018;67:64–71. https://doi.org/10.1016/j.nedt.2018.05.002.

30. Frick E, Theiss M, Recchia DR, Büssing A. Validierung einer deutschsprachigen Skala zur Messung von Spiritual Care Kompetenzen. Spirit Care. 2019;8(2):193–207. https://doi.org/10.1515/spircare-2018-0066.
31. Pastrana T, Frick E, Recchia DR, Krikorian A, Ascencio L, Galeazzi F, Büssing A. Translation and validation of the Spanish version of the Spiritual Care Competence Questionnaire (SCCQ). J Relig Health. 2021;60(5):3621–39. https://doi.org/10.1007/s10943-021-01402-7.
32. Büssing A, Giebel A, Roser T, editors. Spiritual Care & Existential Care interprofessionell. Handbuch spiritueller und existentieller Begleitung in der Gesundheitsversorgung. Stuttgart: Springer; 2024.

Challenges and Approaches to Assessing and Addressing Palliative Patients' Spiritual Needs

Bella Vivat

Abstract Considerable attention continues to be paid to debating spirituality and related concepts: both the term itself, and also spiritual wellbeing, and how the latter relates to psychological, emotional, existential, or social wellbeing, needs, and distress. Alongside these debates, it is also generally agreed that palliative care patients' spiritual needs are frequently not well met, and spiritual care overall is suboptimal. This may be partly due to difficulties with reaching conceptual agreement, which often stagnates in the position that consensus on definitions is impossible, since spirituality is always individual. Yet, there is some common understanding of spiritual care, with shared broad dimensions, while also usually highlighting the individuality of each person's needs, and therefore of the care they require.

The nature of needs and care in this area also unsettles the customary approach to health and social care interventions, which is usually sequential: assessing need/s, planning intervention/s, implementation, and then evaluation (often through re-assessment), enabling planning for next steps. Thus, assessments generally occur before, and separately from, any intervention. However, assessing spiritual needs entails enquiry into the person's spiritual concerns, which of itself is (or initiates) an intervention, so, a spiritual assessment is always also a spiritual intervention, and an initial assessment is simultaneously an initial intervention. Uncertainty around this phenomenon may also contribute to suboptimal provision of spiritual care. Conversely, use of a suitable assessment tool may enable and support palliative care professionals to at least begin to identify and engage with palliative patients' spiritual concerns.

B. Vivat (✉)
Marie Curie Palliative Care Research Department, Division of Psychiatry, University College London (UCL), London, UK
e-mail: b.vivat@ucl.ac.uk

M. C. Best (ed.), *Spiritual Care in Palliative Care*,
https://doi.org/10.1007/978-3-031-50864-6_4

Keywords Assessment · Existential needs · Implementation · Intervention Palliative care · Quality-of-life · Questionnaire · Spiritual care · Spiritual wellbeing Spirituality

1 Introduction

This chapter addresses the ongoing debates regarding the meaning of terms such as spirituality, spiritual needs, and how these relate to, and the consequences for, the provision of the spiritual aspect of care and addressing spiritual needs, particularly those of people with life-limiting conditions. Next, the chapter considers what it means to assess a person's spiritual needs, how this is or might be done, whether the typical separation and distinction made in models of professional care between assessment and intervention, as sequential steps [1], applies in the case of spiritual care, and whether a spiritual assessment can ever be distinct from a spiritual intervention.

It has been, and continues to be, frequently stated [2–5] that growth of interest in spirituality has been rapid. Unfortunately, however, some of this involves the revisiting of issues which have been exhaustively addressed in previous years, often seeking to derive universally acceptable definitions, frequently via small-scale qualitative studies. Publications discussing this topic therefore frequently comprise debates over meanings and definitions [6–8]. However, some issues around definitions are irreconcilable, e.g. whether relationships belong in the spiritual or the psychological domain, and so reaching any consensus is challenging, and the attempt to do so can stall or sidetrack any progress [8].

Studies also frequently observe that spiritual care for patients is suboptimal, or even absent [9–11], e.g. a study with terminally ill people which distinguished between existential, spiritual, and emotional issues states that respondents commented that it was rare for the care they received to address the existential, spiritual, familiar, and emotional aspects of their illness [9].

Fisher et al. [12] point out that the concept of 'spiritual health' is not straightforward, because both terms have expanded. The term 'spiritual' is now understood as much broader than matters relating to the soul, and, similarly, the understanding of 'health' has widened to include the whole person, and not only the treatment of disease, but a sense or state of wellbeing. Yet, interestingly, at the same time as general understandings of 'spiritual' and 'health' are becoming broader, theoretical conceptualisations of spirituality and related issues seem to be becoming narrower.

Key debates concern the term spirituality, and similarities or distinctions between it and its various linked concepts: spiritual wellbeing, spiritual distress, and spiritual needs, and spiritual, emotional, psychological, existential, and social needs and wellbeing. These debates over definitions of concepts echo those regarding definitions of quality of life, and also regarding distinctions in the wider field, between constructs such as palliative care, end-of-life care, supportive care, and palliative medicine [8].

A particularly prevalent strand of the considerable debate over the definition of spirituality/spiritual wellbeing and the related issue of the content of measures of these and related concepts, is the relationship or distinction between the psychological and the spiritual, particularly whether one subsumes the other. Resolution in these debates still seems remote; instead, the fragmentation between different concepts continues, and is, if anything, increasing, although they nevertheless seem fundamentally rather closely related.

The chapter outlines key points of debates around definition and conceptualisation, and then discusses the implications for spiritual assessments and spiritual care interventions.

2 Context: Concepts and Definitions

The term 'palliative care' is just 50 years old, having been introduced by Balfour Mount in 1973 [13]. It grew from Cicely Saunders' theory of 'total pain' [14–19] that the pain of a dying person had four aspects: physical, social, emotional, and spiritual (initially understood as solely religious), which are inextricably interwoven, and all had to be met, via 'total care', for the pain to be addressed. 'Total care' in palliative or hospice care has therefore always been understood to include spiritual care.

However, from early in the construction and professionalisation of this field, the interrelationship between these four aspects of palliative care, and the nature of the non-physical aspects, have been unresolved questions, with the spiritual aspect the most marginalised [20].

Palliative medicine was established as a subspecialty of general medicine in the United Kingdom in 1987, and as a specialty in its own right in 1994 [14]. In the interim, and almost simultaneously, similar concerns were expressed in both the United Kingdom [21] and the United States [22] that palliative medicine could become merely 'symptomatology', offering an expertise which comprised solely the effective management of physical symptoms. Derek Doyle argued that palliative care providers should not be 'merely symptomatologists', but 'have no choice but to be alert to and responsive to human spiritual needs' [21].

Thus, almost from the beginning, palliative care and palliative medicine have existed as two related but somehow distinct terms, and the meaning of both has been contested, explicitly or otherwise, as continues to date [23]. Pastrana et al. have argued that the continuing contestation is due not to a lack of conceptual clarity, but is rather somewhat the opposite, resulting from attempts to achieve precision in meaning [23]. They point out that the multiplicity of terms for related and overlapping fields such as palliative care, terminal care, end-of-life care, hospice care, 'do not simply reflect a jumble of terms but point to the diversity of meanings' [23, p. 222].

Amidst this focus on terminology, what is also a continuing situation is the marginalisation of the spiritual dimension, and this despite the early expressions of concern that palliative medicine could become 'just another specialty' [21, 22] and repeated national and international statements of definition and policy. For example, from the United Kingdom's National Institute of Health and Care Excellence (NICE) in 2019 [24], or the repeated emphasis of the World Health Organization (WHO) on palliative care including and integrating spiritual issues with physical and psychosocial, or, later, dividing the latter into psychological and social (in 2012 the WHO used both, see last line of the following quote) [25–28]. The WHO 2012 definition of palliative care stated:

> Palliative care is an approach that improves the quality of life of patients and their families [...] by means of early identification and impeccable assessment and treatment of pain and other problems, physical, psychosocial and spiritual. Palliative care [...] integrates the psychological and spiritual aspects of patient care [25].

WHO Resolution 67.19 in 2014 [26] states:

> [...] it is the ethical duty of health care professionals to alleviate pain and suffering, whether physical, psychosocial or spiritual, irrespective of whether the disease or condition can be cured [...] [26, p. 2]

The revised 2020 definition emphasises the ethical dimension, and also separates 'psychosocial' into psychological and social [27, 28]:

> Palliative care is a crucial part of integrated, people-centred health services. Relieving serious health-related suffering, be it physical, psychological, social, or spiritual, is a global ethical responsibility.

However, despite these repeated statements of policy explicitly referring to spiritual needs, there continues to be a degree of rather strange reticence to engage with spiritual issues in palliative medicine. The European Association of Palliative Care (EAPC) was founded in 1988, but an EAPC 'Task Force' for spiritual care in palliative care was only established in April 2010 [29], while spiritual care has continued to be lacking or even completely absent in some end-of-life/palliative care contexts [10, 11, 19, 30–32].

This lack has been ascribed to various factors, such as anxiety and uncertainty by some staff concerning how to address patients' spiritual needs, a felt lack of expertise on the part of staff [10, 11, 19] and/or lack of time [31], or patients being reluctant to initiate relevant conversations [32, p. 286], although this latter finding emerged from a study with family physicians in the United States, which did not explore their actual practices, but rather asked them about hypothesised acts. Other studies have found reticence around initiating these kinds of discussions on the part of both staff and patients [10, 19, 32].

In the last few decades, growing numbers of research studies relating to spiritual issues have been published, and research studies in hospices or other palliative care settings increasingly explore what 'total' or holistic care actually means in practice (e.g. [19, 33–35]).

It has been, and continues to be, frequently argued that there is a need for suitable, high-quality measures of spirituality or related issues for people receiving end-of-life or palliative care [4, 36, 37]. Associated with this, frequent research activities, often concurrent with attempts to construct definitive definitions, involve reviews of the literature (systematic and otherwise) for measures of spirituality or related issues, such as spiritual wellbeing, as well as papers reporting on new measures.

2.1 *Spirituality*

Spirituality can seem an amorphous concept, usually considered multidimensional, and, more often in recent years—accompanying increased secularisation in the global North [38]—to be broader than religious beliefs or affiliations, or Saunders' more narrowly religious understanding [16, 17]. People generally have particular, individual understandings of the meaning of spirituality [39], and, since sociocultural factors shape understandings of religion and spirituality, and the conceptual relationship between them, these are diverse within and between cultures [40]. A frequent argument relating to this is that, if spirituality is only what an individual ascribes to it, then so too are spiritual issues and concerns, and it is therefore impossible to make any generalised statements about anything in this field. Some argue further that any attempt to produce a universal definition of spirituality will inevitably exclude some groups [41].

Relatedly, people's responses to measures of spirituality or related concepts must always be understood in the context of their own personal ways of understanding these concepts, and their own understandings of their own spirituality [42]. This can lead to the claim that no standardised measure can capture any person's spirituality. A further argument is that measuring spirituality or spiritual concerns is per se a contradictory activity since the concepts are by their nature impossible to measure [43].

Despite these challenges, some in the field have still attempted to reach a workable definition of spirituality, broadly acceptable by all, which acknowledges the diversity, breadth, and richness, and the tensions between various conceptualisations, while still finding common ground for research and practice in the field [29, 44].

In 1997, Hall said that the link between religion and spirit is the search for meaning, which can culminate in an understanding of self, others, God, and the meaning of one's life [45]. Sawatzky et al. [42] argue that, while definitions of spirituality are diverse, it is possible to extract some common characteristics: defined by subjective experiences; having a relationship to something that lies beyond the physical, psychological, or social; an existential search for meaning and purpose; and being distinct from religion. Similar core factors are identified in other conceptual analyses, which often centre relationship, with oneself, others, the environment and the significant or sacred [4, 29, 44, 46]. The Scottish Government's document *Spiritual Care and Chaplaincy* [47] argues 'that the spiritual dimension is a natural dimension of what it means to be human' and that this dimension includes an awareness of self, and of relationships with others and with creation. Others call relationship connectedness [39], and define spirituality as connectedness, finding meaning in life and the ability to transcend current circumstances [39].

2.2 Quality of Life (QOL)

As noted, the WHO definition of palliative care includes the term 'quality of life', and from early on the National Hospice Organization in the United States also stated that a goal of palliative care is to improve or enhance patients' quality of life (QOL) [48], a term which is now much less problematic than when first introduced on a wide scale in the early 1980s [8]. Many QOL measures have been developed over the past few decades, most particularly for people with cancer, and, although contested by some [49] the term is now common, often simply with the abbreviation 'QOL', and no explanation.

Current debates in the field of spirituality strongly parallel previous debates concerning QOL which were prevalent in the 1990s (and still persist in some quarters). One key issue has always been whether it is possible to have standardised measures of QOL, or whether QOL is always, unavoidably, subjective and specific to each individual [50, 51]. Other debates concerning QOL generally revolve around how the concept is defined, including arguments over whether it is a single construct or multi-dimensional [52], which specific domains or dimensions are relevant, and whether it is appropriate to explore those dimensions collectively, or whether they should be examined separately.

Early research on quality of life was mostly conducted in relation to serious or chronic illness, particularly cancer [53, 54], but this work seldom addressed the spiritual domain. There is no spiritual domain in either of the two widely used general quality of life measures developed in the 1980s, neither the EORTC QLQ-C30 (developed by the European Organisation for Research and Treatment of Cancer (EORTC) Quality of Life Group (QLG) in Europe) [53] nor FACT-G (developed in the United States by the Functional Assessment of Cancer Therapy (FACT) group, later the Functional Assessment of Chronic Illness Therapy (FACIT) group) [54].

2.3 Spiritual Wellbeing

It took some years for either of these large QOL-focused organisations to address the spiritual dimension, and to begin developing measures which took account of spiritual issues. However, in the 1990s, spiritual wellbeing was increasingly highlighted as a discrete domain, equally as important as physical wellbeing when assessing quality of life for people with cancer [55], and distinct from quality of life and other domains: psychological, social (or psychosocial), and emotional [55–57]. Definitions of spiritual wellbeing linked closely with those of spirituality, often emphasising that spiritual wellbeing is the functional aspect of spirituality [4]. In the United States, Ferrell et al. [58] developed a definition of QOL which included spiritual wellbeing, together with three other domains: physical wellbeing, psychological wellbeing, and social wellbeing. In 1996, the WHO defined QOL as having six domains: physical health, psychological state, levels of independence, social relationships, environmental features, and spiritual concerns, and the 100-item WHOQOL (World Health Organization Quality of Life questionnaire) was developed to include all six [59]. The McGill Quality of Life Questionnaire, developed contemporaneously, included an existential domain [60].

The WHOQOL was later reduced from 100 items to 26, the WHOQOL-BREF, with four domains: physical health, psychological health, social relationships, and environment, thus removing the spiritual domain (along with independence). Later, a separate WHO measure of spirituality, religion, and personal beliefs (SRPB) [61] was developed to address this domain alone. Several other standalone measures were developed in the United States in the late 1990s, including the Functional Assessment of Chronic Illness Therapy—Spiritual Well-being Scale (FACIT-Sp) [56], while the EORTC QLG in Europe had also begun developing a measure of palliative care, which was to include a spiritual dimension [4], work which later evolved into developing a single stand-alone measure of spiritual wellbeing for people receiving palliative care for cancer, the EORTC QLQ-SWB32 (SWB32) [4, 62, 63]. This latter project ran from 2002 to 2017, and I was co-Principal Investigator with Teresa Young throughout. We followed the standard, cross-cultural, multilingual QLG approach to developing quality of life measures [64], and developed the SWB32 internationally from the outset, with collaborators in multiple countries using multiple languages. The final validation study included 451 patient participants, in 14 countries, using 10 languages [63].

At the outset, we agreed that the measure would be functional, that is, assess spiritual wellbeing rather than spirituality, and originally hypothesised three broad domains for spiritual wellbeing: relationships with self and others, religion, and existential [4]. These link with the generally understood conceptualisations of spirituality outlined above (e.g. [29, 42, 44, 46]), with relationship being core. The final validated measure, the SWB32, has four scales: relationship with self, relationships with others (the factor analysis split the single hypothesised domain into two), relationship with someone or something greater, and existential, plus an item for global spiritual wellbeing, and a single-item scale for relationship with God, for respondents with a religious faith including a personal God [63]. It has since been translated into another 12 languages including Bengali, Croatian, Finnish, Swahili, and Vietnamese [65–69], and validated in other countries and with people with illnesses other than cancer and with non-terminal diseases (e.g. [66]).

Studies continue to highlight the importance of spiritual wellbeing for people living with advanced disease [70–72]. Higher levels of spiritual wellbeing are associated with improved outcomes [73], including protecting against distress and despair [74, 75], depression and anxiety [76], and helping acceptance and adjustment and even personal growth [74, 77] for patients. Higher spiritual wellbeing benefits informal carers too [78–80]. Many more randomised controlled trials have been conducted in the last decade (40 in 2011–2022) [81] than in the previous 25 years (five in 1985–2011) [82], and 26 of the 40 used spiritual wellbeing as an outcome [81]. However, wide variations in study designs, which outcomes are assessed, and which outcome measures are used, limit meaningful comparisons between studies [81], and details of the mechanisms and causal relationships for these associations are still lacking [83]. More research is needed, from all perspectives and methodologies [83–85], and greater consistency between studies [81].

2.4 Debates over Distinctions and Boundaries Between Spiritual and Other Terms and Concepts

As noted, debates in this field regarding terminology and definitions of concepts are prominent and take much energy and attention. These debates echo those regarding definitions of quality of life, and also concerning distinctions between constructs such as palliative care, end-of-life care, supportive care, and palliative medicine [8]. They focus on similarities or distinctions between spiritual and existential, psychological, or emotional, and occasionally social, needs, wellbeing, distress, care, and assessments, all of which are central concerns and considerations for practice. Interestingly, there is much less debate over the distinction between spiritual and religious, and it seems more generally accepted that spiritual care is not necessarily religious, but religious care may be part of spiritual care, and should always itself be spiritual [47].

Existential

One strand of debate in this area concerns whether existential and spiritual are the same or separate categories [86, 87]. Some argue that existential concerns include loss of personal meaning, whereas spirituality is general beliefs about the meaning of life [88], but proponents of separation are not often clear on how they wish to distinguish between these concepts. Mount et al. [86] discuss 'the relevance of the existential and spiritual domains to suffering, healing and quality of life', pointing out that suffering does not solely equate with lack of physical wellbeing, and stating that the two extremes of QOL are suffering and subjective wellbeing. As noted above, the McGill Quality of Life Questionnaire, developed by Mount and colleagues in Canada, has an existential domain [60]. However, it is not clear how they consider that the existential and spiritual domains are distinct, nor how they contribute differently to suffering.

The Last Acts Task Force in the United States has also distinguished between the spiritual and the existential, stating:

> Palliative care refers to the comprehensive management of the physical, psychological, social, spiritual and existential needs of patients [...] The goal of palliative care is to achieve the best possible quality of life [89].

Yet, similarly, despite presenting spiritual and existential needs as separate, this document provides no clarity on how they are considered to differ from one another. In their review of the palliative care literature on existential suffering, Boston et al. [87] argued that the concepts of spiritual and existential issues are sometimes used interchangeably and conflated with one another, that the meanings of the two terms are not always clearly defined, and that spiritual measures are unsuitable for addressing existential needs. However, they also do not clearly define their own understanding of either concept, nor how they distinguish them from one another.

Psychological

As outlined earlier, since the 1990s, when definitions of QOL began to include a dimension relating to the spiritual, all have clearly distinguished this from the psychological or emotional, and of course, the concept of the spiritual long pre-dates any concept of the psychological. Nevertheless, another ongoing debate centres on whether spiritual issues are distinct from psychological issues, and, again paralleling debates concerning whether quality of life subsumes spirituality or vice versa, how spiritual wellbeing and psychological wellbeing relate to one another, and whether one subsumes the other. Those making this argument usually take the position that psychological wellbeing subsumes spiritual (e.g. [2, 3, 41, 90]).

Some authors categorise feelings of meaning and purpose in life, positive relations with others, and personal growth as psychological wellbeing, and distinguish these from spiritual perceptions [91]. It has also been argued that measures of spiritual wellbeing which include positive psychological traits are flawed, since they are tautological (i.e. wellbeing is a positive psychological trait), so positive outcomes will necessarily correlate with positive mental health [2, 91].

Bekelman et al. [94] sought to address criticisms (e.g. [92]) that the FACIT-Sp measures psychological rather than spiritual wellbeing, and to identify whether the FACIT-Sp [56] and another measure, the Ironson-Woods Spirituality/Religiousness Index [93], obtained the same or different information from respondents. Bekelman et al. point out that instruments that claim to be measuring the same spiritual domains may in fact be measuring different concepts, and argue that their data demonstrate that, while there is some overlap between psychological and spiritual wellbeing, they are distinct phenomena [94].

Coping

Linked to the explicit or implicit claim that psychological wellbeing subsumes spiritual wellbeing, another rather reductionist perspective identifies spiritual beliefs and practices as one coping process among others [95], i.e. holds that finding a positive meaning in one's experiences is simply a way of coping psychologically, rather than one outcome of connection with someone or something beyond or greater than oneself.

Relatedly, some studies use terms such as 'negative religious coping' for religious struggle, such as questioning God's love [96, 97]. But spiritual or religious doubt or uncertainty is much broader than simply an indication that someone is not coping; rather than spiritual wellbeing being a way of coping, therefore, it is rather the opposite, i.e. that coping may be an outcome of spiritual wellbeing. In contrast, Mako et al. [98] argue that spiritual struggles are connected with psychological distress, but do not equate the two.

Others respond to the problem of definitions/domains by collapsing spiritual and psychological wellbeing into a single concept, such as 'psycho-spiritual wellbeing', which Lin and Bauer-Wu [99] define as including both emotional health and meaning-in-life concerns. This then links to yet another point of focus, meaning in life [100], which, again, some identify as distinct from spirituality or spiritual wellbeing, while some claim that meaning in life is not a dimension of, but an outcome of, spirituality [101]. Others distinguish between quality of life and meaning in life, arguing that the latter is related to spirituality and self-transcendence, whereas quality of life reflects current, subjective wellbeing [100].

Distress

The tendency of some to perceive psychological concepts as subsuming all others, even when citing other authors who do make a clear distinction between psychological and other issues, is also evident with regard to distress. The United States National Comprehensive Cancer Network has defined distress as:

> ...a multifactorial unpleasant emotional experience of a psychological (cognitive, behavioral, emotional), social, and/or spiritual nature... Distress extends along a continuum [...] to problems [...] such as depression, anxiety, panic, social isolation, and existential and spiritual crisis. [102]

A systematic review of psychological distress [103] frames the study by referring to this definition, yet collapses all these clearly distinguished psychological/emotional and spiritual or existential issues into a single, psychological, dimension, and states that 'distress' refers to emotional or psychological problems. Similarly, an Italian study [104] of the 'psychological and symptom distress' of terminal care patients, identified patients' needs using a semi-structured interview, which sought to explore five areas: physiological needs, safety needs, love and belonging needs, self-esteem needs, and self-fulfilment needs, and identify which of these were most frequently not met. Over 50% of the respondents spoke of unmet needs for what the study calls 'emotional support', and the study classified all these needs, and related needs for emotional closeness and self-fulfilment, as psychological, with no other distinction between them, despite referencing a prior study [9] with terminally ill people in the United States, which clearly distinguished between existential, spiritual, and emotional issues.

2.5 *Spiritual Needs*

Amidst, and despite, all this theoretical complexity, it is still widely agreed that patients' spiritual needs exist and require care and support, and these needs are widely identified, theoretically [105] and empirically [106–108], as multi-dimensional, broadly concerning suffering associated with relationships, environment, and the search for meaning and peace. Some systematic reviews and surveys also indicate an overlap between patients' spiritual and social needs [109, 110], in domains such as relationship and connectedness. So social workers as well as chaplains, nurses, psychologists, and other allied health professionals may all be involved in addressing these overlapping needs, and a multi-disciplinary approach may be recommended [44], particularly if chaplain services cannot fully meet existing need.

Policy statements also identify these needs and the multi-professional responsibilities for meeting them. The Scottish Government's *Spiritual care and chaplaincy*, published in 2009, states:

> among the basic spiritual needs that might be addressed within the normal, daily activity of healthcare are: giving and receiving love; being understood; being valued; finding forgiveness, hope and trust; exploring beliefs and values; honestly expressing feelings; finding meaning and purpose in life. [47, p. 2]

In 2011, the End-of-Life Care Strategy of the United Kingdom Department of Health (covering England and Wales) published *Route to Success: The Contribution of Nursing to End of Life Care* [111]. This document states that one of the core principles for end-of-life care is to 'Recognise and respect an individual's spiritual and religious needs' (p. 7), and that nurses should 'Ensure that access to spiritual care is available' (p. 22), and 'Ensure that spiritual and religious needs are addressed and appropriate referrals made' (p. 23).

However, the gaps between policy, stated goals, and practice are often evident, and guidance in concrete details often lacking, so this report contains only brief notes in a single page appendix on how nurses might recognise or distinguish between spiritual and religious needs, or how they should address these needs once recognised. It says nothing else. So, what happens in practice with regard to addressing these needs?

3 Spiritual Care and Spiritual Assessment

Despite these multiple debates over definitions of spirituality and spiritual needs and wellbeing, and although it seems difficult to find a single definition of spirituality with which everyone can agree, there does seem to be more consensus and shared understanding over spiritual care, with threads evident in the literature from the earliest days [37, 112–114]. The widespread lack, or inconsistent and/or suboptimal provision, of spiritual care in palliative care may however be associated with the pursuit of definitions, and, in the absence of any single accepted definition, a particular uncertainty regarding what comprises spiritual care.

However, spiritual care is usually understood as recognising and supporting patients' spiritual wellbeing in some way, extending over time. It has been suggested [35] that in the absence of a clear definition of spirituality, nurses might think of caring for the spiritual dimension of a person, rather than for their spirituality, and focus their assessments on key elements of the spiritual dimension: sense of meaning; hope; forgiveness; self-transcendence; and relatedness/connectedness with other people, and, for many people, also with a higher power. This resonates with arguments for using functional measures to assess spiritual wellbeing, rather than substantive measures of spirituality [4], as discussed earlier, and growing numbers of measures for use in spiritual care are being developed and validated [37].

It has been said that it may be difficult to distinguish between spiritual screening, spiritual history-taking, and spiritual care [115], which may be conflated. This is in part because spiritual discussion or history-taking can itself develop into a therapeutic intervention, that is, spiritual care, although this may not necessarily apply with spiritual screening, which can be minimal. If spiritual care is understood as active listening and engagement with patients (and others) who are expressing their spiritual concerns and struggles, then administering a tool which enquires about those spiritual concerns initiates spiritual care, i.e. is a spiritual intervention [63]. Some tools have been developed as clinical assessments, which can initiate discussion of spirituality with patients, such as HOPE [116], or FICA [117], mnemonics which remind the clinician of the key areas of importance to address with the patient. In HOPE, H stands for sources of hope, strength, comfort, meaning, peace, love, and connection, O the role of organised religion, P personal spirituality and practices, E effects on medical care and end-of-life decisions [116]. FICA [117] covers similar ground but in a slightly different way: F stands for Faith, belief or meaning, I for the importance of spirituality in a person's life, and the influence their belief system or values has on their decision making, C is spiritual community, and A is interventions to address spiritual need.

These are not all easy areas for inexperienced generalist staff to frame as questions or otherwise find ways to broach them with patients. Administering these kinds of interventions requires skill and experience, plus training, as do interventions such as Dignity Therapy [118] and Meaning-Centred Psychotherapy [119]. Brief tools or single questions, such as 'are you at peace?' [108] may be discussion openers, but again require skill to manage responses, not least because, again, they do not by themselves cover all the issues which may be important, as a more structured measure can do. A self-completion measure which has questions or items laid out for the patient to answer (or not) as they wish, asks the patient the questions, rather than the clinician having to frame them themselves [63] (see Chaps. 27 and 30 for more discussion of engaging with patients about their spirituality).

Some measures of spiritual wellbeing explicitly acknowledge that discussing a patient's responses to a measure with them should be recognised as a first step in an intervention (e.g. [63]). A measure like this prompts reflection by the respondent, and exploring and engaging with their responses, particularly those areas where the person has indicated poor wellbeing, and associated needs, is the first step in supporting the patient with addressing those needs, i.e. a spiritual care intervention [63].

Administering this kind of measure is thus associated with a specific ethical obligation, beyond the general ethical responsibility in palliative care to address patients' spiritual needs stated by the WHO [26–28]. The person who has administered it has a responsibility to engage with the respondent and their responses afterwards, as the respondent may need support with their related thoughts and feelings, and the provider must allow time to do this appropriately. However, this does not necessarily require any lengthy engagement at the outset; following the initial interaction, time can be scheduled for a return discussion, and/or the professional can make relevant referrals to colleagues. It is important also to note that appeals to lack of time can sometimes be an avoidance strategy [31].

It is always important to be clear about the aim of using any measure; seeking to 'measure' spirituality may be difficult, and substantive assessments of spirituality can produce variable results, even for the same individual, which can at times appear contradictory. In contrast, levels of spiritual need or wellbeing may require and be more amenable to meaningful measurement or assessment, and functional assessments of spiritual wellbeing, or, conversely, spiritual needs, that is, addressing the functions of a person's spirituality, rather than its components, or substance, are more useful as outcome measures [4].

4 Conclusion

Palliative care is interwoven with spirituality, and has been from its beginnings, as is explicit in most definitions of palliative care, but not necessarily in its provision. This interweaving is also evident in struggles seeking to reach generally agreed conceptual definitions. The pursuit of a single agreed definition has resulted in some stagnation in research around spirituality, and perhaps also, and more importantly, with the provision of spiritual care. As observed over 10 years ago [8], the fragmentation of terminology for palliative care-related fields [23] seems also to continue to be happening for spirituality and related issues, resulting in ever narrower and smaller categories being produced.

Around a decade ago, I suggested that it might be necessary, as in the early days with debates regarding the meaning of QOL, to grasp and acknowledge the imperfection and lack of overall consensus regarding spirituality, and, while recognising that any understanding is incomplete and imperfect, act despite it [8]. There is still not a generally accepted single definition of QOL, but the concept seems to now be in general use, and debates over definitions seem to have been at least partially resolved not through reaching general agreement on definition, but rather because the term began to be used by sufficient numbers of people (albeit with individual interpretations of its meaning) for it to become generally accepted. I suggested that it might be better to have an imperfect measure of spirituality than no measure at all, and that, rather than (or while) waiting for the 'perfect' measure to be developed, a possible strategy would be to select a measure from those currently available which seems to address the key elements of relevance to a particular health care setting, while bearing in mind the inevitable limitations of all such measures [8].

The first seems to have happened, but not the second; the diversity of definitions is accompanied by a growing number of measures, and an accompanying diversity of study design, but consideration of associated limitations is often lacking. Spirituality research therefore is not being consolidated. More consistency between designs would help with that. Meanwhile, in practice, despite this diversity of measures or assessment tools, which could potentially offer a range of help to enable staff to initiate spiritual care interventions, practitioners are still hesitant to engage with such conversations. Further, some tools require particular skills, experience, and training, which many staff, particularly generalists, do not have. Other tools, however, are available to use with minimal training. This is perhaps a route to improving and increasing spiritual care provision. Whichever tool is used, it's important to always bear in mind that, since both assessments and interventions relating to spiritual needs entail enquiry into those needs and concerns, a spiritual assessment is always also a spiritual care intervention, at least the initial step in beginning such an intervention and starting to address spiritual needs.

References

1. Ajibade B. Assessing the patient's needs and planning effective care. Br J Nurs. 2021;30(20):1166. https://www.britishjournalofnursing.com/content/clinical/assessing-the-patients-needs-and-planning-effective-care. Accessed 22 Nov 2023.
2. de Jager ME, Garssen B, van den Berg M, van Dierendonck D, Visser A, Schaufeli WB. Measuring spirituality as a universal human experience: a review of spirituality questionnaires. J Relig Health. 2012;51(2):336–54.
3. Monod S, Brennan M, Rochat E, et al. Instruments measuring spirituality in clinical research: a systematic review. J Gen Intern Med. 2011;26(11):1345–57.
4. Vivat B. Measures of spiritual issues for palliative care patients: a literature review. Palliat Med. 2008;22:859–68.
5. Weaver AJ, Pargament KI, Flannelly KJ, Oppenheimer JE. Trends in the scientific study of religion, spirituality and health: 1965–2000. J Relig Health. 2006;45:208–14.
6. Reinert KG, Koenig HG. Re-examining definitions of spirituality in nursing research. J Adv Nurs. 2013;69:2622–34.

7. Tanyi RA. Towards clarification of the meaning of spirituality. J Adv Nurs. 2002;39:500–9.
8. Vivat B. Quality of life. In: Cobb M, Puchalski C, Rumbold B, editors. Spirituality in healthcare. Oxford: Oxford University Press; 2012. p. 341–6.
9. Greisinger AJ, Lorimor RJ, Aday LA, Winn RJ, Baile WF. Terminally ill cancer patients: their most important concerns. Cancer Pract. 1997;5:147–54.
10. Vivat B. "Going down" and "getting deeper": physical and metaphorical location and movement in relation to death and spiritual care in a Scottish hospice. Mortality. 2008;13(1):42–64.
11. Carr T. Mapping the processes and qualities of spiritual nursing care. Qual Health Res. 2008;18(5):686–700.
12. Fisher JW, Francis LJ, Johnson P. Assessing spiritual health via four domains of spiritual wellbeing: the SH4DI. Pastor Psychol. 2000;49(2):133–45.
13. Billings JA. What is palliative care? J Palliat Med. 1998;1:73–81.
14. Clark D. From margins to centre: a review of the history of palliative care in cancer. Lancet Oncol. 2007;8:430–8.
15. Clark D. 'Total pain', disciplinary power, and the body in the work of Cicely Saunders 1958–67. Soc Sci Med. 1999;49:727–36.
16. Saunders CM. The founding philosophy. In: Saunders C, Summers DH, Teller N, editors. Hospice: the living idea. London: Edward Arnold; 1981. p. 4.
17. Saunders C, Summers DH, Teller N, editors. Hospice: the living idea. London: Edward Arnold; 1981.
18. Saunders Dame CM. The management of terminal illness. London: Edward Arnold; 1967.
19. Vivat B. The whole and the parts: spiritual aspects of care in a West of Scotland hospice [Unpublished PhD thesis]. University of Edinburgh; 2004.
20. Byock I. Hospice and palliative care: a parting of the ways or a path to the future? J Palliat Med. 1998;1(2):165–76.
21. Doyle D. Have we looked beyond the physical and psychosocial? J Pain Symptom Manag. 1992;7:302–11.
22. Kearney M. Palliative medicine: just another specialty? Palliat Med. 1992;6(1):39–46.
23. Pastrana T, Jünger S, Ostgathe C, Elsner F, Radbruch L. A matter of definition – key elements identified in a discourse analysis of definitions of palliative care. Palliat Med. 2008;22: 222–32.
24. National Institute for Health and Care Excellence (NICE). End of life care for adults: service delivery (NG142). 2019. http://www.nice.org.uk/guidance/ng142. Accessed 22 Nov 2023.
25. World Health Organization. WHO 2012 definition of palliative care. 2012. https://archive.li/p1C8. Accessed 22 Nov 2023.
26. World Health Organization. WHO Resolution 67.19. 2014. https://apps.who.int/gb/ebwha/pdf_files/WHA67/A67_R19-en.pdf?ua=1&ua=1. Accessed 22 Nov 2023.
27. World Health Organization. WHO 2020 definition of palliative care. 2020. http://www.who.int/health-topics/palliative-care. Accessed 22 Nov 2023.
28. World Health Organization. Fact sheet 5 August 2020. 2020. https://www.who.int/news-room/fact-sheets/detail/palliative-care. Accessed 22 Nov 2023.
29. Nolan S, Saltmarsh P, Leget C. Spiritual care in palliative care: working towards an EAPC task force. Eur J Palliat Care. 2011;18(2):86–9.
30. Williams JA, Meltzer D, Arora V, Chung G, Curlin FA. Attention to inpatients' religious and spiritual concerns: predictors and association with patient satisfaction. J Gen Intern Med. 2011;26(11):1265–71.
31. Best M, Butow P, Olver I. Doctors discussing religion and spirituality: a systematic literature review. Palliat Med. 2016;30:327–37.
32. Saguil A, Fitzpatrick AL, Clark G. Are residents willing to discuss spirituality with patients? J Relig Health. 2011;50:279–88.
33. Egan R, MacLeod R, Jaye C, McGee R, Baxter J, Herbison P, Wood S. Spiritual beliefs, practices and needs at the end of life: results from a New Zealand national hospice study. Palliat Support Care. 2017;15:223–30.

34. Edwards A, Pang N, Shiu V, Chan C. The understanding of spirituality and the potential role of spiritual care in end-of-life and palliative care: a meta-study of qualitative research. Palliat Med. 2010;24:753–70.
35. Lemmer CA. Recognizing and caring for spiritual needs of clients. J Holist Nurs. 2005;23(3):310–22.
36. Mularski RA, Dy SM, Shugarman LR, et al. A systematic review of measures of end-of-life care and its outcomes. Health Serv Res. 2007;42(5):1848–70.
37. Nissen DR, Falkø E, Viftrup DT, Hvidt EA, Søndergaard J, Büssing A, Wallin JA, Hvidt NC. The catalogue of spiritual care instruments: a scoping review. Religions. 2020;11(5):252. https://doi.org/10.3390/rel11050252.
38. Norris P, Inglehart R. Sacred and secular: religion and politics worldwide. 2nd ed. Cambridge/New York/Melbourne: Cambridge University Press; 2012.
39. Weathers E, McCarthy G, Coffey A. Concept analysis of spirituality: an evolutionary approach. Nurs Forum. 2016;51(2):79–96. https://doi.org/10.1111/nuf.12128.
40. Hanssen I, Pedersen G. Pain relief, spiritual needs, and family support: three central areas in intercultural palliative care. Palliat Support Care. 2013;11(6):523–30.
41. Moberg DO. Assessing and measuring spirituality: confronting dilemmas of universal and particular evaluative criteria. J Adult Dev. 2002;9(1):47–60.
42. Sawatzky R, Pesut B. Attributes of spiritual care in nursing practice. J Holist Nurs. 2005;23(1):19–33.
43. NHS Education for Scotland. Spiritual care matters: an introductory resource for all NHS Scotland staff. Edinburgh: Scottish Government; 2009, revised 2021. https://www.nes.scot.nhs.uk/media/xzadagnc/spiritual-care-matters-an-introductory-resource-for-all-nhsscotland-staff.pdf. Accessed 22 Nov 2023.
44. Puchalski C, Ferrell B, Virani R, Otis-Green S, Baird P, Bull J, Chochinov H, Handzo G, Nelson-Becker H, Prince-Paul M. Improving the quality of spiritual care as a dimension of palliative care: the report of the consensus conference. J Palliat Med. 2009;12(10):885–904. https://doi.org/10.1089/jpm.2009.0142.
45. Hall BA. Spirituality in terminal illness. J Holist Nurs. 1997;15(1):82–96.
46. Sulmasy DP. A biopsychosocial-spiritual model for the care of patients at the end of life. The Gerontologist. 2002;42(suppl_3):24–33. https://doi.org/10.1093/geront/42.suppl_3.24.
47. Scottish Government. Spiritual care and chaplaincy. Edinburgh: Scottish Government; 2009. https://www.nes.scot.nhs.uk/media/5zjf1gog/cel_2008.pdf. Accessed 22 Nov 2023.
48. National Hospice Organization. Standards of a hospice program of care. Arlington: National Hospice Organization; 1993.
49. Grant M, Sun V. Advances in quality of life at the end of life. Semin Oncol Nurs. 2010;26(1):26–35.
50. Joyce CRB, McGee HM, O'Boyle CA. Individual quality of life: approaches to conceptualization and assessment. Amsterdam: Harwood Academic Publishers; 1999.
51. Waldron D, O'Boyle CA, Kearney M, Moriarty M, Carney D. Quality-of-life measurement in advanced cancer: assessing the individual. J Clin Oncol. 1999;17(11):3603–11.
52. Bush SH, Parsons HA, Palmer JL, Li Z, Chacko R, Bruera E. Single- vs. multiple-item instruments in the assessment of quality of life in patients with advanced cancer. J Pain Symptom Manag. 2010;39(3):564–71.
53. Aaronson NK, Ahmedzai S, Bergman B, for the European Organization for Research and Treatment of Cancer, et al. The QLQ-C30: a quality-of-life instrument for use in international clinical trials in oncology. J Natl Cancer Inst. 1993;85:365–76.
54. Cella DF, Tulsky DS, Gray G, et al. The Functional Assessment of Cancer Therapy (FACT) scale: development and validation of the general measure. J Clin Oncol. 1993;11(3):570–9.
55. Brady MJ, Peterman AH, Fitchett G, Mo M, Cella D. A case for including spirituality in quality-of-life measurement in oncology. Psycho-Oncology. 1999;8(5):417–28.
56. Peterman AH, Fitchett G, Brady MJ, Hernandez L, Cella D. Measuring spiritual well-being in people with cancer: the Functional Assessment of Chronic Illness Therapy-Spiritual well-being scale (FACIT-Sp). Ann Behav Med. 2002;24(1):49–58.

57. Steinhauser KE, Christakis NA, Clipp EC, McNeilly M, McIntyre L, Tulsky JA. Factors considered important at the end of life by patients, family, physicians, and other care providers. JAMA J Am Med Assoc. 2000;284(19):2476–82.
58. Ferrell BR, Dow KJ, Leigh S, et al. Quality of life in long-term cancer survivors. Oncol Nurs Forum. 1995;22:915–22.
59. WHOQOL Group. What is quality of life? The World Health Organization quality of life assessment. World Health Forum. 1996;17:354–6.
60. Cohen SR, Mount BM, Bruera E, et al. Validity of the McGill quality of life questionnaire in the palliative care setting: a multi-centre Canadian study demonstrating the importance of the existential domain. Palliat Med. 1997;11:3–20.
61. WHOQOL SRPB Group. A cross-cultural study of spirituality, religion, and personal beliefs as components of quality of life. Soc Sci Med. 2006;62:1486–97.
62. Vivat B, Young T, Efficace F, et al. Cross-cultural development of the EORTC QLQ-SWB36: a stand-alone measure of spiritual wellbeing for palliative care patients with cancer. Palliat Med. 2013;27(5):457–69.
63. Vivat B, Young TE, Winstanley J, et al. The international phase 4 validation study of the EORTC QLQ-SWB32: a stand-alone measure of spiritual well-being for people receiving palliative care for cancer. Eur J Cancer Care. 2017;26(6):12697.
64. Wheelwright S, Bottomley A, Bjordal K, on behalf of the EORTC Quality of Life Group, et al. EORTC Quality of Life Group guidelines for developing questionnaire modules. 5th ed. 2021. https://www.eortc.org/app/uploads/sites/2/2022/07/Module-Guidelines-Version-5-FINAL.pdf. Accessed 22 Nov 2023.
65. Biswas J, Islam N, Afsar N, Mroy WW, Chandra BP. Validation of Bengali version of EORTC QLQ-SWB32: a standalone measure of spiritual wellbeing for advanced cancer patients receiving palliative care. Heliyon. 2024;10(9):e29927. https://doi.org/10.1016/j.heliyon.2024.e29927. PMID: 38699031; PMCID: PMC11064144.
66. Dabo I, Skočilić I, Vivat B, Belac-Lovasić I, Sorta-Bilajac TI. Spiritual well-being for Croatian cancer patients: validation and applicability of the Croatian version of the EORTC QLQ-SWB32. Int J Environ Res Public Health. 2021;18(22):11920.
67. Goyarrola R, Lipsanen J, Saarelainen SM, et al. Spiritual well-being correlates with quality of life of both cancer and non-cancer patients in palliative care – further validation of EORTC QLQ-SWB32 in Finnish. BMC Palliat Care. 2023;22:33.
68. Poyhia R, Mwalumuli E, et al. (unpublished) https://qol.eortc.org/questionnaire/qlq-swb32/
69. Huong Pham TT, Dau VV, Tam NB, et al. Validation of the Vietnamese version of the EORTC QLQ-SWB32: a measure of spiritual well-being in cancer patients. Kurdish Studies. 2023;11:2350–8.
70. Cobb M, Dowrick C, Lloyd-Williams M. What can we learn about the spiritual needs of palliative care patients from the research literature? J Pain Symptom Manag. 2012;43(6):1105–19.
71. Mesquita AC, de Cássia Lopes Chaves E, Moreira de Barros GA. Spiritual needs of patients with cancer in palliative care: an integrative review. Curr Opin Support Palliat Care. 2017;11(4):334–40.
72. Bandeali S, des Ordons AR, Sinnarajah A. Comparing the physical, psychological, social, and spiritual needs of patients with non-cancer and cancer diagnoses in a tertiary palliative care setting. Palliat Support Care. 2020;18(5):513–8.
73. Koenig H, King D, Carson VB. Handbook of religion and health. Oxford: Oxford University Press; 2012.
74. McClain CS, Rosenfeld B, Breitbart W. Effect of spiritual well-being on end-of-life despair in terminally ill cancer patients. Lancet. 2003;361(9369):1603–7.
75. Wasner M, Longaker C, Fegg MJ, Borasio GD. Effects of spiritual care training for palliative care professionals. Palliat Med. 2005;19(2):99–104.
76. McCoubrie RC, Davies AN. Is there a correlation between spirituality and anxiety and depression in patients with advanced cancer? Support Care Cancer. 2006;14(4):379–85.

77. Yanez B, Edmondson D, Stanton AL, Park CL, Kwan L, Ganz PA, Blank TO. Facets of spirituality as predictors of adjustment to cancer: relative contributions of having faith and finding meaning. J Consult Clin Psychol. 2009;77:730–41.
78. Best MC, Butow P, Olver I. Creating a safe space: a qualitative inquiry into the way doctors discuss spirituality. Palliat Support Care. 2016;14(5):519–31.
79. Delgado-Guay MO, Parsons HA, Hui D, de la Cruz MG, Thorney S, Bruera E. Spirituality, religiosity, and spiritual pain among caregivers of patients with advanced cancer. Am J Hosp Palliat Med. 2013;30(5):455–61.
80. O'Callaghan C, Seah D, Clayton JM, Welz M, Kissane D, Georgousopoulou EK, Michael N. Palliative caregivers' spirituality, views about spiritual care, and associations with spiritual well-being: a mixed methods study. Am J Hosp Palliat Med. 2020;37(4):305–13.
81. Vivat B, Speck P, Jones L, Uddin I, White N, Rohde G, White C, Candy B, Tookman A, King M. What do research studies identify as spiritual and religious interventions at the end-of-life? Findings from a Cochrane review. Palliat Care Soc Pract. 2022;16:1–119.
82. Candy B, Jones CL, Varagunam M, Speck P, Tookman A, King M. Spiritual and religious interventions for well-being of adults in the terminal phase of disease. Cochrane Database Syst Rev. 2012;5:CD007544. https://doi.org/10.1002/14651858.CD007544.pub2.
83. Best M, Vivat B, Gijsberts M-J. Spiritual care in palliative care. Religions. 2023;14(3):320.
84. Steinhauser KE, Fitchett G, Handzo GF, Johnson KS, Koenig HG, Pargament KI, Puchalski CM, Sinclair S, Taylor EJ, Balboni TA. State of the science of spirituality and palliative care research. Part I: definitions, measurement, and outcomes. J Pain Symptom Manag. 2017;54(3):428–40.
85. Selman LE, Brighton LJ, Sinclair S, Karvinen I, Egan R, Speck P, Powell RA, Deskur-Smielecka E, Glajchen M, Adler S, Puchalski C, Hunter J, Gikaara N, Hope J. Patients' and caregivers' needs, experiences, preferences and research priorities in spiritual care: a focus group study across nine countries. Palliat Med. 2018;32(1):216–30.
86. Mount BM, Boston PH, Cohen SR. Healing connections: on moving from suffering to a sense of well-being. J Pain Symptom Manag. 2007;33(4):372–88.
87. Boston P, Bruce A, Schreiber R. Existential suffering in the palliative care setting: an integrated literature review. J Pain Symptom Manag. 2011;41(3):604–18.
88. Henoch I, Danielson E. Existential concerns among patients with cancer and interventions to meet them: an integrative literature review. Psycho-Oncology. 2009;18:225–36.
89. Last Acts Task Force. Precepts of palliative care. Princeton: Robert Wood Johnson Foundation; 1997.
90. Moreira-Almeida A, Koenig HG. Retaining the meaning of the words religiousness and spirituality: a commentary on the WHOQOL SRPB group's "a cross-cultural study of spirituality, religion, and personal beliefs as components of quality of life". Soc Sci Med. 2006;63:843–5.
91. Greenfield EA, Vaillant GE, Marks NF. Do formal religious participation and spiritual perceptions have independent linkages with diverse dimensions of psychological well-being? J Health Sci Behav. 2009;50(2):196–212.
92. Koenig HG. Concerns about measuring "spirituality" in research. J Nerv Ment Disord. 2008;196(5):349–55.
93. Ironson G, Solomon GF, Balbin EG, et al. The Ironson-woods spirituality/religiousness index is associated with long survival, health behaviours, less distress, and low cortisol in people with HIV/AIDS. Ann Behav Med. 2002;24(1):34–48.
94. Bekelman DB, Parry C, Curlin FA, Yamashita TE, Fairclough DL, Wamboldt FS. A comparison of two spirituality instruments and their relationship with depression and quality of life in chronic heart failure. J Pain Symptom Manag. 2010;39(3):515–26.
95. Folkman S. Positive psychological states and coping with severe stress. Soc Sci Med. 1997;45(8):1207–21.
96. Hills J, Paice JA, Cameron JR, Shott S. Spirituality and distress in palliative care consultation. J Palliat Med. 2005;8(4):782–8.
97. Pargament KI, Koenig HG, Perez LM. The many methods of religious coping: development and initial validation of the RCOPE. J Clin Psychol. 2000;56:519–43.

98. Mako C, Galek K, Poppito SR. Spiritual pain among patients with advanced cancer in palliative care. J Palliat Med. 2006;9(5):1106–13.
99. Lin H-R, Bauer-Wu SM. Psycho-spiritual well-being in patients with advanced cancer: an integrative review of the literature. J Adv Nurs. 2003;44(1):69–80.
100. Fegg MJ, Brandstätter M, Kramer M, Kögler M, Haarmann-Doetkotte S, Borasio GD. Meaning in life in palliative care patients. J Pain Symptom Manag. 2010;40(4):502–9.
101. Meraviglia M. Critical analysis of spirituality and its empirical indicators. Prayer and meaning in life. J Holist Nurs. 1999;17:18–33.
102. National Comprehensive Cancer Network. Clinical practice guidelines in oncology. 2007. http://www.nccn.org/professionals/physician_gls/PDF/distress.pdf. Accessed 22 Nov 2023.
103. Thekkumpurath P, Venkateswaran C, Kumar M, Bennett MI. Screening for psychological distress in palliative care: a systematic review. J Pain Symptom Manag. 2008;36(5):520–8.
104. Morasso G, Capelli B, Viterbori P, et al. Psychological and symptom distress in terminal cancer patients with met and unmet needs. J Pain Symptom Manag. 1999;17(6):402–9.
105. Kellehear A. Spirituality and palliative care: a model of needs. Palliat Med. 2000;14(2):149–55.
106. Hermann CP. Spiritual needs of dying patients: a qualitative study. Oncol Nurs Forum. 2001;28(1):67–72.
107. Grant E, Murray SA, Kendall M, Boyd K, Tilley S, Ryan D. Spiritual issues and needs: perspectives from patients with advanced cancer and non-malignant disease. A qualitative study. Palliat Support Care. 2005;2(4):371–8.
108. Steinhauser K, Voils C, Clipp E, Bosworth H, Christakis N, Tulsky J. "Are you at peace?" One item to probe spiritual concerns at the end of life. Arch Intern Med. 2006;166(1):101–5.
109. Lormans T, de Graaf E, van de Geer J, van der Baan F, Leget C, Teunissen S. Toward a socio-spiritual approach? A mixed-methods systematic review on the social and spiritual needs of patients in the palliative phase of their illness. Palliat Med. 2021;35(6):1071–98.
110. Gijsberts M-JHE, van der Steen JT, Hertogh CMPM, Deliens L. Spiritual care provided by nursing home physicians: a nationwide survey. BMJ Support Palliat Care. 2020;10(4):e42.
111. National End of Life Care Programme. Route to success: the key contribution of nursing to end of life care. London: Royal College of Nursing/NHS; 2011. https://www.england.nhs.uk/improvement-hub/wp-content/uploads/sites/44/2011/06/End-of-Life-Care-Route-to-Success-Nurses.pdf. Accessed 22 Nov 2023.
112. Vivat B, Lodwick R, Garcia-Baquero Merino MT, Young T. What do palliative care professionals understand as spiritual care? Findings from an EAPC survey. Religions. 2023;14(3):298.
113. Gijsberts M-JHE, Liefbroer AI, Otten R, Olsman E. Spiritual care in palliative care: a systematic review of the recent European literature. Med Sci. 2019;7(2):25.
114. Hvidt NC, Nielsen KT, Korup AK, et al. What is spiritual care? Professional perspectives on the concept of spiritual care identified through group concept mapping. BMJ Open. 2020;10:e042142.
115. Cobb M. The dying soul: spiritual care at the end of life. Maidenhead: McGraw-Hill Education; 2001.
116. Anandarajah G, Hight E. Spirituality and medical practice: using the HOPE questions as a practical tool for spiritual assessment. Am Fam Physician. 2001;63(1):81–9.
117. Puchalski C, Romer AL. Taking a spiritual history allows clinicians to understand patients more fully. J Palliat Med. 2000;3:129–37.
118. Chochinov HM, Hack T, Hassard T, Kristjanson LJ, McClement S, Harlos M. Dignity therapy: a novel psychotherapeutic intervention for patients near the end of life. J Clin Oncol. 2005;23:5520–5.
119. Breitbart W. Spirituality and meaning in supportive care: spirituality- and meaning-centered group psychotherapy interventions in advanced cancer. Support Care Cancer. 2002;10(4):272–80.

Part II
Diversity

The Role of Religious Beliefs in Palliative Patients

Kate L. Bradford, Helena De la Cruz, and Marvin Omar Delgado-Guay

Abstract Spiritual care is part of holistic care in the person-centred biopsychosocial–spiritual model. In addition to meeting patients' physical and medical needs and social and emotional needs, holistic care entails a commitment to meet the spiritual needs of all patients. Spiritual care is particularly concerned with how a person makes sense of circumstances and events, finding meaning and purpose through a web of connections including family, friends, pets, institutions, nature, the cosmos, or a higher power. Religious care in contrast to spiritual care operates out of a distinct religious framework, including particular beliefs, values, rituals, structures, communities of practice, or perspectives on reality. Religious care and spiritual care are intimately related; however, neither can substitute for the other as a person approaches the boundaries of life. For a religious person, as death approaches, there will be an increasing asymmetry between more general concerns of spirituality and more specific attention paid to faith or religious belief and ritual. Recognition of the role spirituality plays in the care of the patient with serious illness is crucial in addressing patient symptoms and suffering.

Keywords Spiritual care · Religious care · Palliative care · Spirituality · Positive and negative religious coping · Stages of faith · End of life · Miracles

---

K. L. Bradford (✉)
Chaplaincy Department, Westmead Hospital, Westmead, NSW, Australia
e-mail: kate.bradford@health.nsw.gov.au

H. De la Cruz
Barnard College, Columbia University, New York, NY, USA
e-mail: hjd2120@barnard.edu

M. O. Delgado-Guay
Department of Palliative, Rehabilitation, and Integrative Medicine, MD Anderson Cancer Center, The University of Texas, Houston, TX, USA
e-mail: Marvin.Delgado@mdanderson.org

M. C. Best (ed.), *Spiritual Care in Palliative Care*,
https://doi.org/10.1007/978-3-031-50864-6_5

1 Introduction

The medicine and art of palliative care represents a commitment to the biopsycho-social–spiritual model of care which welcomes a person, body and soul, intellect and imagination, individual and community member, past and future. The European Association for Palliative Care (EAPC) has suggested that 'Spirituality is the dynamic dimension of human life that relates to the way persons (individuals and community) experience, express and/or seek meaning, purpose and transcendence, and the way they connect to the moment, to self, to others, to nature, to the significant and/or the sacred' [1]. From the inclusion of the terms *transcendence* and *sacred* in this definition, it becomes clear that the spiritual domain of care includes both spiritual and religious care.

Globalisation, mass migration, rapid economic growth and free trade have all ensured that vastly different cultures now encounter each other. As a result, many societies are multicultural and multifaith which is reflected within healthcare systems leading people to construct different meanings and perceptions of severe illness, end of life, and death [2]. The World Health Organization (WHO) emphasises the responsibility of healthcare providers to be culturally and personally sensitive to the needs and beliefs of patients and their families who are facing the problems associated with life-threatening illness, and asserts the importance of attending to not only the physical and psychosocial needs of patients, but also to patient spiritual needs [3]. The assertions of the WHO reflect the scientific literature from the past decade, increasingly affirming that spiritual care is an essential component of end-of-life (EOL) care, indicating the need for spiritual care training for all healthcare professionals [1, 3–5].

A comprehensive palliative care service that seeks to provide holistic care will attend to both patients' spiritual and religious needs where neither is neglected, nor one substituted for the other, and recognises that for many patients, for whom their spirituality is a religious spirituality, it will be expressed through a particular religious tradition. For patients for whom religious faith forms a significant part of their identity, the decision to accept palliative care and the approach to the end of life may well be apprehended through their existing religious framework. As well as patients who have differing spiritual and religious needs, a multidisciplinary team has staff members with different levels of expertise in responding to spiritual and religious needs. For a religious person, there may be an increasing asymmetry between more general concerns of spirituality and more specific attention paid to the specifics of faith or religious belief and ritual as death approaches, often seen in the saying of particular prayers, preparation of the body after death and funeral arrangements.

2 Spirituality and Religiosity

The key components of spirituality can be summarised by the broad concepts of meaning, belonging, purpose, and transcendence. Everyone has a spiritual outlook which may be deep and coherent or conversely, thinner and less cohesive, and yet, for each person, it includes how they make sense of life, drawing on different resources and anticipating the future. A religious framework includes an existing stock of language, terminology, concepts, and patterns of processing life events guided by the religious belief system. For example, a patient may speak of prayer, the will of Allah, miracles, karma, a cross to bear, the soul, an act of self-emptying, the path of suffering, or life after death. Members of the multidisciplinary team must have a working knowledge of the difference between spirituality and religiousness.

Formal religions differ from spiritualities in that they can be summarised more concisely as having four Cs: creeds, codes, cult, and community. The creeds are widely accepted beliefs, the codes relate to conduct, and the cult is expressed through ritual by which people of a community locate themselves in the world concerning ordinary and extraordinary powers, meanings, and values [6]. Religion as a concept is somewhat broader and more concrete than spirituality and has been summarised by Friedrich von Hugel as having three main elements: the institutional, the intellectual and the mystical [7], which provides an overview of religious adherence including historic establishments, shared doctrines and personal belief. From this perspective, religions are more wide-ranging than personal spiritualities as they may include all of life. Religions encompass culture and traditions, constellations of belief, communities of shared practices, values, rituals, and institutions.

However, intrinsic and extrinsic aspects of religion are more circumscribed and narrower than the broader and more nebulous concept of spirituality. In contrast to the cultural and codified aspects of religion, there is a considerable overlap between intrinsic or mystical elements of religion particularly in areas of contemplation, interiority (a focus on inner life or identity), personal habits and practices including prayer, meditation, and rituals. The language of spirituality tends to be more fluid, borrowing eclectically from a range of disciplines including psychology, philosophy, wisdom traditions, and indigenous spiritualities. From this perspective, spirituality and religiosity have a shared concern with how each person makes sense of their life. For the religious and spiritual alike, sense-making is an interconnected relational web which in turn has the possibility of opening avenues for hope and creativity, which for many people open discussions concerning the boundaries of life.

The shared aspects of spirituality and the inward mystical elements of religion were identified by Liselotte Frisk. She demonstrated marked similarities between the attitudes of people who described themselves as spiritual but not religious and the mystical tenets of the major religions. Frisk identified six characteristics that bore a resemblance to mystical rather than formal religion [8]. These are (1) a shift from particular to eclectic—rather than relying on one source or one religion, world religions are viewed as resources; (2) a shift from dogma to experience; (3) a shift from collective to personal with an emphasis on healing, wellbeing, and relationality; (4) a shift from hierarchical to egalitarian religious views, where God, or Other, is not regarded as above but rather infused through everything; (5) a further shift from theological to anthropological that emphasises subjective feeling and a personal growth dimension. The final shift mentioned by Frisk is (6) a shift in focus from life after death to this-worldliness with more emphasis on a spiritual life now, rather than life after death. Frisk's analysis indicates an underlying shared basis of intrinsic religiosity and a more eclectic account of spirituality, and by implication, the importance of providing religious care that considers a person's intrinsic spirituality as well as more extrinsic aspects of religious faith. Such intrinsic aspects may include facilitating the patient's reflection on the source of their faith, how they experience their faith personally, how their faith fits with other aspects of their life and their formation, and the place of faith when facing a life-limiting condition.

3 The Spiritual Care Matrix

One way of envisaging the provision of spiritual and religious care by a multidisciplinary team employs four quadrants in a two-by-two matrix [9]. By using the matrix, the patients' spiritual needs are allocated to the categories of *broad spiritual* or *narrow religious* on the *x*-axis, then on the *y*-axis the staff's expertise in offering spiritual care is classified as *generalist* or *specialist* (see Fig. 1). In this system, the four quadrants of spiritual care are understood as follows:

1. *Broad Generalist Spiritual Care* can be practised by all staff providing a compassionate presence to all patients by attending to the person, accompanying, and attuning with them through life events and circumstances. All other quadrants assume the knowledge and skills of this quadrant as a minimum requirement for offering any form of more specific or specialised spiritual care.
2. *Narrow Generalist Religious Care* is intentional religious care which may include praying, bible reading, talking about religion. The offer of religious care arises out of the patient's presenting needs, is offered seeking permission, is other person led, and does not provide counsel or offer advice. Those offering religious care at a generalist level include multidisciplinary staff, volunteers, or visitors from the particular religious tradition of the patient.
3. *Broad Specialist Spiritual Care* is a professional level of care conducted by certified spiritual care practitioners. A spiritual care practitioner is a professional who understands spirituality, spiritual distress, techniques of deep listening, and is qualified to accompany a person through a spiritual conversation, facilitating

SPIRITUAL CARE MATRIX

	Broad Meaning, Purpose & Belonging	Narrow Specific Religious Tradition
General Connect and understand	Broad General Spiritual Care Attends to and accompanies a patient through the event happening Compassionate Presence	Narrow General Religious Care Responds to patient's requests Does not offer spiritual or religious counsel
Specialist Explore and respond	Broad Specialist Spiritual Care Is offered by a certified Spiritual Care Practitioner, who provides spiritual counsel in areas of existential and personal questions of meaning, purpose and belonging	Narrow Specialist Religious Care Is offered by an authorised religious representative qualified to explore complicated and complex spiritual and religious questions within a specific religious tradition

Fig. 1 Spiritual care matrix

deeper insight into circumstances and experiences. Such conversation includes existential and personal questions of meaning, purpose, and belonging.

4. *Narrow Specialist Spiritual Care* is a professional level religious care offered by an authorised religious representative who ideally has expertise in all the above and is also qualified to explore complicated and complex spiritual and religious questions within a specific religious tradition including theological discussions, prayer, Bible reading, reflection on readings, communion, and other services.

The Spiritual Care Matrix provides a model of spiritual care that accommodates the strengths of the generalist-specialist model of whole person care within the interprofessional model of biopsychosocial–spiritual care [10]. In this model, all team members are trained in spiritual care commensurate with their scope of practice and all provide care through a lens of compassionate practice and have the training to identify spiritual distress and recognise when referral to a specialist spiritual care practitioner is required [11]. The Spiritual Care Matrix extends the interprofessional model by differentiating in greater detail the overlaps and distinctions between spiritual and religious care. A second model that reviews the integration between spirituality, religion, and medicine is the existential function model [11] with a focus on aspects of wisdom, contemplation, integration, and transformation which provides a valuable summary of types of areas for which specialist spiritual care practitioners and specialist religious carers would be skilled, and able to discern between spiritual and religious distress and disorders of mental and emotional health and refer appropriately if present.

The Spiritual Care Matrix works from a basis of open pluralism which acknowledges the multicultural multifaith culture of many societies and most hospitals [11, 12]. The specialist spiritual care practitioner is qualified to provide specialist counsel in areas of existential distress and personal questions of meaning, purpose, and belonging and transcending current circumstances, recognising that many people do not belong to formal spiritual or religious communities. The designation of 'narrow specific religious tradition' refers to the beliefs of a patient who identifies as belonging to a formal spiritual or religious community and a religious representative who may be a hospital chaplain, or a religious visitor. This person has been authorised by that community as qualified to explore complicated and spiritual and religious questions within a specific religious tradition, often within specific cultural and linguistic communities.

Specialist spiritual care is concerned with the general ways in which a patient makes sense of life and finds meaning, the presence or absence of supportive relationships in various forms of friendship, family and faith communities and the extent to which the patient is able to be honest about events, their sense of control in the situation, or sense of peace amid turmoil [13]. In moving from a broad spiritual care assessment to a more specific religious care assessment, the spiritual care practitioner would be interested in the strength and depth of the patient's religious faith and the extent to which a person depends upon their religious faith to face challenges and changes, and also the maturity of their religious community to help them through transitional periods of challenge and change.

4 The Role of Religious Coping

The term 'religious coping' refers specifically to the ways in which individuals make use of their religious beliefs in order to understand and adapt to stress [14]. In light of the high number of patients to whom religious spirituality is important, many patients and families turn to religious coping when struggling with life-threatening illness. Religious coping can include individual activities such as prayer, meditation, and religious study (e.g. reading religious texts) [14, 15] and may also include involvement with a religious or spiritual community. A person's religiosity alone does not indicate whether a person will cope better or more poorly with a palliative diagnosis, as demonstrated by research that suggested that relying upon religion to cope with terminal cancer may contribute to receiving more aggressive medical care near death [14]. This highlights the importance of specific religious care and the need for good religious assessment, and an understanding of the positive and negative valance that religion can cast over decision-making processes.

Religious coping can be divided into two major categories: positive religious coping and negative religious coping. Positive religious coping is 'characterised by a constructive reliance on faith to promote healthy adaptation', and there is clear evidence of a correlation between a sense of coherence and spirituality and religiosity suggesting that there are religious and spiritual pathways to a strong sense of coherence [16]. However, Pargament et al. noted that 'several indicators of poorer physical health (e.g. number of medical diagnoses, functional status, cognitive status, Post Traumatic Stress Disorder) were associated with higher levels of both positive and negative religious coping' [17]. This indicates that religious coping needs to be held in tension with a person's religious maturity (see Fowler's stages of faith below) and their openness to enter into religious and spiritual struggles [18], and the wisdom and maturity of the person's surrounding religious community.

4.1 Miracles as an Example of Religious Coping

A common expression of religious faith encountered by staff when a patient or family member is confronted with a life altering diagnosis is, 'I'm still hoping for a miracle' [15, 19]. Miracles are commonly understood as extraordinary events 'not applicable to the laws of nature', and contrary to scientific 'facts' [20]. This view of miracles and the spiritual and/or religious can give the impression that the gravity of a prognosis and/or the concrete limitations of medicine has been misunderstood. 'Hoping for a miracle is an example of spiritual or religious speech, and it is important to understand more fully what the speaker means by the expression.

Myrick Shinall et al. [21] have classified the motivation for hoping for a miracle into four broad categories [20] summarised as:

1. *Innocuous*, when patients use 'miracles' to represent hoping for the best while preparing for the worst, allowing for both simultaneous denial and acceptance.
2. *Shaken*, when hope for a miracle specifically and faith in general are challenged by unfavourable clinical outcomes. This does not usually cause conflict between patients and clinicians but has the potential to cause great spiritual and existential pain affecting the patient's quality of life if not addressed.
3. *Integrated*, when belief in miracles is based on religion and can be in discord with health professionals which can create conflict in the doctor-patient relationship as events are being viewed through different levels of explanation; in such cases the patient or family are deeply embedded in a cohesive world view of a religious community.
4. *Strategic*, when the belief in a miracle functions as a way for patients or their families to maintain power and control over their situation while impeding deeper discussions about medical intervention and decisions, commonly interpreted by staff as a negation of reality.

It can be seen from this brief overview of hope for a miracle that understanding a patient's spiritual and religious interpretation of events affects their relationship with the medical team and compliance, or otherwise, with their treatment. For many people, religion is an important factor during the medical decision-making process, whether it is conscious or unconscious. It shapes individuals' beliefs, and the kinds of decisions patients (and their families) might make. Factors that will affect a person's religious coping will include their faith development, their spiritual struggles, and the wisdom of the religious community in which they are embedded. Their relationships with these factors all have the potential to affect their treatment and their relationship with their multidisciplinary team.

5 Religious Assessment

More in-depth religious assessments are best made by a religious representative of the patient's faith group (or as near as possible), taking language and culture into consideration and working with a certified translator as necessary. A religious assessment would seek to ascertain the place of the four Cs of religion in the person's life: the creeds, codes, cult, and community. It would also explore whether religion is held intrinsically and personally or whether the more extrinsic cultural and communal aspects of religion are more prescient, and the extent to which religion is a part or the whole of their life. Which elements of religion come to the fore for this patient: the institutional, intellectual, or mystical? A scale, such as Fowler's 0–7 stages of faith scale [22], is helpful in evaluating intrinsic religiosity or spiritual maturity which gives an indication of how much weight a person's spirituality may be able to bear in the face of challenge or change. Such scales are not designed to determine the genuineness or sincerity of a person's faith position. Their value lies in providing an assessment of how a person thinks about their religion and the extent to which a person's faith is integrated into all aspects of their life. This in turn will affect the extent to which a person's faith can accommodate difficult and complex change and reminds the spiritual or religious care practitioner to work within a person's existing understanding, vocabulary, and concepts before trying to extend their understanding, bearing in mind that personal faith may be held implicitly with little explanatory language around it. Conversely explicit faith is where a person is well able to articulate their faith.

Fowler's scale of the progressive stages of faith may be summarised as follows:

0—represents a child's undifferentiated faith, characterised by trust, or conversely mistrust and often related to absence or presence of primary caregivers;

1—faith at this stage is experiential and develops through encounters with stories, images, and the influence of others but cannot be used to reason through problems;

2—the person has belief in justice and fairness in religious matters, a sense of reciprocity in the workings of the universe, but has difficulty working through contradictory facts;
3—identification of the adolescent/adult with a religious institution, belief system, or authority, and the growth of a personal religious or spiritual identity, but may ignore challenges that threaten one's faith identity;
4—often characterised by angst and struggle as the individual takes personal responsibility for her beliefs or feelings and they may find herself at variance with members of her religious group;
5—acknowledges paradoxes and the mysteries attendant on transcendent values; and
6—able to reflect on events from a perspective of compassion or love.

Fowler developed his framework in a Christian environment with input from other multicultural and multifaith perspectives [23], and other researchers have employed his framework in other contexts including sub-Saharan Africa [24].

The second factor in a religious assessment is the maturity or otherwise of the religious or faith community in which the patient is embedded. A religious community can be summarised as having shared beliefs and narrative, practices, and rituals, providing wisdom and belonging. Such beliefs and narratives scaffold a person through the difficulties of life, suffering, illness, injustice, evil, death, and the frailties and ambiguities of life. Practices and rituals provide rhythms of life including prayer, thanksgiving, celebrations, births, deaths, marriages, and funerals. Wisdom is the time-tested weighing of the presenting reality by elders in discussion with ancient texts and traditions to perceive how to live with liminality, the in-between places, and to discern the best way forward. The community provides belonging, a worldview and network to help people walk these ancient paths with wisdom and holds a person as such, so they are not walking this path alone.

Studies of religious and spiritual struggles provide an insight into the way in which personal and community beliefs and practices are challenged and reconfigured. A person's spirituality and religiosity are valanced, and much depends upon the wisdom in which a life is envisaged. Drawing on Paul Ricoeur's study of emplotment [25], it is important to consider how life is *pre*figured, *con*figured, and *re*figured. When considering *pre*figuring, we are exploring what were the *givens*: was there generational security or trauma, war or peace, indifference or love, alienation or community integration? *Con*figuring; how does the patient construct the narrative of their world and identity now? *Re*figuring; what emergent possibilities exist into the future? It is this area of emergent possibility that represents an area of potential resolution or hope for the patient, and as such it is important that the religious carer has the skills to guide such a conversation. From the field of psychology, Kenneth Pargament and Julie Exline [18] have developed an excellent resource in which they detail six areas of religious or spiritual struggles: struggles of ultimate meaning, struggles with the Divine and doubt, and the experience of struggles with moral, interpersonal, and demonic dimensions. Religious care employs cognition and works with conversation, when possible, but is not limited to these facets. Religious care is deeply embodied and works with signs, symbols, rituals, prayer, meditation, and presence.

If holistic care is to be provided there is little doubt that it includes the personal, existential, spiritual, and religious aspects of a person's life. However, when endeavouring to meet a person's deepest spiritual and existential needs, it is important to appreciate that spirituality and religion are complex multivalent constructs which may, or may not, materially alter the health outcome for the patient. However, attempting to meet a patient's deepest needs and to accompany them through their suffering are acts of compassion that honours the dignity and humanity of the whole person.

6 Bringing the Various Threads Together: A Case Study of a Palliative Care Patient

Anita was a softly spoken, shy 38-year-old woman from Peru who had migrated to Australia during her high school years to join her father who had migrated 10 years earlier. Anita's mother left the family when she was three, her father then moved away, and Anita was sent to live with her grandmother in a regional town. Anita's grandmother was a Christian and Anita was absorbed into her grandmother's extended Christian community. She volunteered that she liked living with her grandmother, and described herself as a Christian believer, but was happy when her father asked her to join him and his new wife in Australia. Anita completed high school in Australia and trained as a disability care worker and was employed by a disability care agency providing home care support. Anita was in a long-term relationship with the father of her 10-year-old son, but her partner was a businessman who lived in Peru. He had never moved to Australia, although Anita was under the impression that he would move as soon as he was able. Anita's main community was a large vibrant Latin Pentecostal church.

When Anita was 35 years, a cervical screen test picked up some abnormalities, and she was referred to a specialist for further tests but did not attend the appointment. A year later, Anita presented to a hospital emergency department with abnormal bleeding and pain in her lower abdomen. Further tests revealed cancer with significant progression of her disease, which now involved her bladder and outer rectum wall. Surgery was performed, but Anita attended very few of her scheduled follow-up radiotherapy appointments and then would not return any calls from the clinic. At 37 years, Anita appeared at the emergency department of another hospital with severe abdominal pain and evidence of advanced cancer in several organs, but again missed two-third of her scheduled treatment appointments, and after three months, Anita's care was transferred to the palliative care team. Anita's treatment team included an oncologist, a psychiatrist, a social worker, and a chaplain who was both a senior spiritual care practitioner and authorised religious representative.

From a biopsychosocial–spiritual perspective, Anita had advanced cancer which had developed from a treatable condition to metastatic disease when Anita repeatedly failed to attend medical appointments. This was further complicated as she moved between different health districts and medical services. During Anita's latter admissions, she was diagnosed with an emotional regulation disorder, this condition complicated the work of the social worker as Anita often refused to speak with the social worker or disclose personal details particularly to do with the care of her son. She was supported from time to time by members of her church. The church seemed to be her only support network as she was estranged from her father and stepmother. Anita's multidisciplinary team provided consistent compassionate presence while referring her to a hospital chaplain who was of a confessional protestant background. The multidisciplinary team spoke together and communicated through the electronic medical records system. The chaplain wrote in the notes, without betraying confidences, providing information on the care that she had been able to offer and how Anita was coping spiritually with her admission.

From a spiritual care perspective, Anita held a conventional if childlike Christian faith. When she spoke of her faith in Jesus, she was congruent, relaxed, maintained good eye contact, and smiled in a gentle way and enjoyed talking about her childhood and living with her grandmother in Peru. There may have been some transference from her grandmother to the chaplain—an older woman who was simply there to care for her. However, this simple Christianity was juxtaposed with her inability to confront the reality of her illness, or the need, in the latter stage of her illness, to consider the possibility of leaving her son. The childlike nature of her faith was a strength in that it was a comfort, but the weakness was that it was so childlike, it was unable to bear the realities of her present life. Despite its genuineness, it lacked an integrated maturity of a 37-year-old, and this provides a clue to some of Anita's struggles if viewed through Fowler's scale of stages of faith. Anita's faith was still at the first stage; her faith was reasonably undifferentiated and seemed closely tied to the dependability of her grandmother. There was a quality of magical thinking in her faith that didn't seek to engage with her illness, her treatment team, or to think through problems. Anita liked being cared for by the chaplain if it didn't involve any challenge, she liked kind Bible verses printed on post cards, being reminded that Jesus loved her, and prayer for her and her son.

When conducting a comprehensive spiritual assessment, it is necessary to review the patient's spirituality through a set of diverse lenses, as a person's spirituality is in a state of dynamic interplay with other aspects of a person's life. In Anita's case, the critical lenses with which to engage were adverse childhood experiences (ACEs), disrupted attachment, cut-offs in her family system, trauma, cross-cultural issues, her mental and emotional health issues, the challenges of serious disease, her support systems through family, faith and friends, and the culture of the religious community in which Anita was embedded. After reviewing these factors, a simple spiritual assessment for Anita could be summarised as follows: her meaning in life was the care of her son, her support community was her church, her hope was to not be separated from her son and she held a transcendent belief that Jesus would somehow 'fix' things or make everything 'right'.

A second part of a religious assessment involved the religious community of which Anita was part. When a religious community is functioning well, it can provide remarkable spiritual support, but it needs to be acknowledged that, while this is often the case, it's not universally the case and religious communities can have either a positive or negative valence on the life of its members. As discussed above, a well-functioning religious community is evidenced by beliefs that help scaffold a person through the difficulties of life, provide practices and rituals that help face realties, draw in the wisdom of elders, and provide a community where people do not suffer alone. However, in Anita's case, the visitors from her church did not help her face the reality of her illness and were at times quite oppositional to suggestions and recommendations made by the treating team.

Towards the end of Anita's illness, the religious visitors demonstrated a pattern of behaviour consistent with Shinall's description of the strategic use of miracles endeavouring to control the situation [21]. The religious visitors always prayed for miraculous healing and asserted strongly that prayer by anyone (including the chaplain) for courage, comfort, and perseverance through Anita's struggles and difficulties was evidence of lack of faith in healing. It was observed that there was an absence of mature elders supporting Anita, and towards the end of Anita's life, the church sisters took over her hospital room, playing high volume sermons on healing, bringing in special soups from home, and feeding Anita even when she was semi-conscious. The staff were nervous about entering the room, and the chaplain asked the church sisters to turn off the sermons as they were disturbing the whole unit. The chaplain also recorded in the EMR that the patient was being spoon fed when she was not fully conscious. Yet, in the previous months, when the social worker had asked if the 'sisters' could help with practical support that would have allowed Anita to return home to be with her son, nobody was willing to help her.

For most of Anita's illness, there had been no contact from her family, but towards the end of her illness, her father visited, and Anita reconciled with her father a few days before she died. At first, he too believed that she would be miraculously spared, and he was praying for a miracle but didn't really engage much with Anita or the church visitors. As her death was approaching, he spoke with the chaplain acknowledging that he realised his daughter was dying. She encouraged him to speak with Anita. He spoke with his daughter; he told her he loved her and wished that he had been there for her for more of her life and they said their goodbyes. This reconciliation was well received by Anita, who by this time seemed to understand she was dying.

In conclusion, without the support of Anita's extended family and faith community engaging with the reality of Anita's illness and latter prognosis it is difficult to imagine a different outcome or to see any new possibilities that may have presented that could have altered the course of Anita's distress or final outcome. Anita's situation was medically, psychologically, socially, and spiritually complex, but if she had one or two mature church elders to walk with her through her illness, people who knew of loss, pain, and a type of hope that can exist together through suffering, things may have been different. Critical interventions that may have altered Anita's trajectory included: people to accompany Anita to medical appointments, people to stay with her at home when she was too weak to care for herself and her son, and working together with the social worker, helping Anita make plans for her son should she be unable to continue to care for him, and for people to walk with her and help prepare her for death as she entered the final palliative stage of her illness and also to help prepare her son for the loss of his mother.

7 Conclusion

Recognition of the role spirituality and religiosity play in the care of the patient with serious illness is crucial in addressing patient symptoms and suffering. Oftentimes, the influence of one's belief in the divine and one's spiritual needs are overlooked. Studies have shown that spiritual distress is associated with physical distress and therefore needs to be explored; however, it is important the recognise that spirituality and religiosity are multivalent concepts that include attitudes of both positive and negative religious coping, spiritual and religious struggles, stages of faith maturity, and the wisdom and cohesion of the surrounding religious community. Ideally, providing good religious care to people of faith will alleviate distress and help people draw deeply on their religious understanding and find support in their extended religious community.

References

1. Best M, Leget C, Goodhead A, Paal P. An EAPC white paper on multi-disciplinary education for spiritual care in palliative care. BMC Palliat Care. 2020;19(1):9. https://doi.org/10.1186/s12904-019-0508-4. PMID: 31941486; PMCID: PMC6964109.
2. Ng PC, Fung GPG. Spiritual and cultural influences on end-of-life care and decision-making in NICU. Semin Fetal Neonatal Med. 2023;21:101437. https://doi.org/10.1016/j.siny.2023.101437. PMID: 37105859.
3. World Health Assembly, 67. Strengthening of palliative care as a component of comprehensive care throughout the life course. 2014. https://apps.who.int/iris/handle/10665/16286.
4. National Consensus Project for Quality Palliative Care. Clinical practice guidelines for quality palliative care. 4th ed. Richmond, VA: National Coalition for Hospice and Palliative Care; 2018.
5. Ferrell BR, Twaddle ML, Melnick A, Meier DE. National Consensus Project clinical practice guidelines for quality palliative care guidelines, 4th edition. J Palliat Med. 2018;21(12):1684–9. https://doi.org/10.1089/jpm.2018.0431. Epub 2018 Sep 4. PMID: 30179523.
6. Albanese CL. America: religions and religion. London: Cengage Learning; 2013.
7. Avis P. The mystical and the institutional. Int J Stud Christ Church. 2004;4(1):1–5.
8. Frisk L. Globalization: an important key factor in contemporary religious change. J Altern Spiritual New Age Stud. 2009;5:4.
9. The Spiritual Care Matrix was developed from my research in presented in an earlier paper. Bradford KL. The nature of religious and spiritual needs in palliative care patients, carers, and families and how they can be addressed from a specialist spiritual care perspective. Religions. 2023;14(1):125.

10. Puchalski C, Ferrell B, Virani R, Otis-Green S, Baird P, Bull J, Chochinov H, et al. Improving the quality of spiritual care as a dimension of palliative care: the report of the consensus conference. J Palliat Med. 2009;12(10):885–904.
11. Balboni MJ, Puchalski CM, Peteet JR. The relationship between medicine, spirituality and religion: three models for integration. J Relig Health. 2014;53:1586–98.
12. Stewart WC, Seiple C, Hoover DR. Toward a global covenant of peaceable neighborhood: introducing the philosophy of covenantal pluralism. Rev Faith Int Aff. 2020;18(4):1–17.
13. At this point I borrow from the work of Snowden A, Karimi L, Tan H. Statistical fit is like beauty: a rasch and factor analysis of the Scottish PROM. J Health Care Chaplain. 2022;28(3):415–30.
14. Phelps AC, Maciejewski PK, Nilsson M, Balboni TA, Wright AA, Paulk ME, Trice E, Schrag D, Peteet JR, Block SD, Prigerson HG. Religious coping and use of intensive life-prolonging care near death in patients with advanced cancer. JAMA. 2009;301(11):1140–7. https://doi.org/10.1001/jama.2009.341. PMID: 19293414; PMCID: PMC2869298.
15. Gradick K, October T, Pascoe D, Fleming J, Moore D. 'I'm praying for a miracle': characteristics of spiritual statements in paediatric intensive care unit care conferences. BMJ Support Palliat Care. 2022;12(e5):e680–6. https://doi.org/10.1136/bmjspcare-2020-002436. Epub 2020 Aug 27. PMID: 32855234.
16. Jeserich F, et al. Sense of coherence and religion/spirituality: a systematic review and meta-analysis based on a methodical classification of instruments measuring religion/spirituality. PLoS One. 2023;18(8):e0289203. ProQuest. 3 Jan 2024.
17. Pargament KI, et al. Patterns of positive and negative religious coping with major life stressors. J Sci Study Relig. 1998;37(4):710–24. https://doi.org/10.2307/1388152.
18. Pargament KI, Exline JJ. Working with spiritual struggles in psychotherapy: from research to practice. New York: Guilford Publications; 2021.
19. Nafratilova M, Allenidekania A, Wanda D. Still hoping for a miracle: parents' experiences in caring for their child with cancer under palliative care. Indian J Palliat Care. 2018;24(2):127–30. https://doi.org/10.4103/IJPC.IJPC_195_17. PMID: 29736112; PMCID: PMC5915876.
20. de Freitas MH, Leal MM, Nwora EI. Praying for a miracle part II: idiosyncrasies of spirituality and its relations with religious expressions in health. Front Psychol. 2022;13:893780. https://doi.org/10.3389/fpsyg.2022.893780. PMID: 35832915; PMCID: PMC9272886.
21. Shinall MC Jr, Stahl D, Bibler TM. Addressing a patient's hope for a miracle. J Pain Symptom Manag. 2018;55(2):535–9.
22. Fowler JW. Faith development and pastoral care. Philadelphia: Fortress; 1987.
23. Fowler JW. Faith development theory and the postmodern challenges. Int J Psychol Relig. 2001;11(3):159–72.
24. Selvam SG. Towards religious-spirituality: a multidimensional matrix of religion and spirituality. J Study Relig Ideol. 2013;12(36):129–52.
25. Blundell B. Paul Ricoeur between theology and philosophy: detour and return. Bloomington: Indiana University Press; 2010.

Māori Spiritual Care During COVID-19 Lockdowns

Tess Moeke-Maxwell, Richard Egan, Ria Earp, and Bobbi Laing

Abstract Tending to *wairua* (spirit) and spiritual aspirations is of the utmost importance for Māori (Indigenous New Zealanders) during the end of life. The significance of wairua was apparent during the New Zealand COVID-19 lockdown periods when, despite many challenges, Māori families provided end-of-life care and adapted their funeral customs. This chapter draws from the Rapua te Mārama COVID-19 study, informed by Kaupapa Māori Research methods. The findings identify what supported families who cared for someone in their 'bubble' before, during, and following death, including conducting funerals and coping with bereavement. The first author and her team interviewed over 100 people, including bereaved *whānau* (extended family), palliative care health professionals, and funeral directors. An inductive thematic analysis found four themes highlighting the importance of wairua: Wairua is fundamental at the end of life; Wairua knows no boundaries and is connected to everything at the end of life; Wairua is a perceived sensation at the end of life; and Wairua is relational at the end of life. Palliative care must prioritise Indigenous cultural safety training and awareness among staff to ensure culturally safe environments for whānau, especially during national crises.

Keywords COVID-19 · Bereavement · End of life · Indigenous · Family · Māori Palliative care · Spirit · Spirituality · Wairua · Spiritual care

---

T. Moeke-Maxwell (✉) · B. Laing
School of Nursing, University of Auckland, Auckland, New Zealand
e-mail: t.moeke-maxwell@auckland.ac.nz; b.laing@auckland.ac.nz

R. Egan
Department of Preventative & Social Medicine, University of Otago, Dunedin, New Zealand
e-mail: richard.egan@otago.ac.nz

R. Earp
Ria Earp Consulting, Wellington, New Zealand
e-mail: ria@riaconsulting.co.nz

M. C. Best (ed.), *Spiritual Care in Palliative Care*,
https://doi.org/10.1007/978-3-031-50864-6_6

1 Introduction

This chapter explores a Māori (Indigenous New Zealander) perspective of *wairua* (the spirit or soul of a person that exists beyond physical death) and its central importance for Māori during and following death [1–3]. Māori view wairua as foundational to being a human, residing everywhere inside a person like a centrifugal force that intertwines and influences a person's physical, emotional/mental well-being, and deeply connected to *whānau* (extended family), *tīpuna* (ancestors), and the environment. It cannot be separated or isolated from the other dimensions of a person. As such, it must be attended to across the lifespan to assist the spirit's safe arrival and departure from the world, particularly at death. *Tohunga* (spiritual leaders and healers) and *rongoā* (natural) practitioners play an important role in supporting people's spiritual well-being at the end of life. It is essential to support the transition of the person's wairua through the *ārai* (veil) [3, 4] to help it return home. Traditionally, Māori *iwi* (tribes) believe the wairua leaves the body at the time of death and travels to a sacred spiritual place where it leaves Aotearoa New Zealand via a portal; 'Te Rerenga Wairua' is one such sacred portal referred to as the 'leaping place of spirits' located at Cape Reinga on the tip of the North Island. The wairua then travels to the underworld where it joins its ancestors.

Within *te Ao Māori* (Māori worldview), *whanongo pono* (values) and *tikanga* (customs) are observed and specific tribal *karakia* (prayers, incantations, and chants) are used to ensure the whole person is protected and to encourage the person's wairua through this transition. This may include *karanga* (traditional calling done by women), *waiata* (singing), *whakanoa* (cleansing rituals), and *whakawātea* (clearing rituals). These are seen as the primary source of spiritual safety [3] keeping whānau spiritually protected and the environment free from negative spiritual forces, particularly at the end of life. These practices reflect the ancient belief in, and practices of *tapu* (spiritual restrictions) and *noa* (to be free from tapu, unrestricted) [5].

1.1 The Health Dimension of Wairua

Te Ao Māori belief is that if wairua is adversely affected by negative forces, e.g. unsupportive spiritual caring, it causes the wairua to become sick and the body ill. Conversely, positive spiritual activities through karakia provide protection, safety, and peace, as they petition well-being for the sick, release the spirit at the time of death, and send the spirit on its way [6–8]. The belief in wairua has traditionally been influenced by *mātauranga* (knowledge) and tikanga, which reflect tribal knowledge and customs [5, 9–11]. Contemporary Māori individuals and whānau have a multiplicity of spiritual beliefs and practices (which may include Christian beliefs—a legacy of colonisation), that incorporate religious or other spiritual affiliations and practices, whanonga pono, and tikanga, and can differ both within and between whānau [12]. However, despite this diversity, the belief in the importance of wairua at end-of-life and the spiritual connections with family and *whenua* (homelands) is maintained, as it is among all first nations peoples [13].

The aim of this chapter is to explain the Māori wairua experiences of end of life during COVID-19. It is based on findings from the Rapua te Mārama study, which aimed to identify those things that helped families to cope with death, post-death care, funerals, and bereavement during this time.

2 Rapua te Mārama Research Methods

The research team used Māori research methods [14–17] and interviewed whānau at eight different geographical places in *Aotearoa* (New Zealand) including the Mid-North, Aotea Great Barrier Island, Auckland, Tauranga, Hawkes Bay, Wellington, Motueka, Central Otago, and Southland.

The first author led this work under the guidance of Te Ārai Kāhui Kaumātua (Te Ārai Palliative Care and End of Life Research Group). Māori participants were involved in the 2-year study and took part in the research processes [18]. The team made sure that participants felt safe to share their stories [19] and to share these publicly if they chose [16].

Between 2020 and 2021, bereaved whānau, health professionals who provided palliative care and funeral directors who provided their services to Māori whānau, were interviewed. A total of 59 kanohi-ki-te-kanohi (face-to-face) interviews were conducted with whānau involving over 100 people. Our goal was to transfer their stories into virtual and hardcopy resources [20, 21]. For example, we created an online virtual reality photographic exhibition using gaming technology, and we published a book of short stories highlighting whānau experiences of life and death during the COVID-19 lockdowns. Whānau were invited to take part in a public exhibition of their stories and professional portraits in an online photographic exhibition. Twenty-three whānau chose to take part in a public photographic and storytelling exhibition.

3 Findings

We adapted four wairua themes identified by Valentine and colleagues [22] to describe how the 23 Rapua te Mārama storyteller families' experienced wairua as a critical end-of-life dimension during COVID-19 lockdown. Valentine and colleagues identified the following four wairua themes:

1. Wairua is fundamental (wairua is foundational and fundamental to the existence of being human throughout the lifecycle).
2. Wairua knows no boundaries (wairua cannot be confined or bound; when one health domain is affected every health domain is affected).

3. Wairua is a perceived sensation (wairua is an internal compass, a particular type of knowing, understanding, or sixth sense).
4. Wairua is relational (wairua has a relationship to everything in existence, past, present, and future, and is linked with Māori ancestors).

We adapted the themes identified by Valentine and colleagues to include an end-of-life perspective:

1. Wairua is fundamental at the end of life.
2. Wairua knows no boundaries and is connected to everything at the end of life.
3. Wairua is a perceived sensation at the end of life.
4. Wairua is relational at the end of life.

3.1 Wairua Is Fundamental at the End of Life

Whānau participants confirmed that wairua was considered foundational and fundamental to the existence of being human throughout their life. They viewed wairua implicitly as an essential element of health and cultural identity and they perceived this essence as becoming more active as someone approached death. They particularly saw wairua as supporting whānau to navigate the challenges they faced when caring for someone critically unwell or dying during the lockdowns. For example, Phil from the Raukawa whānau recalled how his whānau let wairua guide them after learning his unborn daughter was likely to die during birth or shortly afterwards. They saw this as fundamental for the end-of-life passage for their daughter. Phil said how they deliberately drew from this spiritual support system:

> I think when we had found out that Bubba was going down this path [life limiting illness] then we put that in God's hands and, and we said 'well no matter what, we're going to let the wairua guide us…' We followed everything that we believed; 'no, we'll put it in God's hands, and we'll believe in all of this'… [O]ur culture was based around the divine so you know having, having a strong sense of belief in God and then in Māori culture… I'd have a prayer and then all of these things would just [resolve]… but if you didn't have that, you're alone.

The Kahi whānau explained how fundamental it was to have the presence and guidance of wairua when they related their experience of preparing to take home their elderly mother with dementia. When the hospital informed them that their mother was dying, Maggie (daughter) commented that her mother knew she was dying because she saw her deceased sons; 'She was saying "You know, your brothers are waiting for me"'. The hospital gave whānau special permission to be with her, which enabled them to support her transition as her wairua left her body:

> First, she had a big *kai* (meal); she ate every single spoonful. She had a beautiful cup of tea. But she went down after her lunch as her oxygen levels dropped badly. Her eyes were tired. I closed them for her and waited for our *tūpuna* (ancestors) to guide her over. Tears fell as we sat in the *mauri* (energy life force) as she passed over to her loved ones.

Whānau perceived wairua as an integral and fundamental part of a person's living essence, and they spoke about how they worked hard to preserve this divine essence within the ill or dying person to ensure their total well-being. Their narratives expressed how important it was that whānau and everyone involved in the person's final days, hours, and moments contributed to this. Caring for the critically ill person meant being completely present with the person and doing whatever was possible to ensure that their physical and emotional states and their wairua essence was flowing peacefully. This was to guarantee an optimal death where the wairua essence was perceived as transitioning across the ārai. A death that went well was marked by a sense of peacefulness, a transcendent experience for the living, and a sense of love and connection with the divine.

In the time leading up to Te Minaora's (their new-born baby) death from a rare heart condition, the Raukawa whānau reflected:

> Phil/father: Yeah, we, we were focussed on what we could do for her to have the best life that she could have and then when she passed, how could we have the best, passing [death] for her.
>
> Racheal/mother: [E]verything… little wee steps, every little wee moment became more important. Every little process, every, every moment became laden with importance. We were just focussed on her in that moment and trying to live in that moment with her, yeah. Yeah, yeah, trying to just be with her. That evening [when she was dying] Te Minaora was peaceful… Karakia were said and waiata sung as Te Minaora rested her head peacefully on my chest. The feeling in the room was beautiful—there was so much joy and love for her. While Nani was singing Te Minaora quietly left her body. Phil and I held her close and cried.

The connection to the whenua (land) was also a fundamental factor in helping peoples' wairua to feel settled. This is evidenced in Baz's experience. He felt at home at his local hospice because it was built on his whenua. Fortunately, Baz had an opportunity to develop a relationship with hospice staff before lockdown and therefore was comfortable receiving support in the community at home during lockdown, which was a great support to him, his wife, and whānau who cared for him:

> Baz could see the [name of] club from the hospice, and he saw people he knew coming and going from the local club. Stephen his son said, 'He loved being on the land there because he was right next to his *awa* (river), so he felt at home. That's where he was brought up—there was no hospice down there then, it was all swamp and that's where he used to hunt for eels (fish). They were on the same paddocks he used to roam over'.

3.2 Wairua Knows No Boundaries and Is Connected to Everything at the End of Life

When COVID-19 arrived and ill people were hospitalised, whānau needed to ensure the person was well taken care of at every level because they understood the importance of the sick person's physical, emotional, and spiritual interconnectedness with whānau and their environment. Participants' reflections of palliative care within the healthcare setting described the need to preserve a sense of total well-being for the loved person receiving care. Whānau spoke about the *mamae* (emotional and spiritual pain) that their elders experienced when their *mana* (authority, status, prestige) felt diminished by hospital staff, or they were separated from whānau. In this sense, wairua was conceived as something that could not be confined or bound. When one health dimension was affected, wairua was also affected.

Racheal reflected on how a lack of paediatric palliative care support at home, poor communication, and inadequate instructions on how to administer morphine-created distress for her dying baby, her husband, and herself. This experience affected every fibre of their being, including their wairua:

> The hospital doctors were kind. They said her oxygen was at 70 per cent. We were given a bottle of morphine. When we got home Te Minaora was struggling to breathe. It was like she was having a heart attack. We gave her some morphine, but we didn't know what we were doing. We rang the number the doctor gave us, but the person said, 'We'll get the doctor to ring you back, I'll try to find them'. Finally, the morphine worked and Te Minaora's breathing relaxed. We didn't know how long it would take. We wished we had this information a lot earlier. We felt traumatised.

Whānau had a sense of knowing that an ill person needed them as they approached death and, in this sense, wairua appeared to have volume or a spaciousness to it. Wairua existed outside normal sensory modalities and operated beyond spatial and temporal boundaries. The whānau recognised that everything was connected to wairua even though it could not be seen with the naked eye or touched with a physical hand. Whānau went to extraordinary lengths to ensure they could be present as the person came near to the end of their life and especially at the time of death when the person was transitioning—they sensed the wairua activity heightening. Whānau tried hard to ensure the connectivity and harmony between the physical, emotional, and wairua dimensions were as optimal as possible. Lisa did a risk assessment on herself as lockdown approached to ensure the aged care facility her ill mother was living in would accept her visiting during lockdown:

> I had to be able to visit Mum, to advocate on her behalf when she was not able to communicate her needs toward the end. It was important Mum had whānau around her… Caring for her was everything. Nothing else mattered. My head was going into overdrive. With my skills and background around control measures, I wrote to the Facility Manager with a risk assessment on myself. Fortunately, families of dying residents were allowed 24/7 entry on compassionate grounds and I will be forever grateful.

As soon as the aged residential care staff informed the Te Moana whānau that their wife and mother had become critically ill during lockdown, Margaret's daughter was assertive in asking staff if she could be with her mother to ensure she got the best holistic care. Margaret's husband reflected:

> By the end of April, I noticed things were getting worse. Margaret couldn't swallow her food. She knew she was crook. She was hiding her pills or spitting them out. The doctor said to me, 'Oh, I think we're going to have to move to palliative care'. I didn't know what the fuck palliative care was. My kids asked, 'What does that mean?' I said, 'Well, from what I can gather, although they didn't put it into words, it's like—there's no hope'. 'Well, how long have we got?' Parani phoned the rest home, 'What does palliative care look like? How do we get access to Mum? What kind of things can we do and not do with COVID-19 being the way it is?'

Whānau did not compartmentalise the ill person physically, emotionally/mentally, or spiritually because they perceived the person in their entirety; they belonged to a whānau, *hapū* (sub-tribe), and *iwi* (tribe), and each dimension of that person was viewed as interconnected.

Wairua, being connected with everything, meant there were consequences for 'everything' when the whole person was not cared for sufficiently. For example, whānau expected that hospital services would provide whole-person-centred care in a health setting particularly if their whānau were absent. When this did not happen, or care was disrupted, trust was broken, and the person and their whānau experienced deep distress. For example, the Sheeran whānau spoke about their wife and mother when she was first admitted to hospital and how she felt unwelcome when she could not have her whānau with her. This affected her sense of well-being, and it also harmed the whānau:

> Mum was admitted to hospital. Twice, we dropped her off at the Emergency Department, but we couldn't be with her because of the [COVID-19] restrictions. One time, a doctor came up and asked, 'What are you doing here? Why don't you go home and let your meds do the job'. That was awful. Mum didn't want to be there, and now she felt like she wasn't meant to be there, and that she wasn't welcome. David was upset and rang her G.P. (primary practitioner). It got sorted, but Mum went downhill from there.

The impact of not feeling wanted in the hospital caused a deep mamae for the older woman and her whānau who could sense her vulnerability. She felt lonely for her whānau and rejected by the hospital staff. The whānau believed this caused her deep distress and pain in the core of her essence—her wairua.

3.3 Wairua Is a Perceived Sensation at the End of Life

Wairua was perceived as a guiding light, directing people towards the best outcome in any situation. People consciously trusted and followed wairua. This meant for many that wairua was positioned as an internal compass, a particular type of knowing, understanding, or sixth sense, and invisible promptings were acted upon. Tau, a spiritual healer's sister, died during lockdown; he spoke about the importance of healing wairua at the end of life:

> So, I think there's this thing of wairua is a beautiful thing. I think it's up to the individual and sometimes they *paru* (soil) their wairua, you know, or they fill it up with dope or alcohol. And sometimes people are traumatised, and it hides the wairua or suppresses it. You know? And sometimes people who have been hurt, act from that sore wairua place... it's really important that when it comes to end-of-life that we're able to clear that for them. So that... their journey back into the wairua world is easier for them because it's been cleansed.

Cynthia reflected on sensing that her husband was dying during lockdown. This helped to prepare herself and her daughter for what was to come. They had the loving responsibility to conduct their cultural customs to ensure their spiritual customs were completed in the absence of their cultural and spiritual leaders:

> Melvyn was admitted to hospital with a urinary tract infection on Monday before lockdown. I stayed with him. Alert Level 4 arrived (COVID-19 restrictions) and restricted visiting to one person. Our daughter Rhonda worked at the hospital so she could also visit. Melvyn had two nurses and a doctor. The nurses massaged him with oils and couldn't do enough for him. On Saturday morning I sensed his time was close; I contacted our son Brad… I held Melvyn's hand as he was dying. 'This is it' I said to Rhonda. We had *karakia* and *waiata* while we prepared his body [washed and dressed him]. I was grateful he was no longer in pain.

Some whānau had a strong awareness of wairua and could sense or articulate these sensations and experiences more easily than others. Tau, from the Huirama family, was able to express the importance of wairua when someone is dying:

> It is exciting when you work with wairua as you are acknowledging that it's an important part of any environment. Our role is always to help other peoples' wairua to flow and for their whānau's wairua to flow. One of the points that I always try to get across, for others to believe, is that everyone has wairua. Everyone has that privilege of being born with wairua, with mana, and *mauri* (energy life force). I believe that wairua comes from within the cosmology of Māori, and it flows through everything. It's important when it comes to the end-of-life that we're able to help clear that mamae up for the dying, so that when they journey back into the wairua world it is easier for them. The spiritual cleansing processes we use are karakia, *whakawātea* [clearing the environment], and *whakanoa* (cleansing people). Spiritual cleansing and clearing mahi is *wairua mahi* (work).

Whānau had a sixth sense when using healthcare services and intuited when something felt wrong. Naomi felt hospital staff lacked a caring attitude when she tried to exercise her cultural prerogative to be with her partner's body following his death:

> Hospital protocols were that we had to go down to the whānau room. When we got told that we had to move I objected and said, 'Why can't we stay here, it's not like people are coming in?' They wrapped Matt up and took him down there [to a cold back room]. I didn't like that; it just didn't seem right to me. It was cold and there was nothing there for us. There could have been coffee, tea, or something, but there wasn't.

Caring for the wairua at end of life is not just about meaning and purpose, as sometimes portrayed in the spiritual care literature [23]. It is connected to everything that happens to the person and whānau; thus, the care Naomi experienced undermined the wairua of the place, the patient, and the whānau.

3.4 Wairua Is Relational at the End of Life

Wairua has a relationship to everything in existence, past, present, and future, and is linked with Māori ancestors. One of the most challenging aspects of COVID-19 was the impact the visiting restrictions had on the person who was ill and on their whānau. It contributed to poor palliative care in the community. Some people chose not to go to hospital to get pain and symptom relief because the risk of not being with their whānau was too great. Lenise explained how the hospital visiting restrictions affected her father:

> COVID-19 arrived. The pandemic was actually quite a scary time for us, particularly in Level 4. Dad was living in the bubble with us… There were times when I said 'Dad do you think you need to go to the hospital? I think we need to ring an ambulance'. And his response to me was, 'If I go, I won't be coming back'. That was his feeling inside. Dad did all he could to stay with us because he knew we couldn't be in hospital with him. He knew if you died you got buried straightaway. He listened to the news. That was the dilemma we were in. He also feared if he went to hospital, he would get COVID-19. I knew that he would rather die here with his whānau than alone in the hospital, so I went with what he wanted.

The Sheeran whānau were upset that health professionals could not determine what was ailing the older woman requiring her to have repeated hospital visits. This produced a sense of powerlessness and a lack of trust in the health professionals during lockdown. The whānau expressed this to the health professionals caring for their mother:

> We said, 'If you can't do anything more to help her, we'll bring her home'. You trust in the white coats. That's their job. We're looking to them as experts of their field. Okay, they're not God, they can't do everything, but when they're saying they're discharging her, and we know how ill she is, that's devastating. We sent Mum to a place to protect life, but because her illness wasn't COVID-19 related, the protection wasn't there.

Naomi reflected on her partner's admission to hospital and the policy requirement for only one person by the bedside with which she disagreed. Providing end-of-life care to someone who is critically ill and dying requires whānau to provide *aroha* (love, care, compassion), *manaakitanga* (reciprocal care), and tikanga appropriate to the care of the wairua. Mere stated:

> At one point, I was told by staff, 'Only one person is allowed to be here; one of you will have to leave'. I said, 'I'm not leaving, and I don't want Matt's son to go either because I need him to support both of us. I'm staying here'. Then I rang a hospital manager I knew and said, 'Look this is what's happening'. I said, 'One of us has been asked to leave, neither of us are going'. In support, Matt's cardiologist wrote a letter to the CE (Chief Executive) signed off by Palliative Care, to say that Matt was at the end of his life and was likely to pass away over the next couple of days. It was a shock; I was trying to be positive, thinking we're going to go home!

Donna commented how hard it was for her grieving process as she wasn't able to be with whānau when her father died. COVID-19 restrictions for tangihanga meant whānau were prevented from having proper tangihanga which deeply impacted their wairua, affecting their grieving process:

> With our tangihanga processes disrupted, the hardest thing was not being physically held. I missed being able to really cry and the laughter and stories people would normally share at these times. I missed the *marae* (ancestral gathering place). I missed the *iwi* (tribe). I missed my friends and whānau who couldn't be there. My brother in New Plymouth and another in Australia. My aunty in England and one in Auckland. I couldn't let go of Dad. My mourning process, incomplete.

4 Discussion

We adapted Valentine and colleagues [22] four wairua themes (wairua is fundamental; wairua knows no boundaries; wairua is a perceived sensation; and wairua is relational) to explore the importance for Indigenous whānau who cared for a family member who died during the COVID-19 lockdowns in New Zealand. These four themes illustrate the fundamental importance wairua holds for Māori at the end of life and following death. These themes display the remarkable diversity of wairua, how its presence encompasses all aspects of life, death, and the afterlife. This profound and authentically holistic belief underscores the necessity for end-of-life care to recognise, acknowledge, and address this integral Indigenous reality. Numerous Indigenous scholars have echoed this sentiment, emphasising the pivotal role of wairua, while simultaneously resisting the Western compulsion to overtly define and quantify it [22]. These strengths-based views from Māori show they are transferable themes for Indigenous peoples across the globe, particularly in relation to understandings of spirit, and experiences of spiritual care, and offer recommendations for improved end-of-life care for Indigenous communities.

The interconnected nature of wairua, evident from the way participants associate it with the entirety of existence, highlights the far-reaching repercussions which occur when comprehensive care is lacking for the individual. Wairua transcends reductionist or biomedical interpretations, existing as an intrinsic and interwoven force intertwined with the full spectrum of life and death. Building upon Durie's Te Whare Tapa Whā framework, [24] from this research we have created a new end-of-life model that centres wairua at the core, recognising its interconnectedness with other dimensions of *hauora* (well-being), including *te hinengaro* (the mind/emotions), *te tinana* (the physical), and *te whānau* (the family). This model also extends to *te taiao* (the environment), underscoring the encompassing influence of wairua, both seen and unseen. We created the following palliative care model, inclusive of all ages, to highlight the fundamental centrality and importance of wairua within Indigenous palliative care in Fig. 1.

Previous Māori experiences within mainstream end-of-life care have highlighted the crucial facets of spiritual and cultural safety for Māori. [25] This significance is starkly exemplified by this study's findings. How Māori experience wairua in dying, death, and mourning, profoundly underscores the pivotal role of wairua in shaping interactions with whānau, healthcare professionals, and institutional systems. Numerous Māori have observed that the prevailing public health system in Aotearoa New Zealand is often perceived as 'hostile and alienating' [26]. Their experience of the palliative care framework is that it predominantly rests upon Westernised conceptions of health, with a primary focus on addressing physical well-being rather than holistic well-being [26]. This study supports this suggestion and emphasises the critical dimensions of wairua care and injury during the end-of-life phase. As one participant aptly described the experience, 'it threw our world upside down', not only in the context of their family member's illness but also in relation to how hospital policies caused restrictions to access the dying person.

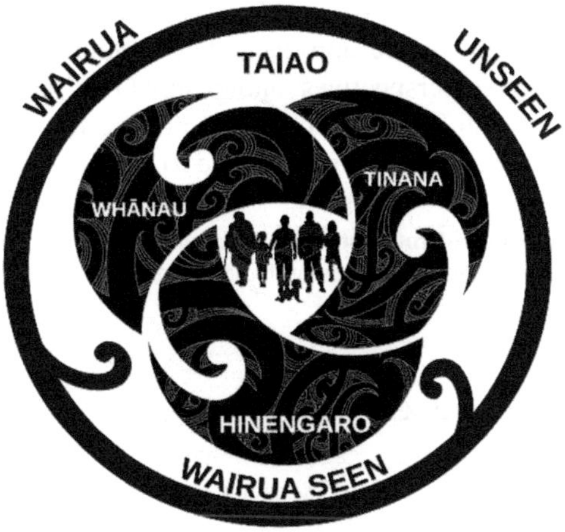

Fig. 1 Wairua palliative care model. (Moeke-Maxwell T, Egan R, Earp R, Laing B. Wairua Palliative Care Model. 2023)

Even under the most favourable circumstances, our hospitals frequently struggle to provide an environment that is culturally safe and appropriate. Such struggles are expressed by participants as having the interconnectedness of wairua with *whanaungatanga* (connectedness) broken. This resulted in their experiencing an 'incomplete mourning process', highlighting the distress that emanates from a system that lacks awareness of a wairua-centric universe. Also evident in the COVID-19 narratives concerning wairua are the tensions that emerge when the health system reduces end of life to biology and medicine and ignores or undervalues peoples lived spiritual experiences and realities [27].

Within Aotearoa, the Health Quality and Safety Commission's Te Ao Māori Framework [28] advocates for an evolution of cultural competence that explicitly encompasses spiritual safety. This policy directive is rooted in evidence-informed positions that underscore the significance of wairua and aligns with the government's commitment to Te Tiriti o Waitangi. Mauri Mate provides a whānau-centric framework to guide to Māori palliative care that is guided by Māori tikanga [29]. Based on the insights provided in this remarkable COVID-19 end-of-life study, two key recommendations are warranted to enhance Māori spiritual care at the end of life:

1. Improved cultural safety training: Healthcare professionals should receive comprehensive cultural safety training that includes a deep understanding of *Te Ao Māori* (a Māori worldview) and other indigenous worldviews. This training should emphasise the significance of wairua and its integral role in end-of-life care.
2. Culturally safe *taiao* (environments): Hospitals and healthcare institutions should prioritise the creation of culturally safe taiao that respect and accommodate Māori cultural practices and beliefs. This includes recognising and addressing tensions between spiritual safety and established hospital protocols.

In essence, effective Māori spiritual care at the end of life requires a holistic and culturally safe approach that honours the significance of wairua, acknowledges diverse perspectives, and ensures that individuals and their whānau feel respected, understood, and supported until the last breath and following death. These important insights are transferable to Indigenous peoples all over the world.

Conflict of Interest All participants gave both verbal and written consent to use their names and information in our research dissemination activities.

References

1. Gott M, Wiles J, Mason K, Moeke-Maxwell T. Creating 'safe spaces': a qualitative study to explore enablers and barriers to culturally safe end-of-life care. Palliat Med [Internet]. 2022;37(4):520–9. Available from: https://doi.org/10.1177/02692163221138621.
2. Moeke-Maxwell T, Mason K, editors. Whānau reflections on life and death during COVID-19 [Internet]. Te Ipu Aronui. 2022. Available from: https://www.teipuaronui.co.nz
3. Ngata P. Death, dying and grief. In: Schwass M, editor. Last words: approaches to death in New Zealand concerning death in New Zealand's cultures and faiths. Wellington: Bridget Williams Books and the Funeral Directors Association of New Zealand; 2005.
4. Nelson-Becker H, Moeke-Maxwell T. Spiritual diversity, spiritual assessment, and Māori end-of-life perspectives: attaining ka ea. Religions [Internet]. 2020;11(10):536–52. Available from: https://doi.org/10.3390/rel11100536.
5. Marsden M. The woven universe: selected writings of Rev. Māori Marsden. Royal TAC, editor. Otaki: Estate of Rev. Māori Marsden; 2003.
6. Moeke-Maxwell T, Mason K, Gott M. New Zealand's indigenous end-of-life customs: a qualitative study on Māori, by Māori, for Māori, with Māori. In: McLaughlin H, Beresford P, Cameron C, Casey H, Duffy J, editors. The Routledge handbook of service user involvement in human services. Abingdon: Routledge; 2021. p. 347–59.
7. Moeke-Maxwell T, Mason K, Toohey F, Wharemate R. He taonga tuku iho: indigenous end of life and death care customs of New Zealand Māori. In: Selin H, Rakoff RM, editors. Death across cultures: death and dying in non-Western cultures [Internet]. Cham: Springer; 2019. pp. 295–316. Available from: https://doi.org/10.1007/978-3-030-18826-9_18.
8. Moeke-Maxwell T, Wharemate R, Black S, Mason K, Wiles J, Gott M. Toku toa, he toa rangatira: a qualitative investigation of New Zealand Māori end of life care customs. Int J Indig Health [Internet]. 2018;13(2):30–46. Available from: https://doi.org/10.32799/ijih.v13i2.29749.
9. Mead SM. Tikanga Māori: living by Māori values. Wellington: Huia; 2003.
10. Beaglehole E, Beaglehole P. Contemporary Māori death customs. J Polyn Soc [Internet]. 1945;54(2):91–116. Available from: https://www.jstor.org/stable/20703006
11. Oppenheim RS. Maori death customs. Wellington: Reed; 1973.
12. Clair S, Piripi H, Reid P. Contemporary perspectives. In: Schwass M, editor. Last words: approaches to death in New Zealand's cultures and faiths. Wellington: Bridgett Williams Books with the Funeral Directors Association of New Zealand; 2005.
13. Duggleby W, Kuchera S, MacLeod R, Holyoke P, Scott T, Holtslander L, et al. Indigenous people's experiences at the end of life. Palliat Support Care [Internet]. 2015;13(6):1721–33. Available from: https://doi.org/10.1017/s147895151500070x.
14. Bishop R, editor. Kaupapa Māori research: an indigenous approach to creating knowledge. In: Robertson N, editor. Maori and psychology: research and practice: the proceedings of a symposium sponsored by the Maori and Psychology Research Unit. Maori & Psychology Research Unit; 1999.

15. Cram F. Rangihau Māori: Tona tika, tona pono: the validity and integrity of Māori research. In: Tolich M, editor. Research ethics in Aotearoa New Zealand: concepts, practice, critique, vol. 35–51. North Shore: Pearson Education New Zealand; 2001.
16. Hudson M, Milne M, Reynolds P, Russell K, Smith B. Te Ara Tika guidelines for Māori research ethics: a framework for researchers and ethics committee members. Auckland: Pūtaiora Writing Group. Health Research Council of New Zealand; 2010.
17. Walker S, Eketone A, Gibbs A. An exploration of kaupapa Maori research, its principles, processes and applications. Int J Soc Res Methodol [Internet]. 2006;9(4):331–44. Available from: https://doi.org/10.1080/13645570600916049.
18. Moeke-Maxwell T, Nikora LW, Mason K, Carey M. Te whakatara! Tangihanga and bereavement COVID-19. Ethnogr Edge [Internet]. 2020;4(1):19–34. Available from: https://doi.org/10.15663/tee.v4i.77.
19. Curtis E, Jones R, Tipene-Leach D, Walker C, Loring B, Paine SJ, et al. Why cultural safety rather than cultural competency is required to achieve health equity: a literature review and recommended definition. Int J Equity Health [Internet]. 2019;18(1):174. Available from: https://doi.org/10.1186/s12939-019-1082-3.
20. Parsons J, Boydell KM. Arts-based research and knowledge translation: some key concerns for health-care professionals. J Interprof Care [Internet]. 2012;26(3):170–2. Available from: https://doi.org/10.3109/13561820.2011.647128.
21. Spagnol GS, Tagami CY, De Siqueira GB, Li LM. Arts-based knowledge translation in aerial silk to promote epilepsy awareness. Epilepsy Behav [Internet]. 2019; 93:60–4. Available from: https://doi.org/10.1016/j.yebeh.2018.12.005.
22. Valentine H, Tassell-Mataamua N, Flett R. Whakaira ki runga: the many dimensions of wairua. N Z J Psychol [Internet]. 2017;46(3):64–71. Available from: https://www.proquest.com/scholarly-journals/whakairia-ki-runga-many-dimensions-wairua/docview/1987344234/se-2
23. Park CL. The meaning making model: a framework for understanding meaning, spirituality, and stress-related growth in health psychology. Eur Health Psychol [Internet]. 2013;15(2):40–7. Available from: https://www.ehps.net/ehp/index.php/contents/article/download/ehp.v15.i2.p40/1041
24. Durie M. Whaiora, Māori health development. Auckland: Oxford University Press; 1998.
25. Egan R, MacLeod R, Jaye C, McGee R, Baxter J, Herbison P. What is spirituality? Evidence from a New Zealand hospice study. Mortality [Internet]. 2011;16(4):307–24. Available from: https://doi.org/10.1080/13576275.2011.613267.
26. Graham R, Masters-Awatere B. Experiences of Māori of Aotearoa New Zealand's public health system: a systematic review of two decades of published qualitative research. Aust N Z J Public Health [Internet]. 2020;44(3):193–200. Available from: https://doi.org/10.1111/1753-6405.12971.
27. Chuengsatiansup K. Spirituality and health: an initial proposal to incorporate spiritual health in health impact assessment. Environ Impact Assess Rev [Internet]. 2003;23(1):3–15. Available from: https://doi.org/10.1016/s0195-9255(02)00037-9.
28. Te Ao Māori framework: Te Anga Ao Māori [Internet]. Te Tāhū Hauora: Health Quality & Safety Commission. 2023 [cited 2023 Aug 21]. Available from: https://www.hqsc.govt.nz/resources/resource-library/te-ao-maori-framework/
29. Te Ohu Rata o Aotearoa. Mauri Mate: Māori palliative care framework for hospices [Internet]. Te Aho O Te Kahu: Cancer Control Agency. Te Kahu Pairuri o Aotearoa, Hospice New Zealand; 2020 [cited 2023 Aug 21]. Available from: https://teaho.govt.nz/publications/cancer-state

Navigating the Soul's Departure: Spiritual Care for Muslim Patients in Palliative Care

Manar Ghamian

Abstract Spiritual care is an integral component of holistic palliative care. Muslim patients in palliative care have specific spiritual and religious needs. This chapter offers care providers four general considerations to better tend to Muslim patients' spiritual needs: privacy, mobility for prayer and ablution, provision of religious items, and inclusion of family in the decision-making process. For spiritual care providers, this chapter presents an Islamic understanding of death and dying and highlights a prophetic model that can help Muslim patients deal with emotions related to death and dying. All *Qur'an* translations from the original Arabic to English are by the author.

Keywords Spiritual care · Palliative care · Muslim patients · Death and dying Grief · Islam and death and dying · Spiritual bypassing

1 Case

Sameera, an elderly Muslim woman, lay in her hospital bed, where it feels like she spends more nights than in her bed at home. This hospital admission was due to her chronic heart failure, which is exacerbated due to several other chronic illnesses. When she is not asleep, Sameera is quiet, reflective, and pensive. Her demeanour does not hide that she has relinquished all potential for meaningful recovery and has accepted reaching a critical and irreversible stage of illness. Her multiple hospital visits in the last year have made it clear to her that she is on the cusp of palliative care. As a Muslim, she credits her faith as an indispensable source of strength and comfort as she comes face to face with her mortality.

M. Ghamian (✉)
Spiritual and Religious Care Provider, Westpark Healthcare Center, Toronto, ON, Canada
e-mail: manar@lighthouseoftherapy.com

M. C. Best (ed.), *Spiritual Care in Palliative Care*,
https://doi.org/10.1007/978-3-031-50864-6_7

Outside Sameera's hospital room, her husband is frantically seeking the attention of the attending physician to follow up on several test results. With admonishment, he repeatedly exclaims to the nurse that his wife must be helped by hospital staff to eat her meals, for when she is left unattended, she barely eats any of her food. Forever hopeful of his wife's return to health, he is insistent on every possible treatment to maintain and prolong his wife's life.

Sitting at her bedside, her son awaits his mother to have a instance of lucidity to steal a moment of connection. As the eldest son, he is ever mindful of his duties and his position as a support not only to his mother, but his father and his siblings. His austere and plain face conceals his anxiety and fear for his mother's deteriorating condition. He has not considered exploring palliative care for his mother with his family, not out of belief for her recovery, but rather to push away the unspeakable discomfort of having to come face to face with his mother's impending death. He recognises that his mother has been and is suffering from her illness. He hopes that she becomes free from suffering but is also fearful of losing her.

2 Overview

According to the latest projections, Muslims are the fastest growing religious group and is currently the second largest religious group globally, accounting for approximately 25% of the world's population [1]. Appearing in the early seventh century of the common era, Islam is considered the last of the Abrahamic religions. Islam is centred around the teachings of the *Qur'an*, believed by Muslims to be the unadulterated and final revelation from God, and the life of Prophet Muhammad, seen by Muslims as an exemplar for emulating in matters of religious practice and daily life. Muslims' understanding of death and dying is shaped by Qur'anic teachings and the collective practices and sayings of Prophet Muhammad, referred to by Muslims as *hadith*. The *Qur'an* speaks about death and its inevitability, while the Prophetic life sheds light on how to interact with death and dying in a wholesome fashion while negotiating its complexities.

Sameera's case above offers an opportunity to explore the unique spiritual needs of Muslim patients in palliative care settings and the various factors that inform their experience at the end of life. This case will also provide a glimpse into what providing spiritual support to families of Muslim patients can look like. First, death and dying as experienced by Sameera and her family is explored through an Islamic lens. Second, a model of dealing with grief is presented based on Prophet Muhammad's exemplary practice. Following that, a short exposition is given on the unique spiritual needs of Muslim patients in palliative care settings. This includes a section on providing psychospiritual care to Muslim patients who are actively dying. Lastly, important notes are provided on post-death care for Muslim patients and their families.

3 Death and Dying from an Islamic Understanding

The attitudes of Sameera, her husband and her son are reflective of the various spiritual, emotional, and religious responses Muslims have to death and dying. Each embodies a characterisation of reactions to end of life that highlight various values, teachings, and understandings common to the Muslim experience.

To start, Sameera's husband's adamant striving to exhaust every possible treatment for his wife is a frequent occurrence among individuals from devout Abrahamic religions. According to the Muslim tradition, life is a gift from God, The Life Giver (*Al-Muhyiy*). To honour The Giver of this gift, Muslims strive to live their life in accordance with God's commands and decree. Furthermore, in respecting this gift of life, not only is it reprehensible to commit suicide, but every effort must be exerted to honour and maintain God's gift of life. Similarly, just as it is God's rightful attribute to be The Life Giver, He is also the One Who Takes Life (*Al-Mumeet*). As such, it is believed that death cannot and, more importantly, should not be hastened before its divinely allotted time [2]. In this, Sameera's husband believes he is upholding the sanctity of life and completely submitting to God's commandment of preserving life and honouring the gift of life to its fullest.

Sameera's approach towards her impending death is representative of the recommended inward attitude towards death in Islam. Death, for the believer, is a long-awaited friend who ushers the believer from this world of struggle, hardships, and rancour into a hereafter of peace, freedom, light, and communion with loved ones. At first glance, Sameera's yielding approach towards her end of life is a stark contrast to that of her husband's active and unremitting hope for her recovery. However, her accepting psychospiritual mindset is equally rooted in Islamic teachings. It is noted that Prophet Muhammad had said 'The ultimate gift for the believer is death' and 'there is no [true] comfort for the believer until [after] death' ([3], p.37). These two hadiths allude to the reality that this world is one of trials, difficulties, and much hardship. The believer lives his/her life with that reality in mind and with the recognition that this life is only a preparation for the afterlife. Just as the runner has to push through until the end of the race, so does the believer exert all his/her efforts until the end. It is only after the race of this world that the believer experiences true comfort and the felicity of the afterlife.

As for Sameera's son, he displays the very human struggle of honouring and holding space for both life and death. His attitude is not based on any Islamic teachings per se, rather it is the human condition to fear the unknowns that death brings about. While it does not escape the son that his mother is terminally ill, it can be very hard to come to terms with accepting it. As such, the Qur'an on multiple occasions asserts the unavoidable reality of death and exhorts believers to prepare for it: '*Every soul shall taste death and then to Us, you shall return*' (Qur'an 29:57) and '*Say: the death that you run away from, it will certainly catch up to you*' (Qur'an 62:8).

4 Reconciliation of Seeking Treatment and Acceptance

Many patients with chronic or life-limiting illness are faced with the question of palliation: whether to continue active treatment or to transition to a palliative-based approach. This question evokes a full range of emotional, psychological, and spiritual responses from not only the patient, but also the family. These responses are informed by the values and religious beliefs of those facing this situation. At first glance, it may appear that the dichotomous nature of the decision (active treatment or palliation) would also reflect equally dichotomous spiritual responses of resilience or acceptance. However, spiritual matters are rarely this clear cut, and the path of reconciliation between the two spiritual responses is interwoven. For Muslim patients, this inward spiritual journey is inseparable from the outward reality.

Islamic teachings relate to two domains of the human experience. The outward domain (*zahir*) relates to priorities, rulings, and a hierarchy of values and concepts that dictate a course of action in a particular situation. This exoteric dimension of Islam may prescribe, in the context of patients, the preferred course of action for a patient with a terminal illness, taking into account the physicians' recommendations. In the case presented above, this is embodied by Sameera's husband, whose drive to continue to seek treatment for his wife is based on the Islamic teaching of preserving life and seeking treatment whenever possible as per the prophetic saying 'Seek treatment for God has not created an illness except that He also created for it a cure, save for old age' ([4], p. 5).

The second domain relates to the inward (*batin*) experience of the believer. This concerns the spiritual dimension of a believer's experience that yearns to find the true purpose and hidden meanings within one's outward experience. The inner dimension of Islamic teachings shape the believer's experience of their outward reality. Referring to the above case, Sameera's acceptance of her mortality reflects her inner spiritual dimension that allows her to surrender her fate to God's decree and accept what God has for her. The Qur'anic verse '*And that which is with God is better and more lasting for those who are mindful of God, those whom upon their Lord rely*' (Qur'an 42:36) gives reassurances to Sameera that her affairs are in good hands.

Thus, the task of the believer is to act upon the exoteric dimension of Islam while embodying the inward spiritual dimension; the two together make one whole. In Sameera's case, she can simultaneously seek treatment while being fully accepting that her lifespan may be measured in days and not years. When the medical professionals' recommendation favours palliation over active treatment, it will fall on ears that have long accepted this as a real possibility. Holding both positions as equally true appears to be a paradox, yet it lies at the heart of the journey of integration of faith.

The role of a spiritual care provider at this junction of a patient's journey is invaluable. A spiritual care provider can help Sameera and her family sort through the emotional and spiritual responses to end of life care. With adequate knowledge of Islam's approaches to death and dying and through thoughtful questions and exploration of her religious tradition, the spiritual care provider can bring the considerations noted above into the family's collective approach. With an understanding of both the outward and inward dimensions of Islamic teachings, the spiritual care provider can journey with the family in navigating these paradoxical stances at the end of life and give validation to Sameera, her husband and her son's attitudes towards death and dying. Furthermore, the spiritual care provider, who supports not only the patient, but also the family, can help each family member understand the value of each emotional and spiritual response and as such, step into the shoes of the other. This facilitates communication between family members and helps the patient and family to be unified in their approach to goals of care.

Walking the nebulous boundary of the exoteric and esoteric dimensions of Islamic teachings, the following prophetic supplication summarises the crux of this delicate act of negotiating the inner and outward realities: '*God, give me life as long as life is good for me. And take my soul [to you] if death is good for me*' ([5], p. 197). This supplication affirms that in some cases continued life is the better option and at other times death, despite its finality, is more favourable. It is worthy to note that many Muslim patients are not aware of this supplication and its spiritual implications for the approach to their own death. Thus, providing patients and family members with religious education in the form of sharing the above supplication with them can help ease tensions regarding differing stances on goals of care. In Sameera's case, she was more inclined towards palliation, while her husband sought active treatment. For their son, the above supplication both validates his desire for his mother's survival and also his wish for her to be free from suffering. In making this supplication, one effectively turns one's affairs inwardly to God, seeking His assistance in facilitating what is best, through the treatment decision or despite it. In actively making a decision and then turning affairs over to God, one relinquishes any illusions of control and as such, is more likely to exhibit higher levels of acceptance to how the patient's journey unfolds.

5 Facing Death, Spiritual Bypassing and the Prophetic Model of Grieving

Naturally, death and dying evoke in patients and their families a strong range of emotions. From anger, sadness, relief, and despair, each emotion is connected to a life of experiences, spiritual beliefs and values related to death and dying. The experiencing and expression of these emotions is significantly informed by cultural norms and, in some cases, religious values [6]. For patients and family members with a strong sense of faith, experiencing and expressing emotions related to death and dying, particularly those of anger or sadness, may be viewed as tantamount to not accepting God's decree or destiny.

For Muslim patients in particular, phrases such as 'lifespans are in God's Hands' or 'they are in a better place' or 'To God we belong and to Him we shall return' are commonly used at the time of death. However, if used to repress or avoid the experiencing of emotions, it is regarded as 'spiritual bypassing', a process where the usage of religious beliefs or practices avoids addressing raw emotions, psychological wounds or traumas [7]. In cases of death, phrases similar to the ones mentioned above are often used to circumvent raw emotions of sadness, sorrow, and anger and instead jump straight to acceptance of the loss. This process, common among Muslims, is in stark contrast to the prophetic model of Muhammad in dealing with loss.

It is recorded that Prophet Muhammad had to contend with the loss of his son, Ibrahim, when he was aged one. The loss of a child is devastatingly tragic for all parents, and this was no exception. As his son passed away in his hands, Prophet Muhammad was seen by his companions crying. Exclaiming to him, his companions asked him 'You cry, and you are God's Messenger?' To this he replied, 'It is a mercy [to show compassion]...the eye sheds tears, the heart trembles with sorrow, and we only say that which pleases our Lord, and we are at losing you, Ibrahim, saddened' (Al-Nawawi, p. 279).

The example set by Prophet Muhammad is a wonderfully holistic approach to dealing with loss of a loved one. In stating that his eyes shed tears, Prophet Muhammad is exemplifying and giving permission to the adherents of his faith that the somatic experiencing and expression of the emotion of sadness is completely valid. In noting the sadness of his heart, he normalises the emotion of sadness at loss, hereby negating any illusion that being a person of faith would separate one from their emotions or make one stoic or insensitive to loss. Loss of loved ones is a deeply human experience, and the Islamic faith does not veil an individual's humanity, but rather makes it whole. The path to becoming whole is found in fully experiencing sadness at times of sadness, and joy at times of joy.

In the prophetic example above, the uninhibited experiencing of sadness through the tearing eyes and saddened heart facilitates the sincere and complete acceptance of God's decree just as in his statement of 'and we only say that which pleases our Lord'. In other words, how could one aim to recognise and accept God's decree regarding loss, when one cannot even acknowledge and accept one's own immediate emotions? Is it even possible to truly accept the loss, if one does not accept the emotions evoked by it? The answer given in the prophetic model would be unequivocally 'no'. Giving oneself permission to fully experience emotions and the corresponding somatic sensations enables a higher spirituality that aspires to 'say that which pleases our Lord'.

Finally, the final statement of Prophet Muhammad sheds important light on relationships post death. In his statement 'we are at losing you, o' Ibrahim, saddened', Prophet Muhammad uses the second person pronoun 'you', clearly addressing his deceased son. From an Islamic perspective, this gives credence to the belief that deceased individuals still have some form of perception that would allow them to perceive what is said by the living. Second, and more importantly for the context of grieving death, the prophetic example encourages those who are mourning to continue to nurture their relationships with their loved ones, even after death. It affirms that even after the passing of loved ones, the relationship does not end, but endures. That is why the Prophet encouraged giving to charity in the name of the deceased one, to visit their friends as a form of duty and honour to the deceased, and to perform certain acts of worship and grant its reward to the deceased.

In the context of palliative care, the above example is relevant for both patients as well as their family members. For patients, it gives them permission, from a religious perspective, to fully experience their emotions, to embrace their humanity and through it, grow spiritually even throughout their dying moments. For family members, the prophetic model gives them a road map that fully validates the range of emotions that they may be experiencing. It also facilitates the grief process by recognising that relationships with loved ones do not end with their death but endure in a changed and new form. The prophetic model also opens the door for Muslims to partake in post-death rituals, often facilitated by spiritual care providers, that invite loved ones at the bedside to speak to the deceased patient to share last words with them, to say a prayer or to simply tell them how they feel. This process is immensely powerful and helps initiate the long journey of grief. The formal rituals relating to death and funeral services further aid family members along this journey of grief.

6 Unique Needs of Muslim Patients in Palliative Care

Given 'improving quality of life' is an essential aim of palliative care, it is imperative for healthcare providers to address the needs of patients holistically, including spiritual and religious needs. This is particularly relevant when caring for Muslim patients in palliative care settings. Muslim patients may require special attention to meet their spiritual and religious needs. Below are four main areas of concern for Muslim patients within palliative care settings: the need for privacy, mobility for ablution and prayer, provision of religious items such as prayer mats and religious scripture, and family involvement in decision-making regarding health needs.

6.1 The Need for Privacy

Privacy holds profound cultural and religious significance with Muslim patients. In palliative care, where patients often face physical and emotional vulnerabilities in an all-encompassing environment, the need to respect privacy is heightened [8]. This is particularly true for female patients who adopt the *hijab* (head covering) and feel uncomfortable if male care providers enter their room without notification. A simple 'This is your nurse, may you please let me know when you are ready for me to enter' can give female patients time to cover themselves as they find necessary. For patient interactions that require touching or examining the body, it is preferred that female patients receive care from female healthcare providers, although it is recognised that this may not always be possible. As such, it becomes more imperative for staff to obtain consent from the patient for intimate patient interactions.

Furthermore, the importance of privacy for Muslim patients is multi-layered. Matters of personal concern, including health issues, are often regarded as private and should not be discussed around individuals not privy to family matters. A study by Tayeb et al. [9] emphasises the importance of preserving privacy and dignity in end-of-life care for Muslim patients.

6.2 *Mobility for Ablution and Prayer*

At the core of the life of every practising Muslim are the five daily prayers. The movements required in the prayer include standing, bowing, prostrating, and sitting on the floor. Inviting the worshipper to be connected to nature, the timing of each prayer is prescribed by the sun's movement through the sky: pre-sunrise, when the sun reaches its zenith, when the sun passes the midway between noon and sunset, immediately after sunset, and lastly when the last rays of light from the sun are no longer visible. The timing of the prayers varies by season, given the sun rises and sets at differing times throughout the year. This should be taken into consideration when caring for Muslim patients as the timing of their daily routines will vary by season. Each prayer is typically preceded by ablution (*wudu*), which consists of washing the face, hands, and feet. For Muslim patients in palliative care, mobility challenges may pose barriers to fulfilling the religious obligation of ablution and prayer. Recognising and addressing this aspect of their spiritual practice is crucial for holistic care [10]. Occupational therapists can help set up patients with specialised equipment to conduct the ablutions without having to go the washroom. Physical therapists can also help develop personalised exercise plans to address mobility limitations, ensuring that patients can engage in prayer and ablution rituals safely and comfortably. For bed-ridden patients, if possible, hospital beds should be directed towards Mecca, to allow patients to be in the correct orientation for prayer. Spiritual care providers can connect Muslim patients with *imams* (religious leaders) who can help patients find religious dispensations regarding how the prayer form and ablution rituals can be adapted to patients' limited mobility. The significance of prayer in Islam extends beyond the physical act; it is a moment of connection with the Divine, providing solace and strength. For patients at end of life, facilitating the prayer, even in the smallest ways, can be the difference between patients fulfilling their religious obligations and meeting their spiritual needs or not.

6.3 *Provision of Religious Items*

Attending to the spiritual needs of patients includes ensuring they have access to scripture, sacred objects or other religious paraphernalia. For patients who do not have access to their own items, hospitals should keep on hand some of the most common religious paraphernalia from various religious and spiritual traditions. In palliative care, the provision of these items contributes positively to the emotional and spiritual well-being of patients. The most common religious items desired by Muslim patients include The Holy Qur'an, a prayer mat, and religious garments for prayer. The Qur'an may be made available in the original Arabic or in other translated languages. Spiritual care providers can help facilitate the provision of religious items to patients within palliative care settings. Local mosques may be contacted to request copies of the Qur'an and other religious items. Communicating with the interdisciplinary care team, the entire team should be mindful of these religious items and be wary of misplacing or unintentionally disregarding them.

6.4 Family Involvement in Decision-Making

In most Muslim cultures, family plays a significant role in the decision-making processes, where decisions are usually collectively made ([11], p. 1235). This is particularly relevant in health matters for elderly parents. In palliative care, where complex decisions are commonplace, involving the family in a culturally sensitive manner is integral to supporting Muslim patients. Spiritual care providers, as essential members of the interdisciplinary care team, can facilitate family discussions, providing emotional and spiritual guidance during decision-making processes [12]. They assist in bridging communication gaps and ensuring that the family's values and preferences are considered. This is particularly relevant if family members espouse different values or attitudes towards death and dying, as presented in the case above. A collaborative approach enhances the overall quality of care by acknowledging the importance of family involvement in the spiritual and medical journey of Muslim patients in palliative care.

7 Spiritual Care for Dying Patients

The provision of effective spiritual care for dying patients is a skill that adapts to the needs of the patient. The psychospiritual needs of patients should dictate the interventions and type of support offered. Muslim patients have spiritual needs that are shared with patients of other and no faith traditions and require common interventions. These include creating a safe space for patients to experience and express their full range of emotions, providing patients with emotional support, helping them identify values that would inform their advanced care planning, and facilitating a 'good death' [13].

End-of-life care aims to provide a good death, often associated with dignity and minimal suffering ([14], p. 24). Spiritually, a good death from an Islamic understanding is a good end, where the doors for returning to God are open until the last breath. For a patient, the experiencing of God and His mercy is accessible even while in the throes of death. The experiencing of God's mercy and compassion is not contingent on external circumstances, such as comfort or pain-free illness. Rather, it is sensing God's proximity as an inward reality that depends on the patient's spiritual framework and practice.

To illustrate this, an incident of Prophet Muhammad visiting an ailing man is explored. In this incident, the Prophet Muhammad visited an ill man and said ‘Do not worry, no harm shall come [out of this]. This [illness] shall be a cleansing of your sins’. For the believer seeking God’s mercy, hearing these words would bring calmness, acceptance of the illness and hope for full recovery as the Prophet himself is promising him a positive turn of events. However, this man was not in the mind-set, or perhaps the ‘spiritual-set’ to see what the Prophet saw. The man exasperatingly replied ‘Cleansing!? No! This an overwhelming burning fever that has ravaged an old frail man and will soon be his escort to the grave’. To this, the prophet merely replied ‘Then, so it will be as you say’ ([15], p. 2143).

For the believer, this incident highlights two important considerations. First, that even amidst severe illness, one can witness God’s gentle mercy within the illness. Experiencing the illness as an expiation of sins, which is a goal for every sincere believer, is a blessing. In another hadith, the Prophet states ‘The believer does not experience discomfort, illness, sadness or [a reason for] anxiety or grief, not even the pricking of thorn, except that God will expiate his/her sins [on account of his/her patience] ([5], p. 29). Second, the story of visiting the sick man affirms that one experiences reality based on one’s cognitive and spiritual framework. A belief about an experience will undoubtedly shape the experience itself. Believing an illness is a punishment, for example, will paint it as a punishment for the one experiencing it. On the other hand, believing an illness presents a doorway to knowing God in a new light will transform a person’s experience and predispose them to seeking God within the illness.

Here, the crucial role that spiritual care providers play in supporting Muslim patients in palliative care settings becomes evident. Conducting a spiritual care assessment can uncover patients’ values and beliefs regarding their palliative care experience. Through reflecting what they share back to patients, spiritual care providers can help patients become aware of: a) their (sometimes implicit) beliefs regarding death and dying; and b) the impact said beliefs have on their current experience in palliative care.

Exploring with Muslim patients their understanding of death and unpacking some of the baggage associated with the death and the dying process can help ease the pain through finding meaning within the suffering. Spiritual care providers can also ask patients to share particulars from scripture that shape their view of death and dying. For Muslims, discussing death and dying puts humanity’s true destiny in the afterlife into focus and urges preparation for it. In palliative care, death and dying is not merely a discussion, but a lived reality, and thus, it is imperative to help patients process it through expressing their emotions and beliefs. The Muslim and Persian philosopher Ibn Miskawayh (d. 1030) ([16], p. 91) notes that the primary method of addressing the anxieties related to death is through normalising it and becoming familiar with all things related to death and the dying process. In doing so, it is hoped that the believer experiences God’s promise ‘*So, surely with hardship there is ease. Surely with hardship there is ease*’ (Qur’an 94:5–6).

To conclude this section on spiritual care for dying Muslim patients, there are a number of practices recommended for patients who are actively dying. The first is giving charity at the time of death in the hope of easing suffering ([15], p. 1008). In the likely scenario where the dying patient is unable to direct the giving of charity, the person holding power of attorney, or a family member may give charity in the patient's honour. Second, it is strongly encouraged that the patient be reminded to utter the Islamic testimony of faith '*la ilaha ila Allah*' (There is no god but God) ([3], p, 108). If the patient is unconscious, a Muslim spiritual care provider or family member can chant the testimony at the bedside. Lastly, the Prophet advised his companions to read from the Qur'an the Chapter of Ya-Sin at the time of death, for it eases the pains of death ([3], p, 108). It is common practice for family members to read the Qur'an out loud at the death bed of patients. It also possible to use recordings of Qur'anic recitations if required.

8 Post-Death Care

Post-death care for Muslim patients involves adhering to Islamic traditions and providing support to the family during this challenging time. As is common with other faith traditions, Islam puts great importance on the dignified handling of the deceased patient. Fundamental to the rights of the body is hastening it to rest in its final abode ([15], p. 442). A general guide to post-death care for Muslim patients is presented below.

As soon as a Muslim patient passes away, it is recommended that the family contact Muslim burial services to arrange for post-death care of the body. Whenever possible, it is encouraged that the deceased is buried on the same day of death or the day following. Conducting an autopsy or organ transplant may be a valid exception to this guideline; however, swiftness of burial should be observed as far as possible. According to some practices, it is recommended for family members or a Muslim chaplain to recite certain verses from the Qur'an, namely the Chapter of Ya-Sin, after the passing of the patient ([3], p, 108). Typically, the body of the deceased must be washed by members of the same gender. This process is known as *ghusl* and is typically performed by family members or individuals with expertise in this ritual at the funeral or burial service. This ritual is immensely powerful for family members in helping process the grief of the loss. After the *ghusl*, the body is wrapped in a simple white shroud known as *kkafan*. The simple shroud symbolises equality in death, as all individuals are dressed in the same manner, regardless of their socioeconomic status in their life. The shrouding is typically perfumed with simple fragrance; a ritual that symbolises hope that God's mercy envelopes the deceased and to make the lasting impression of the deceased a fragrant one for those in the procession.

Prior to the burial, the *janazah* prayer, which is a collective prayer for the deceased, is performed by the Muslim community either in the mosque or at the burial site. If needed, hospital staff should facilitate a designated area for this prayer, ensuring that family and friends can participate in the ritual. As noted earlier, Islamic practice emphasises burying the deceased as soon as possible. Certain guidelines dictate that the body should be buried in an orientation towards Mecca. Typically, Muslim patients are buried in Muslim cemeteries, or cemeteries that have dedicated areas for Muslims. Barring any legal requirements, the body is to be buried wearing only the shrouding. In some countries, a coffin is a legal requirement, and as such, a simple plain wooden coffin may be used. Hospitals should work closely with local Muslim burial services to arrange for a timely burial while respecting any legal requirements.

Providing post-death care for a Muslim patient in a hospital setting involves a combination of adherence to Islamic rituals and cultural sensitivity. Spiritual care providers and other trained staff should be able to help navigate the specifics of Islamic traditions surrounding death and work collaboratively with the family to ensure a dignified and respectful farewell to their loved one. By integrating these practices into the hospital's standard procedures, healthcare providers can contribute to the well-being of Muslim patients and their families during a challenging time.

9 Conclusion

This chapter has provided a basic guide for healthcare workers, with a particular focus on spiritual care workers, to understanding and addressing the unique spiritual needs of Muslim patients in palliative care. As has been shown, Muslims' approach to death is based on religious teachings found in the *Qur'an* and Prophetic sayings. As such, for spiritual care providers to be effective in supporting Muslim patients, they must have an adequate understanding of Islam's view of death, and the various approaches and rulings associated with the dying process. Acknowledging the Islamic perspective on death and dying lays the foundation for a culturally sensitive and holistic approach to end-of-life care for Muslim patients.

The exploration of the four distinct spiritual needs—privacy, the need for mobility, access to religious items such as the *Qur'an*, and the importance of family inclusion in the decision-making process—highlights critical facets of caring for Muslim patients in palliative care. The entire interdisciplinary care team should be cognisant of these needs when attending to their Muslim patients.

By highlighting a prophetic model that allows for the full experiencing and expressing of the somatic, emotional, and spiritual responses to death, patients have a blueprint for what spiritually grounded and healthy responses to death can look like. Enriched with this knowledge, spiritual care providers can support their Muslim patients by relying on frameworks of grief from within their patients' religious tradition. Culturally competent spiritual care providers who have a basic understanding of Islamic tradition regarding death and dying can immensely help patients achieve a 'good death' and assist family members with their grief.

The final section shed light on some of the actively dying and post-death rituals for Muslim patients. A competently trained spiritual care provider can facilitate some of these rituals and help the family respond to their loss. In consultation with the family, it may be advisable to contact an Imam to help facilitate some of the ritualistic practices associated with death and dying. Addressing the rituals and practices associated with the Muslim burial process is crucial for ensuring a dignified and respectful transition for the deceased and providing solace to the family as it embarks on its journey of grief.

References

1. Pew Research Center. The future of world religions: population growth projections, 2010–2050 [Internet]. Pew Research Center's Religion & Public Life Project; 2015 [cited 2023 Dec 3]. Available from: https://www.pewresearch.org/religion/2015/04/02/religious-projections-2010-2050/
2. Sachedina A. End-of-life: the Islamic view. Lancet. 2005;366(9487):774–9.
3. Ibn Abi Al-Dunya. Remembering death [Internet]. Al-Salman AUM, editor. Al Furqan Publishing; 2002 [cited 2023 Dec 3]. Available from: http://archive.org/details/zikralmout
4. Abi Dawud. Sunan Abi Dawud [Internet]. Arnā'ūṭ S, Kurahbilli, Muhammad Kamel, editors. Vol. 6. Dar Al-Risalah Al-Alamiyah; 2009 [cited 2023 Dec 3]. Available from: http://archive.org/details/waq105201
5. Al-Nawawi YR. As-Saliheen [Internet]. Damascus; 2007 [cited 2023 Dec 3]. Available from: http://archive.org/details/waq85745waq
6. Benbenishty J, Bennun M, Lind R. Qualitative analysis of European and Middle East intensive care unit nursing death rituals. Nurs Crit Care. 2020;25(5):284–90.
7. Masters RA. Spiritual bypassing: when spirituality disconnects us from what really matters. Berkeley: North Atlantic Books; 2010. 206 p.
8. Kennedy G. The importance of patient dignity in care at the end of life. Ulster Med J. 2016;85(1):45–8.
9. Tayeb MA, Al-Zamel E, Fareed MM, Abouellail HA. A "good death": perspectives of Muslim patients and health care providers. Ann Saudi Med. 2010;30(3):215–21.
10. Boucher NA, Siddiqui EA, Koenig HG. Supporting Muslim patients during advanced illness. Perm J. 2017;21(3):16–190.
11. Abdullah R, Guo P, Harding R. Preferences and experiences of Muslim patients and their families in Muslim-majority countries for end-of-life care: a systematic review and thematic analysis. J Pain Symptom Manag. 2020;60(6):1223–1238.e4.
12. Klitzman R, Di Sapia NG, Garbuzova E, Sinnappan S, Al-Hashimi J. Muslim patients in the U.S. confronting challenges regarding end-of-life and palliative care: the experiences and roles of hospital chaplains. BMC Palliat Care. 2023;22(1):28.
13. Leget C. Art of living, art of dying: spiritual care for a good death. London: Jessica Kingsley Publishers; 2017.
14. Cipolletta S, Oprandi N. What is a good death? Health care professionals' narrations on end-of-life care. Death Stud. 2014;38(1):20–7.
15. Al-Bukhari MII. Sahih Al-Bukhari [Internet]. 5th ed., Bugha MD, editor. Damascus: Dar Ibn Khathir; 1993. Available from: https://archive.org/details/20191204_20191204_0610/page/n2/mode/1up
16. Ghaly M. End-of-life care, dying and death in the Islamic moral tradition, Studies in Islamic ethics, vol. 4. Leiden: Brill; 2023.

Spiritual Care for Buddhist Palliative Care Patients in Taiwan

Ben-Liang Shih, Pu-An Shih, Mei-Ling Huang, Shao-Yi Cheng, Huimin Bhikshu, Rong-Chi Chen, Ching-Yu Chen, and Jaw-Shiun Tsai

Abstract Facing death is an inescapable reality which has long been a core concern in Buddhism. This chapter focuses on exploring how to guide terminally ill patients in facing life and death issues through clinical approaches in the dying process, based on Buddhist teachings and the spiritual care model in Taiwan. It provides an integrated view of theoretical foundations and practical methods related to Buddhism, aimed at promoting the development and application of end-of-life care and spiritual care. The spiritual care of Buddhist patients involves correct understanding of Buddhist doctrines. It helps in correctly comprehending the true meaning of life, assisting terminally ill patients in facing life and death issues and enhancing their inner spiritual strength. The role of a clinical Buddhist chaplain is

B.-L. Shih
Department of Family Medicine, Taichung Tzu Chi Hospital, Buddhist Tzu Chi Medical Foundation, Taichung, Taiwan

P.-A. Shih
Department of Family Medicine, Dalin Tzu Chi Hospital, Buddhist Tzu Chi Medical Foundation, Chia-Yi, Taiwan

M.-L. Huang
Nursing Department, Taichung Tzu Chi Hospital, Buddhist Tzu Chi Medical Foundation, Taichung, Taiwan

S.-Y. Cheng · C.-Y. Chen · J.-S. Tsai (✉)
Department of Family Medicine, College of Medicine and Hospital, National Taiwan University, Taipei, Taiwan
e-mail: cycchen@ntu.edu.tw; jawshiun@ntu.edu.tw

H. Bhikshu
Dharma Drum Institute of Liberal Arts, New Taipei City, Taiwan

R.-C. Chen
Department of Neurology, En Chu Gong Hospital, New Taipei City, Taiwan

M. C. Best (ed.), *Spiritual Care in Palliative Care*,
https://doi.org/10.1007/978-3-031-50864-6_8

not to proselytise but to conduct a comprehensive assessment of the patient's physical, mental, and spiritual well-being, identifying potential spiritual distress. Through the six Buddhist care approaches, patients learn wisdom to transcend death, reducing their fear and suffering with hope for a peaceful passing. Companionship and guidance are provided based on Buddhist assessment at the dying stage to reduce the fear of death and guide the patient along the four pathways leading to a peaceful ending. Thus, the goal of care for the well-being of both the living and the dying can be achieved.

Keywords Buddhist patients · Spiritual distress · Spiritual care · Buddhist view of life and death · Clinical Buddhist chaplain · Six Dharma approaches · Palliative care · Buddhism

1 Introduction

Death is a topic that everyone must face, and it is also one of the core issues for Buddhism. Therefore, Buddhism has proposed a doctrine that helps sentient beings to overcome the suffering from vicissitudes between life and death, to culminate in *Nirvāṇa* (a state transcending life and death and free from suffering).

This chapter will describe the theory and practice of spiritual care for terminal Buddhist patients and end-of-life care in Taiwan, based on Buddhist doctrines and methods, according to an 'Indigenous spiritual care model', in order to adapt to the needs of modern society and to provide professional care for Buddhist patients with the goal of improving quality of life and enabling a peaceful passing.

We hope to provide an integrated framework and a practical reference to promote the development of theory and practice in the spiritual care for Buddhist patients, and to inspire more research, discussion, and social services for spiritual care based on Buddhist teachings.

2 Fundamental Buddhist Doctrines Related to Life and Death

Buddhism is a religion that has a deep and profound comprehension of life and death, encompassing teachings such as the Three Dharma Seals, the Four Noble Truths, the Twelve Links of Dependent Origination, and the concept of karma. These teachings are intricately connected to the cycle of birth and death, and the attainment of *Nirvāṇa*.

2.1 The Three Dharma Seals

The Three Dharma Seals are the three basic truths of Buddhism and include impermanence (*Anicca*), non-self (*Anatta*), and Nirvāna (*Nibbana*).

- Impermanence—People may perceive a pleasant environment as happiness or consider a state of equanimity without suffering or happiness as peacefulness. However, Gautama Buddha pointed out that even these comfortable and happy states are still considered suffering because they too will eventually come to an end. Thus, the recognition of 'impermanence leads to suffering' is the first mark.
- Non-self—Gautama Buddha referred to suffering as 'non-self' because the concept of 'self' implies a notion of control and autonomy. However, sentient beings are subject to the impermanent changes of aggregates, sense bases, and realms, and fundamentally lack true autonomy.
- *Nirvāna*—Due to the attachment to the idea of self, sentient beings generate delusions (defilements) and create karma. By realising the concept of 'non-self', one can eliminate the various causes of suffering and understand the true nature of being [1], which is known as '*Nirvāna*' or 'cessation and tranquillity'.

2.2 The Four Noble Truths

The Four Noble Truths are the four truths that lead to the end of suffering. They are:

- *Dukkha* (suffering)—The unavoidable realities of suffering and dissatisfaction in life.
- *Samudaya* (origin of suffering)—Suffering arises from the presence of defilement and karma.
- *Nirodha*—Suffering can be ended by eliminating defilements.
- *Marga*—There is a path to end suffering. Through ethical conduct (*sila*), mental discipline (*samadhi*), and wisdom (*panna*), one can overcome defilements and attain *Nirvāṇa*.

Buddhist teachings explain that the arising and cessation of suffering are dependent on causes and conditions. Understanding the dependent origination of suffering guides individuals to practice and achieve their goals. Therefore, only by comprehending dependent origination and cessation can one reasonably allow what needs to arise to come into being and what needs to cease to be eliminated.

2.3 The Twelve Links of Dependent Origination

Dependent Origination explains how suffering arises. The twelve links are: Ignorance, Formation, Consciousness, Name-and-form, The six sense bases (the eyes, ears, nose, tongue, body, and mind), Contact, Feeling, Craving, Clinging, Becoming, Birth, Ageing, and Death. The process of birth to death of sentient beings unfolds within the development of the twelve links [2, 3].

2.4 Karma

To name three types of Karma:

1. Fixed Karma and Unfixed Karma: Fixed karma refers to deliberate actions with definite consequences [4]. Whether an action will have definite consequences depends on oneself. One can counteract negative karma through the cultivation of wholesome actions [5, 6].
2. Individual Karma and Shared Karma: Individuals coexist. One's action and words have direct or indirect implications on others. Karma that primarily affects us is individual karma, while karma that affects others is known as shared karma. According to the law of shared actions and shared results, the collective karma of society requires everyone's participation to bring about change.
3. Directive Karma and Particularising Karma: The aggregate results of a strong karma that manifests in a particular life, leading to the rebirth of certain sentient beings (the 'aggregates, abodes, and realms'), are known as Directive karma. Some types of karma determine various aspects of our present life and are called Particularising karma. For instance, physical appearances would be different, some look solemn, some unattractive, etc.

The Twelve Links of Dependent Origination can be divided into three periods (the past, present, and future) and are characterised by dual causality: past causes (ignorance and formation) lead to present effects (consciousness, name and form, six sense bases, contact, and feeling), while present causes (craving, clinging, and becoming) lead to future effects (birth, ageing, and death) [3, 7]. Furthermore, before this life, there were past lives, and after this life, there will be future lives, if one has not transcended the cycle of reincarnation. The three periods and dual causality explain the complete process of infinite reincarnation.

The cycle of birth and death of sentient beings continues endlessly from one life to the next. Thus, the Buddhist concept of karma and dependent origination does not involve a self-entity or soul in the cycle of rebirth, nor does it consider karma as separate from body and mind. Instead, it operates based on the law of cause and effect, similar to ripples in flowing water or flames in a burning candle.

3 Spiritual Distress in Buddhist Patients in Taiwan

Regarding spiritual care, spirituality is not equivalent to religion, but the purpose of religious care is to meet spiritual needs, as religions provide important methods and guidance for self-transcendence, spiritual growth, and transcending the challenges of life and death [8, 9].

Indigenous Spiritual Care Research shows that the most common spiritual distress for terminal cancer patients is 'fear of death', followed by 'reluctance to let go' [10]. Clinically, most Buddhist patients have spiritual issues such as fear of death, pain before death, dreams about fear of death, and a sense of meaninglessness and worthlessness in life. Some commonly observed spiritual issues in clinical practice are described as follows.

3.1 Loss of Self-Respect

Loss of self-respect can result from the frustration caused by illness, damage to one's self-image, a sense of punishment from a higher power, value conflicts with family leading to fear of being abandoned by family members, or feelings of unfairness and uselessness. Additionally, the fear and dread of illness and death can cause self-isolation and withdrawal, leading to a lack of interaction with others.

From a clinical perspective, the problem of loss of self-respect is often manifested in terminal patients as loneliness caused by changes or damage to their appearance or disability, leading to self-isolation. Especially when death approaches gradually, when tangible (body) or intangible (psychological, role, identity) meaningful things and dignity are lost, the sense of loss leads to distress and frustration in patients [11].

3.2 Self-Abandonment

Self-abandonment is characterised by believing that death is inevitable with a passive and negative attitude, not seeking solutions to problems or perhaps adopting an uncooperative attitude towards the medical team, making it difficult to establish relationships. Symptoms of depression or suicidal tendencies and hopelessness may be observed.

Terminal patients often experience unbearable physical suffering during their terminal illness, leading them to perceive life as valueless and meaningless. Some patients may feel they become a burden to their families due to the care and financial support required [11]. Such feelings lead to self-abandonment in order to avoid becoming a burden to others. Lack of encouragement in the family support system is an important factor contributing to the emergence of suicidal thoughts in terminal patients.

3.3 Reluctance to Let Go

During the end-of-life stage, terminal patients often experience a diminishing sense of self-control, and the most common distress is the reluctance to let go. Driven by the thought 'I cannot die', they find compelling reasons to continue living. Clinically, this reluctance can be categorised into four types.

1. Unwillingness: During the treatment process, there is a sense of unwillingness, repeatedly thinking 'why me?' believing that there are still ways to live and it's not the end yet. As a result, they spend time and money seeking alternative treatments, hoping for a miraculous cure. Spiritual distress may arise from the disparity between their efforts and pay-offs.
2. Worry: Due to concerns about their family's abilities and circumstances, patients are worried about their loved ones, which leads them to cling to life despite their condition.
3. Unable to let go: Patients may have personal attachments to their bodies, wealth, family, reputation, etc., making it difficult for them to accept death.
4. Regrets and Guilt: Patients may experience regret for their life, or the consequences of wrong choices made during the treatment process. This may lead to a sense of irreparable loss and a feeling of regret. They may feel angry and resentful due to their suffering, feeling unfairly treated or guilty for past misdeeds.

3.4 Fear of Death

When patients face internal illness or external threats to life, their usual coping mechanisms may not address the issue of death and uncertainty of the future. This can lead to spiritual distress involving doubts, panic, and avoidance at the physical, emotional, and social levels during the dying process. Patients may worry about what will happen after death, whether they will go to hell, what the afterlife will be like, and if there will be any suffering [12].

In addition to fear of the dying process and death itself, many terminal patients' fear of death comes from unwillingness to be separated from their loved ones. They may also experience death-related nightmares or worry about losing all their possessions after death, or where they will go in the afterlife.

3.5 Unfulfilled Wishes

Unfulfilled wishes refer to the unfinished matters related to a peaceful death. It is possible that unfulfilled wishes may prevent a patient from finding peace until their last moment. This topic encompasses both unresolved desires and the reinterpretation of the meaning of life.

In clinical settings, some patients often express regrets about not having enough time to realise their dreams, such as spending more time with their parents or visiting places they've always dreamed of. To assist patients in fulfilling their wishes, healthcare providers may assess the feasibility of achieving them and, if possible, make concrete efforts to fulfil the patient's wishes. If fulfilling the wish is not feasible, symbolic assistance may be offered to help the patient find vicarious or compensatory satisfaction regarding their unfulfilled wishes.

3.6 *Incorrect Understanding of Dharma*

'Dharma' refers to the wisdom of facing life and death, and any method that can assist patients in their spiritual growth and help them confront the reality of life and death before the end of life.

Incorrect understanding of Dharma refers to the situation where patients still adhere to worldly laws and past coping mechanisms when facing death. They may engage in actions contrary to medical advice in an attempt to avoid facing death and refuse to learn correct coping methods and attitudes. They may struggle to comprehend that life and death are natural laws of the universe, governed by the law of causality. When unable to accept death and resort to avoidance, spiritual distress can arise.

4 Formation and Operation of the Buddhist Spiritual Care System in Taiwan

4.1 *The Framework of Spiritual Care*

Since its establishment in 1994, the Buddhist Lotus Foundation has been committed to promoting palliative care and the integration of Buddhism and end-of-life care. In 1998, at the invitation of Dr. Rong-Chi Chen, Dr. Ching-Yu Chen and Master Huimin jointly served as project leaders for the 'Research on the Application of Buddhism in Hospice Care/Palliative Medicine'.

In 1999, research entered the stage of clinical application, focusing on the 'Study of Spiritual Care Model' and developing an 'Indigenous Spiritual Care Framework'. The framework encompasses both the passive aspect, which aims to alleviate suffering and enhance vitality, and the assertive aspect, which involves spiritual growth and mental maturity. It follows the course of 'Suffering, Origination, Cessation, and Path'. Spiritual care is roughly divided into stages such as 'relieving patients' overall pain, informing patients of their condition, accepting death, sensing spiritual existence, relying on Buddhism, and eventually becoming a 'Buddha' [13–15], to help patients deal with physical, mental, and spiritual problems. Thus, an indigenous spiritual care model that combines medicine and Buddhism in the context of the Taiwanese religious culture and responds to contemporary care trends has been established [16, 17].

This model has been in use for more than 20 years with analysis on factors and outcome indicators [18, 19], and it has gradually become a prominent feature of hospice palliative care in Taiwan.

4.2 Training and Functions of Clinical Buddhist Chaplains

Compared to Western medical chaplains, the involvement of 'clinical Buddhist Chaplains' in hospice care is a pioneering move in Buddhist history and a major characteristic of the indigenous spiritual care model.

'Spiritual care' calls for professional caregivers to work with patients in exploring ultimate life issues and affirming meaning of life. It assists in promoting mindfulness, addressing various spiritual issues (life-and-death distress) [12], even learning to face and perhaps transcend death to achieve a peaceful end (or what Buddhism calls 'rebirth in the Pure Land'). These trained Buddhist chaplains have been shown to fit in and support Chinese culture and customs.

1. *Buddhist Chaplains' Participation in End-of-Life Care Through the Facilitation of the Buddhist Lotus Foundation*

   The key promoter of the birth of Clinical Buddhist Chaplains was Professor Rongji Chen, hailed as the 'Helmsman of Palliative Care in Taiwan'. Professor Chen noticed that a Western palliative care team often includes clergy or spiritual leaders. However, while 65% of Taiwan's population is Buddhist or has affiliations with Buddhist beliefs, no Buddhist chaplains were involved in palliative care. Consequently, when the palliative care unit was established at National Taiwan University Hospital, he invited willing Buddhist chaplains to join in patient care. After a 2-year pilot, it was confirmed that Buddhist chaplains were indeed needed.
2. *Training for 'Clinical Buddhist Chaplains'*

   Since Buddhist monks do not receive medical training in their education, to meet the needs of Buddhist chaplains participating in palliative medicine and spiritual care, the training for 'Clinical Buddhist Chaplains' officially began at National Taiwan University Hospital in 2000 and was subsequently expanded to establish a 'Clinical Buddhist Chaplain Training Centre' at Dalin Tzu Chi Hospital led by Master Pu'an in 2018 [20].

   The training for clinical Buddhist Chaplains is based on clinical medicine and Buddhist teachings [19]. It adopts a problem-oriented, self-learning approach similar to the training of resident physicians. Buddhist chaplains must complete three stages of training: basic, advanced, and internship. After passing an examination, they participate in 15 weeks of clinical training [13, 21]. Finally, they must pass another examination to be awarded the certificate of 'Clinical Buddhist

Chaplain' and become qualified to provide physical, mental, social, and spiritual care for patients [13]. Strict training and requirements represent lofty expectations and care [22].

3. *The Main Responsibilities of Clinical Buddhist Chaplains*

   Clinical Buddhist Chaplains regard preparation for death as their core professional role. Combining practice and care, they use wisdom on life and death to assist patients in facing spiritual distress (the dilemma of life and death). They inspire patients' inner strength, encourage the awakening of compassion, help patients let go of attachments, overcome the fear of death, and guide patients in 'preparing for imminent death' (learning Dharma teachings) and 'preparing for the next life'. They elevate the definition of 'life' for patients to include not only the current one but also the future ones (reincarnation), completing end-of-life practice to complement the shortcomings of current medical and other health care professions. Additionally, they provide life and death education to families, transforming obstacles into assistance, reducing anticipatory grief, and boosting the morale of the palliative care team.

   During the uncertain journey of facing death at the end of life, when patients are hesitating in the transition between life and death, clinical Buddhist chaplains act as guides. If they can closely connect with the patient's mind and soul at this moment, they can achieve deep empathy and internal transformation.

5 Practice of Buddhist Spiritual Care in Taiwan

5.1 Dharma Based on Buddhist Beliefs

Buddhist end-of-life care requires the study and application of Buddhist teachings that connect the present to the future. For these purposes, six major care approaches have been developed in the indigenous spiritual care model, based on common practices in Buddhism, each with its unique value and significance.

(a) *Practice of Benevolence (Zhong Shan Fa Men)*

   Also known as the 'Compassion Practice', it serves as the foundation for other practices. In clinical settings, inspiring patients with benevolence, compassion, positive thoughts, and beliefs can affirm the meaning of life, elevate inner strength, and help them let go of grievances and confront the issues of life and death. It reduces physical and mental suffering and opens a new perspective on the reality of life.

(b) *Practice of Taking Refuge (Gui Yi Fa Men)*

   Taking refuge is an important ritual in becoming a Buddhist disciple. It signifies a new milestone in life, representing the first step of 'rebirth'. This practice can provide patients with hope and faith, eliminate doubts and confusion, and enhance their sense of security and belongingness. In clinical settings, the Practice of Taking Refuge helps terminal patients establish a direction and goal for cultivating a firm and pure resolution. Patients shift their focus from seeking physical comfort or healing to pursuing the growth of their minds and natures, learning the wisdom of life and death, enhancing inner strength, and preparing for their future destination without fear of death.

(c) *Practice of Repentance (Chan Hui Fa Men)*

Repentance is the power of purifying mind and soul and eliminating afflictions from past wrongdoings and karmic consequences [23, 24]. It helps patients or family members release inner worries and regrets and find solace in their hearts. Clinically, during the retrospective review of their lives, patients recount the difficulties in their past and present lives; sometimes they attribute their illness to punishment and experience spiritual unease. In such situations, the 'Practice of Repentance' is employed to guide patients to come to terms with themselves and others, leaving no regrets or grudges.

(d) *Practice of Reciting Buddha's Name (Nian Fo Fa Men)*

Clinically, terminal patients who suffer from physical pain, emotional anxiety, nightmares, perceived heavy karma, death fear, and uncertainty about the future can benefit from the 'Practice of Reciting Buddha's Dharmic title'. This practice helps alleviate patients' fear of suffering and death, enhances their confidence and joy, enables them to let go of attachments, and lives fully in each moment.

(e) *Breath Counting Meditation (Shu Xi Liao Fa)*

Clinically, if a patient's wheezing or coughing is due to psychological reasons or even spiritual issues, breath counting therapy, meditation, or observation of the pain points may be used depending on their wheezing or pain condition to help them relax and practice concentration. As their anxious emotions subside or become tranquil, they often perceive a significant relief in breathing difficulties.

(f) *Pre-death Dharma Teachings and Chanting (Lin Zhong Shuo Fa and Zhu Nian)*

This practice includes taking a retrospective look with patients at their lives, affirming the meaning and purpose of life; teaching patients how to adjust their consciousness to cope with imminent organ failure and death; explaining the meaning of life and the vicissitudes in life; and forewarning the patient of possible physical and mental transformations during the dying process. It reminds patients to adhere to the teachings that help them to face death calmly and achieve a peaceful death. This practice also has a comforting effect on family members, making it 'a mutual comfort of the living and the dying'. Therefore, it is vital for end-of-life patients to receive Dharma teachings from clinical Buddhist chaplains.

'Chanting assistance' involves helping individuals on the verge of death to induce positive thoughts. As each stage of spiritual growth directly affects the next destination, guiding the mind and heart during the process of imminent death is crucial. Chanting assistance is meaningful only after the patient understands its benefits following Dharma teachings. It serves two main purposes: continuing the benefits of Dharma teachings and involving family members, which helps the family's bereavement.

5.2 *End-of-Life Care*

Buddhism views death as a process of reincarnation. The end-of-life stage involves various phenomena resulting from organ failure, which Buddhism explains as the 'disintegration of the four elements'.

Assessment of End-of-Life Phenomena

As terminal patients' bodies weaken and their organs gradually wear out, they experience changes and suffering in body, mind, and spirit. Once they enter the end-of-life stage, what changes will occur in their body, mind, and spirit?

1. *End-of-Life Symptoms (Physiological)*

   During the end-of-life stage, the following symptoms or phenomena can be observed clinically: increasing fatigue, weakness, and drowsiness; reduced appetite; indifference towards the surroundings; decreased vision and hearing; confusion about time, location, and people; restlessness; cold extremities and discoloration of the skin, appearing bluish or purple; urinary incontinence or changes in urine colour and volume, possibly leading to no urine output; increased difficulty in controlling pain or other symptoms; gurgling sounds during breathing, known as the 'death rattle'; irregular breathing patterns or temporary cessation of breathing, etc.

   It is important to note that solely relying on medical vital signs such as body temperature, pulse, respiration, and blood pressure or physiological conditions to determine likelihood of death or survival may not always be accurate, as patients may hold on due to unresolved spiritual concerns.
2. *Delirium (Agitation Before Death)*

   End-of-life delirium is commonly observed in clinical settings and may include the following symptoms: rapid changes in the patient's personality with emotional disturbances, seemingly becoming a different person; exhibiting strange or disorganised behaviours, excessive alertness, restlessness, fear, irritability, outbursts, yelling, cursing, or even aggressive behaviour; incoherent speech, muttering, with difficulty in understanding what the patient is saying; abnormal sleep patterns—sleeping during the day and restlessness or insomnia at night; hallucinations or illusions—seeing or hearing things that others cannot perceive.

   When symptom control or sedative medication is ineffective, and physiological causes are ruled out, delirium may be of psychological origin. In such cases, clinical Buddhist chaplains intervene. We attempt to understand the patient's life experience and context, often discovering suppressed subconscious issues, inner thoughts, unresolved concerns, significant negative experiences or psychological complexes from the past.

3. *Decomposition of the Four Elements—Earth, Water, Fire, Wind*

   Buddhism believes that the human body is composed of elements such as 'earth, water, fire, and wind', [25, 26] collectively referred to as the Four Elements. During the process of dying, the body transitions from a state of imbalance or deterioration of the Four Elements to a state of disintegration or collapse of the Four Elements, which is equivalent to the gradual failure of the body's organ systems, as described in medical terms.

   A. Decomposition of Earth—pressure from all directions

      In clinical settings, the disintegration of the Earth element is the most easily noticeable. Patients may exhibit signs of wanting to step on the ground or sit up. Some patients may feel that they are sinking when they get out of bed and refuse to go back to bed. Others may wave their hands in the air, as if trying to grab something, a phenomenon colloquially referred to as 'climbing a muddy slope'. Some patients may become restless and agitated, sit unstably, lean forward or sway from side to side. They may request more pillows or remove blankets and clothing or diapers.

   B. Decomposition of Water—cold pressing

      Clinically, during water decomposition, patients may experience involuntary flow of saliva, nasal secretions, and tears. Some patients may have urinary or faecal incontinence. Due to increased secretions in the mouth and nose, patients may feel sticky or as if their airways are blocked. Some patients may have drooping lips and nasal collapse or feel dryness in their eyes. Patients may tremble or have muscle spasms. Some may exclaim that they are 'falling into water' or about to drown.

   C. Decomposition of Fire—like a raging fire

      Clinically during fire decomposition, patients may experience dryness in the mouth and nose, with a parched and burning sensation. However, the tumour within the body may be warm or hot, creating a feeling of internal heat with external coldness. At times, patients may feel sudden hot flashes, as if being burned alive.

   D. Decomposition of Wind—changes in breathing patterns

      During the decomposition of Wind, some patients may exhibit laborious breathing, starting with shallow, slow breaths that gradually become deeper and faster, then gradually returning to shallower and slower breaths, repeating this pattern. This is known as 'Cheyne-Stokes respiration'. Some patients may feel chest tightness, as if their chest is full and produce heavy, panting sounds. Others may experience a long, deep inhalation followed by an exhalation like a sigh, called 'agonal breathing'. Some patients may make gurgling sounds in their throats during breathing, known as the 'death rattle'.

4. *The Awareness of Imminent Death*

As a result of prolonged illness and declining physical strength, patients may sense that their death is approaching or feel a gradual detachment from their family. According to our clinical experience, this awareness may be more accurate in predicting imminent death than end-of-life symptoms or vital signs.

The awareness of imminent death may manifest in various forms but is often overlooked or labelled as 'delirium or imagined'. Consequently, the opportunity for final interaction may be missed. The following are some common manifestations of the awareness of imminent death in clinical settings.

A. I want to go home

The most common and typical manifestation of the awareness of imminent death is when patients insist on going home. However, a thorough assessment by the medical team and consideration of family care is needed.

B. Seeing deceased relatives

It is common for terminally ill patients to see their deceased relatives or loved ones appearing before them and even having casual chats. Seeing the deceased loved ones signifies that the patient has been acknowledged by their family [27]. This acknowledgment allows their ancestors to personally welcome them, indicating that their contributions to the family have been recognised.

C. Going on a trip or seeing transportation vehicles

During the end-of-life stage, some patients may suddenly express a desire to go to a distant place and request immediate preparation, as if for travel. They may mention or imagine various forms of transportation. If the patient is a believer in Pure Land Buddhism, they may see the symbolic means of transportation to the Western Pure Land—the lotus flower, which is indicative of their imminent departure.

D. Predicting death time (self-knowledge)

In some cases, patients may explicitly state the time of their imminent death or indirectly express or imply it in different ways. Sometimes, the expression may not be clear or easily understood by the listener.

E. Seeing the desired destination

Some terminal patients, fearing they may not be believed, may cryptically describe seeing extraordinary scenes, such as lights, bright glare, grasslands, the Western Pure Land or out-of-body experiences.

F. Manifestation of religious symbols before death

During the end-of-life stage, patients may encounter religious symbols, such as Buddha, Bodhisattvas, lotus flowers, God, Jesus Christ, deities or other divine figures [28]. It is referred to as the 'manifestation of religious symbols'. When patients encounter any religious symbols, we encourage them to strengthen their beliefs. This often alleviates the fear of death and instils confidence in facing death and the afterlife.

Care and Companionship Before Death

During the dying stage, terminally ill patients experience various changes in their physical, mental, and spiritual states. They may exhibit different dying phenomena, and the fear of death looms large, particularly when pain and symptoms become challenging to manage, even causing unrelieved emotional and spiritual distress.

1. Explain the decomposition of the four elements to reduce fear of death

   In the process of spiritual accompaniment or care, we will explain the possible situations arising from the decomposition of the four elements. It may not necessarily happen but allows patients and family members to be psychologically prepared. Therefore, they will not panic or fear when facing sudden physical, mental and spiritual changes.

   A. Companionship during earth decomposition

      We may gently hold the patient's hand or provide a light hug when appropriate to make the patient feel comfortable and secure. We should also try to observe or understand if the patient is concerned about anyone or anything and provide assistance accordingly.

      Some patients may continuously want to stretch their legs under the bed, indicating their desire to have a firm grounding and prevent a sensation of continuous descent. It may also symbolise the desire to 'bid farewell to the earth', and placing something under their feet to simulate stepping on the ground can give them a sense of security and reassurance.

   B. Companionship during water decomposition

      If patients experience situations like water rushing down or flooding up, in addition to guiding them with positive thoughts or religious beliefs, we can also resolve crises by turning off faucets or pulling them from water surfaces. Some patients may exhibit tearful eyes (scleral oedema or 'lychee eyes') or tears may flow. Family members may mistakenly interpret this as spiritual unrest or a reluctance to leave loved ones. However, it is a normal phenomenon associated with water decomposition.

   C. Companionship during fire decomposition

      In most cases, patients will exclaim, 'It's very hot inside; I want to eat something cold'. In principle, we should follow the patients' feelings. We can offer them ice cubes to suck on. If the patient complains of a burning sensation in his throat and is conscious enough to swallow, we can moisten a cotton-tipped applicator with ice-cold water and let him gently suck it to quench his thirst.

      In the later stages of the Fire element decomposition, patients may find it challenging to speak. We may notice dry lips, and sometimes they may appear cracked. If the patient can still open his mouth, we can moisten a cotton-tipped applicator with ice-cold water and gently apply it inside the mouth, similar to brushing the teeth, to provide moisture or just moisten the lips directly if the patient cannot open the mouth.

D. Companionship during wind decomposition

We raise the head of the bed and adjust the patient's position to make him feel comfortable. Depending on the situation, we use indoor air conditioning, small fans or open windows to ensure air circulation, as cool air can help the patient breathe more comfortably. Some patients may develop the 'death rattle'. Elevating the head of the bed by about thirty degrees or having the patient lie on his side can reduce the sound of the rattle. At this stage, companionship focuses on whether the patient can mentally accept his condition. Techniques such as 'mindfulness of breath' or 'mindful recitation of Buddha's name' or gently holding his hands can be used to soothe. The purpose of mindfulness is not to cure or alleviate shortness of breath but to guide the patient's focus on his breath and help ease his restlessness and anxiety.

2. Guiding the Four Pathways: Gratitude, Apology, Love, and Farewell

Zhao Keshi proposed the 'Four Pathways' of life, emphasising family relationships in Taiwanese society. These 'Four Pathways' are Gratitude, Apology, Love, and Farewell. Subsequently, some have suggested the addition of 'Forgiveness' or 'Life' to form the 'Five Pathways' or 'Six Pathways'. Regardless, the core essence remains the same—to lead towards a good ending [11].

Regarding the indigenous spiritual care model, the Four Pathways mainly involve bidding farewell to karmic relationships in this lifetime. Afterwards, we guide patients to focus on preparing for the next life and acquiring wisdom about life and death. By striving to make a good transition, one can find peace in both life and death.

6 A Clinical Case

A clinical case is provided to illustrate application of these principles. The patient is 43 years old and suffers from head and neck pain due to hypopharyngeal cancer. He is not able to rest well because of the unbearable pain. Despite various treatments, the condition doesn't improve. The patient is depressed and loses the motivation to live.

His wife not only feels sorry to see the patient suffering but is also concerned about whether the patient is mentally ready to die. She is lacking the knowledge to accompany the patient and maintain spiritual stability. Therefore, she hopes to take refuge in Buddhism.

The patient has been admitted to the hospital many times, and his body has become weaker and weaker. In the end, he can no longer interact with people nor communicate. His wife said: 'I am afraid that when he passes away, he is not mentally ready and does not know where to go'. She cries a lot and feel helpless and worried because she does not know how she can help the patient.

6.1 Intervention Measures

1. Taking Refuge (Buddhism Conversion)

   After explaining the meaning of taking refuge, the ceremony was held in 'Bodhi House' in the ward. After the ceremony, a 'Buddhist certificate' and prayer beads were given to encourage the patient and the wife to study and practice hard in Buddhism.
2. Counting Breaths

   In addition to medical intervention for the pain, attempts were made to guide the patient in mindfulness and focusing on breathing, relaxation, and other methods to relieve pain.
3. *Nian Fo* (Reciting Buddha's name)

   The patient and his wife were provided with the *Diligent Nian Fo Record* guide and encouraged to use it together. The wife was guided to understand the changes in the patient's state of mind and encouraged to continue guiding the patient through scriptures and Buddha's names in daily interactions to establish a clear direction for the afterlife.

6.2 Outcome Evaluation

During the taking refuge ceremony, the patient was conscious and completed the conversion procedures with guidance. The wife said that they found a common direction after conversion. During guided breathing relaxation practice, although pain still existed, the patient was able to focus on his own breathing and gradually felt comfortable and at ease. He also reminded himself of Nianfo which made him feel more peaceful.

After understanding the changes in the patient's inner world, the wife was more willing to try accompanying him by reading scriptures and reciting Buddha's names with him, strengthening his faith in seeking rebirth in Amitabha's Pure Land, even when he did respond.

7 Conclusion

Through this chapter, we have gained an understanding of how the Taiwanese perceive Buddhist beliefs, including core concepts such as the Three Seals, Four Noble Truths, and Twelve Links of Dependent Origination. We have also observed the spiritual distress faced by Buddhist patients in Taiwan. This spiritual distress often causes fluctuations in the patients' inner world and can impact their overall well-being.

This chapter has explored how to guide terminally ill patients to face life and death issues through the clinical approach and care of the dying process, from the perspective of core Buddhist teachings and an indigenous spiritual care model. It provides an integrated view of theoretical foundations and practical methods related to Buddhism, aimed at promoting the development and application of end-of-life care and spiritual care.

However, we also recognise certain limitations in this research. The observation of spiritual distress among Buddhist patients requires further in-depth study. Therefore, we encourage future research to look deeper in this area and strengthen the training of professionals to provide more specialised and effective spiritual care services. Through continuous efforts, we believe that we can bring spiritual comfort and support to more patients, helping them better face health challenges and achieve physical, mental, and spiritual balance and peace.

References

1. Sheng Yan Master. Commentaries on the heart sutra. Taipei: Dharma Drum Culture; 2020. p. 51.
2. Yin Shun Master. Exploring the origin of emptiness. 1st ed. Hsinchu: Zhengwen Publishing House; 1944. p. 50.
3. Sheng Yan Master. Comparative study of religion. Taipei: Dharma Drum Culture; 2021. p. 394.
4. Madhyama-āgama Volume 3, CBETA, T01, no. 26, p. 437b26–28.
5. Yin Shun Master. The origin and development of early Mahayana Buddhism. 1st ed. Hsinchu: Zhengwen Publishing House; 1980. p. 573.
6. "Abhidharma Mahāvibhāṣā Śāstra" Volume 69, CBETA T27, no. 1545, p. 359b20–26.
7. Yin Shun Master. Notes on the Madhyamaka Shastra lecture. 1st ed. Hsinchu: Zhengwen Publishing House; 1952. p. 516.
8. Shih H-Z, Shih P-A, et al. Real cases of spiritual guidance on palliative care. Taipei: Sanying; 2023. p. 65–333.
9. Zongdun S, Qingyu C, Huimin S. The role and service status survey of clinical religious chaplains in hospice palliative care. J Life Death Stud. 2007;5:65–97.
10. Chen C-Y. Clinical scenarios of fear of death in patients with terminal cancer: clinical Buddhist chaplains participate in spiritual care. Formosan J Med. 2014;18(1):115–25.
11. Byock I, translated by Wen Bizhun. The courage to face death directly. Taipei: Gao Bao International; 2018. p. 130.
12. Huang W-H, Cheng Y-R, Yang Y-T, Chang C-Y, Huang S-C. How to face terminal death anxiety: who should be responsible for their own death? Taiwan J Hospice Palliat Care. 2017;22(2):202–12.
13. Chen C-Y. Clinical buddhist chaplain based spiritual care in Taiwan. Taiwan J Hospice Palliat Care. 2012;17(3):300–9.
14. Chen R-C. Clinical buddhist chaplaincy training program: history of the development of Taiwan's clinical buddhism. J Sci Discov. 2017;1(1):1–5.
15. Chen C-Y. Clinical buddhology and hospice: Buddhist chaplain based spiritual care. Taipei: Hungyeh Culture; 2022. p. 160–1.
16. Tsai C-h. Humanistic Buddhism in practice hospice care and Buddhist chaplaincy in Taiwan. Humanis Buddh J Arts Cult. 2016;5:154–73.

17. Chen C-Y. Clinical Buddhology and hospice: Buddhist chaplain based spiritual care. Taipei: Hungyeh Culture; 2022. p. 159.
18. Chen C-Y, Chiu T-Y, Wen-Yu H, Bhikkhuni T-T, Huang F-Y, Bhikkhu H-M. Clinical Buddhist Chaplain's care enhanced the good death index of terminal cancer patients. Taiwan J Hospice Palliat Care. 2003;8(1):13–27.
19. Bhikkhuni M-S, Bhikkhuni T-T, Chen C-Y, Chiu T-Y, Huang F-Y, Bhikkhu H-M. Investigation of the role and service of clinical Buddhist Chaplains in a palliative care unit. Taiwan J Hospice Palliat Care. 2001;6(4):1–12.
20. Chen R-C. The spirit of humanism in terminal care: Taiwan experience. Open Area Stud J. 2009;2:7–11.
21. Chen C-Y, Chiu T-Y, Bhikkhuni T-T, Bhikkhu H-M. The indigenous culture of spiritual care in Taiwan. Taiwan J Hospice Palliat Care. 2002;7(1):20–32.
22. https://www.lotus.org.tw/service/buddhist
23. "Dharmagupta-vinaya" Volume 35, CBETA, T22, no. 1428, p. 817c10–11.
24. "Bodhisattvapitaka Sūtra", CBETA, T24, no. 1491, p. 1087c1–3.
25. "Satyasiddhi Śāstra" Volume 2, CBETA, T32, no. 1646, p. 251a8–10.
26. Yin Shun Master. "The way to Buddhahood" (annotated edition). 1st ed. Hsinchu: Zhengwen Publishing House; 1960. p. 152–3.
27. "Kṣitigarbha Bodhisattva Pūrvapraṇidhāna Sūtra" Volume 2, CBETA, T12, no. 374, p. 785b11-c1.
28. Shih H-Z, Shih P-A, et al. Real cases of spiritual guidance on palliative care. Taipei: Sanying; 2023. p. 377.

Spiritual Aspects of End-of-Life Care for Christian Patients

Ian Olver and Benji Callen

Abstract Christianity aligns well with the principles of palliative care which respects the dignity of individuals and provides holistic care, embracing their physical, psychosocial, and spiritual needs, as did Jesus' healing ministry. Although Christians comprise groups which differ in their interpretations of the teachings of Jesus Christ and they observe different rituals and practices, their spiritual beliefs, which influence their end-of-life care, align. Following the example of Christ, they believe in an afterlife where they may dwell with the eternal God. As a response to God's grace, Christians aspire throughout life and at the end of life to love God, and others, discern with humility and submit to God's will, and repent for wrongdoings to seek God's forgiveness. The promise of eternal life is the source of great hope for Christians as death approaches. This will guide what is required at the end of life to achieve their spiritual wellbeing, which is beyond secular spiritual support and results in finding meaning and achieving peace.

Keywords Spirituality · Christianity · Palliative care · End-of-life · Death
Healing · God · Jesus Christ · Eternal life · Grace · Spiritual care

I. Olver (✉)
University of Notre Dame, Sydney, NSW, Australia

B. Callen
Burnside City Uniting Church, Adelaide, SA, Australia
e-mail: benjic@burnsidecityuc.org.au

M. C. Best (ed.), *Spiritual Care in Palliative Care*,
https://doi.org/10.1007/978-3-031-50864-6_9

1 Introduction

The end of life (EOL) is perhaps the ultimate nexus between medicine and spirituality. Historically there has been a close relationship between the two. Although the emphasis on spirituality has changed over time, the relationship persists. The Biblical Old Testament records that Moses was ordered by God to wrap a copper snake around a pole so the people could look at it and be cured of the snake bites they suffered when turning against God. The symbol of medicine, the rod of Aesculapius, the Greek God of healing, has a serpent entwined around it, where one of the interpretations is that it represents the ambiguity of the doctors' roles between managing both healing and death [1].

Christians are encouraged to care for others and have done so over the centuries. In the West, the Christian church built the first public hospitals in the fourth century and trained medical practitioners right up until the Reformation [2]. It is worth noting that Dame Cicely Saunders, who is credited with founding modern hospice care, with St Christopher's Hospice opening London in 1967, was a committed Christian, as were many of her successors [3]. Palliative care embraces holistic care which not only focuses on relieving physical suffering but provides emotional, social, and spiritual care. For centuries, spiritual EOL care for many Christians involved last rites or the commendation of the dying, especially in Roman Catholic, Orthodox, and Lutheran traditions [4].

Christianity, however, encompasses a diverse range of beliefs and this needs to be recognised in providing appropriate EOL care to Christian patients. Spiritual beliefs certainly can assist patients to cope with their illnesses, and spiritual wellbeing, independent of other factors, contributes to overall quality of life [5].

2 The Diversity of Christianity

It is estimated that Christianity has around 2.6 billion followers or just under one third of the world's population, which makes it the world's largest religion. Approximately one-half are Roman Catholic, just over a third are Protestant (although there are many denominations within that grouping), and 12% are Eastern Orthodox with the remainder in an 'other' category which includes Christian Scientists and the Church of Jesus Christ of Latter-Day Saints [6]. We will explore how the different beliefs may impact on the practice of palliative care for Christians.

Christians believe in one God, the Creator, and in Jesus Christ, the incarnation of God who was born as a man some 2000 years ago. Jesus taught about the nature of God, His grace, and love for His creation and about human mortality. He performed many miracles of healing to teach us how we should respond to God's grace. Christians believe that Jesus was the Messiah, the anointed one prophesied in the Jewish Bible, who came to be saviour of the Jews (the Greek for Messiah being *Khristos* or Christ). Christianity is a religion practised as a worshipping community of the faithful who support each other, and individual Christians practice private prayer as well.

As recorded in the Christian Bible, Jesus attracted a large following to His ministry of preaching and healing, which was threatening to the Jewish leadership and the Roman rulers, and He was crucified [7]. He was entombed, but on the third day rose from the dead. After appearing to several of his followers, He subsequently ascended to be with God. Christians believe that in dying for the sins of humanity, He saved humanity, defeating death and showing the path by which humankind can also join with the eternal God after death. Jesus Christ, then, is the source of human hope. Most Christians believe in a Trinity where the third expression of God is the Holy Spirit as an ongoing personal connection to God.

One approach to understanding Christian belief and practice was formulated by John Wesley as a method for theological reflection, but it also helps with understanding the diversity of Christian views. In what became known as the Wesleyan Quadrilateral, there are four inputs into interpretation of Christian beliefs and practice [8]:

1. The primary source is the Bible.
2. When there is difficulty with interpretation, there is an appeal to the tradition of a denomination based on creeds and traditional interpretation.
3. This must be assisted by reason, which means that we are empowered to use our intellect to arbitrate between contrary views.
4. Finally, we bring our own experience of God and the Spirit.

Christians don't need to prove the existence of God, they experience God [9].

So, interpretation between different Christian denominations may be partly explained by putting a different emphasis on those four components. For example, Pentecostals put more emphasis on the experiential whereas Roman Catholics appeal more to the traditions of their Church. Different denominations will also differ on who they see has the authority to offer Christian spiritual care at the EOL. In general, it is Christian practitioners. However, Catholics will traditionally look specifically to priests to administer last rites. For many Protestant denominations who put primary emphasis on the Bible, it requires a minister or elder of the church who has studied scripture. Those emphasising the experiential will want a person with the greatest experience, whereas someone driven only by reason may simply require a reasonable person.

3 Christian Views of Death

Nearly all Christian denominations believe that after the death of our earthly bodies there is an afterlife [7]. This is grounded in the belief of the bodily and spiritual resurrection of Jesus and is often viewed as existence with the eternal God. Jesus Christ showed the way that this could be achieved. God is seen as sovereign over life and death, with life being a gift from God to God's people. Mortal life is therefore sacred, but we are created to also be able to achieve eternal life with God. It is the source of Christian hope, when faced with death, that our salvation lies in having faith in God, repenting, and achieving a new life beyond death as an experience of God's grace. Death has lost its sting [10].

Even with faith in an afterlife, the concept of death and dying still holds a sense of dread. It can involve finally abandoning a hope for physical healing. It is the end of a life that is known, a loss of identity, and transition to an existence that is not known, but is a matter of faith. It is separation, at least temporarily, from valued personal relationships. It often comes with a sense of regret for things left undone. In our experience, the regret of missed opportunities can be a great source of sadness and distress towards the end of life. There can be distress over who will care for others for whom the dying person has had responsibility. There may be a need to ponder what legacy a person's life will leave. Certainly, it is a process involving a spiritual journey from fear to acceptance which can result in achieving peace in God's presence.

The range of beliefs has implications for how Christians approach end-of-life care and emphases can evolve over time. For example, Julia Neuberger reports Rt Rev Richard Harries' views that with Anglicans the emphasis has changed over the centuries from focussing on judgement after death to living well in this world and dying well in terms of giving back to God because of loving God and reflecting that love to other people in your life [7]. However, if a Christian sees their disease and death as a punishment from God, they may feel intense anger towards God. In that situation, pastoral counselling as part of end-of-life care needs to help patients work through those feelings [11].

Christian beliefs about eternal life depend on their understanding of God's grace. God's grace is the unmerited or undeserved favour of God. It is a gift from God that cannot be earned but is given because of God's love for us. Many believe that the response to grace requires repentance and seeking God's forgiveness as part of the pathway to continued existence with the eternal God. This has consequences for a Christian's attitudes to death and on a number of aspects of end-of-life care [12]. Some Christians may not want a sudden death in their sleep, which many other people regard as an ideal way of dying, because they prefer knowing that death is pending, thereby providing a chance to prepare for it and seek forgiveness. The concept of death with dignity is replaced by death with repentance. Some may refuse sedation in the terminal phase of life because they see it as removing a last opportunity for repentance. Others may seek aggressive treatment to postpone death for a similar reason. Those Christians who have submitted to God's will in the way they have lived their lives may not experience the same need to know that death looms, or to try to postpone death. They would consider that they were born into a new relationship with God at baptism and this is reinforced during Holy Communion (*Eucharist*). They lovingly and humbly submit to God, as Christ did on the cross. They have achieved peace.

If, as some Christians believe, repentance to God can occur after death, then the urgency of repentance before death is mitigated. This view is often couched in terms of people of other faiths who have not had the opportunity to know Jesus before death and yet in the presence of a loving God can still achieve eternal life.

There is nothing in Christian belief that says that earthly life must be pursued at any cost. Burdensome treatments which will not alter impending death need not be maintained or introduced. St Basil the Great in the fourth century saw medicine as a gift from God, but it should not be an end in itself to be pursued at all costs when salvation should be to what the Christian is committed [13]. This may be seen as part of a humble submission to God.

This belief may be a point of difference with relatives who hold secular views that the end of mortal life is the end of all life and may wish to pursue treatments at any cost. This is where advance care directives may be very helpful in demonstrating to family members that the palliative care team is following the patient's wishes.

Decisions about medical treatments that have to weigh the likely benefit with the likely toxicity of a treatment are commonplace throughout medicine, not just at the end of life. Even if a treatment may have an undesirable side effect or even hasten death when the intent is a positive outcome such as controlling pain or distress, the treatment may still be permitted under the Roman Catholic doctrine of double effect where the intention is to achieve only a positive treatment outcome and the risk of the unintended outcome is justified [14].

The concept of advance care planning itself may reveal a divergence in Christian views [15]. Concerns have been expressed that advance care planning and a discussion of dying may itself herald death or undermine prayers for healing and represent 'giving up' [16]. It may be seen as not seeking God's will and be subject to the judgement of God. However, as Grace Johnston argues, there are examples of Jesus' advance care planning such as showing how He wanted to be remembered at the Last Supper, asking the disciples to pray with Him in the Garden of Gethsemane and arranging for John to care for His mother [17]. Advance care planning certainly does not preclude discerning God's will in the EOL phase but forms part of the process for Christians.

3.1 Rituals

One of the important aspects of end-of-life care that palliative care teams need to know when caring for Christians is the differences in rituals surrounding death between the different Christian groups. When a Roman Catholic patient is dying, a priest should be called in to administer a sacrament known as the *last rites* (Commendation of the Dying) which includes Holy Communion, anointing with oil and prayers to grant the patient absolution from past sins and God's forgiveness [4]. This is a path to repentance. Patients may wish to have a rosary, medallions of saints or the Virgin Mary and a crucifix at their bedside. Catholics often pray through Mary as a mediator.

Likewise, the families of Orthodox patients ask the local Orthodox priest to visit before death, hear a final confession and anoint with oil and give communion. Patients may derive comfort from having a valued family icon at their bedside [7].

Protestants do not have the formality of last rites. Chaplains, if called, may simply provide assurance of God's presence in the here and now, showing that we are never alone. They may simply sit with the patient or offer the comfort of the familiar and the hope and encouragement of the promises of God, often echoed in prayers such as the Lord's Prayer or Holy Communion, or having hymns played or reciting psalms (like the 23rd Psalm) if requested. Holding a cross may provide an assurance of God's presence. Increasingly in healthcare, chaplains are ecumenical in this role rather than denomination specific [7]. With smaller denominations it is best to ask the family what will be required if it has not been specified during advance care planning.

In general, with Christian patients, there are no restrictions on how nursing staff should handle the body to lay it out after death. There may be specific requests like Catholics wanting a Rosary in the hands of the deceased [7]. Some may want to have the funeral as soon as practical; others may want the deceased to be available for viewing in the coffin for some days before the funeral occurs. The funerals may range from Roman Catholic funerals with a full Requiem Mass to more a more informal Protestant service with Bible readings, prayers, and eulogies. Often after the funeral there will be a gathering of friends and relatives over food and drink to share memories of the departed. Christian families are often comforted by their belief that their loved one has moved beyond the grave to an eternal life with God.

There are certainly divergent views of Christians on whether the body is buried or cremated. Some Christians have a more literal interpretation of resurrection of the body in a physical sense rather than a spiritual sense and want the body to be buried as is. This may also influence decisions on organ donation. Michael Waterhouse interprets this as an identity issue of not being able to imagine ourselves without our bodies [18]. It is much like the concept of heaven and hell pictured as places characterised by images like beautiful gardens or fiery furnaces rather than heaven meaning existence in the presence of God and hell being separated from God.

4 Palliative Care

Palliative care is a subset of supportive care for a patient and also describes a professional discipline [19]. The World Health Organisation definition is: Palliative care is an approach that improves the quality of life of patients and their families facing the problem associated with life-threatening illness, through the prevention and relief of suffering by means of early identification and impeccable assessment and treatment of pain and other problems, physical, psychosocial, and spiritual [20]. An holistic approach is taken because the complexity of the human persons makes them irreducible to single components such as only physical or only psychological. For example, even if physical pain is well controlled, the patient may still be suffering existential distress.

A palliative care team can include clinicians from many disciplines: nurses, allied health practitioners including psychologists, social workers, physiotherapists, and chaplains and pastoral counsellors [21]. The person who is sick and dying continues to be valued, which aligns with the Christian view that they continue to embody God's image.

Palliative care was initially regarded as occurring after active treatment for a disease had been completed and was most identified with EOL care [22]. However, with their expertise in symptom control, palliative care specialists, when consulted earlier in the course of an illness, have been shown to improve quality of life in several randomised trials in patients with cancer [23].

5 Spirituality

We are all spiritual beings who ponder questions of the purpose of our lives. Spirituality is a nebulous concept with no one clearly accepted definition. The elements were captured by Rentzky when he described, 'the need to find meaning, purpose, and fulfilment in life, suffering or death. The need for hope and the will to live. The need for belief and faith in self, others and a power beyond self or God as defined by the individual'. [24] It is often confused with religiosity but that is really a subset of spirituality where answers to spiritual questions are sought using organised religious frameworks.

Spiritual wellbeing is a subjective experience where a sense of peace has been achieved, often by finding meaning in challenging times, like nearing the end of life [25]. Alternatively, spiritual distress can compromise quality of life, even if other symptoms have been adequately managed [25]. Christians may be spiritually distressed if they feel separated from God, or believe that they are not forgiven by God, or have failed to reconcile past disputes with family or friends [26]. Alternatively, they may gain a sense of peace with a heightened sense of God's presence through familiar spiritual practices.

Tools have been devised for both research and clinical care to assess spirituality, spiritual needs, and spiritual distress. To give an example, the Functional Assessment of Chronic Illness Therapy–Spiritual Well-being (FACIT-Sp) tool uses broad questions to assess the domains of meaning, peace, and religiosity [27]. It has been employed to assess the impact of spiritual interventions [28].

6 Spiritual Dimensions of Palliative Care and Christianity

Palliative care at the end of life accepts dying as a normal process [21]. It seeks to reduce physical suffering and attend to psychosocial needs to maximise quality of life. It embraces ordinary treatments and hydration and often nutrition but does not seek to continue futile or extraordinary treatments. The ethos of palliative care is that if a patient can't be physically healed, they can still be shown love, and the endpoint of healing focuses on the relief of suffering rather than cure. The dignity of the person continues to be respected despite their physical state and their closeness to death. Their vulnerability is embraced with compassion. Presence is the willingness of the carer to come to know the person who is suffering to the point of becoming vulnerable to that person's suffering. It is a dynamic healing relationship between the two which includes listening, non-verbal communication at the bedside and respecting that the patient makes the decisions about their path ahead [29].

The spiritual dimension of palliative care may need to address fear, grief, guilt, feelings of being isolated, emotional issues, concern for the spiritual and general wellbeing of those left behind and helping a patient discover meaning in their situation so that they may achieve peace, as well as providing support for facing physical symptoms [21]. The palliative care focus on spirituality embraces hope and also includes trying to bring peace to the patient's relatives through spiritual care [30].

The palliative care aim to promote human flourishing at the end of life is counter to the trend to reduce modern medicine to its technical capabilities. Despite what we presented about the utility of scales of measurement of spiritual wellbeing, it is far from adequate to attempt to purely medicalise spiritual wellbeing. It is, however, important to document spiritual care interventions as part of the management plan of a patient. It is interesting that when a group of patients with cancer were asked about the role of the doctor in the provision of spiritual supportive care, they wanted doctors to ask about the source of their spiritual support and facilitate access to it, but did not necessarily expect the doctor to provide that support [31]. In a further study of palliative care clinicians, it was found that they were more likely to recognise the importance of spiritual care and report more positive self-reported ability to provide it than other clinicians engaged in supportive care in general. This was attributed to the greater likelihood of the palliative care workers being trained in spiritual care [32].

The Christian ethos of care very much embraces that of palliative care. Caring for others and healing reflects the examples of Jesus in demonstrating God's love for us [33]. However, for Christians, human flourishing at the end of life is to know, love and serve God and others and this is what Christians would see as their responsibility in helping others to achieve [29]. The Christian patients will need more than just someone providing human comfort. As chaplains respond to more secular work environments and health units are considering more generic non-denominational spiritual counsellors, it should be recognised that chaplains ministering to Christian patients will, through prayer and insight into God's word as recorded in the Bible, want to walk beside the patient in their spiritual journey at the EOL reassuring them on issues such as repentance, salvation and eternal life and the hope that this brings. Patients will expect theologically based spiritual care in addition to the secular comfort offered by other members of the palliative care team [21]. Christians believe that this spiritual care would benefit all. Chaplains report that they gain strength from their faith in God for their work, and their work engaging with the spiritual journey of their patients influences their own spirituality [34].

7 What Is a Good Death?

In a systematic review of systematic reviews on what constitutes a 'good death', 13 of 275 papers initially identified by Zaman et al. were analysed and reflected the views of patients, family members and health practitioners [35]. They identified 11 common themes. At the top of the list was the relief of pain and other physical symptoms. However, only two more of the themes that followed required medical interventions. The other themes were effective communication and relationship with healthcare providers, performance of cultural, religious or spiritual rituals, relief from emotional distress or psychological stress, patient autonomy in deciding treatments, dying at the preferred place, not prolonging life unnecessarily, awareness of the deep significance of dying, emotional support from family and friends, not being a burden on anyone, and the right to terminate one's life.

Some of these responses require further investigation. We would probably add that being assured of the ongoing wellbeing of surviving family members will relieve that anxiety. Also, patients often state that they want to die at home rather than a hospital but if the human resources are not available at home they may well prefer dying in hospital where loved ones can stay with them throughout the day rather than trying to be of comfort to them as well as taking on the role that three shifts of nurses would do in a hospital. In terms of the relative importance of the conditions for a good death, we learned during COVID-19 how devastating it was to be separated from loved ones who in turn were unable to offer final farewells [35].

We know that palliative care can improve the quality of life of dying patients by clarifying the aims of palliation, reducing unnecessary medical interventions or investigations, and caring for the psychosocial and spiritual needs of the patients and relatives. With the relatives this should extend beyond the death of the patients to embrace bereavement counselling [34].

As we have discussed, these elements of a good death that palliative care seeks to deliver, are totally compatible with Christian ideals. Christians take the example of Jesus' healing ministry which emphasised helping the neediest of our neighbours. Through healing He was able to reveal the loving nature of God to humanity and God's compassion for our physical lives [33]. The healing ministry of Jesus restored people to their communities but for Christians restoring the relationship with God is paramount.

We have already discussed the Christian's need for repentance and seeking God's forgiveness through life and at the end of life. Priests, chaplains or Christian pastoral counsellors may help reveal God's word and join with patients in prayer to help discern God's will and enable a good Christian death. This may not involve a cure, but it does constitute a healing. It counters the fear of death, addresses the meaning of the final phase of someone's life and creates the conditions to achieve peace.

Moreover, it allows the Christians to embrace the hope that comes from faith in God and an afterlife in the presence of the eternal God, which was demonstrated to them through Jesus Christ.

8 Challenges for Christians at the End of Life

The spiritual care of Christians at the end of life is set against the background of changing societal values. The most challenging recently is legislation across many countries to legalise voluntary euthanasia or voluntary assisted dying (VAD) which allows the lawful administration of a lethal medication by a physician to end a life in order to end suffering [36]. Roman Catholics will not accept VAD based on an understanding of God's sovereignty over life and death and believing that in approaching the end of life the focus should not be on self and controlling the end of one's life but in humility and with repentance, seeking to focus on loving God and loving others [12]. As we have discussed, withdrawing burdensome treatments that will not change an impending death is not euthanasia but is a recognition of a time to die. Many Protestants also share the position against VAD, but some believe that VAD as a means of relieving suffering can be justified if the patient requests it. The physician managing end-of-life care needs to ascertain the patients' beliefs but also must act as an independent moral agent in terms of his or her own beliefs. There is an ongoing debate about whether a physician opposing VAD must refer to a colleague who is prepared to offer this option.

9 Conclusion

The practice of palliative care with its focus on the dignity of the person who is dying and the practice of holistic care closely align with Christian values. The attention to spiritual well-being is vital, but for the Christian, this goes well beyond secular support. Christians seek to understand God's will for them, submit to loving God and repent, seeking forgiveness for wrongdoing in this life. Following the example of Jesus Christ of how to live life to the full and achieve peace in dying, they understand that after death they can achieve ongoing life with the eternal God. This is the great source of hope for Christians facing death and aids them in achieving the peace which is part of a good death.

References

1. Schouten J. The rod and serpent of Asclepius. Symbol of medicine. Amsterdam: Elsevier; 1967.
2. Koenig HG. Religion, spirituality, and medicine: how are they related and what does it mean? Mayo Clin Proc. 2001;76:1189–91. https://doi.org/10.4065/76.12.1189.
3. Stephenson J. Being a Christian in palliative care. 2004. https://www.cmf.org.uk/resources/publications/content/?context=article&id=726. Accessed 18 July 2023.
4. Wikipedia Last Rites. https://en.wikipedia.org/wiki/Last_rites#. Accessed 4 Aug 2023.
5. Whitford HS, Olver I. The multidimensionality of spiritual wellbeing: peace, meaning, and faith and their association with quality of life and coping in oncology. Psycho-Oncology. 2012;21:602–10. https://doi.org/10.1002/pon.1937.

6. Wikipedia. Christianity by country. 2023. https://en.wikipedia.org/wiki/Christianity_by_country. Accessed 18 July 2023.
7. Neuberger J. Caring for dying people of different faiths. Oxon: Radcliffe Medical Press; 2004.
8. Bounds C. The Wesleyan Quadrilateral. 2022. https://weslyan.org/the-wesleyan-quadrilateral. Accessed 19 July 2023.
9. Joseph T. Care at the end of life: what orthodox Christianity has to teach. 2020. http://ww1.antiochian.org/node/21291. Accessed 19 July 2023.
10. Reynolds AG. Life and death. A study of Christian hope. London: Lutterworth Press; 1960.
11. Exline J, Park CL, Smyth JM, Carey MP. Anger toward God: social-cognitive predictors, prevalence, and links with adjustment to bereavement and cancer. J Pers Soc Psychol. 2011;100:129–48.
12. Engelhardt HT Jr, Iltis AS. End-of-life; the traditional Christian view. Lancet. 2005;366(9490):1045–9.
13. St Basil. The long rules. Sister Monica Wagner, trans. Washington, DC: Catholic University of America Press 1962: 330–331.
14. Boyle JM Jr. Toward understanding the principle of double effect. Ethics. 1980;90:527–38.
15. Mack JW, Weeks JC, Wright AA, Block SD. Prigerson HG> End-of-life discussions, Goa attainment and distress at the end of life: predictors and outcomes of receipt of care consistent with preferences. J Clin Oncol. 2010;28:1203–8.
16. Coyne HL. End-of-life care considerations for the Pentecostal patient #449. J Palliat Med. 2022;25:1877–8.
17. Johnston G. Jesus practiced advance care planning: biblical basis and possible applications. Palliat Med Rep. 2020;1:242–5.
18. Waterhouse M. Staying close: a positive approach to dying and bereavement. London: Constable; 2003.
19. Hui D, Mori M, Parsons HA, et al. The lack of standard definitions in the supportive and palliative care literature. J Pain Symptom Manag. 2012;43:582–92.
20. World Health Organisation. WHO definition of palliative care. https://www.who.int/cancer/palliative/definition/en/. Accessed 28 July 2023.
21. Jayard SS, Irudayadason NA, Davis JC. Healing ministry and palliative care in Christianity. Indian J Med Ethics. 2017;2:238–43.
22. Olver I, Keefe D, Herrstedt J, Warr D, Roila F, Ripamonti CI. Supportive care in cancer- a MASCC perspective. Support Care Cancer. 2020;28:3467–75.
23. Haun MW, Estel S, Rücker G, et al. Early palliative care for adults with advanced cancer (review). Cochrane Database Syst Rev. 2017;6(6):CD011129. https://doi.org/10.1002/14651858.CD011129.pub2.
24. Renetzky L. The fourth dimension: applications of the social sciences. In: Moberd D, editor. Spiritual wellbeing: sociological perspectives. Wasington: University Press of America; 1979. p. 215–54.
25. Holloway M, Adamson S, McSherry W, Swinton J. Spiritual care at the end of life: a systematic review of the literature. 2011. https://www.gov.uk/government/publications/spiritual-care-at-the-end-of-life-a-systematic-review-of-the-literature. Accessed 29 July 2023.
26. Hinshaw DB. The spiritual needs of the dying patient. J Am Coll Surg. 2002;4:565–8.
27. Peterman AH, Fitchett G, Brady MJ, Hernandez L, Cella D. Measuring spiritual well-being in people with cancer: the functional assessment of chronic illness therapy-spiritual well=being scale (FACIT-Sp). Ann Behav Med. 2002;24:49–58.
28. Olver IN, Dutney A. A randomized, blinded study of the impact of intercessory prayer on spiritual Well-being in patients with cancer. Altern Ther Health Med. 2012;18:18–27.
29. Perkins I. Human flourishing in Christ; a journey of hope in the Christian Community. Linacre Q. 2001;88:175–83.
30. Batstone E, Bailey C, Hallett N. Spiritual care provision to end-of-life patients; a systematic literature review. J Clin Nurs. 2020;29:3609–24.

31. Best M, Butow P, Olver I. Spiritual support of cancer patients and the role of the doctor. Support Care Cancer. 2014;22:1333–9.
32. Best M, Butow P, Olver I. Palliative care specialist's beliefs about spiritual care. Support Care Cancer. 2016;24:3295–306.
33. O'Brien D. Palliative care: the biblical roots. Health Prog. 2014;95:42–9.
34. Chang B-h, Stein NR, Trevino K, Stewart M, Hendricks A, Skarf LM. End-of-life spiritual care. Palliat Support Car. 2012;10:273–8.
35. Zaman M, Espinal-Arango S, Mohapatra A, Jadad AR. What would it take to die well? A systematic review of systematic reviews on the conditions for a good death. Lancet Healthy Longev. 2021;2:e593–600.
36. Treleaven L, Komesaroff P, LaBrooy C, Olver I, Kerridge I, Philip J. A review of the utility of prognostic tools in predicting 6-month mortality in cancer patients, conducted in the context of voluntary assisted dying. Intern Med J. 2023. https://doi.org/10.1111/imj.16081. Online ahead of print.

A Hindu Perspective of Spiritual Care in Palliative Care

Avinash Kumar Tiwari and Santosh Kumar Chaturvedi

Abstract Hinduism has been considered as a synthesis of various Indian cultures and traditions with diverse origin and no single founder. Hinduism, also known as *Sanatan Dharma,* is a religious and universal order or way of life by which followers abide. Spiritual care is an important part of palliative care and end-of-life care among Hindus. Palliative care settings do give some informal attention to this aspect; however, formal spiritual care is missing. Spirituality and religion are strongly associated in Hinduism in different tenets. Hindus with chronic illnesses utilise the concept of *karma* to reconcile to this distress. There are different theologies, practices, and sacred texts in Hinduism. Practice and beliefs near and after death differ region to region. The cultural and religious dynamics in India have been changed drastically over time after reform movements and colonisation of Asia by the western world. There are many formal and informal ways of assessing spiritual distress among Hindus. The Spiritual Distress Scale for Palliative Care in India tool (SpiDiScI-PC) is a new development for assessing spiritual assessment in Indian population.

Keywords Spiritual Care · Palliative Care · Hinduism · India · Karma · *Sanatan Dharma* · *Samsara* · *Bhagavad Gita*

A. K. Tiwari (✉)
Department of Pain, Palliative Medicine and Supportive Oncology,
Sanjeevani CBCC USA Cancer Hospital, Raipur, Chhattisgarh, India

S. K. Chaturvedi
Jagadguru Kripalu Chikithsalaya, Vrindavan, Uttar Pradesh, India

M. C. Best (ed.), *Spiritual Care in Palliative Care*,
https://doi.org/10.1007/978-3-031-50864-6_10

1 Introduction

Hinduism is often called the 'oldest religion' in the world [1] and has been considered as a synthesis of various Indian cultures and traditions with diverse origin and no single founder [2]. Hinduism, also known as *Sanatan Dharma,* is a religious and universal order or way of life by which followers abide. *Sanatan* means eternal. The meaning of *Dharma* is more profound but is often translated as 'duty', 'religion' or 'religious duty'. The word itself comes from the Sanskrit root '*dhri*', which means 'to sustain'. Another related meaning is 'that which is integral to something'. For example, the dharma of sugar is to be sweet, and the dharma of fire is to be hot. Therefore, a person's *dharma* consists of duties that sustain them, according to their innate characteristics. Such characteristics are both material and spiritual [3]. As a religion, Hinduism is the world's third largest, with over 1.2–1.35 billion followers, or 15–16% of the global population, known as Hindus [4]. Spirituality and religion are strongly associated in Hinduism in different tenets. Hinduism has various cultural and religious practices influencing followers' spiritual needs and practice. Assessment of spirituality and managing spiritual issues can be challenging in a country like India with diverse cultural, religious and social practices. Spirituality is a core component of Hinduism, and attention to detail is important in the spiritual care of Hindus. In this chapter, we will discuss spirituality for Hindus both in India and in other countries.

2 Spirituality in Hindus

Traditionally, Hinduism identifies three *marga* (ways) of spiritual practice, namely *Jnana*, the way of knowledge; *Bhakti*, the way of devotion; and *Karma* yoga, the way of selfless action. It defines spiritual practice as one's journey towards *moksha*—awareness of self, the discovery of higher truths, the true nature of reality, and a consciousness that is liberated and content [5].

For most Hindus, spirituality cannot be separated from religiosity. Religious beliefs and practices form their spirituality. Those persons who are considered religious are also considered spiritual. Often, spirituality and religiosity are used interchangeably among Hindus. There is also an impact of religiosity and culture on spirituality, i.e. how people understand spirituality. There is a challenge of space and privacy in Indian settings, and hence, it is a tricky conversation to start and a hugely challenging area of care in healthcare. Spirituality in Hinduism is not a concrete concept, and hence, there is no standard practice across the country, and each practitioner develops their own unique style of addressing the patient's spiritual distress over time. The spirituality of the care providers cannot be fully distanced from the spiritual care they provide.

3 Driving Principles (Core) of Spirituality in Hinduism

Hinduism has no traditional ecclesiastical order, no centralised religious authorities, no governing body, no prophet(s), nor any binding holy book. Hindus can choose to be polytheistic, henotheistic, pantheistic, monotheistic or atheistic [6]. Spiritual distress is almost universally defined by the question, Why did this happen to me? What will happen to me after I die? Why would God allow me to suffer this way? Will I be remembered? Will I be missed? Hindus with chronic illnesses utilise the concept of *karma* to reconcile to this distress. Teachings in Hinduism reiterate that for any individual, *karma* can influence the future by their present actions [2].

3.1 Karma

This is a vital concept in *Sanatan Dharma* and means an action *(Kriya)* of a *Karta* (person performing the action) and its associated result (cause and effect) [7]. Understanding *karma* and its source are vital to interpreting this concept and are very important in addressing spiritual distress in Hinduism.

3.2 Concepts of Paap, Punya, Prayaschitha

Paap, though widely interpreted as sin, these concepts are explained in *Sanatan Dharma* literature as an experience of the *Jiva* (living creature) as a result of *dush:karma* (bad deeds), and *punya* as an experience of *sat:karma* (*good or saintly deed*). These concepts are inherent in Hinduism and Buddhism. In the form of *paap,* the *Jiva* experiences *dush:karma* through some sort of unavailability or suffering, and *punya* through some sort of availability or happiness. *Punya* and *paap* both get exhausted over time. As and when suffering and happiness get exhausted, the *Jiva* tends to accumulate both based on its current actions, which is nothing but *karma,* making it a never-ending cyclic loop called *saṃsara* [8]. There is also a belief that the effects of bad deeds can be removed or minimised by *prayaschitha* (atonement). Hence, people perform various religious activities to undo their past karma.

4 Purpose of Existence

The purpose of life for Hindus is to achieve four aims, called *Purusharthas (*object of human pursuit). These are: *Dharma* (righteousness, moral values); *Artha* (prosperity, economic values); *Kama* (pleasure, love, psychological values) and *Moksha* (liberation, spiritual values) [9]. These provide Hindus with opportunities to act morally and ethically and lead a good life. Throughout their lives, Hindus attempt to end the cycle of *samsara* (aimless wandering) and behave in a way that provides good *karma* in this life and the next.

5 Meaning of Death (Mṛtyu) in Hinduism

Hinduism subscribes to a belief in *samsara* (the cycle of life, death, and reincarnation), until liberation *(moksha)* is achieved. Death is a hugely significant life event signalling either the attainment of liberation or the continuation on the pilgrimage of life. According to the *Vedas* (the earliest body of holy scripture among Hindus), all beings are souls (*aatma*) and thus are spiritual in nature. Though the body is temporary and eventually dies, the soul is eternal. After death, the soul is reincarnated, taking birth in another physical body or form. Passing from one life to the next, each soul is on a journey of spiritual development facilitated in part by *karma*, the concept that every thought and action has a corresponding reaction. This belief in the reincarnation (*punarjanma*) of the soul is probably helpful in coping with death or loss of a loved one—as the person has taken birth elsewhere. In clinical practice, one does not encounter severe abnormal or morbid grief reactions as in other parts of the world, because it is accepted that one experiences the results of both good and bad deeds over a series of lives.

5.1 The Soul (Aatma)

Aatma is uplifted through every good action performed and degraded with every bad action. Stuck in this cycle of birth and death (*samsara*) the soul experiences the results of its *karma*, through which it becomes more aware of how its actions affect the world and others around it. This growth of awareness enables one to become a more selfless and loving being, until enough progress has been made to attain *moksha*, or liberation from *samsara*, resulting in complete spiritual existence.

6 Death Rituals for Hindus

Shamshan refers to the cremation ground of Hindus, usually located near a river. Those who can afford it may go to special sacred places like Kashi (Varanasi), Haridwar, Prayagraj (formerly Allahabad), Srirangam, Gaya or Puri [10].

6.1 The Cremation (Antyesti)

Known also as 'the last rites', *Antyesti* are usually completed within a day of death and vary from place to place and between believers. Generally, the body is washed; sandalwood paste and turmeric are applied to the body, and it is wrapped in a *dhoti* (a cotton white cloth) for a man and a *saree* for woman. The big toes are tied together with a string and a *Tilak* (red, yellow or white mark) is placed on the forehead. A bed is made out of bamboo sticks on which the deceased is taken to the *Shamshan* [11]. As well as the cremation method, several sects in Hinduism follow the practice of burial of the dead. For example, followers of the *Ayyavazhi* sect bury the body. The only Hindus not typically cremated are babies, children, and saints, who are believed to be pure and unattached to their bodies; therefore, they may be buried instead of cremated.

6.2 Post-antyesti Rituals (Niravapanjali)

It is a sacred ritual in Hinduism where, after the cremation rites, the ashes are ceremonially immersed in holy water, usually in the River Ganges, by the closest relatives' (usually) elder son, so that the soul may rise to heaven.

6.3 The Chautha (4th Day) and Terahvin (13th Day of Death)

The *Chautha* ceremony usually takes place on the fourth day after the last rites. Families of the deceased perform this ritual in a place of worship, and those gathered offer flowers and tributes to a picture of the deceased. *Terahvin* is a ritual performed in Hinduism on the 13th day of death. This ritual is performed to place the departed soul with the ancestors and God. It is believed that before the ritual, the departed soul is a *preta (*evil spirit), and after performing this ritual, the soul will become *pitr* (good spirit) and will go to be with the ancestors [12].

Among the Hindus, there is a belief that the spirit is in the *Pret yoni* for 13 days, after which it is re-born and hence no longer dangerous (some *preta* (non-harmful evil) becomes *pishachi* (harmful evil) and is considered dangerous to the person's own family and possibly others). Fasting and offerings are made to expedite the passage through the *Pret yoni*. These culturally determined rituals and customs serve defensive functions to deal with allaying anxiety, guilt and grief and are considered as cultural defence mechanisms [13].

Purpose of the Chautha and Tehravin Ceremonies

The *Chautha* and *Tehravin* ceremonies allow members of the family to come together, to talk about the deceased, to re-live their life with the deceased and thus relinquish him. This is recommended in the treatment of grief and the death ritual permits this treatment at a group level to permit an optimal resolution of the bereavement [13]. These ceremonies are beneficial as they help the bereaved family to recognise the reality of death, they testify to the life of the deceased, they encourage expression of grief according to cultural values and they help family members cope with the grieving process.

6.4 Hospice Towns and Cities

Sannyasa is one of the four stages/*ashramas* of a Hindu's life. Over the course of one's life, in the last years, one may abandon the world entirely for a life of contemplation. A sacred place (*tirtha*) is meant for accomplishment of spiritual progress. According to *Garuda Purana* (holy scripture primarily centring around the Hindu god Vishnu), there are seven cities (Ayodhya, Mathura, Haridwar, Varanasi (Kashi), Kanchipuram (Kanchi), Ujjain (Avantika), and Dwarka) known as the givers of *moksha* (liberation from the cycle of birth and death) and have been considered as *SannyasaTirth*, which translates as a kind of hospice town.

7 Assessment of Spiritual Distress in Hinduism

Distress is a multifactorial, unpleasant, emotional experience of a psychological (cognitive, behavioural, and emotional), social, and/or spiritual nature. The Hindu conceptualisation of suffering is that suffering in any form does not occur at random but is the consequence of past inappropriate actions (thoughts, words, deeds) in the current life or past life. Suffering is not punishment, but rather a consequence of one's actions. Hindu philosophy views suffering as atonement for one's actions and urges individuals to accept full responsibility for the suffering without blaming others [14]. Assessment of spirituality in Hindus can be done in formal and informal ways.

7.1 Informal Assessments of Spirituality

Hindu priests (*Pundit, purohit*) assess one's suffering by their *Janmapatri/ Janmakundali:* they assess the patient's astrological document based on the date and time of birth in order to find out the cause of suffering and they then offer a solution based on their finding. Palmistry is another form of foretelling one's suffering and pain in Hinduism.

7.2 *Formal Assessment*

For clinical assessment of patient, the following can be pointers for assessment of Spirituality in Hindus.

History, Personal and Family History

- Attitudes of the self and family: How does a patient and their family think, feel, and behave? Assessing their state in response to the distressing situation.
- Beliefs held by self and family: Assessing faith, attitude, and opinion about ongoing suffering.
- Context: cultural, religious, and spiritual—exploring contextual factors which may affect spirituality.
- Decision-making process in family: Functionality and dynamics of family.

Environment—Family and Sociospiritual Activities of Daily Living

- Religious/spiritual activity during the day: Assessing routine religious and spiritual tasks for a day, e.g. prayers, chanting, and mantras, visiting temples or religious places, performing pujas, fasting, and rituals. Expressing gratitude is also a routine practice for Hindus.
- Assessing view on forgiving and being forgiven.
- Asking about any act of receiving blessings from elders, gurus, and teachers.
- Some Hindus use holy water from the River Ganges or any other sacred river. They usually drink or sprinkle it on themself.

Observations/Examination of Behaviours

- Signs and signals giving idea of spiritual distress like being angry with God.
- Symbol denoting any religious meaning may give an idea about whether the person has been religious or has specific faith.
- Rings, necklaces, bands, and sacred threads. Sometimes, objects like charms and amulets are carried.
- Signs on forehead—e.g. Chandan (sandalwood paste), bindi (a decorative mark worn on forehead).
- Touching feet is also a common practice among Hindus.
- Leaving slippers outside the room.
- Offering *prasadam*: food offered to a devotee after worship.

Spiritual Distress

How great is the spiritual distress and what is the possible cause of spiritual distress? There is no specific universally valid tool to assess severity or quantification of spiritual distress, but one can explore its impact on the patient and family, on decision making, adherence to treatment, etc. The cause of ongoing spiritual distress can be (for example) diagnosis, prognosis, symptoms, treatment or disability related, and needs to be explored.

Recent Updates in Spiritual Care in Indian Perspectives with the SpiDiScI-PC (Spiritual Distress Scale for Palliative Care in India)

Palliative Care professionals in India have recently developed a tool taking regional cultural and religious concerns into account to assess spiritual distress. The Department of Onco-Anaesthesia and Palliative Medicine at IRCH-AIIMS (Institute Rotary Cancer Hospital–All India Institute of Medical Science), New Delhi, together with collaborators from India and abroad have developed a Hindi-language scale that has been specifically designed to assess spiritual distress in palliative care patients in India. The original Hindi version of SpiDiScI along with an English translation is available. SpiDiScI may be used, free of charge, for non-commercial research purposes. The spiritual distress score is calculated by coding the answers as 1 for *sahmat/agree* and 0 for *asahmat/disagree*. Neutral responses are not coded and are not considered while calculating the distress score, so the outcome will be a score between 0 and 100. There was an immense need for such culturally accepted tools in Indian settings [15].

Unfortunately, the amount and quality of the available data on spirituality among Indian Palliative Care patients are limited. 'How to recognise spiritual distress at the end of life?' is a question frequently voiced in palliative care meetings. We need other approaches, such as theology and philosophy, that explore the domains of religion and belief systems, and sociology and psychology, with their resources to make sense of life experiences, to help us see the whole picture [16].

8 Aspects of Spiritual Practice Around Death in Palliative Care in Hinduism

There are some practices around death in Hinduism which vary from family to family and where family is available, their preferences should be acknowledged. However, when the family knows that the patient is approaching death, they often start the customary preparations for the end-of-life rituals and may not be at the bedside. In the event that the patient's family are not immediately available, healthcare staff should only conduct essential tasks such as closing the eyes of the deceased, removing any tubes and cleaning any excretions.

There are different theologies, practices, and sacred texts within Hinduism. Professionals working in palliative care settings employ many different methods to improve quality of life for patients including suggesting prayer, devotion, yoga, meditation, or philosophical pursuits. Apart from these, patients may seek to perform fire rituals (*homa/havan*), fasting (*vrata*), chanting (*japa*), sacrifice (*yajña*), charity (*dāna*), selfless service (*sevā*), learning and knowledge (*jñāna*), recitation and exposition of scriptures (*pravacana*), and homage to one's ancestors (*śrāddha*). A concept unique to India is when the patient seeks refuge in holy or religious places, akin to hospice towns or cities, to obtain mental and spiritual solace while awaiting death [17].

8.1 Activities Prior to Death (When Death Is Imminent)

Family members or patients may wish to contact a priest in order to receive proper guidance and so they can be available for a ceremony if desired. In India, if a patient is in the hospital, family work with medical staff to see that the desired activities are performed.

Prokshana

Usually, both family members and patients ask for holy water (Ganga water, i.e. water from the Ganges River) to be placed in the mouth of the patient or put holy basil (*Ocimum tenuiflorum*) into the mouth, and chant divine names (such as Ram, Krishna, Shiva) while administering or sprinkling the holy water. If the Ganga water is not available, purified water can be used.

Chanting of Divine Names

The family typically chants the names of God, plays appropriate *Bhajans* (devotional songs with religious theme) usually into the right ear. Usually, this is done by close family members; however, anyone attending can join in the chanting. They usually chant at 108 times or more: '*Hare Rama Hare Rama Rama Rama Hare Hare Hare Krishna Hare Krishna Krishna Krishna Hare Hare*'.

Following this, a family may also wish to read the 7th, 12th, and 15th chapters or the entire *Bhagavad Gita* or any selected chapter(s) of *Ramayana* or other sacred scripture.

9 Spiritual Issues for Caregivers

Spiritual issues for the caregivers of the terminally ill person are equally, if not more, important, due to the length of time during which they may suffer. The spiritual concerns and distress in caregivers are likely to continue from the period of anticipatory grief to the grieving period, that is, from onset of distressing symptoms or from diagnosis of the life limiting condition in their loved one to grief after loss, i.e. the death of loved one.

The assessment and management of spiritual distress in caregivers could be similar to that of patients [18]. After noticing any verbal or nonverbal cues suggesting distress among carers, they may be helped by offering spiritual support within their own faith, empathetic conversation, active listening, joining their prayers, sharing thoughts, and connecting them to a spiritual support group or spiritual care provider.

The spiritual issues related to professional caregivers and healthcare providers are another important area, which can either facilitate the spiritual care or cause spiritual conflict. Healthcare professionals should avoid causing any spiritual conflict or distress such as expressing ignorance of one's belief, miscommunication, misunderstanding, competitiveness, perceived bias and above all by expressing a sense of superiority.

10 Cultural and Ethical Issues/Challenges in Providing Spiritual Care to Hindus

Among Hindus, certain customs and rituals for a dying person include putting the person on the ground (and not the bed), pouring holy water (of the Ganges or any other holy river) into the person's mouth, and chanting hymns. The risk of aspiration and interference with ventilator efforts are overlooked at such a time [19, 20].

It is known that patients at the end of life are vulnerable to suggestion, and counsellors must refrain from imposing their own beliefs on patients. Most hospices in India provide nursing care through Christian missionaries, who do a tremendous selfless service, but this may create a conflict with the predominant religious groups of Hindus [19]. For example, in our clinical experience, we have come across patients seeking religious conversions (for example to Christianity) during their last days of life, creating conflict within the family and community. On the other hand, religious groups have successfully participated in community palliative care programmes [21].

Are religious ethics equivalent to medical ethics, one may ask? India has many systems of alternative and unorthodox medicine that have some link with spirituality. Examples include applying curcumin, basil extract on wounds or use of magic (*jhad fuk*) services offered by unorthodox practitioners. Hospice professionals recommend that these are best tried outside the hospice unless they are in fully studied clinical trials [22].

10.1 Cultural and Religious Dynamics in India

Cultural and religious dynamics in India have changed drastically over time, especially after historical reform movements. These reforms have broken the traditional orthodox way of practising Hindu spirituality and have influenced various geographical areas in India differently, so that Hindu practice now has more heterogenicity. One practising in Southern compared to the Northern part of India, for example, may face a different set of Hindu beliefs.

A major influence began in the nineteenth century. Major representatives of 'Hindu modernism' are Ram Mohan Roy and Swami Vivekananda, who were involved in creating much diversity and heterogeneity in *Sanatan Dharma* as described in the following:

Sanatan Dharma: The term is used in Indian languages alongside the more common *Hindu Dharma* for Hinduism. See Sect. 8.1

Vaidika dharma: Traditional scholars employed the terms *Vaidika* and *Avaidika* for those who accept the Vedas as a source of authoritative knowledge and those who do not, to differentiate various Indian schools from Jainism, Buddhism, and Charvaka. According to Klaus Klostermaier, the term *Vaidika dharma* is the earliest self-designation of Hinduism [23].

***Neo-Vedanta* (Hindu modernism):** An important influence on western spirituality was Neo-Vedanta, also called *neo-Hinduism* and *Hindu Universalism*, a modern interpretation of Hinduism which developed in response to western colonialism. It aims to present Hinduism as a homogenised ideal of Hinduism with *Advaita Vedanta* as its central doctrine. Due to the colonisation of Asia by the western world, since the nineteenth century, an exchange of ideas has been taking place between the western world and Asia, which also influenced western religiosity. Unitarianism and the idea of Universalism were brought to India by missionaries and had a major influence on neo-Hinduism via Ram Mohan Roy's Brahmo Samaj and Brahmoism. Roy attempted to modernise and reform Hinduism from the idea of Universalism. This universalism was further popularised, and brought back to the west as neo-Vedanta, by Swami Vivekananda [24].

Since the various reforms have influenced cultural and religious practices as well as other important contextual aspects differently among Hindus, Hinduism as a religion is now heterogeneous. Practice in one Hindu community can be different from another community. Therefore, in providing spiritual care to Hindus, it will be important to perform a formal assessment and communicate with the patient and family regarding the care that best aligns with their own beliefs.

11 Conclusion

Spiritual care in palliative care among Hindus is enmeshed with numerous traditions, rituals, religious actions and symbolism. Most life, death, and religious functions are achieved symbolically. The symbolism makes spiritual care possible in palliative care. The vast spirituality in Hinduism is well defined in the numerous ancient scriptures. As well, there are numerous gurus, saints, swamis, and learned persons with thousands of followers, who are both spiritual and religious and guide the common man. Among Hindus, there is a big overlap between religiosity and spirituality—religious people are spiritual, and those with high spirituality are religious. Religious activities are a part and parcel of many devout Hindus. Health, illness, disease, death, and afterlife are a mix of spiritual and religious thoughts. At the end of life, people expect peace of mind and a satisfactory spiritual quality of life [25]. Hinduism, with such vast diversity and ways of seeking fulfilment of spiritual need, should be assessed in-depth for each patient, and a care plan should be tailored accordingly.

References

1. Fowler JD. Hinduism: beliefs and practices. Brighton/Portland: Sussex Academic Press; 1997. 162 p. (The Sussex Library of religious beliefs and practices).
2. Kitagawa JM, editor. The religious traditions of Asia: religion, history, and culture. London: RoutledgeCurzon; 2002. 375 p.
3. https://iskconeducationalservices.org/HoH/concepts/key-concepts/sanatana-dharma/
4. https://en.wikipedia.org/wiki/Hinduism_by_country
5. Sivaraman K, Sundararajan KR, Mukerji B, editors. Hindu spirituality. New York: Crossroad; 1989. 2 p. (World spirituality).
6. Lipner J. Hindus: their religious beliefs and practices. 2nd ed. Abingdon: Routledge; 2010. 426 p. (The library of religious beliefs and practices).
7. https://www.holy-bhagavad-gita.org/chapter/9/verse/21/hi
8. Śrīmad Bhagavād Gita, Chapter 9 of Rajavidya Rajaguhya Yoga, Sloka 21, wherein Gitacharya (Śrī Kṛiṣṇa) says: [Internet]. [cited 2023 Aug 7]. Available from: https://www.holy-bhagavad-gita.org/chapter/9/verse/21/hi
9. Pal. Leading a balanced life though pursuit of Purushartha. https://timesofindia.indiatimes.com/readersblog/leading-a-balanced-life-though-pursuit-of-purushartha/leading-a-balanced-life-though-pursuit-of-purushartha-12089/. 2020 Apr 16.
10. Justice C. Dying the good death: the pilgrimage to die in India's Holy City. Albany: State University of New York Press; 1997. p. 268.
11. Olson C. The many colors of Hinduism: a thematic-historical introduction. New Brunswick: Rutgers University Press; 2007. 395 p.
12. Ramey SW. Hindu, Sufi, or Sikh: contested practices and identifications of Sindhi Hindus in India and beyond. 1st ed. New York: Palgrave Macmillan; 2008. 222 p.
13. Varma KV. Cultural psychodynamics in health and illness. Indian J Psychiatry. 1986 Jan;28(1):13–34.
14. Kaufman W. Karma, rebirth, and the problem of evil. Philosophy East and West. 2005;55:15–32. https://doi.org/10.1353/pew.2004.0044.

15. Gielen J, Kashyap K, Singh SP, Bhatnagar S, Chaturvedi SK. Psychometric assessment of SpiDiscI: spiritual distress scale for palliative care patients in India. Indian J Palliat Care. 2022;28:13–20.
16. Inbadas H. The philosophical and cultural situatedness of spirituality at the end of life in India. Indian J Palliat Care. 2017;23(3):338.
17. Chaturvedi SK. Exploration of concerns and role of psychosocial intervention in palliative care – a study from India. Ann Acad Med Singap. 1994;23(2):256–60.
18. Chaturvedi S. Spiritual issues at end of life. Indian J Palliat Care. 2007;13(2):48.
19. Chaturvedi SK, Chandra PS. Palliative care in India. Support Care Cancer. 1998;6(2):81–4.
20. Chaturvedi SK. Ethical dilemmas in palliative care in traditional developing societies, with special reference to the Indian setting. J Med Ethics. 2008;34(8):611–5.
21. Sallnow L, Chenganakkattil S. The role of religious, social and political groups in palliative care in Northern Kerala. Indian J Palliat Care [Internet]. 2005 [cited 2023 Aug 6];11(1). Available from: https://link.gale.com/apps/doc/A137290142/HRCA?u=anon~697d909f&sid=googleScholar&xid=3dd03f8b
22. de Souza LJ, Lobo ZM. Symptom control problems in an Indian hospice. Ann Acad Med Singap. 1994;23(2):287–91.
23. Klostermaier KK. A concise encyclopedia of Hinduism. New York: Oneworld Publications; 2014.
24. King R. Orientalism and religion: post-colonial theory, India and "the mystic east". Routledge [Internet]; 1999. Available from: https://foldxx.files.wordpress.com/2011/02/orientalism-and-religion-post-colonial-theory-india-and-the-mystic-east.pdf
25. Chaturvedi SK. What's important for quality of life to Indians – in relation to cancer. Soc Sci Med. 1991;33(1):91–4.

He Heals the Broken-Hearted and Binds Up Their Wounds: A Jewish Approach to Spiritual Aspects in Palliative Care

Yaffa Naomi Stokar and Gil Goldzweig

Abstract This chapter explores concepts from Jewish theology and traditions relevant to the spiritual dimensions of palliative care. The chapter is based on the view of Judaism as a holistic way of life that guides ethical perspectives and practical decisions, including in healthcare contexts. The chapter explores the sanctity of life principle in Judaism, rooted in the Jewish concept of *Pikuach–Nefesh* (a Hebrew term that means 'saving a soul'), which emphasises preserving and saving life. This concept guides medical ethics and care for the terminally ill. Other key topics in this chapter include the caring for body and soul, visiting the sick, end-of-life rituals, grief, and bereavement customs. The chapter highlights the possible contribution of Jewish teachings to patient-centred palliative services, emphasising the infinite value of human life while accepting death as a natural part of existence. Integration of these ideas and the Jewish view of the soul's journey at life's end, guided by contemplative rituals, prayers, and community, can pave the way to respectful end-of-life care that enables connection to the divine while easing suffering.

Keywords Palliative Care · Judaism · Jewish funeral · End-of-life Care · Jewish Spirituality · Spiritual Care

Y. N. Stokar
Hadassah Medical Center, Hebrew University of Jerusalem, Jerusalem, Israel

The Paul Baerwald School of Social Work and Social Welfare, Hebrew University of Jerusalem, Jerusalem, Israel
e-mail: yaffa.stokar@mail.huji.ac.il

G. Goldzweig (✉)
School of Behavioural Sciences, The Academic College of Tel-Aviv Jaffa, Tel-Aviv, Israel
e-mail: giligold@mta.ac.il

M. C. Best (ed.), *Spiritual Care in Palliative Care*,
https://doi.org/10.1007/978-3-031-50864-6_11

1 Introduction

He heals the broken-hearted and binds up their wounds. (Psalm 147:3)

Judaism is more than a religion; Judaism is a multifaceted entity encompassing aspects of religion, nationhood, and tradition. Most of all, Judaism is a way of life that significantly influences the experiences and practices in various life aspects [1, 2]. Even Jews who declare themselves as secular, particularly in Israel but also in other countries, maintain traditional Jewish practices and approach ethical dilemmas and various life aspects through the lens of Judaism [3, 4].

The Jewish tradition sanctifies life. The sanctity of life in Judaism is not just an inherent attribute of life but is significantly influenced by the values and actions of the individual living that life [5, 6]. In Judaism, the value of innocent life is considered limitless, and it cannot be compromised under any circumstances. This perspective is crucial in ethics and *Halacha* (Jewish law).

The sanctity of life in Judaism is not just a theological concept but a practical guideline that influences decisions and actions, especially in situations where life and death are at stake. The sanctity of life in Judaism is related to the Hebrew concept of *Pikuach–Nefesh*, which literally translates to 'saving a soul' or 'watching over a life', and is rooted in the *Talmud* (the primary source of Jewish religious law) interpretation of Leviticus 18:5, which states, '*Ye shall therefore keep my statutes, and my judgments: which if a man do, he shall live in them…*' ([7], Levictus 18:5). The commandments are meant to promote life, not cause death. In practical application, the principle of Pikuach Nefesh permits the overriding of nearly all Jewish laws when essential to save a life.

This doctrine highlights the immense importance Judaism assigns to the sanctity of human life, positioning the preservation of life as a paramount moral duty [8]. *Pikuach–Nefesh* serves not merely as a legal directive but also as a guiding ethical and moral framework, profoundly shaping Jewish perspectives and practices. This is especially evident in the realms of medical ethics and end-of-life care, where the principle of *Pikuach–Nefesh* plays a critical role in decision-making processes, emphasising the priority of life preservation in complex ethical scenarios, particularly in the context of medical ethics and end-of-life care [8]. In Judaism, death is seen as an integral part of the life cycle, a transition rather than an end. This view is reflected in the rituals and traditions surrounding death and mourning in Jewish culture [9].

In Judaism, death is not merely a biological event but a moment that carries profound spiritual and communal significance. The rituals and beliefs surrounding death in Judaism are deeply connected to the values of the community and the individual, reflecting a holistic view of life where death is a natural and respected part of the human experience [9]. This perspective is further shaped by Jewish law, ethics, and cultural practices, which emphasise the importance of pain management, care for the dying, and post-death rituals [10]. For example, there is an important Jewish principle that one must not be so arrogant as to think that God is somehow required to provide what one asks for. Thus, one always needs to be active in life and not just wait, trusting that God will act. Similarly, accepting palliation does not mean losing faith in God as a healer. One can have total faith that God will heal and still must do what is best to reduce pain and suffering [11].

In this chapter, we aim to demonstrate several important aspects of Judaism which are relevant to palliative care. It is beyond the limits of this chapter to cover all relevant aspects in Judaism, but we hope that what is covered here will inspire the readers to further investigate the concept of palliative care in Judaism.

2 The *Neshama* (Soul)

The body and soul are deeply intertwined in Judaism, with the body serving as the vessel for the soul. The twelfth-century Jewish philosopher Maimonides further emphasises this unity, highlighting the role of the soul in guiding the body and its importance of observing commandments for maintaining health [12]. In Judaism, life is represented by the *Neshama* or *Ruach*, the Hebrew terms for soul; both of these terms are related to the Hebrew word for breath or wind. In Genesis, it is described that when God created Man, God '*…formed man of the dust of the ground and breathed into his nostrils the breath of life; and man became a living soul*' ([7], Genesis 2:7). This breath is how Man got his soul, the very essence of life. It is also the Jewish tradition that once a person stops breathing, his or her Neshama leaves their body along with their last breath, reversing the way the Neshama entered the body at the beginning of life. '*Then shall the dust return to the earth as it was: and the spirit shall return unto God who gave it*' ([7], Ecclesiastes 12:7).

The early Jewish sages depicted the idea that every night, when going to sleep, the Neshama leaves the body, going up to the Heavens to be in the Godly presence, returning down to earth and the body as the person awakes. This belief reflects the idea that people experience a bit of death every night, '*Sleep is one-sixtieth part of death*' ([13], Mas. Berachoth 57b). This notion is also represented in the daily morning Jewish prayers, beginning with the prayer *Mode Ani* (I thank thee). '*I give thanks before you, King living and eternal, for You have returned within me my soul with compassion; abundant is your faithfulness'*. Life is a God-given gift, not only at birth but every single day thereafter. And this gift of life should be cherished, as it can easily be taken away at any time. This belief is reflected in the emphasis on the power of choice, which is seen as a gift from God and is crucial for the continuation of life [14, 15]. These ideas are repeated in the daily morning prayers, confirming one of the basic tenets in traditional Judaism, that life is transient and should be cherished as such:

> My God, the soul you have placed within me is pure. You created it; You formed it; You have breathed it into me, and you preserve it within me. Ultimately, you will take it from me, and restore it within me in the Time to Come. As long as the soul is within me, I thankfully acknowledge You, my Lord, and Lord of my fathers, Master of all works, Lord of all souls. Blessed are You, God, who restores souls to lifeless bodies. [16, 17]

3 Caring for Body and Soul

Preserving life, caring for both body and soul, is considered one of the highest values in Judaism. In health, one should take care to maintain both physical and mental health. When falling ill, it is a *Mitzvah* (action mandated by God) to strive towards wellness [18]. As part of that same mitzvah, medical professionals are mandated to facilitate healing, and family and friends to tend to the ill person through *Bikur-Cholim* (visiting the sick). Visiting the sick does not merely mean spending some time at the bedside of an ill person, helping them pass the time. In traditional Judaism, visiting the sick is a divine commandment, an act of loving kindness and an example of true *chesed* (act of human kindness or good deeds) [19]. Chesed is done for the sake of another person out of love or generosity of heart; it is not done out of coercion, but with the intention of receiving nothing in return [20]. In the Mishna, the first major written collection of the Jewish oral traditions, acts of chesed are viewed as one of the three pillars that support the world [21]. The early sages explain that acting in the ways of chesed is an imitation of God's ways in this world. Divine grace accompanies all life on earth. Just as God shows loving kindness to all creatures, so should people show kindness to one another. The mitzvah can be expressed in different ways, for example, acting with kindness towards others, giving charity (monetary or other), striving to make peace between conflicted people, or assisting people who feel they are at a low point in life. In the context of this chapter, it also includes visiting the sick, tending to the funeral and burial of the dead, and comforting mourners [22]. In Judaism, all acts of chesed are a mitzvah, including any kind of assistance to others—whether it is by use of one's body, money, or soul. The body refers to any assistance lent by using the body. It can be tending to the ill, lifting or showering them, replacing them in daily chores, or other actions requiring physical ability. Assistance by money can mean covering medical costs but also just helping with grocery shopping or paying the electricity bill instead of the ill person. Applying the soul directs one to engage with the ill person wholeheartedly; supporting their spiritual and emotional needs as they arise; being that partner for difficult conversations, a shoulder to cry on, and someone to carry fears with [23–25].

In the earlier stages of an illness, visiting the sick focuses on giving the ill person strength and encouragement, offering support in whatever way will help weather the illness and heal when possible. In the case of a more severe and persistent illness, visiting the sick includes assistance with both the physical and spiritual needs of the ill. This includes providing a comfortable environment, preparing any special food or drink, and assisting with any other physical needs. It is also important to tend to the spiritual needs of the ill person, and their sorrows or worries, whether by engaging in conversation, prayer, song, reading together, or any other activity that brings solace to the Neshama [24]. As the illness progresses, the needs of the ill person grow, and the burden of caring for the ill person naturally grows as well. In these instances, caring for the ill person has even more merit, and is considered an even greater act of chesed [26].

4 Palliative Care

In the past, treatment of the mortally ill, including during the last months and weeks of life up until death, regularly took place at home. The family members were entrusted with carrying out most of the treatment, tending to all needs. Medical professionals, even if available, were called in just for brief consultation visits. Today, most patients with advanced diseases, especially those suffering from severe physical symptoms, receive help and support from healthcare professionals who have dedicated training. These treatments can take place at home or at hospitals and hospices [27].

Both preserving life and tending to the ill are highly valued in Judaism and precede almost all else. This lays first and foremost on each person to honour and preserve their life and take care of their body as well as possible. However, once a person has fallen ill, much of the responsibility is passed on to medical professionals. Treating and caring for the ill is considered a mitzvah, even though it is done as part of the professional's job. This includes offering a cure whenever possible, but also easing pain and suffering, including through palliative care to the severely ill and dying [28]. Though there are traditions within Judaism that view pain and suffering as occurrences that are brought on for a reason, the accepted traditional approach is that illness and death are not considered God-given decrees or punishments; therefore, there is no merit in prolonging the suffering of the soul. On the contrary, since suffering and pain can themselves hasten death, providing palliative care is, in fact, seen as part of the commandment of preserving life [29].

Safeguarding the soul, honouring the gift of life, is considered so important that actively shortening life, for instance, by removing life support, is prohibited according to Jewish law. However, since God created man in his image, it is also important to regard the souls of the severely ill and dying with respect. This includes respecting the wishes of the dying and allowing them to dictate which treatments are desirable and which are not. It also leads to preferring a course of natural death. Jewish law does not mandate the use of invasive or life-prolonging measures in order to extend life, though it does allow them if one requests the use of such measures, or when it is medically advised [30]. In fact, when a person is nearing death, there is an obligation to treat and ease their suffering as much as possible [31]. This includes the use of medications to ease pain and suffering. It also includes permission to stop any medical care that might be causing or enhancing inconvenience or suffering, since the belief is that they might prevent the soul from leaving the body. Thus, unnecessary routine tests such as blood tests, measuring blood pressure or temperature or more drastic invasive procedures, if they are causing inconvenience to the dying person, are prohibited [30].

5 Nearing Death

When it is apparent that a person is nearing death, they enter the special state of *Goses*. In the Jewish law, a *goses* is someone who is moribund, or actively dying [32]. According to traditional Judaism, that is the time to turn to God and pray. At times, death happens suddenly, and there is no time to engage in prayer. In other situations, the hours before the actual death are long, and family members, and perhaps also the dying person, are free to devote time to prayer. These prayers are not said as a statement that the end has come and should not be seen as an omen. Rather, the prayers are viewed as an offering, and in the case that the person does die, the prayers are offered as their final words. There are dedicated prayers reserved for these special hours [33]. The first part is called the *Viduy* (confession). If possible, it is to be recited by the dying person, provided they are still able to do so. In situations where it is no longer possible, family members or other people surrounding the dying person may say it in their stead. The viduy is a significant aspect of end-of-life care in Judaism, particularly in Orthodox Jewish tradition. It is a time for the dying person to reflect on their life and seek forgiveness for any wrongdoings. This practice is deeply rooted in the Jewish emphasis on the preservation of life and the importance of spiritual preparation for death [30]. The idea of the *viduy* is to express the importance of the relationships in a person's life, with God and the community, as opposed to the person's accomplishments or material success. It is the final repentance of any wrongdoings within those relationships throughout one's life. Some also add prayers recited on *Yom Kippur,* the Jewish day of atonement.

It is the custom that once the viduy is recited and death seems imminent, there should continuously be someone at the bedside, so that the dying person does not die alone [34]. This practice is rooted in the belief that life is sacred and should be preserved, but that the agony of a moribund person should not be prolonged. This tradition is held as it is believed that someone at the bedside can prevent additional sorrow from the dying person. It is even recommended that if grief overcomes family members during these moments, and the need to cry arises, they step out for a bit. It is believed that crying near the dying person symbolises the difficult imminent parting. Therefore, crying next to the dying loved one may cause them great sorrow, making it difficult for the soul to leave, needlessly extending the suffering of the dying person [35].

6 As the Soul Leaves the Body

At the time of death, when the Neshama leaves the body, it is a custom to open a window as a symbolic act, assisting the soul on its journey (Jewish Funeral, Burial, and Mourning). This is the time for the second part of the prayers called *Tziduk–HaDin* (justification of ordinance), which begins with the words 'blessed is the judge of truth'. It is a custom from the *Kabala* (Jewish mysticism) to close the eyes of the deceased, as it says in the book of Exodus: '*For you cannot see my face, for no one can see me and live*' ([7], Exodus 33:20). However, once a person has passed, they can see the glory of God, and eyes that have seen such glory should not look back on earthly things [36]. Once the death of a loved one has been determined, traditionally, all who are present are to make a small tear at the top of their shirt, near the collar. This was then expanded as a custom that family members perform even later when receiving the news of the passing of their family member. Today, this custom is usually reserved for immediate family members, and performed at the time of burial [37]. The tear symbolises the divide in a person's life caused by the death of their beloved family member. This symbolic mark is carried for the seven days of mourning following the burial. There are various approaches providing insights into this custom [38]. The first, tearing, is due to the loss of the inherent potential in a person that will not be realised, focussing on the future. The second approach focuses on the past. The tearing is a result of the meaning that a person has created for themselves through their good deeds: studying the *Torah* (Jewish code of law, but also guidance) and keeping its commandments. Another aspect of this explanation focuses on the person's actions and achievements. In this sense, the tearing is an expression of sorrow for the loss of a person whose life was full of positive content. According to the third approach, the tearing is necessary because a Neshama has been lost, a great loss in itself. One of the ways God is revealed in this world is through the miraculous unification of the soul and body. When the Neshama separates from the body and returns to the heavens, the world loses a bit of God's revelation in the world.

7 Pre-burial: Between Heaven and Earth

After the ill person's death, when the Neshama has separated from the body, it is a mitzvah not to leave the body unaccompanied; this is called *shemira* (literally, guarding). The body may be covered or in a closed casket. As being close to a lifeless body causes some to feel uneasy, shemira can be done by sitting right outside the door in the room next to the body. There are different ideas behind the notion of shemira. The first reason is a physical reason. Out of respect for the deceased they are not left alone so that it should not seem as though they are no longer important and have been abandoned. Historically, in the first centuries AD, shemira was instituted in order to protect the body against rodents and other harmful conditions that might violate the body [39]. The second reason for shemira is based on spiritual beliefs. Traditionally, it is believed that the Neshama continues to hover over the body until burial, before returning to the heavens. Some believe there exists a liminal space between death and burial; the human soul finds itself in a state of disorientation and uncertainty. The people performing the shemira are, therefore, entrusted with guiding the departed soul through its transition after death. It is believed that reciting Psalms and other prayers helps the Neshama on this journey [40]. When sitting by the deceased reciting Psalms, one is encouraged to adopt an attitude of loving connection with the departed Neshama as if to say, 'You are free to relinquish this earthly realm and continue your spiritual journey' [41, p. 418].

Traditionally, the shemira is not performed by immediate family members, but rather by grandchildren, friends, and community members, and can even be performed by hired help. In the time preceding burial, the immediate family (parents, siblings, children, and the spouse) is in a unique state, inhibiting them from partaking in the shemira. This state is called *Aninut* (the status of a bereaved person in the period between the death and the burial of a close relative). Persons in the state of aninut are exempt from observing the Jewish code of law, and from keeping the *mitzvot* (actions mandated by God), such as the prayers or blessings said before or after eating, and observing the Sabbath [42]. This is so the bereaved family can focus solely on the deceased and all the preparations needed for the funeral in order to hasten the burial. It is also a display of respect towards the deceased; taking care of their final needs on this earth supersedes all else. There may also be a psychological reasoning behind aninut. Family members, amidst profound sorrow, find themselves abruptly thrust into a state of emotional upheaval as they grapple with the overwhelming impact of loss. Experiencing the death of a close family member causes many to feel emotional disarray and disorientation, sometimes temporarily overshadowing their ability to engage in coherent and structured thinking. This emotional and cognitive state is recognised as a unique spiritual time in the lives of the bereaved family members. Being in a state of aninut, disengaging from the daily actions, signifies to themselves and the community that it is a sacred time.

The final act to take place before the burial is the ritual of *tahara* (purity). In Judaism, the purification of the dead, the tahara, is the process of washing, both internal and external cleaning, which is done to the body of the deceased before it is dressed in white linen or cotton shrouds for burial. Today the purification procedure is usually carried out at the funeral home or special room at the cemetery [43, 44].

During the purification process, the deceased is treated with all due respect, as if they were still alive, able to watch their actions and hear them. Therefore, it is customary to refrain from engaging in casual everyday conversations. Some recite prayers while performing the purification. Men purify men, and women care for the women. Each organ is washed separately, and then nine buckets of water are poured over the whole body of the deceased to signify the observance of another mitzvah, ritual purification at the *mikvah* (traditional ritual baths). Rabbi Kaplan, a modern sage and community leader, has suggested the idea that immersion in the mikvah symbolises a spiritual rebirth and the mikvah itself the womb [45], p. 77]. Thus, the pouring of the waters together with the entire tahara ceremony signifies completion of the life cycle as the soul prepares for the journey back to the Heavens.

8 Burial

The soul is the focus of the Jewish burial ceremony. In accordance with the belief that the soul is in a liminal state until burial, it is the custom to perform the burial as soon as possible, often not more than 24 hours after the passing ([40, 46]. It is a simple ceremony focused on showing respect to the deceased and accompanying the soul in beginning its journey up to the heavens once the body is laid in the ground. Partaking in the burial ceremony, accompanying a person to their final resting place, is considered one of the greatest acts of kindness in Judaism [47]. The Hebrew word for funeral is *levaya*, literally meaning 'companion' or 'to accompany'. Another name for the Jewish funeral is *Chesed Shel Emet,* which means 'charity of true loving kindness'.

The early sages explained that generally, when acting in kindness, there is always the chance that the recipient of the kindness will someday repay the favour somehow. However, when doing something for a deceased person, there is no expectation of ever receiving reciprocation from them. Thus, it is considered the ultimate kindness for the sake of kindness itself [34, 48].

In every Jewish community, there is a group of volunteers called the *Chevra–Kadisha* (literally 'holy society'). They are the local Jewish burial society that take care of the burial process, starting with the tahara mentioned above, sometimes beginning with the shemira when there is no one else that can guard the body. They bear the responsibility of overseeing the entire funeral and burial process. Family members or friends who wish to participate may join them at any stage. However, the Chevra–Kadisha are the ones entrusted with the final operations in a person's life, even when there is no one else to partake in the deceased's funeral. The idea that there is always someone who will take care of a person once they pass brings great comfort to those lying on their deathbeds and is another testament to the phrase 'act of loving kindness' which is the essence of a Jewish burial [49, 50].

In Judaism, traditional burial means placing the body directly in the earth. This is informed by the verse in Genesis 3:19 [7] '*With the sweat of your face you shall eat bread, until you return to the ground, for you were taken therefrom, for dust you are, and to dust you will return*'. When circumstances do not enable direct burial in the ground, a simple closed wooden casket is used. Ornate open coffins are not the Jewish custom. If one wants to honour the deceased, the custom is to donate to a charitable cause in merit of the deceased, instead of putting the money towards a funeral of means. If using a casket, it should be made from biodegradable material that will disintegrate in the ground. This allows the body to return to earth as quickly as possible, enabling the soul to attain true and final peace. In some opinions, metal, even in the shape of nails, should not be used in the casket. It is a symbol of weapons of war and has no place in the ceremony that sends off the deceased to their final resting place [51].

Jewish burial customs differ from other belief systems in that a Jewish individual is not buried in their usual clothing. Similarly, jewellery or other adornments are not worn. Jewish funerals highlight the spiritual and transcendent aspects rather than the physical and material ones. In accordance with Jewish tradition, the deceased is clothed in plain white burial furnishings: *tachrichim,* the traditional shrouds carefully crafted from linen or cotton. These garments are deemed appropriate for an individual who is soon to face divine judgment [52]. Another rationale for using simple shrouds is to ensure that individuals who cannot afford extravagant clothing are not made to feel 'embarrassed' due to their lack of resources. The symbolism associated with tachrichim underscores the adherence to this practice. These burial garments serve as a physical manifestation of respect, purity, and equality in death. The act of carefully dressing the deceased in tachrichim reflects the community's commitment to honouring the departed and treating every individual with dignity, even in their final journey. In Jewish law, it is mandated that the funeral should be delayed until appropriate tachrichim are obtained or crafted, despite the general principle of avoiding unnecessary delays in burial [53].

In the past, the departure of the funeral procession would typically occur from the home of the deceased. However, in modern times, it has become more customary for the departure to take place from the cemetery or funeral home. According to some customs, the funeral procession departs from the *synagogue* (house of community prayer) the deceased attended. If family and loved ones wish to eulogise the deceased, this is usually done before the departure of the funeral procession. Psalms are recited during the procession. Throughout the procession towards the gravesite, there are intermittent brief pauses, symbolising a reluctance to part with the presence of the deceased.

The procession ends at the burial site. Throughout the funeral, a few prayers and Psalms are recited. Before the body is laid in the ground, one of the Chevra Kadisha leading the funeral recites the following text from the Mishna, intended for the deceased, but also for all who are present. '*Rabbi Akavia, the son of Mahalalel, would say: Reflect upon three things, and you will not come to the hands of transgression. Know from where you came, where you are going, and before whom you are destined to give judgement and accounting*' [54]. As the body is being laid in the ground, the Chevra Kadisha ask for forgiveness of the deceased. '*In the name of the Chevra Kadisha, in the name of those who took care of you, in the name of your family and friends: I am asking for your forgiveness. If heaven forbid, we've corrupted something during your purification, or while caring for your funeral, or in carrying your bed here or in the preparation of the grave. Please forgive us, as it was unintentional. Everything we did was to honour you according to the customs of the place… Go in peace and rest in peace in your final resting place and ascend to your destiny until the end of time. Be a good advocate for your family and friends, and life and peace will be upon us and to all Israel forever. Amen*'. [55]

Afterwards, the body is laid in the ground, symbolically returning it to its source. The grave is filled with earth. All who choose are invited to approach the grave and add a shovel of dirt. This is the final act of compassion and caring. Prayers are recited while the filling of the grave takes place, including *Tziduk HaDin* (justification of ordinance), which was recited first as the soul left the body. Once the grave is filled, the soul is free to move on, no longer linked to its earthly bond. It is customary to place a pebble on the filled grave, bringing together all who have come to accompany the deceased. The pebble continues the idea of burial in the earth and allows for all to participate in the kindness of the burial, even when the funeral is attended by many people. The pebble is also a symbolic gesture as it is everlasting, remaining on the grave long after the funeral, signifying the eternal connection with the deceased. This concludes the funeral [56].

9 Grief and Bereavement

The ill person is at the centre of the palliative care. However, from a palliative approach, care for the patient also entails caring for the family members. In Judaism, this care for the family continues also after the death and burial.

In Judaism, the purpose of the burial ceremony is not to provide immediate consolation to the mourners. The early sages recognised the inherent futility of offering comfort to grieving individuals while their departed loved one remains visibly present. Therefore, the Jewish bereavement customs, pertaining to the immediate family, begin only at the end of the ceremony once the body has been completely covered.

A mourning process commences immediately following the burial within the confines of the cemetery. Attendees of the funeral create two rows, side by side, while the mourners, having removed their leather shoes symbolising their state of mourning, walk through this supportive assembly. As the mourners pass through, those standing in the two lines express traditional words of comfort, extending solace and support to the grieving individuals. Once the funeral ceremony is finished, the mourners begin a seven-day mourning period known as the *Shiva* (literally seven). Throughout the Shiva period, mourners observe a custom of staying at home, while friends and family come to offer condolences and support, following a tradition dating back to biblical times. This structured practice facilitates the natural process of facing and navigating grief. Shiva allows individuals to openly express their sorrow and engage in discussions about their loss with others as they gradually start adjusting to a new reality without their loved one [57].

Traditionally, when the mourners return home, they begin the Shiva with a special meal called *Seudat–Havra'ah* (healing meal or meal of comfort or consolation). This meal is the first meal during the seven days of mourning. This meal is provided by the neighbours or relatives of the bereaved family. The reason for this is that the mourners are often consumed with grief directly after the funeral and do not think or pay attention to their bodily needs and their hunger. Another reason may be that the mourners are in such grief that they wish to join their loved one in death, and any thought of food and self-care is beyond them. Providing the meal, the second mandated act of condolence, allows for a more active role. In the first act, the comforters played a passive role, by creating a wall of comfort, as providing a meal allows them to further engage with the mourners. Customarily, the meal includes round food such as rolls, hard-boiled eggs, and lentils or other round foods. The round foods represent the cycle of life and death and renewal [58].

The third act of condolence, which is carried out for the entire week, is the Shiva visitation. This is the time when the mourners begin to verbalise their feeling of loss. It is customary for the visitors to sit in silence until the bereaved themselves desire to speak and engage the visitors in conversations of their choice. Sometimes, sitting in silence is more desirable to the mourners; other times, stories and pictures form the deceased life are shared.

10 Conclusion

This exploration of Jewish perspectives on palliative care underscores a deeply spiritual and holistic approach to end-of-life issues that can enrich palliative services. The multifaceted nature of Judaism, intertwining religion, nationhood, and tradition, manifests profoundly in its approach to palliative care, emphasising both the sanctity of life and the acceptance of death as a natural part of existence. Core Jewish values highlight the duty to preserve and cherish each living moment while accepting mortality. Traditions of visiting and caring for the sick model practical acts of loving kindness that support body, mind, and soul. The Jewish emphasis on spiritual preparation for death through rituals like confession also offers inspiration for patient-centred end-of-life care focused on healing relationships and easing the transition of the soul. Overall, Jewish customs reveal an integrated, holistic paradigm that does not compartmentalise the physical and spiritual but attends gracefully to both dimensions. Jewish traditions around death, mourning, and the afterlife reflect a comprehensive view of life, acknowledging death as a spiritual and communal event. While modern medical systems often isolate the dying in sterile hospital rooms, Jewish tradition brings community and connection around the soul's departure.

Palliative care in Judaism goes beyond mere symptom management; it encompasses a profound respect for the patient's wishes and spiritual needs. This approach integrates medical, emotional, and spiritual care, ensuring a dignified journey towards life's end. In applying such wisdom to modern palliative contexts, both Jewish and secular, the core relational ethic stands out. The acts of bikur cholim or shemira require presence and togetherness, facing mortality with courage and care. Reflecting on this Jewish approach offers valuable insights for patient-centred palliative care across cultures and belief systems. It challenges us to consider the balance between preserving life and honouring the natural process of dying, urging a compassionate and holistic approach to palliative care. This Jewish perspective invites us to view palliative care not just as a medical practice but as a spiritual journey, honouring the sacredness of life and the dignity of death.

References

1. Marom, M. S. (2020). A second exodus: Ethiopian Jews in Israel between religion, nation and state. Croat J Educ/Hrvatski Casopis za Odgoj I Obrazovanje, 22:171-191.
2. Merrick J, Gabbay Y, Lifshitz H. Judaism and the person with intellectual disability. J Relig Disabil Health. 2001;5(2–3):49–63.
3. Creese J. Secular Jewish identity and public religious participation within Australian secular multiculturalism. Religions. 2019;10(2):69.
4. Troen I. Secular Judaism in Israel. Society. 2016;53:153–62.
5. Jakobovits Y, Tendler MD, Rosner F. Sanctity of life. Tradition. 1994;28(4):131–3.
6. Rosner F. Jewish perspectives on issues of death and dying. J Halacha Contemp Soc. 1986;11:50–69.
7. Official King James Bible online. 2023. https://www.kingjamesbibleonline.org/
8. Kinzbrunner BM. Jewish medical ethics and end-of-life care. J Palliat Med. 2004;7(4):558–73.
9. Lamm M. The Jewish way in death and mourning. Rev. and exp. ed. Middle Village: NY David; 2000. https://swbplus.bsz-bw.de/bsz260129771kla.htm
10. Prosser R, Korman D, Feinstein A. An orthodox perspective of the Jewish end-of-life experience. Home Healthcare Now. 2012;30(10):579–85.
11. Schultz M, Baddarni K, Bar-Sela G. Reflections on palliative care from the Jewish and Islamic tradition. Evid Based Complement Alternat Med. 2012:2012.
12. Mizrahi A. The soul and the body in the philosophy of the Rambam. Rambam Maimonides Med J. 2011;2(2):e0040.
13. Halakhah.com Babylonian Talmud Online in English. 2023. https://halakhah.com/
14. Caplan R. Therefore choose life. Iowa Med J Iowa Med Soc. 1993;83(7):266.
15. Mendes-Flohr P. In the shadow of death: Jewish affirmations of life. Religions. 2021;13(1):26.
16. Modeh Ani: it's not just about gratitude | My Jewish Learning. 2023. https://www.myjewishlearning.com/article/modeh-ani-its-not-just-about-gratitude/
17. velveteenrabbi. Prayers for the morning, part 2: soul. 2023. https://velveteenrabbi.blogs.com/blog/2015/06/prayers-for-the-morning-part-2-soul.html
18. Bleich JD. The obligation to heal. In: Judaism and healing: halakhic perspectives. KTAV Publishing House, Brooklyn, NY, US; 2002. p. 1–10.
19. Bleich JD. Visiting thesick. In: Judaism and healing: halakhic perspectives. KTAV Publishing House, Brooklyn, NY, US; 2002. p. 44–7.
20. Sheer C. Bikkur Holim: the origins of Jewish pastoral care. J Health Care Chaplain. 2008;15(2):99–113.
21. Tzvi. Three pillars – Pirke Avot 1:2 – Aish.com. 2009, May 09. https://aish.com/48884852/
22. Shapiro RM. Amazing chesed: living a grace-filled Judaism. Woodstock: Jewish Lights Publishing; 2012.
23. Ben-Sefer E. Gemilat chesed and moral behaviour at Westerbork: lessons from the past to remember for the future. In: Remembering for the future: the holocaust in an age of genocide. London: Palgrave Macmillan UK; 2001. p. 962–79.
24. Cedar S. From ministry to hospitality: welcoming the stranger in Judaism as a practical model for contemporary healthcare chaplaincy. Pract Theol. 2020;13(5):480–92.
25. Friedman HH. Human dignity and the Jewish tradition. 2008. Available at SSRN 2295178.
26. Meyerstein I, Ruskin G. Spiritual tools for enhancing the pastoral visit to hospitalized patients. J Relig Health. 2007;46(1):109–22. https://doi.org/10.1007/s10943-006-9085-y.
27. Lowey SE. A historical overview of end-of-life care. In: Nursing care at the end of life. 2015.
28. Jotkowitz A, Zivotofsky AZ. "Love your neighbor like yourself": a Jewish ethical approach to the use of pain medication with potentially dangerous side effects. J Palliat Med. 2010;13(1):67–71. https://doi.org/10.1089/jpm.2009.0182.
29. Weiss RRB. Pain management at the end of life and the principle of double effect: a Jewish perspective. Cancer Investig. 2007;25(4):274–7.
30. Baeke G, Wils JP, Broeckaert B. Orthodox Jewish perspectives on withholding and withdrawing life-sustaining treatment. Nurs Ethics. 2011;18:835–46.

31. Sanhedrin veha'Onashin haMesurin lahem – Chapter 13. 2023. https://www.chabad.org/library/article_cdo/aid/1172736/jewish/Sanhedrin-vehaOnashin-haMesurin-lahem-Chapter-13.htm
32. Lessons from a "Goses"--a Dying Person | jewishideas.org. 2023. https://www.jewishideas.org/article/lessons-goses-dying-person
33. Popovsky MA. Jewish ritual, reality and response at the end of life: a guide to caring for Jewish patients and their families. Durham: Duke Institute on Care at the End of Life; 2007.
34. Ross HM. Jewish tradition in death and dying. Medsurg Nurs. 1998;7(5):275–9.
35. Linzer RD. Treatment of terminally ill patients according to Jewish law. AMA J Ethics. 2013;13(12):1081–7.
36. The Jewish Burial. 2023. https://www.chabad.org/library/article_cdo/aid/368092/jewish/The-Jewish-Burial.htm
37. The Basics of Kriah, or Tearing a Piece of Clothing | My Jewish Learning. 2023. https://www.myjewishlearning.com/life/Life_Events/Death_and_Mourning/Burial_and_Mourning/Kriah.shtml
38. Jerome OM, Uroko FC. Tearing of clothes: a study of an ancient practice in the old testament. Verbum et Ecclesia. 2018;39(1):1–8.
39. Zivotofsky AZ. Government regulations of Shechita (Jewish religious slaughter) in the twenty-first century: are they ethical? J Agric Environ Ethics. 2011;25:747–63.
40. Matz M. Judaism and bereavement. J Relig Health. 1964;3:345–52.
41. Raphael SP. Jewish views of the afterlife. Rowman & Littlefield; 2019.
42. Rubin SS. Loss and mourning in the Jewish tradition. OMEGA-J Death Dying. 2014;70(1):79–98.
43. Chafetz PK. Jewish practices in death and mourning. Death Stud. 1979;3:363–9.
44. Goldberg H. Funeral and bereavement rituals of Kota Indians and orthodox Jews. OMEGA J Death Dying. 1982;12:117–28.
45. Kaplan A. Waters of Eden: the mystery of the mikvah. New York: National Conference of Synagogue Youth, Union of Orthodox Jewish Congregations of America; 1982.
46. Epstein S, Robinson SL. The soul, evil spirits, and the undead: vampires, death, and burial in Jewish folklore and law. Preternature. 2012;1:232–51.
47. Hitchcock J. "Leveiya": the process of the Jewish funeral service. Verbum. 2004;1:41–8.
48. Sharp C, Randhawa G. Altruism, gift giving and reciprocity in organ donation: a review of cultural perspectives and challenges of the concepts. Transplant Rev. 2014;28(4):163–8.
49. Handbook for Hevra Kadisha Members "Kavod v'Nichum". Jewish Funerals, Burial and Mourning. For shrouds and 7 day- candles US: Rose Solomon, CANADA: Hesed Shel Emes Brooklyn Naval Yards Winnipeg, Manitoba 718-855-1788 Rena Boroditsky. https://www.jewish-funerals.org/handbook-for-hevra-kadisha-members/
50. Heílman SC. When a Jew dies: the ethnography of a bereaved son. Berkeley: University of California Press; 2001.
51. A Jewish Burial and Procession. 2023. https://www.chabad.org/library/article_cdo/aid/281569/jewish/A-Jewish-Burial-and-Procession.htm
52. Geus CHJ d, Bloch-Smith E. Judahite Burial practices and beliefs about the dead. J Econ Soc Hist Orient. 1991;37:331.
53. Delaying a Funeral – Dalet Amot of Halacha – OU Torah. 2021. https://outorah.org/p/86096/
54. Three Times Three – Avot 3:1. 2023. https://www.chabad.org/therebbe/article_cdo/aid/4015147/jewish/Avot-31-Three-Times-Three.htm
55. Chevra Kadisha and the Ritual Care of the Dead. 2022. https://www.talkdeath.com/chevra-kadisha-and-the-ritual-care-of-the-dead/
56. Placing a Stone | Shiva, Jewish Mourning. 2023. https://www.shiva.com/learning-center/death-and-mourning/placing-a-stone
57. Maoz B, Lauden A, Ben-Zion IZ. [A psychosocial view of a number of Jewish mourning rituals during normal and pathological grief]. Harefuah, Israel Medical Association. 2004;143(4):287–90, 317.
58. Brensel A. Jewish meals of condolence & Shiva food traditions – Beth El Mausoleum. 2021. https://bethelmausoleum.org/2021/07/21/jewish-meals-of-condolence-shiva-food-traditions/

Spiritual Care by Nurses for Non-Religious Patients in Japan

Sayaka Takenouchi, Keiko Tamura, and Tatsuya Morita

Abstract Patients at the end of life experience existential suffering regardless of their religious beliefs; thus, spiritual care appropriate for non-religious patients may be required. Nurses often provide spiritual care unrelated to a particular religion or belief system. This chapter illustrates the non-religious spiritual care nurses provide in Japan by providing examples of how non-religious spiritual care has been provided, assessing patients experiencing spiritual pain and the essentials of care. Finally, strategies for spiritual care for non-religious persons aimed at spiritual healing are discussed using case examples.

Keywords Non-religious · Spiritual care · Nurse · End-of-life care · Spiritual but not religious · Spiritual well-being · Serious illness · Palliative care

1 Introduction

Spiritual well-being is one of the most important outcomes for patients at the end of life [1–3]. Originally derived from religious well-being, the interpretation of spiritual well-being has expanded in recent years [1]. Spiritual well-being is currently

S. Takenouchi (✉)
Department of Human Health Sciences, Kyoto University, Kyoto, Japan
e-mail: takenouchi.sayaka.6u@kyoto-u.ac.jp

K. Tamura
Osaka Dental University, Osaka, Japan
e-mail: tamura-k@cc.osaka-dent.ac.jp

T. Morita
Seirei Mikatahara General Hospital, Hamamatsu, Japan
e-mail: tmorita@sis.seirei.or.jp

M. C. Best (ed.), *Spiritual Care in Palliative Care*,
https://doi.org/10.1007/978-3-031-50864-6_12

understood as a state of being free of existential pain, in which one feels a sense of meaning, value, and purpose in life and is free from the burdens and dependence on others. In countries where most of the population follows a particular religion, regularly attends church or temple services, participates in religious rituals, and consults with pastoral professionals on life issues, pastoral professionals play an essential role in alleviating spiritual distress [4].

The percentage of the population with a particular religion is declining worldwide, and Japan is no exception [5]. According to one survey, only one in four Japanese professes a specific religion, and over 70% do not believe in any religion [6]. In Japan, spirituality is seldom preached or established as a doctrine. Instead, spirituality is a moral code, a way of living almost indistinguishable from Japanese social and cultural values [6]. Most people also have a sense of reverence and awe for nature and their deceased ancestors. Many Japanese perceive spirituality as 'living in harmony with nature and the people surrounding you'. [7] Thus, Japanese people are classified as 'spiritual but non-religious'. [8, 9]

Terminally ill patients experience existential suffering regardless of their religious beliefs, and spiritual care is recognised as necessary in Japan [9–11]. The development of spiritual care in Japan started in the late 1970s with the hospice care and death studies movement, as Christian hospitals established pioneer hospices [12]. Later, Buddhist hospices (*Vihara*) and clinical religious workers covering all religions began to operate in some institutions. However, spiritual care has not been fully integrated into healthcare settings, and combined with a lack of systematic multidisciplinary education, resources for spiritual care are lacking in Japan [9].

Nevertheless, spirituality is deeply rooted in Japanese culture, and nurses most frequently provide spiritual care and are more competent than other staff, partly because they have better opportunities than other professionals to receive education and training in spiritual care as part of their palliative care nursing education [12]. Therefore, if nurses can better alleviate patients' spiritual distress in their daily nursing practice, they can significantly contribute to patients' spiritual well-being and quality of life. For example, spiritual care training provided to nurses has been reported to be effective in improving their knowledge and confidence in providing care [13, 14].

In light of the above, we introduce a way to alleviate the spiritual pain experienced by seriously ill or terminally ill patients in daily nursing practice in Japan, which does not have the custom of consulting a specific religious leader or chaplain.

2 Spiritual Pain and Care for Patients Who Are Spiritual But Not Religious

The concepts of 'spiritual' and 'spirituality' tend to be more religious in Western contexts, and the question of how spirituality differs from religion has been debated in Japan. Non-religious patients in Japan tend to be reluctant to have their spiritual needs approached religiously [15], but this does not mean they reject spiritual care

[16]. Alternatively, religious people seek a religious approach, and providing spiritual care that meets their needs is essential [15, 16]. Direct importation of spiritual care with a strong religious component into Japan runs the risk of overshadowing the supernatural spirituality handed down in Japan since ancient times [9].

In 2004, the Research Group for the Development of Palliative Care Programs to Improve the Quality of Life of Cancer Patients, funded by a Grant-in-Aid for Scientific Research on Cancer from the Ministry of Health, Labour, and Welfare of Japan, began to address the issue of establishing and implementing spiritual care in palliative care in Japan.

Initially, experts debated the definition of spiritual pain. Amid the muddled discussion, experts proposed that research be conducted from the perspective of 'what is useful for patients' rather than 'what is the correct definition'. This proposal led to an agreement to use Murata's [17] concept of spiritual pain as a tentative, unified concept and interdisciplinary research on spiritual care was initiated and expanded. Even today, Japan has no unified definition of spiritual pain, and the term remains ambiguous. Notably, palliative care physicians and psychiatrists recognise the importance of differentiating spiritual pain from psychological distress, such as depression, and most physicians believed that spiritual pain and psychological distress should be distinguished [18].

2.1 Definition and Structure of Spiritual Pain

Murata's theory is widely recognised as the most clinically applicable for clinicians providing spiritual care in Japan. Hisayuki Murata, a professor of philosophy, defined spiritual pain at the end-of-life stage as 'pain that arises from the extinction of the being and the meaning of self'. [17] Murata's theory is based on the concept that 'the thought of one's death' strongly impacts the patient and causes various spiritual pains to emerge, depending on the orientation of the patient's consciousness at the time.

Based on the 'structure of human existence' and focusing on the orientation of consciousness, Murata proposed that spiritual pain can be categorised into three structures: relational, autonomous, and temporal (Table 1) [17, 19].

1. *Relational* (*kankei sonzai*): When thoughts of one's death are directed towards the severance or separation of relationships with others and the world, the patient loses support for their existence and experiences spiritual pain, such as the loss of a sense of existence and meaning, loneliness, and emptiness. This orientation of consciousness indicates a relational aspect based on a raw existential structure that views relationships with others as necessary to establish existence and meaning.
2. *Autonomous* (*jiritsu sonzai*): The body is active and autonomous, always seeking to live independently. It also has a private nature and does not share perceptions with others. However, when the body's activity and autonomy are

Table 1 Spiritual pain from the perspective of consciousness orientation: relationality, autonomy, and temporality

Spiritual pain as relational beings (emptiness/loneliness)	When you die, there's nothing left I'm alone. I feel like I'm the only one left behind My daughter is with me, but I feel alone When I'm alone and looking at the ceiling, I don't feel alive No one understands me What will happen to me now? Where am I going? My sins will never disappear
Spiritual pain as autonomous beings (worthlessness/nonsense)	There is no value in living in the care and to the annoyance of others If I cannot take care of myself, I am no longer a human being I am of no use. I am not alive or worthy
Spiritual pain as temporal beings (meaninglessness/purposelessness)	It doesn't matter if I do this Hospice is boring. There is nothing to do I don't know what to do Nothing makes sense anymore I just want them to make me comfortable as soon as possible I can't wait to go to heaven I don't know how I got into this mess What was my life all about?

interrupted by the approach of death, the patient loses productivity owing to the self's inability and experiences of worthlessness or being of no use to others. Furthermore, spiritual pain manifests as a feeling of nuisance and burden owing to one's need to depend on others. This orientation of consciousness indicates the autonomy of the structure of life's existence, in which independence (autonomy and privateness) and productivity are necessary to establish one's existence and meaning.

3. *Temporal* (*jikan sonzai*): When faced with the death of the self, if the orientation of the patient's consciousness is towards the interruption of life and the loss of the future, in which the patient perceives 'there is no future' and 'it is over'. Per this orientation of consciousness, spiritual pain will then appear as 'meaninglessness, purposelessness, and absurdity'. This orientation of consciousness indicates the temporality of the existential structure of life in which a future is necessary to establish one's existence and meaning.

2.2 Assessment of Spiritual Pain

To provide spiritual care for spiritual pain, nurses must first assess the spiritual pain. Figure 1 describes the Spiritual Pain Assessment Sheet (SpiPas) developed in Japan based on Murata's theory [20, 21]. Clinical trials conducted in Japan with 46 advanced cancer patients showed that spiritual care using SpiPas, delivered by trained nurses, was associated with significant improvements in the Functional Assessment of Chronic Illness Therapy-Spiritual (FACIT-Sp) and the Hospital

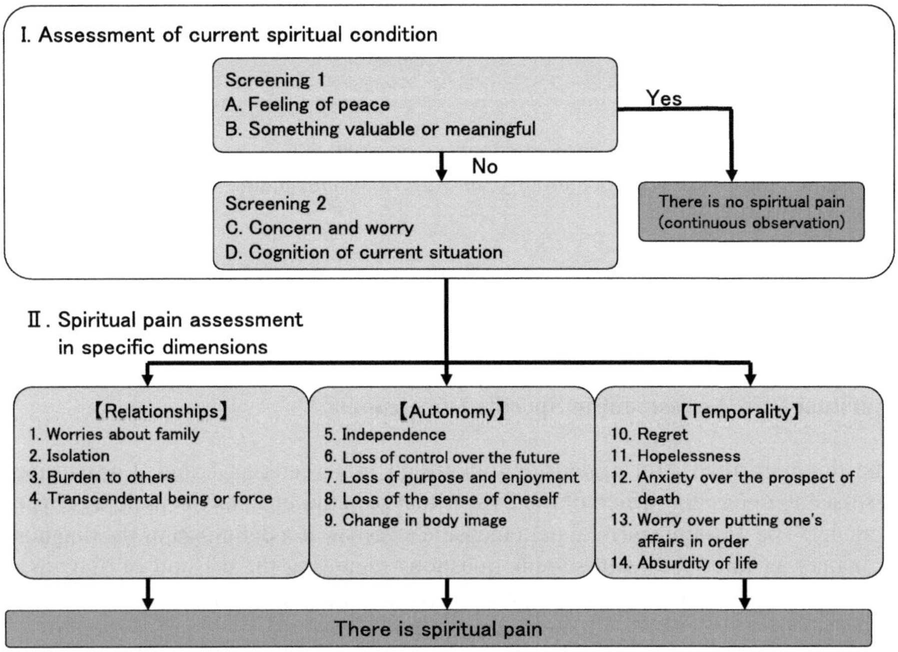

Fig. 1 Spiritual Pain Assessment Sheet (SpiPas)

Anxiety and Depression Scale (HADS) scores during a 2-week period in palliative and hospice care settings [22, 23].

SpiPas has a two-step structure. The first step involves identifying the patient's current spiritual state. If a patient was assessed as having experienced spiritual pain, the second step was identifying the pain dimension. Spiritual pain was evaluated in a conversational format that can be adopted in conversations in medical settings to minimise the burden on patients and healthcare professionals. Given that this tool requires verbal communication, it cannot be applied to patients with impaired consciousness or severe cognitive impairment.

Assessment of Current Spiritual Condition

The *Spiritual Status Assessment* [22] comprises four items, with two questions each for screenings 1 and 2, as described below.

Screening 1

Question A: Are you feeling peaceful at this moment?

Question B: What do you find most important/supportive/meaningful/valuable right now?

Screening 1 assesses the patient's spiritual state and concerns using questions A and B. If the patient feels calm and has a support system, it can be concluded that they are not experiencing apparent spiritual pain. The interview is terminated, and the patient's condition observed. Assessment using the SpiPas is resumed as the patient's situation changes.

Screening 2

Question C: What are your current concerns or worries?

Question D: How do you feel about your current situation, and what do you think is happening to you?

Screening 2 determines the dimensions of pain (relational, autonomous, and temporal) experienced by the patient based on their responses to questions C and D.

Spiritual Pain Assessment in Specific Dimensions

The three spiritual pain dimensions identified in screenings 1 and 2 are further assessed to determine which of the 14 spiritual pain dimensions the patient is experiencing. The 14-item spiritual pain measure consists of a definition of the diagnostic name, an interview with sample questions regarding the method of diagnosis, and an example of the patient's expression for the diagnostic index.

2.3 *Planning Spiritual Care*

General Spiritual Care

The World Health Organisation's concept of spiritual support states that 'relationships in care that include spiritual aspects have the power to promote healing of the heart'. The etymology of the word 'healing' is the same as 'wholeness'. When one is healthy, one lives with a sense of wholeness, as one's connection to the world gives rise to notions of all-ness and immortality. However, illness robs a person of his or her connection to the world, causing them to lose their sense of being whole. The essence of healing is regenerating a person's connections and restoring their wholeness. Healing renews relationships and restores wholeness. Specifically, general spiritual care must be practised to create a foundation for patients to regenerate their connections with others and regain wholeness.

General spiritual care includes the following types of support:

- Providing care that strengthens the meaning of life, peace of mind, and dignity
- Building a trusting relationship between healthcare professionals and patients
- Supporting acceptance of reality
- Providing emotional support
- Facilitating changes in the patient's perception of their situation and self
- Reinforcing social support, including that of family, friends, and support groups
- Providing a comfortable environment and a way to relax
- Providing symptom relief
- Coordination of care teams

Individualised Spiritual Care in the Relational, Autonomous, and Temporal Dimensions

Spiritual Care for Relationships Patients experience spiritual pain after losing their relationships with others, such as loss of identity, loneliness, and emptiness. When providing spiritual care, it is essential to rebuild relationships with others. Table 2 shows the key points in providing care for the following spiritual pain: [1] worry about family and loved ones, [2] loneliness, [3] feeling of or apologising for being a burden, and [4] anguish about things and beliefs beyond human beings.

Spiritual Care for Autonomy Spiritual suffering may be inevitable, such as when patients feel a burden and annoyance owing to their dependence, which exposes them as helpless to others. Thus, spiritual care for autonomy is vital to encourage the maintenance and reacquisition of a sense of control and self-worth. This type of spiritual care helps patients feel independent in their daily lives. Table 3 shows the key points in providing care for each of the following spiritual pain types: [5] the pain of not being able to do one's own thing, [6] loss of control over the future, [7] loss of role and enjoyment, [8] loss of sense of self, and [9] change in body image.

Spiritual Care for Temporality Given that patients feel the meaninglessness, purposelessness, and absurdity of the present due to the loss of the future with the approach of their death, spiritual care for temporality is essential to help patients

Table 2 Spiritual care for relationships

Spiritual pain	Key points in providing spiritual care
1. Worries about family and loved ones Ramifications	• Helping patients prepare for what happens after their death • Caring for grieving family members • Identify specific conflicts • Encourage the patient's own forgiveness • Promote reconciliation with others
2. Loneliness	• Discuss the fundamental human feeling of "loneliness" • Respect the patient's desires for the way they relate to their family and others • Create opportunities for patients and families to spend time together • Minimize factors that keep family members away from the patient
3. Feel burdened/sorry	• Understand the patient's values • Coordinate with the patient and family to communicate feelings of burden/apology • Design care that reduces the patient's sense of burden/remorse • Present new perspectives • Ease the burden on the family • Advocate for patient coping
4. Beyond human existence Distress about faith	• Understand the patient's view of life and death • Discuss life, death, and afterlife with patients, if they wish • Work with religious leaders

Table 3 Spiritual care for autonomy

Spiritual pain	Key points in providing spiritual care
1. The pain of not being able to take care of oneself as one would like The pain of not being able to think clearly	• Minimise loss by helping patients to do things for themselves • Maximise the patient's sense of control by facilitating their own choices • Support patient coping • Minimise loss by using methods of pain relief that are less likely to affect consciousness • Maximise the sense of control by sharing what is important to the patient
2. Loss of control over the future	• Encourage patients to verbalise their fears and maximise their sense of control, including addressing vague fears • Discuss options for delegating or letting go of what cannot be controlled
3. Loss of role and enjoyment	• Create an environment in which the patient can continue to do things they value as they wish
4. Loss of self	• Create an environment that allows the patient to make the most of their abilities • Consider introducing rehabilitation • Alleviate symptoms according to the patient's wishes
5. Change in body image	• Provide support according to the patient's wishes and values • Take into account beauty, sexuality, and aesthetics • Be supportive of the patient's coping

Table 4 Spiritual care for temporality

Spiritual pain	Key points in providing spiritual care
1. Unfinished business	• Support the patient in accomplishing unfinished business • Support patients to write down their feelings in a letter, even if it is difficult to accomplish immediately
2. Lack of hope	• Support the search for specific, achievable goals • Support the patient's hope • Support the search for hope that continues after death • Understand and support patient coping
3. Death anxiety	• Uphold the patient's anxious feelings about death and assure support • Understand and support the patient's coping • Endorse coping in the face of defences, such as denial and avoidance
4. Concerns about personal affairs	• Assist in putting important things in order • Care for grieving family members
5. Absurdity of life	• Provide emotional support and care for the patient's sense of self-worth • Engage to understand anger and underlying expectations expressed as "anger" • If the anger is real, take steps to remedy the problem

feel a sense of generational legacy, hope, and commitment to the anxiety of death. Table 4 shows the key points in providing care for the spiritual pain of [10] regret, [11] hopelessness, [12] death anxiety, [13] concerns about personal affairs, and [14] absurdity of life.

2.4 Example of Spirituality Assessment and Care Practice Using the SpiPas

This section presents an example of spiritual pain assessment and care according to SpiPas through a case study.

Mrs. Aoki (a woman in her 70 s) was hospitalised for pain control because of worsening pain during body movements caused by bone metastases from end-stage breast cancer. After 5 days of hospitalisation, pain management was successful, and her pain level had decreased, but when the nurse asked how she was doing, the patient only stated, 'The pain is better. I'm fine'.

The nurse asked Mrs. Aoki, using the SpiPas (Fig. 1), 'I'm glad your pain has eased, but how are you feeling?' Mrs. Aoki replied, 'The pain is much better, but I am very anxious about whether my husband and I will be able to live together as we did before. When I started thinking about what would happen next, I got increasingly depressed'; the nurse replied, 'You are worried about the future. You have a son, don't you?' Mrs. Aoki replied, 'I do, but my son and husband don't get along. I no longer have the strength to hold on to their relationships'. Mrs. Aoki was unable to ask her children for help.

Based on the conversation with Mrs. Aoki up to this point, the nurse assessed that rather than psychological distress, Mrs. Aoki was more likely to be experiencing spiritual distress in the relational dimension, stemming from existential losses, including the loss of personal relationships at the end of life [21]. After reviewing the four dimensions of spiritual pain in the relational dimension, the nurse believed that Mrs. Aoki's spiritual pain was worries about her family and loved ones. The nurse asked Mrs. Aoki, 'What concerns do you have about your husband?' Mrs. Aoki responded, 'I have taken care of everything at home and am very worried about whether my husband can live independently. I won't be able to do anything for him anymore…' Based on what Mrs. Aoki said, the nurse diagnosed her spiritual pain as worry about family and loved ones.

When planning Mrs. Aoki's care, the nurse initially considered determining the necessary spiritual support. Although Mrs. Aoki's physical pain was alleviated, and she had a good relationship with her nurses, her relationship with her husband and son prevented her from being at peace. The nurse first checked her family background and support systems to strengthen her social support. The nurse also developed a plan to support Mrs. Aoki in preparing herself so that her most significant concern—her anxiety about her husband, who would be left behind—that is, could be eased as much as possible. For example, listening and acknowledging Mrs. Aoki's feelings, supporting her in developing a plan to help her husband become capable of self-care, and reassuring her that she can always seek help when she needs it.

3 Case Study of Spiritual Care for a Non-Religious Patient

In the previous section, we discussed spiritual care strategies for patients without a specific religion, along with examples of how to assess and provide care based on the Japanese cultural background and SpiPas. In this section, we illustrate how nurses recognise and respond to spiritual pain when the temporal, relational, and autonomous dimensions of spiritual pain are not expressed in an orderly fashion in clinical practice but emerge in response to the constantly changing orientation of the patient's consciousness.

3.1 Ms. Iwata's Case

Patient: Ms. Tomoko Iwata, a woman in her 60s

Medical history: In 20xx, when Ms. Iwata underwent excisional surgery for left breast cancer, uterine cancer was discovered, and she underwent further surgery and chemotherapy. Four years later, the cancer recurred, and she underwent radiation therapy. Ten years later, multiple lymph nodes and skin metastases were found, and she was told that continuing treatment would be difficult. Ten years and three months after the initial diagnosis, a gene panel test was conducted at the patient's request, which revealed a candidate drug for treatment. However, treatment was postponed due to the deterioration of her general condition. A few days before Nurse T met Ms. Iwata, she became immobile and was hospitalised urgently.

3.2 Meeting with Ms. Iwata

The day after Ms. Iwata's admission to the hospital, the ward nurse contacted the author, KT (hereafter referred to as 'I' and 'my'), saying, 'Ms. Iwata would like to talk to you. Please come to her room as soon as possible'. I met Ms. Iwata once at the Consultation Support Centre while waiting for the results of the gene panel test, but we had not had a chance to meet since then. I visited Ms. Iwata at her hospital bed the next day without knowing why she had requested a meeting.

Ns (nurse)	*Hello, this is Nurse T. I came to see you because one of the nurses from the floor contacted me.*
Pt (patient)	*Oh, Ms. T, I've been waiting for you. Thank you.* (Smiles)
Ns	*I see you were admitted to our hospital. It must have been difficult suddenly becoming very sick like that.*
Pt	*Yes, I suddenly got stuck at the entrance of my house. I was hospitalised in an emergency.*
	Ms. Iwata was lying in bed with severe oedema throughout her body, making it difficult for her to turn over, and she appeared to be deterio-

rating. When she saw my face, she said, 'I've been waiting for you! Thank you for pointing this out'. I was puzzled, not knowing what her 'thank you' meant, but Ms. Iwata continued to speak.

Pt *I didn't have any expectations for genomic medicine. However, a miracle happened. I felt like saying, 'Thank you!' When I learned they could treat me, I wanted to do whatever it took to get a cure.*

Ns (Nods silently)

Pt *Nonetheless, the other day at the doctor's office, they said it was no good because of my condition. I was thrown into the abyss in one fell swoop. I asked my doctor repeatedly, 'What do you mean when you say that the medicine capable of treating my condition is unsuitable for me?' He kept saying 'no'.*

When Ms. Iwata began to speak, her breathing became laboured, and she seemed distressed. However, she said, 'I'm fine because I'm not having trouble breathing. I'm happy I get to talk to you', and continued to talk about her story.

I assumed that Ms. Iwata was frustrated when told by her doctor that she could not undergo therapy because of her declining physical strength, even though she had been waiting for the gene panel test with a glimmer of hope. I felt that it was understandable that she was dissatisfied with the current situation.

These thoughts floated in my mind during our conversation; *she probably did not call me to express this 'unconvinced' feeling.* What *does she want to talk to me about?* I was at a loss regarding Ms. Iwata's thoughts and what to do about them. At the same time, I sensed from Ms. Iwata's condition that she did not have much time left. I decided to sit down and listen to her story, thinking the 'here and now' was important.

3.3 Wanting to Believe in Miracles

Ms. Iwata told her life story before her hospitalisation and then said the following, as her voice rose slightly:

Pt *I know that many people are worried about me. But I want to believe in miracles until the very end. Do you know what I mean?*

Ns *Yes, I understand. Surely miracles can happen.*

Pt *Isn't that right? However, they keep discussing how they cannot cure me or that hospice is the way to go. The head nurse and the social worker, too. While listening to them, I started feeling sick, like I was going to throw up. I still feel nauseous when I think about it.*

Ns (Nods)

Pt *I know you all are worried about me, but I want to live more. I know, but I want to believe in miracles.*

Ns *You want to believe in miracles.*

Pt (Nodding broadly) *Yes, I do. Tomorrow, the doctor will talk to me (about future treatment and where I will receive care). My brother will be with me. I'm getting depressed thinking about it.*

I realised that Ms. Iwata wanted to discuss her treatment options with me. From Ms. Iwata's expressions, I understood that she was aware of her condition but strongly wished to continue her treatment, hoping for a miracle. I assumed this was due to her lack of conviction that she could not be treated simply because of her deteriorating health after finding a drug that could be used for her condition.

The medical team believed that further treatment would be too physically intensive. They repeatedly tried to persuade Ms. Iwata to accept her condition: Ms. Iwata seemed angry at the medical team's response; I sensed her resenting this harsh reality. In my eyes, it seemed that Ms. Iwata was expressing her uncontrollable anger, knowing that she understood the situation and that it was no one's fault. If I were in Ms. Iwata's shoes, I knew that I would also feel uncontrollable resentment, and I knew that I could not let this slide.

3.4 Together We Stand in the Situation

To respond carefully, I wanted to know more about Ms. Iwata, such as what values and beliefs she cherished, what her life was like, and why she wished to 'believe in miracles' so much in the first place. When Ms. Iwata had finished talking about her thoughts and feelings and looked slightly relieved, I asked her questions.

Ns *I understand the course of your illness very well, but other than that, I know very little about you. May I ask you a few questions? Is it hard for you to talk?*
Pt *No problem.* (nodding)

Through the dialogue that followed, I learned that Ms. Iwata had been working and living independently, that she wanted to be a novelist after she retired but had to give it up when diagnosed with cancer, and that she had had to take care of her elderly mother. I also learned from her hospital visits that she had acquired a strong sense of wisdom regarding survival. However, I still could not see how a miracle would happen to Ms. Iwata, as her condition left little hope for a miracle.

3.5 Suggestion to Play the Queen

As the dialogue continued, Ms. Iwata expressed concern about the next day's conversations with her physician.

Pt *By the way, what should I do tomorrow? I'm going to feel sick again.*
Ns *Ummm...*

Pt *Just thinking about it makes me feel bad. I still want to stay here. Is that a bad idea?*

Ms. Iwata believed a mistake could have occurred and wanted to continue her treatment at the hospital. Nonetheless, I knew her family and the medical team were concerned about her and suggested a transfer to a hospice. I knew that for the miracle Ms. Iwata believed would happen, the scheduled discussions would likely end without agreement if the medical team proceeded as they had in the past. In this situation, I realised that it was important for Ms. Iwata to feel that her decision to transfer to a hospice was her own. As we continued our dialogue, I considered how to proceed and what kind of proposal would make Ms. Iwata feel better. I decided to convey my ideas to her.

Ns *Ms. Iwata, why don't you consider becoming a queen? I think a queen would go along with the suggestions of those around her if she felt that her retainers were doing something for her, even if it was something she disagreed with.*
Pt *What, a queen?*
Ns *Yes, I was wondering if you would like to play the role of queen when we discuss the care plan at the doctor's appointment tomorrow.*
Pt *Well, that sounds interesting. Do you mean I play the role?*
Ns *Yes, that's right. Could you play the role of queen and tell everyone to do what they think is best? You have said that people are concerned about you and have told you about the hospice. Thus, the queen would think, 'Why don't I agree with that suggestion?' and leave the details to everyone else.*
Pt *Okay, I'll play along. I'll try to play the role of a queen. It's fun.*
Ns *Okay, I'm glad.*
Pt *However, doesn't 'queen' seem a bit overbearing?*
Ns *Yes. I think the queen has a high status. Do you have a problem with being high and mighty?*
Pt *Ummm, it makes me old, doesn't it?*
Ns *Well, shall we make her a princess? How about Princess Tomoko?*
Pt *Well, that's good. Okay, I'll play it tomorrow.*
Surprisingly, Ms. Iwata was immediately enthusiastic about this suggestion, and we discussed how to perform this role.
Pt *It's getting more and more fun. You are such an interesting person, Ms. T. It's amazing.*
Ns *Really? I am a good wizard. Didn't you know that?*
Pt *Oh, really? Then please make me your apprentice.*
Ns *Of course, I will make you my first disciple. Then, from now on, let's ride on a broomstick. Flying in the sky, you can see much further and have peace of mind, right?*

I suggest that Ms. Iwata rides on a broomstick to look peacefully ahead of the future, including her imminent death.

3.6 It Is Just the Beginning

The next day, Ms. Iwata and her family discussed with the doctor and decided to transfer her to a hospice. She told the social worker about her thoughts at that time as follows:

Pt *It was a very shocking story. A miracle was about to happen, but they couldn't use that medicine on me. My doctor did his best, but after discussing it with the department, they concluded that it was too risky for me physically. If I had not been able to talk to Ms. T yesterday, I am sure I would not have been able to recover from my confusion. Yesterday's talk made me express myself in a world that fits me perfectly [queen and wizard], and today I tried to act out a different version of myself as the wizard's apprentice. Everyone was very surprised, but I hid my true feelings and followed obediently. The nurse wanted to ask me what I talked with Ms. T. about, but I didn't tell her. [Performing] felt good. I do want to make a miracle happen and become Mr. T's number one disciple. That's what I'm going to do now.*

The social worker told me that although Ms. Iwata expressed frustration and concerns about her mother, her expression remained calm, and I was relieved to hear that.

3.7 I Will Come Back Here

The nurses in the unit contacted me to request a meeting with Ms. Iwata. I visited her bed 4 days after her appointment with the doctor. She was started 24-h oxygen therapy.

Ns *Hello, Ms. Iwata. I'm here after receiving a call from your nurse.*

Pt *Thank you very much. I am so happy. I enjoyed it. The doctor, the head nurse, and my brother were all very surprised. They thought I would say I didn't want to do it and wondered, 'What happened?' I hid my true feelings and played along. It looks like we will look for a hospice as soon as possible. The social worker asked me which hospice I preferred, but I told her I didn't care and would leave it up to my brother. It seems my brother will go to the hospice [to apply]. I don't care which one because I am sure I will come back here with a miracle. I called my mother to tell her how it happened, and she said it was good. She was relieved.*

Ns *Therefore, you have become Princess Tomoko. You are notably my best disciple.*

Pt *Isn't that right? I think it was perfect. All I need to do now is to make a miracle happen. I'll be back, so please wait here for me.*

Ns *Yes. Of course, I'll wait for you here.*

Pt *Excellent!*

I promised Ms. Iwata that I would see her again and leave the room. A few days later, Ms. was transferred to a hospice near her home and peacefully passed away about a month later.

In this case study, Ms. Iwata understood that her incurable disease was progressing but resisted accepting it. She was trapped when her doctor recommended that she stop anticancer treatment and be transferred to hospice or palliative care. It was then that a nurse approached her and brought hope for the future. Ms. Iwata was aware that her condition was severe and that her death was imminent. However, simultaneously, she believed in miracles and wished to be the master of her own life until the end. The nurse carefully assessed the patient through detailed dialogues and made suggestions based on a well-targeted care plan to gain the patient's trust. The nurse supported Ms. Iwata's attempt to live her life to the fullest in her way and aimed to bring spiritual healing to her through care practices that encouraged her spiritual work.

4 Efforts Expected of Healthcare Professionals in Spiritual Care

4.1 Provide Care That Creates Spiritual Healing

The patient–caregiver relationship, the force that promotes spiritual healing, is woven through a process of care in which caregivers devote themselves to understanding patients' anger, sadness, and despair behind their stories by being present and listening to them. A compassionate relationship is created where the patient feels 'known', and the caregiver seeks to further understand by taking a genuine interest in the patient. The caregiver must be willing to stand beside and share the patient's experiences to understand what is important to them. However, in palliative care settings, patients and professionals often have different values that can pose a dilemma for healthcare professionals. Caregivers must quietly listen to their inner voices and try to understand themselves without denying their feelings. Thus, spiritual care providers must always provide patient care while seeking to understand themselves more deeply.

4.2 Spiritual Care Through a Team Approach

Patients with serious illnesses are forced to confront their illnesses, re-examine their values, and search for ways to live their remaining time, which is a worldwide experience. Some patients feel that professional care is essential for their spiritual pain, whereas others may not wish to address it. Therefore, the following careful care delivery is desirable in any country or regional setting in the world: 1. the ability to appropriately assess the patient's spiritual pain along with unique circumstances and cultural or religious backgrounds; 2. careful consideration of what spiritual care should be provided to the patient according to the results of the assessment; and 3. a system in which doctors, nurses, chaplains, and other healthcare professionals can collaborate to provide a tailor-made multidisciplinary team approach.

In Japan, several academic societies and associations have collaborated to prepare for certification of 'spiritual caregivers'. Nonetheless, the system for them to engage as professionals in the medical field has not yet fully developed. In many countries, such as Japan, the positions of professionals who provide spiritual care may be uncertain.

All professionals involved in palliative care worldwide should be aware of the roles they can play in their positions, regardless of whether they have professional qualifications to provide spiritual care. Healthcare providers should devote more efforts in the future to further improve the practice of healing spiritual pain experienced by their patients, whether they are religious or not. Such diversity-aware individual professionalism will enhance the quality of spiritual care and thus palliative care, worldwide, ensuring equal access and well-being for patients. It is hoped that there will be more active discussions on who, when, and how to provide quality spiritual care to those who need it.

References

1. McClain CS, Rosenfeld B, Breitbart W. Effect of spiritual well-being on end-of-life despair in terminally-ill cancer patients. Lancet. 2003;361(9369):1603–7.
2. Breitbart W, Rosenfeld B, Pessin H, Applebaum A, Kulikowski J, Lichtenthal WG. Meaning-centered group psychotherapy: an effective intervention for improving psychological Well-being in patients with advanced cancer. J Clin Oncol. 2015;33(7):749–54.
3. Balboni TA, VanderWeele TJ, Doan-Soares SD, Long KNG, Ferrell BR, Fitchett G, et al. Spirituality in serious illness and health. JAMA. 2022;328(2):184–97.
4. VandeCreek L, Burton L. Professional chaplaincy: its role and importance in healthcare. The Journal of pastoral care. 2001;55(1):81–97.
5. Inglehart RF. Giving up on god: the global decline of religion. Foreign Aff. 2020;99(5):110.
6. Kavanagh CM, Jong J. Is Japan religious? Journal for the Study of Religion Nature and Culture. 2020;14(1):152–80.
7. Shirahama K, Inoue EM. Spirituality in nursing from a Japanese perspective. Holist Nurs Pract. 2001;15(3):63–72.
8. Ammerman NT. Spiritual but not religious? Beyond binary choices in the study of religion. J Sci Stud Relig. 2013;52(2):258–78.
9. Benedict TO. Spiritual ends – religion and the heart of dying in Japan. Oakland: University of California Press; 2023.
10. Delgado-Guay MO, Hui D, Parsons HA, Govan K, De la Cruz M, Thorney S, et al. Spirituality, religiosity, and spiritual pain in advanced cancer patients. J Pain Symptom Manag. 2011;41(6):986–94.
11. Sakashita A, Kizawa Y, Kato M, Akizuki N, Nakazawa Y, Kaizu M, et al. Development of a standard for hospital-based palliative care consultation teams in Japan using a modified Delphi method. J Pain Symptom Manag. 2018;56(5):746–51.e5.
12. Shimazono S. Development of spiritual care in cancer treatment in Japan. Gan To Kagaku Ryoho. 2017;44(1):1–6.

13. Morita T, Murata H, Kishi E, Miyashita M, Yamaguchi T, Uchitomi Y. Meaninglessness in terminally ill cancer patients: a randomized controlled study. J Pain Symptom Manag. 2009;37(4):649–58.
14. Morita T, Tamura K, Kusajima E, Sakai S, Kawa M, Imura C, et al. Nurse education program on meaninglessness in terminally ill cancer patients: a randomized controlled study of a novel two-day workshop. J Palliat Med. 2014;17(12):1298–305.
15. Okamoto T, Ando M, Morita T, Hirai K, Kawamura R, Miyashita M, et al. Religious care required for Japanese terminally ill patients with cancer from the perspective of bereaved family members. Am J Hosp Palliat Care. 2010;27(1):50–4.
16. Ando M, Fau KR, Morita T, Fau MT, Hirai K, Fau HK, Miyashita M, Fau MM, Okamoto T, Fau OT, Shima Y, et al. Value of religious care for relief of psycho-existential suffering in Japanese terminally ill cancer patients: the perspective of bereaved family members. Psychooncology. 2010;19(7):750–5.
17. Murata H. Spiritual pain and its care in patients with terminal cancer: construction of a conceptual framework by philosophical approach. Palliat Support Care. 2003;1(1):15–21.
18. Naito AS, Morita T, Tamura K, Oya K, Matsuda Y, Tagami K, et al. Beliefs about spiritual pain among palliative care physicians and liaison psychiatrists: a nationwide questionnaire survey. Palliative Care Research. 2021;16(2):115–22.
19. Murata H. Spiritual pain and its care in patients with terminal cancer. Journal of Japan Society of Pain Clinicians. 2011;18(1):1–8.
20. Tamura K, Maetaki E, Ichihara K. Assessing and care planning for spiritual pain. In: Tamura K, Kawa M, Morita T, editors. Kango ni ikasu spiritual care no tebiki. 2. 2 ed. Tokyo, Japan: Seikai sya; 2017. p. 27–49.
21. Tamura K, Ichihara K, Maetaki E, Takayama K, Tanisawa K, Ikenaga M. Development of a spiritual pain assessment sheet for terminal cancer patients: targeting terminal cancer patients admitted to palliative care units in Japan. Palliat Support Care. 2006;4(2):179–88.
22. Ichihara K, Ouchi S, Okayama S, Kinoshita F, Miyashita M, Morita T, et al. Effectiveness of spiritual care using spiritual pain assessment sheet for advanced cancer patients: a pilot non-randomized controlled trial. Palliative and Supportive Care. 2019;17(1):46–53.
23. Ichihara K, Nishiyama C, Kiyohara K, Morita T, Tamura K. Nursing care for spiritual pain in terminal cancer patients: a non-randomized controlled trial. J Pain Symptom Manage. 2024;67(2):126–37. https://doi.org/10.1016/j.jpainsymman.2023.10.016.

Part III
Impact

Impact of Spiritual Care on Patient Outcomes at the End of Life

Winifred Belk and Tracy A. Balboni

Abstract Spirituality plays an important role in the experience of illness for most patients, including its influence on patient well-being and the frequent presence of spiritual needs. Furthermore, spirituality impacts end-of-life medical decision-making. As a result of its multifaceted role in serious illness, spiritual care—recognition of and attention to patient spirituality within care—is a core domain of palliative care. Spiritual care is the responsibility of the multidisciplinary care team that is based on the generalist-specialist spiritual care model. Spiritual care, when present, is associated with improved outcomes for patient and families. Spiritual care is associated with better patient and family quality of life, and care satisfaction. It is also associated with a greater rate of transition to hospice care and less aggressive interventions at the end of life. Spiritual care remains infrequent at the end of life, with the frequent lack of spiritual care training for clinicians being a key factor. Further efforts are required to improve education in spiritual care and its integration into the care of patients and families with serious illness.

Keywords Palliative care · Spirituality · Religiousness · Spiritual care · Chaplaincy Medical decision-making · Quality of life

---

W. Belk (✉)
University of Rochester, Rochester, NY, USA

T. A. Balboni (✉)
Department of Radiation Oncology and Department of Psychosocial Oncology and Palliative Care, Dana-Farber, Brigham and Women's Cancer Center, Harvard Medical School, Boston, MA, USA
e-mail: tbalboni@bwh.harvard.edu

M. C. Best (ed.), *Spiritual Care in Palliative Care*,
https://doi.org/10.1007/978-3-031-50864-6_13

1 Introduction

Dame Cicely Saunders, founder of the palliative care movement in the United Kingdom in the 1960s, proposed a novel, multifaceted conception of pain in serious illness as impacting the physical, psychological, social, and spiritual aspects of the human person. This conceptualisation of 'total pain' necessitates care that recognises and addresses each of the four domains [1]. Research has shown spirituality, one of these four core domains, to play a crucial role in patient health outcomes [2]. Furthermore, spirituality plays a multifaceted role in the experience of serious illness. This includes helping patients find meaning, deepen their connectedness to self and community, and cope with serious illness [3]. Additionally, patients commonly experience spiritual needs [4], including spiritual/existential distress that has been demonstrated to have a detrimental effect on quality of life [5, 6]. And yet, only a minority of patients report having their spiritual needs met by medical teams [7].

The following chapter highlights the role of spirituality in patient experiences of illness by examining how it affects quality of life and medical decision-making, and how having unmet spiritual needs affects quality of life. Next, modes of recognition of and attention to spirituality in illness—or spiritual care—will be considered, including current spiritual care guidelines and delivery models. Also considered will be extant barriers to spiritual care provision that need to be addressed in order to render spiritual care a standard aspect of care in serious illness. Finally, research highlighting the impacts of spiritual care on end-of-life outcomes will be discussed.

2 Role of Spirituality in Serious Illness for Patients and Families

2.1 Importance of Spirituality in Serious Illness

Spirituality is important to most patients facing serious illness, with studies across various populations demonstrating its importance ranges from 71% to 99% [2]. Furthermore, spirituality functions in multiple ways within illness including: (1) as a means of coping; (2) fostering helpful and/or meaningful spiritual practices, such as prayer and meditation, in illness; (3) conferring spiritual beliefs that frame the understanding of illness; (4) bringing transformation in spiritual beliefs through illness; and (5) through the important supportive role of spiritual communities in illness [4]. Furthermore, measures of spirituality and spiritual well-being are associated with better patient quality of life [2, 8]. Spirituality and spiritual well-being have also been found to be positively associated with better mental health outcomes, including less anxiety, depression, end-of-life despair, and reduced desire to hasten death [9]. A number of studies have also shown positive associations between spirituality, physical health, and social well-being [10]. Though spirituality can often function in positive ways within illness, it can also be associated with negative impacts on well-being, in particular through spiritual needs, discussed next.

2.2 *Spiritual Needs in Serious Illness*

Spiritual needs—needs related to spirituality, including spiritual questions, concerns, or distress [2]—are common in serious illness, with rates among diverse populations of seriously ill patients ranging from 23% to 98% [2]. Unmet spiritual needs among seriously ill patients (e.g. seeking meaning in life, seeking forgiveness) have been found to be associated with poorer patient and family quality of life [9]. Negative religious coping, a form of religious struggle, has been associated with reduced patient quality of life [9]. Finally, a body of evidence examining 'spiritual pain' in both patients and family caregivers has shown it to be associated with poor quality of life outcomes [5, 10].

2.3 *Spirituality and Medical Decision-Making in Serious Illness*

A growing body of evidence indicates that patient spirituality affects healthcare decision-making, influencing the types of care seriously ill patients choose as well as the actual end-of-life care received [2]. Most typically, the influence of spirituality on decision-making has been associated with measures of religious beliefs and/or identification. For example, a multi-site study of 275 advanced cancer patients demonstrated that 87% endorse at least one of seven religious beliefs in end-of-life medical care [11]. Furthermore, endorsement of these beliefs was associated with reduced acceptance of the terminal nature of illness. Another large, multi-site cohort study of advanced cancer patients found that patients exhibiting high positive religious coping at baseline were more likely to receive aggressive medical interventions in the last week of life (e.g. hospitalisation in an intensive care unit, resuscitation) [12]. Furthermore, a study including 317 intensive care unit patients from Czech Republic, Israel, Sweden, Portugal, The Netherlands, and United Kingdom found that religious patients more frequently wanted all measures to prolong life [13]. Similarly, in a study of 144 haemodialysis patients, religious activities were associated with greater preference for continued dialysis [14].

3 Spiritual Care Guidelines and the Generalist-Specialist Model of Spiritual Care in Serious Illness

Spiritual care is recognition of and attention to spirituality, including spiritual needs, within patient care [2, 3]. Despite the importance of spirituality, the frequency of spiritual needs, and the role of religious beliefs within illness, spiritual care is infrequent, with studies reporting that 9–51% of seriously ill patients do not receive any spiritual care. In contrast, 50–96% of seriously ill patients report desiring the integration of spiritual care within healthcare [2]. Herein, extant spiritual care guidelines will be described, including the generalist-specialist model of spiritual care, and then barriers to implementing the core element of care in serious illness will be considered.

3.1 Spiritual Care Guidelines

The United States' National Consensus Project for Quality recognises spiritual care as one of eight core palliative care domains, framing a comprehensive guideline for integrating spiritual care within medicine [15]. The generalist-specialist model undergirds these guidelines and includes spiritual care specialists, professionally trained spiritual care practitioners (e.g. chaplains), and other healthcare team members (e.g. doctors, nurses, social workers, etc.) who act as spiritual care generalists.

3.2 Generalist Spiritual Care

The role of the spiritual care generalist involves spiritual history-taking and screening; recognising and addressing patient spirituality, values, and needs within their experience of illness; making referrals to professional spiritual care where required; and supporting a patient's spiritual care plan. Caring for the patient's spirituality also requires the clinician to recognise their own spiritual beliefs and how they might impinge on the patient's. Spiritual care must always be patient-centred, honouring the patient's spirituality and beliefs and must never involve imposition of the healthcare practitioners' own beliefs.

3.3 Specialist Spiritual Care

Specialised spiritual care providers (e.g. chaplains, clergy) receive dedicated training in spiritual care provision. In North America and some other settings, healthcare chaplains in particular receive dedicated training for spiritual care in healthcare settings, termed 'clinical pastoral education' (CPE), though some clergy and other religious community leaders also undergo such dedicated training for spiritual care in this setting (see Chap. 31). Specialised spiritual care providers perform dedicated spiritual assessments of patients, craft spiritual care plans, provide spiritual practices, work with religious communities, and provide counsel and support to patients, families, and healthcare staff. Notably, there are other clinicians that have some overlapping roles with chaplains, for example, social workers and psychologists/psychiatrists with spiritual care training may also provide spiritual interventions to patients.

Chaplains' and other spiritual care providers' spiritual care assessments explore a patient's spiritual, religious, and existential concerns within their experience of illness. Furthermore, chaplains' spiritual care plans and spiritual interventions aim to address spiritual distress and support a patient's spiritual strengths. The most frequent spiritual interventions found in one study in the United States include prayers, blessings, faith affirmations, empathic listening, life review, and emotional support [16]. Additionally, chaplains play important roles in goals-of-care discussions, family meetings, palliative care meetings, and difficult conversations. Spiritual care providers also offer support for patient families. In order to integrate spiritual care into medical care, chaplains record spiritual assessments and spiritual plans and share these guides with the patient's medical team.

3.4 Barriers to Spiritual Care

Spiritual care is critical to improving patient experience of illness and helping them make decisions that are consistent with their core values. However, there are barriers to spiritual care provision in healthcare settings, and it is crucial to address these in order to continue improving patient experience.

Regarding barriers to generalist spiritual care provision, the clinician's perception of their role within patient care may sometimes come into conflict with spiritual care provision. For example, in a study of 339 nurses and physicians providing care to cancer patients, perceptions of their role in spiritual care were predictive of their actual spiritual care provision to cancer patients [17]. Fear of overstepping their professional role as well as a concern about unequal power dynamics between clinicians and patients were also found to be frequent barriers preventing spiritual care provision [18]. These concerns were more frequently reported by physicians than nurses. Lack of time and lack of private space were also often named as barriers impacting the clinicians' ability to provide spiritual care to patients. These barriers reflect how institutional structures can devalue spiritual care. These findings highlight how the integration of spiritual care requires the attention, not only of palliative care teams, but also of hospital administration. It is therefore crucial to consider the availability of time, facilities, and related financial issues when developing a spiritual care delivery model (see Chap. 43). Of all these barriers, the most commonly endorsed and strongest predictor of actual spiritual care provision is spiritual care training [7]. It is hence critical to incorporate appropriate training in medical education. Standard inclusion of spiritual care training in medical disciplines, and most importantly palliative care, is a crucial means of ensuring that the future spiritual needs of the patient can be provided for by clinicians (see Chap. 27).

Provision of specialist spiritual care also is wrought with barriers. Most notably is the frequent lack of professional spiritual care practitioners. The American Hospital Association 2021 survey of hospitals notes that in the United States about

30% of hospitals lack any spiritual care services [19]. Even among those 70% of hospitals, chaplaincy services are most typically limited to inpatient settings.

4 Spiritual Care and Outcomes in Serious Illness

Spiritual care is considered an integral component of palliative care, as illustrated by the American National Consensus Project guidelines [11]. However, spiritual care is frequently absent despite being desired by majorities of seriously ill patients [2]. Addressing barriers to spiritual care is one critical step towards spiritual care provision. Another key step is evidence that illustrates the impact of spiritual care on patient outcomes, and hence characterises the implications of the absence of spiritual care on quality of life and care outcomes. These include the relationship of spiritual care to quality of life in serious illness and spiritual care and medical care outcomes in serious illness.

4.1 Spiritual Care, Quality of Life, and Medical Care Outcomes

Evidence suggests that spiritual care provision by medical teams is associated with improved quality of life, greater satisfaction with care, and reduced futile, aggressive medical interventions at the end of life [2]. A large prospective multi-site study of advanced cancer patients in the United States found that patients reporting a higher support of their spiritual needs by medical specialists had better quality of life at the end of life ($p = 0.007$) [20]. Another large study of religiously diverse cancer patients found that patients whose spiritual needs were met had higher ratings of their care quality and care satisfaction, whereas correspondingly those whose spiritual needs were not met had lower ratings [4]. A prospective study of advanced cancer patients in South Africa found that patients receiving spiritual care in the clinical setting (only 40%) had less pain and were more likely to die at home [21]. Family members of patients who died in the intensive care unit setting also reported greater satisfaction with care when their loved ones had received spiritual care from a chaplain during the intensive care unit stay [22]. Additionally, as previously described, spirituality influences medical decision-making and care received at the end of life. Spiritual care, recognition of the role of spirituality in illness and attention to spiritual needs, appears to interface with this relationship and be conducive to transitions to more quality-of-life focused care. One study of 343 advanced cancer patients from seven hospitals across the United States demonstrated that patients reporting high support of their spiritual needs by their medical team (e.g. physicians, nurses, chaplains) had greater transitions to hospice care and less aggressive medical interventions (e.g. intensive care unit admission and death) at the end of life [7].

4.2 Spiritual Care Interventions and Patient Outcomes

Studies demonstrating associations of spiritual care with quality of life and medical care outcomes have led to studies examining spiritual care interventions as means of improving patient outcomes in the setting of illness. Such studies can be broadly categorised as studies examining: (1) the integration of spiritual care within clinical care, (2) psychotherapeutic, and (3) mind–body interventions.

Interventions Examining Spiritual Care within Clinical Care Studies have examined the integration of spiritual care elements (e.g. spiritual histories, chaplain referrals, etc.) within clinical care. For example, one study examined the impact of structured assessments of patients' spiritual concerns by oncologists at the time of an office visit [23]. In total, 118 patients were alternately assigned to receive the semi-structured intervention or to receive usual care, with 76% indicating that the inquiry was at least somewhat useful. At 3 weeks post-intervention, the intervention group had greater reductions in depressive symptoms ($p < 0.01$), more improvement in quality of life ($p < 0.05$) and improved sense of interpersonal connection with the physician ($p < 0.05$).

Additionally, a body of literature has examined spiritual care as a core component of palliative care intervention studies, consistently showing improved quality of life and decreased healthcare utilisation among seriously ill patient populations [10]. For example, one prospective study examined an interdisciplinary palliative care intervention that addressed patient physical, psychological, social, and spiritual well-being, in comparison to usual care, among 491 lung cancer patients. The study found that the intervention group had better quality of life ($p < 0.001$), lower psychological distress ($p < 0.001$), better spiritual well-being ($p < 0.001$), and better symptom control ($p < 0.001$). The intervention group also had greater completion of advance directives ($p < 0.001$). Given that spiritual care is integrated within a larger framework of palliative care provision, the specific impact of spiritual care on these outcomes is unclear. However, these studies do suggest that spiritual care is a core component of palliative care provision that impacts these patient well-being outcomes.

Psychotherapeutic Interventions Psychotherapeutic interventions that have been studied among patients include meaning-based psychotherapy and life review intervention. Meaning-based psychotherapy, such as Breitbart and colleagues' Individual Meaning-Centred Psychotherapy, is an intervention based on Viktor Frankl's existential logotherapy [24] aiming to enhance patient meaning. Studies of this intervention have shown positive associations with patient quality of life. For example, a prospective study of 120 cancer patients randomly assigned to receive the Individual Meaning-centred Psychotherapy intervention versus therapeutic massage control showed improvements in spiritual well-being ($p < 0.001$) and quality of life ($p = 0.01$) for the intervention group at 2 months [25]. Life review is a psycho-spiritual intervention that involves the recalling, evaluating, and integrating life experiences to preserve and enhance dignity. A meta-analysis of various life review intervention studies among international populations (Australia, Canada, China, Iran, Japan, Netherlands, Norway, Portugal, United Kingdom, and the United States) found that interventions were associated with improved existential well-being for advanced cancer patients [26]. Similarly, a meta-analysis of randomised trials examining life review interventions among seriously ill patient populations from China, Japan, United Kingdom, and the United States showed improvements in measures of depression, self-esteem, and purpose in life among patients receiving the intervention [27].

Mind–body Interventions Mind body interventions largely involve the testing of mindfulness-based stress reduction (MBSR) or other forms as meditation to improve patient well-being. Such interventions have had inconsistent outcomes. A Cochrane review of MBSR interventions among ill patients found no improvements in quality of life outcomes among intervention versus control patients [28]. Another study randomly assigned 83 cancer patients to spiritually focused meditation as compared to secularly focused meditation, with the spiritually focused meditation patients having reduced depression ($p = 0.02$) and increased positive affect ($p < 0.001$) compared with the control group [29].

5 Conclusions and Future Directions

In summary, spirituality has a critical role in serious illness, with implications for quality of life, frequent spiritual needs, and a role in influencing end-of-life medical decision-making. Spiritual care guidelines informing care at the end-of-life call for the standard integration of spiritual care into medical care for the seriously ill. Spiritual care provision is based on the generalist-specialist model, where non-professional practitioners of spiritual care (e.g. physicians, nurses, social workers) play the role of spiritual care generalists, including spiritual history-taking and screening. Spiritual care specialists are trained spiritual care practitioners who provide in depth spiritual assessment, build and implement spiritual care plans, and interface with spiritual communities outside the healthcare settings. Spiritual care, despite extant guidelines, is infrequent in the care of seriously ill patients. However, when spiritual care is present, it is associated with better quality of life and improved medical care outcomes for patients and families. The most common and influential barrier to spiritual care provision is the frequent lack of spiritual care training for clinicians. The evidence base examining the impact of spiritual care interventions on outcomes demonstrates that these interventions improved patient's quality of life outcomes. Future efforts are required to improve education in spiritual care and to determine best models for the standard integration of spiritual care in the care of patients with serious illness.

References

1. Saunders C. The symptomatic treatment of incurable malignant disease. Prescribers J. 1964;4(4):68–73.
2. Balboni TA, VanderWeele TJ, Doan-Soares SD, et al. Spirituality in Serious Illness and Health [published correction appears in JAMA. 2022;328(8):780]. JAMA. 2022;328(2):184–97. https://doi.org/10.1001/jama.2022.11086.
3. Alcorn SR, Balboni MJ, Prigerson HG, et al. "If God wanted me yesterday, I wouldn't be here today": religious and spiritual themes in patients' experiences of advanced cancer. J Palliat Med. 2010;13(5):581–8. https://doi.org/10.1089/jpm.2009.0343.
4. Astrow AB, Kwok G, Sharma RK, Fromer N, Sulmasy DP. Spiritual Needs and Perception of Quality of Care and Satisfaction With Care in Hematology/Medical Oncology Patients: A Multicultural Assessment. J Pain Symptom Manag. 2018;55(1):56–64.e1. https://doi.org/10.1016/j.jpainsymman.2017.08.009.
5. Delgado-Guay MO, Palma A, Duarte E, et al. Association between Spirituality, Religiosity, Spiritual Pain, Symptom Distress, and Quality of Life among Latin American Patients with Advanced Cancer: A Multicenter Study. J Palliat Med. 2021;24(11):1606–15. https://doi.org/10.1089/jpm.2020.0776.
6. Delgado-Guay MO, Chisholm G, Williams J, Frisbee-Hume S, Ferguson AO, Bruera E. Frequency, intensity, and correlates of spiritual pain in advanced cancer patients assessed in a supportive/palliative care clinic. Palliat Support Care. 2016;14(4):341–8. https://doi.org/10.1017/S147895151500108X.
7. Balboni MJ, Sullivan A, Amobi A, et al. Why is spiritual care infrequent at the end of life? Spiritual care perceptions among patients, nurses, and physicians and the role of training. J Clin Oncol. 2013;31(4):461–7. https://doi.org/10.1200/JCO.2012.44.6443.
8. Steinhauser KE, Christakis NA, Clipp EC, McNeilly M, McIntyre L, Tulsky JA. Factors considered important at the end of life by patients, family, physicians, and other care providers. JAMA. 2000;284(19):2476–82. https://doi.org/10.1001/jama.284.19.2476.
9. Steinhauser KE, Fitchett G, Handzo GF, et al. State of the science of spirituality and palliative care research part I: definitions, measurement, and outcomes. J Pain Symptom Manag. 2017;54(3):428–40. https://doi.org/10.1016/j.jpainsymman.2017.07.028.
10. Balboni TA, Fitchett G, Handzo GF, Johnson KS, Koenig HG, Pargament KI, Puchalski CM, Sinclair S, Taylor EJ, Steinhauser KE. State of the Science of Spirituality and Palliative Care Research Part II: Screening, Assessment, and Interventions. J Pain Symptom Manag. 2017;54(3):441–53.
11. Balboni TA, Prigerson HG, Balboni MJ, Enzinger AC, VanderWeele TJ, Maciejewski PK. A scale to assess religious beliefs in end-of-life medical care. Cancer. 2019;125(9):1527–35. https://doi.org/10.1002/cncr.31946.
12. Phelps AC, Maciejewski PK, Nilsson M, et al. Religious coping and use of intensive life-prolonging care near death in patients with advanced cancer. JAMA. 2009;301(11):1140–7. https://doi.org/10.1001/jama.2009.341.
13. Bülow HH, Sprung CL, Baras M, et al. Are religion and religiosity important to end-of-life decisions and patient autonomy in the ICU? The Ethicatt study. Intensive Care Med. 2012;38(7):1126–33. https://doi.org/10.1007/s00134-012-2554-8.
14. Pruchno RA, Lemay EP Jr, Feild L, Levinsky NG. Predictors of patient treatment preferences and spouse substituted judgments: the case of dialysis continuation. Med Decis Mak. 2006;26(2):112–21. https://doi.org/10.1177/0272989X06286482.
15. National Consensus Project for Quality Palliative Care. Palliative care guidelines. 4th ed. https://www.nationalcoalitionhpc.org/ncp/. Accessed 21 Sept 2023.
16. Handzo GF, Flannelly KJ, Kudler T, et al. What do chaplains really do? II. Interventions in the New York Chaplaincy Study. J Health Care Chaplain. 2008;14(1):39–56. https://doi.org/10.1080/08854720802053853.

17. Rodin D, Balboni M, Mitchell C, Smith PT, VanderWeele TJ, Balboni TA. Whose role? Oncology practitioners' perceptions of their role in providing spiritual care to advanced cancer patients. Support Care Cancer. 2015;23(9):2543–50. https://doi.org/10.1007/s00520-015-2611-2.
18. Balboni MJ, Sullivan A, Enzinger AC, et al. Nurse and physician barriers to spiritual care provision at the end of life. J Pain Symptom Manag. 2014;48(3):400–10. https://doi.org/10.1016/j.jpainsymman.2013.09.020.
19. American Association of Medical Colleges. Is there a chaplain in the house? Hospitals integrate spiritual care. November 20, 2017. https://www.aamc.org/news/there-chaplain-house-hospitals-integrate-spiritual-care. Accessed 21 Sep 2023.
20. Balboni TA, Paulk ME, Balboni MJ, et al. Provision of spiritual care to patients with advanced cancer: associations with medical care and quality of life near death. J Clin Oncol. 2010;28(3):445–52. https://doi.org/10.1200/JCO.2009.24.8005.
21. Ratshikana-Moloko M, Ayeni O, Tsitsi JM, et al. Spiritual care, pain reduction, and preferred place of death among advanced cancer patients in Soweto, South Africa. J Pain Symptom Manag. 2020;60(1):37–47. https://doi.org/10.1016/j.jpainsymman.2020.01.019.
22. Johnson JR, Engelberg RA, Nielsen EL, et al. The association of spiritual care providers' activities with family members' satisfaction with care after a death in the ICU*. Crit Care Med. 2014;42(9):1991–2000. https://doi.org/10.1097/CCM.0000000000000412.
23. Kristeller JL, Rhodes M, Cripe LD, Sheets V. Oncologist assisted spiritual intervention study (OASIS): patient acceptability and initial evidence of effect. Int J Psychiatry Med. 2005;35(4):329–47.
24. Frankl VE. The doctor and the soul: from psychotherapy to logotherapy. New York: Vintage Books; 1986.
25. Breitbart W, Poppito S, Rosenfeld B, et al. Pilot randomized controlled trial of individual meaning-centered psychotherapy for patients with advanced cancer. J Clin Oncol. 2012;30(12):1304–9.
26. Bauereiß N, Obermaier S, Özünal SE, Baumeister H. Effects of existential interventions on spiritual, psychological, and physical well-being in adult patients with cancer: Systematic review and meta-analysis of randomized controlled trials. Psychooncology. 2018;27(11):2531–45. https://doi.org/10.1002/pon.4829.
27. Chen Y, Xiao H, Yang Y, Lan X. The effects of life review on psychospiritual well-being among patients with life-threatening illness: a systematic review and meta-analysis. J Adv Nurs. 2017;73(7):1539–54. https://doi.org/10.1111/jan.13208.
28. Candy B, Jones L, Varagunam M, Speck P, Tookman A, King M. Spiritual and religious interventions for well-being of adults in the terminal phase of disease. Cochrane Database Syst Rev. 2012;(5):CD007544.
29. Cole BHC, Spiegel J, Tisak J, Agarwala S, Kirkwood JM. A randomised clinical trial of the effects of spiritually focused meditation for people with metastatic melanoma. Ment Health Relig Cult. 2012;15(2):161–74.

Spirituality and Pain Management in Palliative Care

Philip D. Austin and Melanie R. Lovell

Abstract Pain is a common symptom in palliative care settings. It can be difficult to control due to the complex interaction of physical, psychological, social, and spiritual dimensions. Spiritual distress can have a profound effect on pain severity. The corollary is that spiritual and religious practices can play a significant role in pain relief. This chapter first explores the impact of spirituality on pain perception and the effects of spiritual distress on pain severity and then discusses spiritual coping strategies and how they positively influence pain outcomes. The chapter explores spiritual and pain outcome tools commonly used in palliative care settings before reviewing current evidence for the use of spiritual care interventions for pain control. It concludes with some reflections arising from current research and the need for further research in this field.

Keywords Spirituality · Spiritual care · Pain management · Analgesia · Palliative care · End-of-life care

1 Introduction

Managing pain is a challenge in all areas of healthcare and is markedly compounded when people are faced with life-limiting disease. Pain is experienced by over 65% of people receiving palliative care and in end-of-life settings [1, 2]. Indeed, current data shows increases in pain prevalence and severity in people with late-stage cancers, renal disease, congestive heart failure and chronic obstructive airways disease

P. D. Austin (✉) · M. R. Lovell
Palliative Care, HammondCare, Sydney, NSW, Australia
e-mail: paustin@hammond.com.au; mlovell@hammond.com.au

M. C. Best (ed.), *Spiritual Care in Palliative Care*,
https://doi.org/10.1007/978-3-031-50864-6_14

[2, 3]. Pain in palliative care remains undertreated across developed and developing regions [4]. Pain is caused by the noxious effects of life-limiting diseases, their treatments including chemotherapy and surgery, comorbid disease such as osteoarthritis and migraine [5] and complications including deep vein thrombosis and pulmonary embolism [6]. In malignant disease, pain is most often associated with neural compression, bone metastases, obstruction, and infiltration of soft tissues [7]. Psychosocial and spiritual factors also significantly contribute to the experience of pain. Psychological morbidity and spiritual factors relating to fear and mood, poor social support and reliance on caregivers are all shown to significantly increase pain severity and pain-related disability. These multifactorial mechanisms further generate acute transient flare ups of ongoing pain known as *breakthrough pain* [8].

Freedom from the burden of pain is constantly rated as one of the most important factors in palliative and end-of-life settings by patients, their families and healthcare workers [9]. Thus, pain management is essential to relieve the physical and psycho-spiritual suffering of people with life-limiting disease. Additionally, palliative care patients with uncontrolled pain often present to Emergency Departments, where nearly one in ten visits are from people in the last months of life [10]. The complexity of the management of people with late-stage disease who are suffering pain is particularly challenging for healthcare professionals, especially when they are at the end of life and require admission to acute care.

Spiritual distress in terminal illness is a stressful experience for patients and their families. Distressing experiences associated with life-limiting disease are felt physically with symptoms including pain, nausea, and dyspnoea but also with negative feelings such as depression, social isolation and spiritual suffering. Although clinical assessment and support for physical, emotional and social suffering are common, attention to spiritual distress is still the most neglected component of palliative care [11, 12]. For people with terminal illness facing early death, spiritual distress is often experienced along with increases in pain severity, a loss of meaning and purpose, and significant disruption to their personal beliefs and values [13, 14].

Spirituality and religious beliefs are important for many people and fundamental to their quality of life. Spirituality involves a person's search for meaning and purpose in life and the experience of the transcendent [15]. People receiving palliative care may experience loss of meaning and purpose in life. Pain and suffering are either hidden or not recognised by caregivers, thus leaving them feeling alone and isolated [16]. People may lose their role at work, in the community or in the family, roles which had previously given them meaning. Impact of illness on the body through surgery, or disfigurement caused by disease or cachexia can be another source of loss of identity. People may question why God has allowed their suffering or experience a sense of abandonment by God causing profound existential distress.

Patients prefer their spiritual needs to be addressed or at least acknowledged by healthcare and pastoral care teams. Recognition and the assessment of a person's spiritual needs are essential in helping care teams to not only understand patients' behaviours but additionally to help guide more suitable options for symptom relief and wellbeing [17]. What is certain is that spirituality is interwoven into every experience of people with life-limiting disease from questioning meaning in their lives to approaching death to caregiver dynamics and pain management.

In clinical settings including palliative care, people with greater levels of spirituality and religiosity show higher levels of wellbeing, lower levels of mood disturbance, lower pain severity and greater tolerance of pain [18]. Indeed, several authors also suggest that spiritual wellbeing is now considered one of the most important positive influences on quality of life and pain management [12, 19]. Therefore, in this chapter, we explore spirituality, pain, patient assessment and the role of spirituality in the management of pain in palliative care settings.

2 Spirituality, Pain Perception and Pain Modulation

Pain is defined by the International Association for the Study of Pain as an unpleasant sensory and emotional experience associated with actual or potential tissue damage [20]. Pain is complex and involves a number of behavioural responses, thoughts, and emotions. Non-physical factors, including psychological and social attitudes, life stressors and cultural beliefs, play key roles in how people experience pain [21]. People living with pain report increases in pain severity that are related to disability, depression, anxiety, and fear. Additionally, the beliefs and attitudes of caregivers towards pain can either positively or negatively affect pain severity in patients [22].

Spiritual and religious beliefs further influence pain perception that at times can either increase or decrease pain severity depending on life's meaning, self-efficacy, acceptance of diagnosis, guilt, conflict, and worry [15]. Many people experiencing pain use spirituality and religious practices including prayer, meditation, and engagement with community members to help cope with their pain experience, reduce pain intensity and decrease the negative effects of pain on daily life [18, 21, 23]. These findings have been shown in longitudinal studies where positive spiritual and religious beliefs are associated with lower pain scores [18, 24]. Conversely, negative spiritual and religious coping such as feeling abandoned by God and other spiritual struggles with life meaning are associated with an increase in pain severity [25, 26]. Interestingly, as people age, they are more likely to engage in spiritual beliefs, religious practices and the experience of forgiveness to manage their pain [21, 25].

Importantly, people with positive religious beliefs have been shown objectively to downregulate the perceived intensity of noxious inputs when presented with religious images. In their seminal work, Wiech and colleagues assessed the intensity of noxious electrical stimulation for practising Catholics and acknowledged atheists and agnostics using functional magnetic resonance imaging (fMRI). The religious group reported being in a calm and meditative state while also reporting significant reductions in subjective pain intensity when shown an image with religious content (the Virgin Mary) compared to being shown a non-religious pleasant image. The non-religious group rated their pain as equally intense for both images. Correspondingly, fMRI imaging showed that the right ventrolateral prefrontal cortex, a key area of the brain implicated in cognitive down-modulation of pain, was specifically activated only when the religious group viewed the religious image [27]. These findings suggest that people with religious beliefs are not intrinsically less sensitive to pain but are able to modulate their experience of pain based on cognitive reappraisal of the negative influence of their pain.

People receiving palliative care often experience uncontrolled and complex pain to the point where they are no longer able to cope. Patients subsequently question their beliefs, the loss of meaning and purpose in life, hope and their faith in others. They suffer spiritual and psychological distress that is often not recognised or addressed. Poignantly, Victor Frankl asserts that 'man is not destroyed by suffering: he is destroyed by suffering without meaning' [28]. It is therefore imperative that healthcare professionals realise that approaches focusing on alleviating physical pain only will no longer be adequate and that managing pain in palliative care settings requires the acknowledgement of individuals' spiritual needs.

3 Spiritual Distress and Pain Severity

Current evidence shows a positive relationship between increased levels of spiritual distress and physical pain severity [29]. However, the physical assessment and management of pain frequently take preference over assessment and interventions for spiritual distress in people receiving treatment across many pain settings [30, 31]. In chronic non-malignant pain settings, spiritual distress is shown to be related not only to the exacerbation of pain, but also to the way people cognitively process pain (*catastrophising*) and how pain interferes in important aspects of their daily lives [30]. Conversely, those people reporting higher levels of meaning and faith with lower levels of pain catastrophising show greater levels of pain reduction in pain management programmes with a meaning-based component [32]. Thus, findings suggest that spiritual distress plays a key role in maintaining chronic pain, impairing daily function and increasing emotional feelings including sadness, hopelessness, regret, anger, guilt, and anxiety [33, 34].

Although it is acknowledged that spiritual distress contributes significantly to the experience of pain in people nearing the end of life, it is inadequately addressed [29]. Cross-sectional data from cancer populations show that at least one spiritual need is reported in up to nearly 80% of patients, while up to 44% report spiritual distress [34, 35]. Unfortunately, current evidence shows that up to 70% of patients receiving end-of-life care receive little or no support for their spiritual needs [36]. Indeed, in palliative care settings, people with greater levels of spiritual distress report more severe physical and emotional symptoms including physical pain [37]. Conversely, intractable pain due to life-limiting disease can also intensify negative psychospiritual distress. Thus, if patients report physical pain, screening of both spiritual and other psychosocial variables is essential for implementation of more effective pain management.

4 Spiritual Coping Practices and Pain Severity

Identifying and addressing spiritual needs helps people with terminal illness to cope with pain and other symptoms, including depression and fatigue, by re-evaluating the experience of their disease [19, 38]. Evidence now shows that certain spiritual and religious factors and practices play a significant role in pain relief by helping people to cope and face their illness and death. Indeed, people in palliative care with higher levels of spiritual wellbeing report lower levels of pain severity and pain interference [8], while importantly, those seeking spiritual care and support report more severe pain, depression, and stress [39].

Spiritual and religious coping strategies shown to positively influence pain outcomes in palliative care settings include connection to religious figures or higher powers, forgiveness, prayer, meditation, relaxation practices and connection with family [40, 41]. These beliefs and connections positively relate to benefits such as meaning and purpose in life, compassion towards others, a source of strength, and, importantly, less uncertainty, feeling informed and experiencing autonomy with decisions relating to care planning [41, 42]. Additionally, positive expectations, especially optimism and/or acceptance, have been shown to be a novel target for spiritually related pain management [24, 43]. For example, Mystakidou and colleagues found that people who are spiritually prepared and welcome their death face their journey in a more relaxed way and thus report increases in pain tolerance and reduced anxiety [43]. Healthcare professionals should be aware of patients' spiritual and religious needs and practices and how they use their spirituality to cope with their pain [44]. For example, some people may favour prayer or meditation as a form of pain relief, while others may prefer connection or finding peace with family and friends [45].

Spiritual and religious beliefs are also associated with maladaptive pain coping strategies. Many people with advanced cancer and/or receiving palliative care struggle with negative spiritual coping (feeling punished or abandoned by God) which is associated with increases in spiritual, physical, and psychological distress [46]. Studies also report several misconceptions including beliefs that: (1) one should refuse pain medication; (2) pain must be addressed with spirituality alone and that taking medication is going against God's will; (3) pain is part of spiritual growth and therefore must not be relieved; and (4) pain is a sign of weak faith [40]. Thus, palliative care clinicians and chaplains should first assess patients' current beliefs and prior coping strategies that increase pain severity before introducing and discussing new cognitive, emotional and existential/spiritual coping strategies that are consistent with patients' spiritual and religious beliefs [47].

5 Assessment of Spirituality and Pain Severity in Palliative Care

To guide pain management, it is important to elicit associations between spiritual domains and pain severity. Many studies show the importance of assessment of spiritual domains. A consensus report from Puchalski and colleagues recommended that spiritual assessments should be considered a vital sign and included in care planning because of the impact on pain and other health outcomes [48]. This report identifies several spiritual factors that are important for patient evaluation including religious beliefs, practices, and values, spiritual goals, and assessment of spiritual distress. Thus, to understand associations between pain severity and spiritual domains, preliminary and subsequent routine screening of symptoms including pain and spiritual domains is recommended [48].

5.1 Evaluation of Pain Severity

Pain severity is difficult to assess as it is purely subjective and thus depends only on a person's perception [45]. Describing pain requires a degree of self-awareness that is influenced by cultural and spiritual background and, in palliative care settings, is compounded by emotional, social, and spiritual challenges [49]. Not surprisingly, there is little consensus on a common pain assessment tool that contains all relevant dimensions defined by palliative care experts [50]. Moreover, pain assessment and management in palliative care is not documented consistently, especially in community settings [51].

In clinical settings, pain severity is usually assessed using numerical and/or verbal pain scales [52, 53]. However, unidimensional pain scales do not elicit the magnitude of effect on emotions, maladaptive beliefs and of course, spiritual distress or vice versa. In chronic non-malignant pain settings, spiritual and religious distresses are shown to be associated with increased pain catastrophising, pain interference and pain self-efficacy [25, 30, 54]. Thus, it is more useful to consider multidimensional pain assessment tools such as the *Brief Pain Inventory* that include scales assessing the impact of pain on constructs such as general activity, mood, wellbeing, and relationships [51, 55].

5.2 Evaluation of Spiritual Factors

There are several assessment tools that evaluate spiritual dimensions that have been used in meaning-based pain programmes for people with non-cancer pain [32, 56, 57]. These include tools such as the *Pain Solutions Questionnaire* that assesses meaningfulness of life despite pain [58] and *Functional Assessment of Chronic Illness Therapy-Spiritual Wellbeing-expanded* [59].

Helpfully, Lee and Newberg also outline several questions that are recommended by the American College of Physicians' Consensus Panel to assist inexperienced or untrained healthcare professionals which could be adapted for use in palliative care settings [60].

- Do you rely on your spiritual beliefs to help you cope with pain?
- How do your spiritual beliefs influence your care?
- Is faith (religion and spirituality) important to you in this illness?
- Are there any religious or spiritual issues that need addressing?
- Would you like to explore religious matters with someone?

Thus, recognising and exploring patients' spiritual needs help clinicians to develop and implement individualised pain management plans. Although current evidence is limited, several studies show significant benefit when integrating spiritual care interventions into the management of pain in palliative care settings [4].

6 Spiritual Care and Pain Management in Palliative Care

Spiritual care has been frequently shown to help people cope with spiritual distress in a range of clinical settings. Examples of religious and/or spiritual forms of coping include prayer, dignity therapy and spiritual support [32, 44, 61, 62]. Spiritual support is also effective in both reducing pain severity and increasing pain tolerance in cancer and non-malignant pain settings [4, 18, 63]. However, there is inadequate evidence regarding the effects of spiritual support for pain relief in people with advanced cancer and/or those receiving palliative care. The majority of studies focus on spiritual pain, spiritual needs, and coping with disease [12, 34, 64, 65], chronic non-malignant pain [25, 30, 44], and people with cancer pain receiving curative treatment [66, 67].

6.1 Spiritual and Religious Care

Spiritual care is defined as a more comprehensive approach where spiritual or pastoral carers try to be present to empower, to bring peace to patients and patients' relatives, while also including a combination of connection, creative, narrative, and ritual work as therapeutic interventions [12]. The analgesic effects of spiritual care have only recently been examined in palliative care settings. Firstly, in a prospective cohort study, Ratshikana-Moloko and colleagues investigated the effects of spiritual and religious care received by people in South Africa with advanced cancer at end of life compared to those who did not. Spiritual and religious needs which were addressed by spiritual councillors in this study included a desire for closer connection with their God(s), feeling abandoned by their God(s) and religious communities, and a desire for forgiveness for their sins. The authors compared baseline and last assessment data prior to death. They found that people who received religious and spiritual care reported significantly less pain, less morphine use, less family worry, and were more likely to die at home compared to people who received no religious and spiritual care [19].

In a further study, Sabet and co-workers investigated the effects of spirituality-based palliative care on pain, nausea, vomiting, and quality of life. In this Iranian study, the treatment group participated in four 120-min spiritual care sessions over one month while the control group received standard care. The treatment group took part in sessions that included individual support to encourage hope and peace through prayer, group sessions including rituals using prayer and meaningful writing, and counselling that encouraged participants to speak about their feelings, strengths, relationships, needs, and spiritual concerns. Findings showed significant within- and between-group differences for reductions in pain severity and interference, nausea, vomiting and quality of life [68]. These findings are consistent with similar work where spirituality is shown to be protective against pain and the burden of other symptoms [24, 69, 70].

6.2 Specific Spiritual Interventions

Only a few studies have investigated the effect of specific spiritual interventions on pain in people receiving palliative care and/or those with advanced cancer. In a recent systematic review, Hindmarsh and colleagues located several quantitative studies reporting significant improvements in cancer pain scores after receiving specific spiritual interventions [4]; however, only six studies recruited people in palliative care settings, of which only two showed meaningful pain relief.

Firstly, Lloyd-Williams and co-workers used a focused narrative intervention where therapists discussed sense of meaning and spiritual wellbeing with advanced cancer patients over an eight-week period. They showed that pain scores significantly improved in association with improvements in anxiety and depression [71]. Secondly, Warth and colleagues, using information from palliative care patient interviews, developed and performed songs with high biographical and religious relevance to each patient in a lullaby style [72]. Their findings showed modest to medium size improvements in pain scores, spiritual wellbeing and worry. Other spiritual interventions, including Dignity Therapy, have been investigated in palliative care settings. However, while these studies show improvements in quality of life, sense of purpose, sense of dignity and reduced suffering, they do not show any reductions in pain severity [62, 73–75].

Although some spiritual interventions show promise and are valued by patients and caregivers, the evidence base is still uncertain. For example, qualitative findings from Poletti and colleagues' mixed-method study suggest that a mindfulness-based stress reduction programme improves the ability to spiritually cope with pain rather than reduce pain severity and frequency [76]. However, given such spiritual interventions are well accepted and are found helpful by participants and caregivers, further high-quality mixed-method research using validated outcome assessment tools are required to gain both measurable and textual data.

Future research is needed regarding the impact of specific spiritual interventions on pain outcomes. The few studies investigating the effects of specific spiritual interventions such as Dignity Therapy and focused narrative interventions in palliative care settings show little or no benefit in reducing pain severity [4]. In contrast, prospective studies examining the effects of spiritual care for people receiving palliative care show significant reductions in pain severity in those receiving spiritual care compared to those who did not [19, 66]. Given these contradictory findings, further research is needed to understand whether specific components of spiritual care are more beneficial than others.

Promisingly, these findings do indicate that patients reporting spiritual needs or showing behaviours associated with spiritual distress would benefit from spiritual screening, assessment and care with the aim of reducing pain severity and improving in quality of life [17, 33]. High-quality research exploring the implementation of spiritual assessment and the effects of spiritual care on pain severity across palliative inpatient and community care settings is now required. Only then will we establish the potential role of therapeutic spiritual approaches for the management of pain in palliative care.

Three case histories are now described to illustrate the potential impact of spiritual care on patient experience of pain.

7 Case Studies

7.1 Case Study 1

Mrs S's pain experience exemplifies the interaction between spiritual and existential distress related to dying and pain. When she came to see the palliative care doctor in clinic, Mrs S completed a symptom distress scale. People are invited to circle the number which best shows how distressed they are about certain symptoms. She had distress from pain rated at 9/10, breathing problems 9/10 and bowel problems 9/10. There is a box for 'other symptoms' and Mrs S had added anxiety 8/10. She was clearly a very distressed woman. She talked with her doctor about her mesothelioma which had been recently diagnosed and for which she was about to start chemotherapy. She explained her pain experience and how it was interfering with almost every aspect of her life. She had two important life events coming up: her son's graduation and her wedding anniversary. She did not have a faith nor any spiritual practices which she regularly undertook. The doctor asked a clinical question proposed by Harvey Chochinov: 'What do I need to know about you as a person to provide you the best possible care?' [62] Mrs S said that when the time came, she wanted to gather friends and family and have the opportunity to access voluntary assisted dying. While this was not available in her country, the doctor discussed what could be offered: someone on the end of the phone 24 h a day, good symptom control, emotional and practical support and that she would care for her until the end of her life. The doctor commenced a low dose of a medication for nerve pain which usually takes effect after about 4 days of treatment.

The next day Mrs S rang the doctor. She said she wanted to let the doctor know that she felt much better. All her symptoms had completely or partially resolved. The next week in clinic she completed the symptom distress scale, and all the scores were 0–1/10. Mrs S's existential distress about the manner of her dying had been addressed. This resulted in improvements in not only pain but also all her other symptoms from severely distressing to causing little or no distress. Further, she was enabled to focus on upcoming life events which were sources of joy and love for her.

7.2 Case Study 2

Mr W came into the palliative care ward for pain management for bone pain from his metastatic prostate cancer. His pain escalated during the admission and his pain relief requirements grew accordingly. He was agitated and distressed. He was married with three adult children, a retired accountant and had a wide network of friends through sporting clubs. He had been brought up Catholic but no longer practised. He said he still believed in God.

He was supported in the palliative care ward by the pastoral care worker. As she listened, he talked of the relationships which had been meaningful to him. He became teary when he discussed one such relationship. He revealed he had a close relationship with a woman from their friendship group. They had had an affair years ago and had stayed close, speaking daily. He felt a deep sense of guilt about this relationship which he had not disclosed to his wife. The pastoral care worker prayed with him as he prayed about the relationship. He asked forgiveness from God and reflected on the best approach to the relationships.

His pain levels dropped, his pain relief requirements dropped, and his agitation reduced. He was able to ask forgiveness from both his wife and the woman. He developed complications of his disease and died during the admission. His pain levels and pain relief requirements remained low for the duration of his illness.

7.3 Case Study 3

Mr S was a 63-year-old non-English-speaking man from Asian background who was admitted to the palliative care ward in an English-speaking country for symptom control. He had abdominal pain related to his gastric cancer and abdominal distension related to ascites. Through the Google Translate App and with professional interpreters, he explained his pain and the other symptoms he experienced. He rated his pain 8/10 in severity. All his family were in his country of origin, including his five siblings.

At the time of admission, the palliative care unit was involved in a study to evaluate a tool to measure psychoexistential distress. Mr S completed the tool, and the assessment revealed a significant lack of meaning, purpose and hope which had previously been undetected. The team suggested to Mr S that he engage with the unit's biography service. A biographer whose first language was the same as Mr S's worked with Mr S. He told of his years growing up, his father who had been moved away from home by the government, and his siblings. He told the story of how he had worked on a large infrastructure project of national importance in his home country in his role as engineer. He included photographs. He was able to discuss his losses and grief in being no longer being able to work. As he talked and felt heard, his pain levels dropped. His siblings came to visit. They were able to connect with him for the first time in many years. He was able to find some solace in Christian music and Bible readings which he had had trouble engaging with when his pain was severe. He was able to re-establish a sense of meaning and purpose in sharing his story, which improved his pain levels enough to be able to find peace and hope in his faith. His siblings provided comfort and support.

7.4 Summary

Pain is very common in people receiving palliative care. Much focus remains on the physical aspects of pain management at the expense of psychosocial and spiritual factors that compound the pain experience [75]. Spirituality is an integral part of life that brings connection, meaning and purpose to people's lives which helps shape quality of life and wellbeing. Indeed, evidence shows that most people receiving palliative care report at least one spiritual need, expressing a need for closer connections to their God and forgiveness of sins [76]. Spiritual care can improve pain outcomes.

8 Conclusion

Spiritual distress has a negative impact on pain severity in people receiving palliative care. Current evidence for the beneficial effects of spiritual care and associated interventions for alleviating pain in palliative care settings is limited. However, given that preliminary findings are encouraging, and spiritual care is well accepted by patients and their caregivers where no adverse effects are reported, further research in this important area is required.

References

1. Doyle KE, Nakib SKE, Rajagopal MR, Babu S, Joshi G, Kumarasamy V, et al. Predictors and prevalence of pain and its management in four regional cancer hospitals in India. J Glob Oncol. 2018;4:1–9.
2. Hagarty AM, Bush SH, Talarico R, Lapenskie J, Tanuseputro P. Severe pain at the end of life: a population-level observational study. BMC Palliat Care. 2020;19(1):60.
3. Murtagh FE, Addington-Hall J, Higginson IJ. The prevalence of symptoms in end-stage renal disease: a systematic review. Adv Chronic Kidney Dis. 2007;14(1):82–99.
4. Hindmarch T, Dalrymple J, Smith M, Barclay S. Spiritual interventions for cancer pain: a systematic review and narrative synthesis. BMJ Support Palliat Care. 2022;12(1):1–9.
5. Broglio K, Cole BE. Pain management and terminal illness. Pract Pain Manag. 2008;8(4). https://www.practicalpainmanagement.com/resources/hospice/pain-management-terminal-illness.
6. Chin-Yee N, Tanuseputro P, Carrier M, Noble S. Thromboembolic disease in palliative and end-of-life care: a narrative review. Thromb Res. 2019;175:84–9.
7. Thorp SL. Pathophysiology of cancer pain. In: Gulati A, Puttanniah V, Bruel BM, Rosenberg WS, Hung JC, editors. Essentials of interventional cancer pain management. Cham: Springer; 2019. p. 13–7.
8. Lee Y-P, Wu C-H, Chiu T-Y, Chen C-Y, Morita T, Hung S-H, et al. The relationship between pain management and psychospiritual distress in patients with advanced cancer following admission to a palliative care unit. BMC Palliat Care. 2015;14(1):69.
9. Meier EA, Gallegos JV, Thomas LP, Depp CA, Irwin SA, Jeste DV. Defining a good death (successful dying): literature review and a call for research and public dialogue. Am J Geriatr Psychiatry. 2016;24(4):261–71.
10. Barbera L, Taylor C, Dudgeon D. Why do patients with cancer visit the emergency department near the end of life? CMAJ. 2010;182(6):563–8.
11. Quinn B, Connolly M. Spirituality in palliative care. BMC Palliat Care. 2023;22(1):1.
12. Gijsberts M-JHE, Liefbroer AI, Otten R, Olsman E. Spiritual care in palliative care: a systematic review of the recent European literature. Med Sci. 2019;7(2):25.
13. Kissane DW. Psychospiritual and existential distress. The challenge for palliative care. Aust Fam Physician. 2000;29(11):1022–5.
14. Abbas SQ, Dein S. The difficulties assessing spiritual distress in palliative care patients: a qualitative study. Ment Health Relig Cult. 2011;14(4):341–52.
15. Steinhauser KE, Fitchett G, Handzo GF, Johnson KS, Koenig HG, Pargament KI, et al. State of the science of spirituality and palliative care research part I: definitions, measurement, and outcomes. J Pain Symptom Manage. 2017;54(3):428–40.
16. Quinn B. Making sense of pain and loss: searching for meaning while living with cancer. Cancer Nurs Pract. 2018;17(5):29–36.
17. Balboni TA, Balboni M, Enzinger AC, Gallivan K, Paulk ME, Wright A, et al. Provision of spiritual support to patients with advanced cancer by religious communities and associations with medical care at the end of life. JAMA Intern Med. 2013;173(12):1109–17.
18. Sollgruber A, Bornemann-Cimenti H, Szilagyi IS, Sandner-Kiesling A. Spirituality in pain medicine: a randomized experiment of pain perception, heart rate and religious spiritual well-being by using a single session meditation methodology. PLoS One. 2018;13(9):e0203336.
19. Ratshikana-Moloko M, Ayeni O, Tsitsi JM, Wong ML, Jacobson JS, Neugut AI, et al. Spiritual care, pain reduction, and preferred place of death among advanced cancer patients in Soweto, South Africa. J Pain Symptom Manage. 2020;60(1):37–47.
20. Raja SN, Carr DB, Cohen M, Finnerup NB, Flor H, Gibson S, et al. The revised International Association for the Study of Pain definition of pain: concepts, challenges, and compromises. Pain. 2020;161(9):1976–82.
21. Dedeli O, Kaptan G. Spirituality and religion in pain and pain management. Health Psychol Res. 2013;1(3):e29.

22. Hackett J, Godfrey M, Bennett MI. Patient and caregiver perspectives on managing pain in advanced cancer: a qualitative longitudinal study. Palliat Med. 2016;30(8):711–9.
23. Wachholtz AB, Keefe FJ. What physicians should know about spirituality and chronic pain. South Med J. 2006;99(10):1174–5.
24. Yang Y, Cui M, Zhao X, Wang S, Wang Y, Wang X. Association of pain management and positive expectations with psychological distress and spiritual well-being among terminally ill cancer patients admitted to a palliative care unit. BMC Nurs. 2023;22(1):96.
25. Rippentrop EA, Altmaier EM, Chen JJ, Found EM, Keffala VJ. The relationship between religion/spirituality and physical health, mental health, and pain in a chronic pain population. Pain. 2005;116(3):311–21.
26. Yang Y, Zhao X, Cui M, Wang S, Wang Y. Longitudinal changes in spiritual well-being and associations with emotional distress, pain, and optimism-pessimism: a prospective observational study of terminal cancer patients admitted to a palliative care unit. Support Care Cancer. 2021;29(12):7703–14.
27. Wiech K, Farias M, Kahane G, Shackel N, Tiede W, Tracey I. An fMRI study measuring analgesia enhanced by religion as a belief system. PAIN. 2008;139(2):467–76.
28. Frankl VE. Man's search for meaning. New York: Simon and Schuster; 1984.
29. Robinson KL, Connelly CD, Georges JM. Pain and spiritual distress at end of life: a correlational study. J Palliat Care. 2022;37(4):526–34.
30. Harris JI, Usset T, Krause L, Schill D, Reuer B, Donahue R, Park CL. Spiritual/religious distress is associated with pain catastrophizing and interference in veterans with chronic pain. Pain Med. 2017;19(4):757–63.
31. Caldeira S, Carvalho EC, Vieira M. Between spiritual wellbeing and spiritual distress: possible related factors in elderly patients with cancer. Rev Lat Am Enfermagem. 2014;22(1):28–34.
32. McCabe R, Murray R, Austin P, Siddall P. Spiritual and existential factors predict pain relief in a pain management program with a meaning-based component. J Pain Manag. 2018;11(2):163–70.
33. Storey P, Knight CF. UNIPAC two: alleviating psychological and spiritual pain in the terminally ill. American Academy of Hospice and Palliative Medicine; 1997.
34. Delgado-Guay MO, Chisholm G, Williams J, Frisbee-Hume S, Ferguson AO, Bruera E. Frequency, intensity, and correlates of spiritual pain in advanced cancer patients assessed in a supportive/palliative care clinic. Palliat Support Care. 2016;14(4):341–8.
35. Hui D, de la Cruz M, Thorney S, Parsons HA, Delgado-Guay M, Bruera E. The frequency and correlates of spiritual distress among patients with advanced cancer admitted to an acute palliative care unit. Am J Hosp Palliat Care. 2011;28(4):264–70.
36. Teno JM, Freedman VA, Kasper JD, Gozalo P, Mor V. Is care for the dying improving in the United States? J Palliat Med. 2015;18(8):662–6.
37. Gielen J, Bhatnagar S, Chaturvedi SK. Prevalence and nature of spiritual distress among palliative care patients in India. J Relig Health. 2017;56(2):530–44.
38. Oliveira SSW, Vasconcelos RS, Amaral VRS, Sousa H, Dinis MAP, Vidal DG, Sá KN. Spirituality in coping with pain in cancer patients: a cross-sectional study. Healthcare (Basel). 2021;9(12):1671.
39. Edman JS, Roberts RS, Dusek JA, Dolor R, Wolever RQ, Abrams DI. Characteristics of cancer patients presenting to an integrative medicine practice-based research network. Integr Cancer Ther. 2014;13(5):405–10.
40. Rush C, Vagnini K, Wachholtz A. Spirituality and religion for pain: empirical evidence, theory and mechanisms, and clinical considerations. Elsevier; 2020. p. 179–99.
41. Rego F, Gonçalves F, Moutinho S, Castro L, Nunes R. The influence of spirituality on decision-making in palliative care outpatients: a cross-sectional study. BMC Palliat Care. 2020;19(1):22.
42. Song M-K, Sereika SM. An evaluation of the Decisional Conflict Scale for measuring the quality of end-of-life decision making. Patient Educ Couns. 2006;61(3):397–404.
43. Mystakidou K, Parpa E, Tsilika E, Pathiaki M, Galanos A, Vlahos L. Depression, hopelessness, and sleep in cancer patients' desire for death. Int J Psychiatry Med. 2007;37(2):201–11.

44. Wachholtz AB, Pearce MJ. Does spirituality as a coping mechanism help or hinder coping with chronic pain? Curr Pain Headache Rep. 2009;13(2):127–32.
45. Givler A, Bhatt H, Maani-Fogelman PA. The importance of cultural competence in pain and palliative care. In: StatPearls. Treasure Island (FL): StatPearls Publishing . Copyright © 2023, StatPearls Publishing LLC.; 2023.
46. Greer JA, Applebaum AJ, Jacobsen JC, Temel JS, Jackson VA. Understanding and addressing the role of coping in palliative care for patients with advanced cancer. J Clin Oncol. 2020;38(9):915–25.
47. Jacobsen J, Kvale E, Rabow M, Rinaldi S, Cohen S, Weissman D, Jackson V. Helping patients with serious illness live well through the promotion of adaptive coping: a report from the improving outpatient palliative care (IPAL-OP) initiative. J Palliat Med. 2014;17(4):463–8.
48. Puchalski C, Ferrell B, Virani R, Otis-Green S, Baird P, Bull J, et al. Improving the quality of spiritual care as a dimension of palliative care: the report of the consensus conference. J Palliat Med. 2009;12(10):885–904.
49. Cavalcanti IDL, Costa DT, Soares JCS, Nogueira MCBL. Benefits of spiritual and religious support in the pain management of cancer patients: a literature scoping review. J Relig Health. 2023;62(3):1998–2032.
50. Hjermstad MJ, Gibbins J, Haugen DF, Caraceni A, Loge JH, Kaasa S. Pain assessment tools in palliative care: an urgent need for consensus. Palliat Med. 2008;22(8):895–903.
51. Hall G, Gregory A. 54 Improving assessment of pain in palliative care. BMJ Support Palliat Care. 2017;7(3):A367-A.
52. Ewing G, Todd C, Rogers M, Barclay S, McCabe J, Martin A. Validation of a symptom measure suitable for use among palliative care patients in the community: CAMPAS-R. J Pain Symptom Manage. 2004;27(4):287–99.
53. Hølen JC, Hjermstad MJ, Loge JH, Fayers PM, Caraceni A, De Conno F, et al. Pain assessment tools: is the content appropriate for use in palliative care? J Pain Symptom Manage. 2006;32(6):567–80.
54. Vasigh A, Tarjoman A, Borji M. Relationship between spiritual health and pain self-efficacy in patients with chronic pain: a cross-sectional study in west of Iran. J Relig Health. 2020;59(2):1115–25.
55. Charak S, Thattil G, Srivastava M, Das P, Shandilya M. Assessment and management of pain in palliative care. In: Marco C, Michael John S, editors. Suggestions for addressing clinical and non-clinical issues in palliative care. Rijeka: IntechOpen; 2021. Ch. 11.
56. Siddall PJ, Lovell M, MacLeod R. Spirituality: what is its role in pain medicine? Pain Med. 2015;16(1):51–60.
57. Siddall PJ, McIndoe L, Austin P, Wrigley PJ. The impact of pain on spiritual well-being in people with a spinal cord injury. Spinal Cord. 2017;55(1):105–11.
58. De Vlieger P, Van den Bussche E, Eccleston C, Crombez G. Finding a solution to the problem of pain: conceptual formulation and the development of the Pain Solutions Questionnaire (PaSol). Pain. 2006;123(3):285–93.
59. Brintz CE, Birnbaum-Weitzman O, Merz EL, Penedo FJ, Daviglus ML, Fortmann AL, et al. Validation of the Functional Assessment of Chronic Illness Therapy-Spiritual Well-Being-Expanded (FACIT-Sp-Ex) across English and Spanish-speaking Hispanics/Latinos: results from the Hispanic Community Health Study/Study of Latinos Sociocultural Ancillary Study. Psycholog Relig Spiritual. 2017;9(4):337–47.
60. Lee BY, Newberg AB. Religion and spirituality in pain management. In: Boswell MV, Cole E, editors. Weiner's pain management: a practical guide for clinicians. 7th ed. Boca Raton: CRC Press; 2005. p. 18.
61. Moreira-Almeida A, Koenig HG. Religiousness and spirituality in fibromyalgia and chronic pain patients. Curr Pain Headache Rep. 2008;12(5):327–32.
62. Chochinov HM, Kristjanson LJ, Breitbart W, McClement S, Hack TF, Hassard T, Harlos M. Effect of dignity therapy on distress and end-of-life experience in terminally ill patients: a randomised controlled trial. Lancet Oncol. 2011;12(8):753–62.

63. Feuille M, Pargament K. Pain, mindfulness, and spirituality: a randomized controlled trial comparing effects of mindfulness and relaxation on pain-related outcomes in migraineurs. J Health Psychol. 2015;20(8):1090–106.
64. Mendes BV, Donato SCT, Silva TLD, Penha RM, Jaman-Mewes P, Salvetti MG. Spiritual well-being, symptoms and performance of patients under palliative care. Rev Bras Enferm. 2023;76(2):e20220007.
65. Pérez-Cruz PE, Langer P, Carrasco C, Bonati P, Batic B, Tupper Satt L, Gonzalez Otaiza M. Spiritual pain is associated with decreased quality of life in advanced cancer patients in palliative care: an exploratory study. J Palliat Med. 2019;22(6):663–9.
66. Lieberman MA, Golant M, Giese-Davis J, Winzlenberg A, Benjamin H, Humphreys K, et al. Electronic support groups for breast carcinoma: a clinical trial of effectiveness. Cancer. 2003;97(4):920–5.
67. Cole BS. Spiritually-focused psychotherapy for people diagnosed with cancer: a pilot outcome study. Ment Health Relig Cult. 2005;8(3):217–26.
68. Sabet P, Karimi S, Dehghan A, Bijani M. Effect of spirituality-based palliative care on pain, nausea, vomiting, and the quality of life in women with colon cancer: a clinical trial in southern Iran. J Relig Health. 2023;62(3):1985–97.
69. Bai J, Brubaker A, Meghani SH, Bruner DW, Yeager KA. Spirituality and quality of life in black patients with cancer pain. J Pain Symptom Manage. 2018;56(3):390–8.
70. Bovero A, Digiovanni Y, Botto R, Leombruni P. End-of-life cancer patients' total pain: the necessity to supplement pharmacology with psycho-socio-spiritual treatments. Pain Manag. 2022;12(8):895–906.
71. Lloyd-Williams M, Cobb M, O'Connor C, Dunn L, Shiels C. A pilot randomised controlled trial to reduce suffering and emotional distress in patients with advanced cancer. J Affect Disord. 2013;148(1):141–5.
72. Warth M, Kessler J, van Kampen S, Ditzen B, Bardenheuer HJ. 'Song of Life': music therapy in terminally ill patients with cancer. BMJ Support Palliat Care. 2018;8(2):167–70.
73. Chochinov HM, Hack T, Hassard T, Kristjanson LJ, McClement S, Harlos M. Dignity therapy: a novel psychotherapeutic intervention for patients near the end of life. J Clin Oncol. 2005;23(24):5520–5.
74. Vuksanovic D, Green H, Morrissey S, Smith S. Dignity therapy and life review for palliative care patients: a qualitative study. J Pain Symptom Manage. 2017;54(4):530–7.e1.
75. Mosher CE, Secinti E, Johns SA, O'Neil BH, Helft PR, Shahda S, et al. Examining the effect of peer helping in a coping skills intervention: a randomized controlled trial for advanced gastrointestinal cancer patients and their family caregivers. Qual Life Res. 2018;27(2):515–28.
76. Poletti S, Razzini G, Ferrari R, Ricchieri MP, Spedicato GA, Pasqualini A, et al. Mindfulness-based stress reduction in early palliative care for people with metastatic cancer: a mixed-method study. Complement Ther Med. 2019;47:102218.

Spirituality and Mental Health

Francisca Rego

Abstract The importance of spirituality and its impact on the mental health of palliative care patients has been reported by various studies. It plays an important role as a coping mechanism, namely as a source of strength and support. The interdisciplinary team is essential to adequately address patients' spiritual and psychological suffering; however, the spiritual dimension is still poorly addressed in the palliative care context. The integration of spirituality into psychological support has emerged as a comprehensive and holistic approach, given the contribution that spiritual assessment can have in psychological care to improve patient wellbeing and quality of life. This approach will enable the mental healthcare professional to identify the patients' values, beliefs, fears, distress, and needs, thus assisting to reduce aspects of psychological distress, such as anxiety and depression.

Keywords Psychological care · Mental health · Spirituality · Spiritual care
Palliative care

1 Introduction

When a life-threatening illness emerges, it disturbs one's interpersonal (biological and psychological) and extrapersonal (physical and interpersonal environment) relationships. Through holistic care, healthcare professionals are able to restore the patient's relationships, whether it is related to treatment of symptoms, or the

F. Rego (✉)
Faculty of Medicine, University of Porto, Porto, Portugal
e-mail: mfrego@med.up.pt

M. C. Best (ed.), *Spiritual Care in Palliative Care*,
https://doi.org/10.1007/978-3-031-50864-6_15

restoration of relationships with family and friends or with the transcendent, e.g. questions about existence, value, and meaning [1, 2].

Sulmasy considered the human person to be intrinsically spiritual [1]. The spiritual experience of the illness may be related to the transcendent dimension, a transpersonal dimension that is related to feelings of being greater and lasting. It may be expressed through bonding with groups or through ideals, but it does not necessarily rely on religion [3]. The religious dimension is considered to be more related to an institutional and social experience that supports closeness with the Divine or transcendent and promotes a relationship to a community [4–7].

Spirituality is a unique and broad concept that encompasses an existential and/or religious dimension [8]. In palliative care, recent studies have considered spirituality as a network connecting all aspects of life, linking in a unique way each dimension - biological, psychological, and sociocultural - of the person [9–11].

Spirituality and religiousness are considered powerful predictors of patient wellbeing and of health status [8, 12–15]. Spirituality enables the search for internal strength and meaning, self-knowledge and reflection and acceptance of the illness [16–19]. Religion is also found to be related to improved quality of life and social wellbeing, due to the presence of the community and social relationships related to the religious practice and spiritual wellbeing [16, 20, 21].

2 The Spiritual and Psychological Dimensions

Spiritual wellbeing is a key component of psychological health. Faith, peace, and meaning of life influence many areas of patients' lives, their own future and family's future, death, livelihood, disability and financial problems. Positive emotions and a better quality of life have been found to be related to the presence of faith, rituals, and social interactions. On the other hand, negative emotions, mainly connected to constraints of the illness, e.g. uselessness and fear about the future, are related to decreasing health status, inability to work and/or inability to pursue leisure activities. This highlights the importance of spirituality as a coping mechanism, as studies found a significant relationship between spiritual wellbeing and greater quality of life, and less depression, anxiety, pain, and fatigue [21–25].

Spiritual suffering is common in palliative care patients. It can be expressed as an intrapsychic conflict, interpersonal loss/conflict or in relation to the Divine. Existential distress may include anxiety related to death, loss and change, dignity of the self, isolation/aloneness, altered relationships, and loss of meaning [26–28].

There are certain risk factors associated with spiritual suffering, such as multiple losses, dependence, poor support networks, high symptom burden, non-acceptance of the condition and excessive rumination. On the other hand, literature highlights certain protective factors such as good family/social support, controlled symptoms, resilience, optimism, and acceptance of finitude. Thus, in order to improve spiritual wellbeing, it is important that healthcare professionals pay attention to early palliative measures, family support and other sources of support present, feeling at peace, sense of meaning in life and coping strategies, namely through regular spiritual assessment as part of the interdisciplinary approach [29–31].

Patients may adopt a positive spiritual/religious coping mechanism, which is associated with positive mental health and physical health outcomes. It is related to a beneficial reliance on faith that enables adaptation to the health circumstances and psychological adjustment to stressors. However, when patients adopt a negative spiritual/religious coping mechanism (understanding the illness as a divine punishment or abandonment by God, which can indicate an existential crisis) or rely solely on a higher power for health without any kind of collaborative problem solving, for example believing that God will save them and denying any kind of care, it can lead to poorer long-term health outcomes [32–36]. Thus, the health-care team should be aware when taking the patient's history and during regular symptom control assessment of how patients are experiencing their faith and the coping strategies used to deal with pain and other symptoms, according to their area of expertise. This will help to identify whether specialised mental health support is needed [36].

The psychology literature describes the spiritual phenomenon of the 'fork in the road', which states that spiritual conflicts may be related to unresolved spiritual issues or religious conflicts [37]. On the one hand, these may result in spiritual growth, but on the other hand, may result in spiritual despair, decline, and loss of meaning, and they may lead to worse quality of life and mental health outcomes [14, 35, 37].

The experience of spiritual distress is related to psychological and physical suffering [3, 9]. Literature has pointed to the relationship between the psychological and spiritual dimensions of the patient, which are predictive of quality of life, physical and social suffering and wellbeing, and of mental health outcomes, such as anxiety, depression, and hopelessness [7, 21, 38–40].

Palliative care patients may experience psychological suffering, such as fear, anxiety, and grief, mostly linked to the patient's previous way of life and changes of functional capacities and social/familial roles, which are a result of the constraints of the illness. It impacts patients' wellbeing, quality of life and is linked to spiritual and religious suffering and loss of meaning [22, 26, 27, 41, 42].

Patients need to be able to give a new meaning to their lives, considering their new reality and its constraints (illness); otherwise, they will despair. Spiritual and existential suffering, such as burden to others, hopelessness, loss of sense of dignity, loss of will to live and desire for death, threaten the psychological, social, and spiritual wellbeing of patients and are linked to desire for hastened death [43, 44]. The presence of meaning and peace, which are subdimensions of spirituality, in palliative care patients improves the treatment of anxiety in these patients, and religious support helps address depression in patients whose spirituality is more related to religion [40, 42].

This points to the importance of assessing the spiritual concerns and suffering of patients, as well as being aware of their coping strategies. The ability to find meaning plays an important role in overcoming despair and minimising psychological distress [38]. See Chap. 17 for more on spiritual care therapeutics for the end of life.

3 Spirituality and Psychological Care

Spirituality influences patients' information processing capacities, by enabling them to build a base of knowledge and information according to their values, interests, and competencies, leading to adaptive problem-solving strategies [45]. A person's spirituality predicts one's functioning and allows one to adapt and solve problems, through skills and resources, such as prayer or transcendence, that enable patients to find meaning in life experiences. These resources are related to the awareness and way one relates to oneself, others, the world and transcendence [45, 46].

Palliative care patients usually don't address spiritual issues during consultations or with the healthcare team, because they may believe these aspects not to be relevant or because they may not be aware of the impact of their spiritual dimension to the illness process and wellbeing. The healthcare team should raise questions to address this topic, so patients to feel comfortable in addressing this during their care. Patients need to be able to understand their internal and life experiences, will and values, so they are able to determine the best course of action and care plan according to their priorities. This can be accomplished by the therapist listening to the patient and creating a safe space for them to explore their fears, hopes, needs, and desires [22, 47–49]. This points to the importance of healthcare professionals having the initiative to address spirituality, thus making patients aware and comfortable to address these issues during consultation, by actively listening to their concerns and needs in a neutral way [22, 48].

3.1 Psychological Care

Palliative care mental health professionals' (psychologists and psychiatrists') expertise includes assessment, intervention, advocacy, and research of psychological distress of both the patient and family, but it also involves spiritual and social matters. Given the relation of spiritual concerns to psychological distress, it is crucial to investigate the patient's spirituality during therapy, in order to collect significant data on how they may overcome difficulties, for instance exploring patients' beliefs and loss of meaning when addressing patient's concerns about illness and facing mortality [50–55].

In psychological care, patients share their history, concerns, and fears. It is considered a comprehensive type of care, as it allows the patient to explore one's life history and to understand one's internal experiences, thus promoting better self-knowledge, relational skills and search for adaptive solutions to the patient's needs and psychological and spiritual processes. Through the patients' narratives, patients are able to assemble meanings, psychological representations and values of the spiritual and/or religious beliefs. Thus, through empathic listening, narratives may help mental health professionals to better understand the meaning of 'total pain' to the patient [36, 56–58].

Discussing more explicit spiritual issues—such as institutionalised religion or forms of spirituality—is not usually considered in psychotherapy, given the ethical and competency boundaries of the psychologist. Thus, in a multicultural society, an implicit integration of spirituality in psychological care is sufficient (addressing these matters only when the patient refers to them in the way the patient wants to address them), however with an added encouragement from the mental health professional to address this dimension during consultation in a non-directive and neutral matter. This overcomes the barrier of not approaching these issues during consultation, but at the same time allowing patients to have the autonomy to address these issues as they feel prepared and in the way it makes sense to them. When a more explicit approach to spirituality is needed, collaborations and referrals to appropriate religious/spiritual professionals are important, such as institutionally based chaplains/spiritual care worker in the palliative care team, or religious leaders within the patient's community, to directly address the religious concerns [36, 53, 59, 60].

Psychologists and psychiatrists have the responsibility to listen in a non-judgmental way, to be aware of the impact the spiritual dimension has in the patient's life, to seek appropriate spiritual/religious support, if needed, and to be aware of one's limitations and competence as professionals and to help the patient determine the actions needed to fulfil their needs [36, 61–63].

3.2 Psychotherapeutic Interventions

Currently, there are three main psychotherapeutic interventions used in the palliative care context to improve patients' psychological and spiritual wellbeing. *Counselling* is the most frequently reported and has demonstrated positive effects on depression, resilience, and anxiety, as well as quality of life and spiritual wellbeing [64].

Life review sessions aim to improve the sense of meaning, purpose, and acceptance through the review of the patient's lifespan and most significant narratives. Patients are able to discuss their legacy, regrets, sense of meaning and unfinished business, helping them to recover their self-esteem through a positive and significant revision of their lives. This intervention has been shown to improve anxiety, depression, functional health and preparation for the end-of-life journey [65, 66].

Dignity therapy is an intervention that aims to increase the sense of dignity, meaning, and purpose for the patient. It generates a legacy document from the patient's narratives and has been found to promote a positive sense of purpose and increased will to live in patients, which leads to reduced suffering. Furthermore, the use of a legacy document has been found to promote a sense of legacy, hope and fighting spirit, and post-intervention measures showed a significant decrease in the presence of depressive symptoms. It has also been found to help the family of the patient [64, 65, 67].

4 Conclusion

In palliative care, spirituality plays an important role as a coping mechanism. It plays a major role in the experience of the illness, namely as a source of strength and support, and has an influence on the emotional and physical wellbeing of the patient [22].

The positive relationship between the spiritual and psychological dimensions is evident, as well as its influence of personal integrity and identity and on spiritual wellbeing of the palliative care patient. Psychological wellbeing has a mediating role in spirituality and health outcomes, namely the stress-buffering effect of beliefs, goals, and meaning [21, 36, 68].

Spirituality can also have a negative impact. Spiritual distress, such as sense of meaningless, hopelessness, and guilt, may lead to psychological (e.g. depression and anxiety) and physical (e.g. acute pain) suffering. Thus, it is important that mental health professionals consider the impact of spiritual and existential needs on the patient's emotional distress, psychological functioning, and wellbeing [38, 42, 69].

By including the assessment of spirituality in psychological care, a more comprehensive and multidimensional understanding and response to the patients' needs is promoted, thus addressing the patient as a whole and promoting patient dignity and autonomy [59, 70].

There should be a regular assessment of spirituality within a larger psychosocial assessment, namely of the spiritual and existential concerns and needs, hopes, fears and sense of meaning, as well as patient's social support and cultural background [9, 21]. This way, interventions would encompass patients' spiritual wellbeing and enable the development of a sense of peace and meaning in life, consequently improving mental health at the end of life [21, 71].

References

1. Sulmasy D. A biopsychosocial-spiritual model for the care of patients at the end of life. Gerontologist. 2002;42:24–33.
2. Egnew TR. The meaning of healing: transcending suffering. Ann Fam Med. 2005;3(3):255–62.
3. Cassel EJ. The nature of suffering and the goals of medicine. N Engl J Med. 1982;306(11): 639–45.
4. Koenig H. Spirituality and health research: methods, measurement, statistics and resources. West Conshohocken, PA: Tempelton Press; 2011.
5. Koenig H, McCullough M, Larson D. Handbook of religion and health. New York: Oxford University Press; 2001.
6. McClement S, Chochinov H. Spiritual issues in palliative medicine. In: Hanks G, Cherny N, Christakis N, MFallon M, Kaasa S, Portenoy R, editors. Oxford textbook of palliative medicine. 4th ed. Oxford: Oxford University Press; 2010.
7. Steinhauser KE, Fitchett G, Handzo GF, Johnson KS, Koenig HG, Pargament KI, et al. State of the science of spirituality and palliative care research part I: definitions, measurement, and outcomes. J Pain Symptom Manag. 2017;54(3):428–40.

8. Best M, Butow P, Olver I. The doctor's role in helping dying patients with cancer achieve peace: a qualitative study. Palliat Med. 2014;28(9):1139–45.
9. Puchalski CM, Ferrel B, Viriani R, Otis-Green S, Baird P, et al. Improving the quality of spiritual care as a dimension of palliative care: the report of the consensus conference. J Palliat Med. 2009;12:885–904.
10. Nolan S, Saltmarsh P, Leget C. Spiritual care in palliative care: working towards an EAPC task force. Eur J Palliat Care. 2011;18(2):86–9.
11. Miccinesi G, Caraceni A, Garetto F, Zaninetta G, Bertè R, Broglia CM, et al. The path of Cicely Saunders: the "peculiar beauty" of palliative care. J Palliat Care. 2019;35(7072):082585971983365.
12. Balboni TA, Vanderwerker LC, Block SD, Paulk ME, Lathan CS, Peteet JR, et al. Religiousness and spiritual support among advanced cancer patients and associations with end-of-life treatment preferences and quality of life. J Clin Oncol. 2007 Feb;25(5):555–60.
13. Roberts JA, Brown D, Elkins T, Larson DB. Factors influencing views of patients with gynecologic cancer about end-of-life decisions. Am J Obstet Gynecol. 1997;176(1 Pt 1):166–72.
14. Balboni TA, Balboni MJ. The spiritual event of serious illness. J Pain Symptom Manag. 2018;56(5):816–22.
15. Krikorian A, Limonero JT, Roman JP, Vargas JJ, Palacio C. Predictors of suffering in advanced cancer. Am J Hosp Palliat Med. 2014;31(5):534–42.
16. Nelson CJ, Rosenfeld B, Breitbart W, Galietta M. Spirituality, religion, and depression in the terminally ill. Psychosomatics. 2002;43(3):213–20.
17. Yong J, Kim J, Han SS, Puchalski CM. Development and validation of a scale assessing spiritual needs for Korean patients with cancer. J Palliat Care. 2008;24(4):240–6.
18. Young WC, Nadarajah SR, Skeath PR, Berger AM. Spirituality in the context of life-threatening illness and life-transforming change. Palliat Support Care. 2015;13(03):653–60.
19. Dobratz MC. "All my saints are within me": expressions of end-of-life spirituality. Palliat Support Care. 2013;11(03):191–8.
20. Vallurupalli M, Lauderdale K, Balboni M, Phelps A, Block S, Ng A, et al. The role of spirituality and religious coping in the quality of life of patients with advanced cancer receiving palliative radiation therapy. J Support Oncol. 2012;10(2):81–7.
21. Rego F, Pereira C, Rego G, Nunes R. The psychological and spiritual dimensions of palliative care: a descriptive systematic review. Neuropsychiatry. 2018;8:484–94.
22. Rego F, Gonçalves F, Moutinho S, Guedes L, Nunes R. The influence of spirituality on decision-making in palliative care outpatients: a cross sectional study. BMC Palliat Care. 2020;19(22):22.
23. Elsner F, Schmidt J, Rajagopal M, et al. Psychosocial and spiritual problems of terminally ill patients in Kerala, India. Future Oncol. 2012;8(9):1183–91.
24. Fegg MJ, Kogler M, Abright C, Hensler M, Lorenzl S. Meaning in life in patients with progressive Supranuclear palsy. Am J Hosp Palliat Care [Internet]. 2014;31(5):543–7. http://ajh.sagepub.com/cgi/doi/10.1177/1049909113492411
25. Rabow MW, Knish SJ. Spiritual Well-being among outpatients with cancer receiving concurrent oncologic and palliative care. Support Care Cancer. 2015;23(4):919–23.
26. Kissane D. The relief of existential suffering. Arch Intern Med. 2012;172(19):1501–5.
27. Asgeirsdottir GH, Sigurbjornsson E, Traustadottir R, Sigurdardottir V, Gunnarsdottir S, Kelly E. In the shadow of death: existential and spiritual concerns among persons receiving palliative care. J Pastoral Care Counsel. 2014;68(1–2):4.
28. Selman L, Siegert RJ, Higginson IJ, Agupio G, Dinat N, Downing J, et al. The 'spirit 8' successfully captured spiritual Well-being in African palliative care: factor and Rasch analysis. J Clin Epidemiol [Internet]. 2012;65(4):434–43. https://doi.org/10.1016/j.jclinepi.2011.09.014.
29. Chochinov HM, Krisjanson LJ, Hack TF, Hassard T, McClement S, Harlos M. Dignity in the terminally ill: revisited. J Palliat Med. 2006;9(3):666–72.

30. Blinderman CD, Cherny NI. Existential issues do not necessarily result in existential suffering: lessons from cancer patients in Israel. Palliat Med [Internet]. 2005;19(5):371–80. http://journals.sagepub.com/doi/10.1191/0269216305pm1038oa
31. Selman L, Beynon T, Higginson IJ, Harding R. Psychological, social and spiritual distress at the end of life in heart failure patients. Curr Opin Support Palliat Care. 2007 Dec;1(4):260–6.
32. Wachholtz A, Pearce M. Does spirituality as a coping mechanism help or hinder coping with chronic pain. Curr Pain Headache Rep. 2009;13:127–32.
33. Phelps AC, Maciejewski PK, Nilsson M, Tracy A, Wright AA, Paulk ME, et al. Association between religious coping and use of intensive life-prolonging care near death among patients with advanced care. JAMA J Am Med Assoc. 2010;301(11):1140–7.
34. Ai AL, Hopp F, Tice TN, Koenig H. Existential relatedness in light of eudemonic Well-being and religious coping among middle-aged and older cardiac patients. J Health Psychol. 2013;18(3):368–82.
35. Pargament KI, Koenig HG, Tarakeshwar N, Hahn J. Religious coping methods as predictors of psychological, physical and spiritual outcomes among medically ill elderly patients: a two-year longitudinal study. J Health Psychol. 2004 Nov;9(6):713–30.
36. Rego F, Nunes R. The interface between psychology and spirituality in palliative care. J Health Psychol. 2019;24(3):279–87.
37. Pargament K. Spiritually integrated psychotherapy: understanding and addressing the sacred. New York: Guilford Press; 2007. p. 115–41.
38. McClain CS, Rosenfeld B, Breitbart W. Effect of spiritual well-being on end-of-life despair in terminally ill cancer patients. Lancet. 2003;361(9369):1603–7.
39. McCoubrie RC, Davies AN. Is there a correlation between spirituality and anxiety and depression in patients with advanced cancer? Support Care Cancer. 2006;14(4):379–85.
40. Bovero A, Leombruni P, Miniotti M, Rocca G, Torta R. Spirituality, quality of life, psychological adjustment in terminal cancer patients in hospice. Eur J Cancer Care (Engl). 2016;25(6):961–9.
41. Seah AST, Tan F, Srinivas S, Wu HY, Griva K. Opting out of dialysis – exploring patients' decisions to forego dialysis in favour of conservative non-dialytic management for end-stage renal disease. Health Expect. 2015;18(5):1018–29.
42. Bovero A, Tosi C, Botto R, Opezzo M, Giono-Calvetto F, Torta R, et al. J Relig Health. 2019;58:2144.
43. Chochinov HM. Dying, dignity, and new horizons in palliative end-of-life care. CA Cancer J Clin [Internet]. 2006 Mar 1 [cited 2021 Nov 17];56(2):84–103. https://pubmed.ncbi.nlm.nih.gov/16514136/
44. Fegg MJ, Brandstätter M, Kramer M, Kögler M, Haarmann-Doetkotte S, Borasio GD. Meaning in life in palliative care patients. J Pain Symptom Manag. 2010;40(4):502–9.
45. Emmons RA. Spirituality and intelligence: problems and prospects. Int J Psychol Relig. 2009;8619(November 2014):37–41.
46. Srivastava PS. Spiritual intelligence: An overview. Int J Multidiscip Res Dev. 2016;3(3):224–7.
47. Bottorff JL, Steele R, Davies B, Garossino C, Porterfield P, Shaw M. Striving for balance: palliative care patients' experiences of making everyday choices. J Palliat Care. 1998;14(1):7–17.
48. Long C. Cultural and spiritual considerations in palliative care. J Pediatr Hematol Oncol. 2011;33(2):96–101.
49. Best M, McArdle MB, Huang YJ, Clayton J, Butow P. How and how much are spirituality discussed in palliative care consultations for advanced cancer patients with and without a question prompt list? Patient Educ Couns. 2019;102(12):2208–13.
50. Carpenter BD. Geropsychological practice with people near the end of life. In: Lichtenberg PA, Mast BT, editors. APA handbook of clinical geropsychology volume 2: assessment, treatment, and issues of later life. Washington, DC: American Psychological Association; 2015. p. 579–99.

51. Connor SR, Lycan J, Schumacher JD. Involvement of psychologists in psychosocial aspects of hospice and end-of-life care. In: Werth JL, Blevins D, editors. Psychosocial issues near the end of life: a resource for professional care providers. Washington, DC: American Psychological Association; 2006. p. 203–17.
52. Gamino LA, Ritter RH. Death competence: an ethical imperative. Death Stud. 2012;36(1): 23–40.
53. Golijani-Moghaddam N. Practitioner psychologists in palliative care: past, present, and future directions. Couns Psychol Rev. 2014;29(1):29–40.
54. Sheldrake P. A brief history of spirituality. Oxford: Blackwell Publishers; 2007.
55. Mako C, Galek K, Poppito SR. Spiritual pain among patients with advanced cancer in palliative care. J Palliat Med. 2006;9(5):1106–13.
56. Alleti M. Atendimento psicológico e direção espiritual: Semelhanças, diferenças integrações e … confusões. Psicologia: Teoria e Pesquisa. 2008;24(1):117–25.
57. Mundle R. A narrative analysis of spiritual distress in geriatric physical rehabilitation. J Health Psychol [Internet]. 2015;20(3):273–85. https://doi.org/10.1177/1359105314566609.
58. Moore K, Talwar V, Moxley-Haegert L. Definitional ceremonies: narrative practices for psychologists to inform interdisciplinary teams' understanding of children's spirituality in pediatric settings. J Health Psychol [Internet]. 2015;20(3):259–72. https://doi.org/10.1177/1359105314566610.
59. Moss E, Dobson K. Psychology, spirituality and end-of-life care: an ethical integration? Can Psychol. 2006;47:284–99.
60. Chappelle W. A series of progressive legal and ethical decision-making steps for using Christian spiritual interventions in psychotherapy. J Psychol Theol. 2000;28(1):43–53.
61. Richards PS, Bergin AE. A spiritual strategy for counseling and psychotherapy. 2nd ed. Washington, DC: American Psychological Association; 2005. xi, 422–xi, 422
62. American Psychological Association (APA). Ethical principles of psychologists and code of conduct. Am Psychol. 2002;57:1060–73.
63. Plante TG. Integrating spirituality and psychotherapy: ethical issues and principles to consider. J Clin Psychol. 2007;63(9):891–902.
64. Rudilla D, Galiana L, Oliver A, Barreto P. Comparing counseling and dignity therapies in home care patients: a pilot study. Palliat Support Care [Internet]. 2016;14(04):321–9. http://www.journals.cambridge.org/abstract_S1478951515001182
65. Vuksanovic D, Green H, Morrissey S, Smith S. Dignity therapy and life review for palliative care patients: a qualitative study. J Pain Symptom Manage [Internet]. 2017;54(4):530–537.e1. https://doi.org/10.1016/j.jpainsymman.2017.07.016.
66. Steinhauser KE, Alexander SC, Byock IR, George LK, Olsen MK, Tulsky JA. Do preparation and life completion discussions improve functioning and quality of life in seriously ill patients? Pilot randomized control trial. J Palliat Med [Internet]. 2008;11(9):1234–40. http://www.liebertonline.com/doi/abs/10.1089/jpm.2008.0078
67. Grijó L, Tojal C, Rego F. Effects of dignity therapy on palliative patients' family members: a systematic review. Palliat Support Care. 2021;19(5):605–14.
68. Park CL, Folkman S. Meaning in the context of stress and coping. Rev Gen Psychol [Internet]. 1997;1(2):115–44. https://doi.org/10.1037/1089-2680.1.2.115.
69. Kearney M, Mount B. Spiritual care of the dying patient. In: Chochinov HM, Breitbart W, editors. Handbook of psychiatry in palliative medicine. New York: Oxford University Press; 2000. p. 357–73.
70. Rudilla D, Soto A, Pérez MA, Galiana L, Fombuena M, Oliver A, et al. Psychological interventions in spirituality: a systematic review in palliative care. Med Paliativa. 2018;25(3):203–12.
71. Mystakidou K, Tsilika E, Prapa E, Smyrnioti M, Pagoropoulou A, Lambros V. Predictors of spirituality at the end of life. Can Fam Physician. 2008;54(12):1720.

Part IV
Practice

Compassion in Palliative Care

Małgorzata Fopka-Kowalczyk

Abstract Compassion for others is an essential attitude for healthcare professionals, especially in palliative care. It provides a huge number of benefits for patients and their loved ones. Although compassion for others among professionals could lead to increased compassion fatigue, emotional cost, and burnout, it is worth being compassionate for patients because of the benefits. Research shows that compassionate care increases the well-being of patients, reduces anxiety and depression, and helps during the treatment process. This chapter will demonstrate what compassion is, how we can be more compassionate in practice in palliative care, and how professionals can prevent compassion fatigue.

Keywords Compassion for others · Benefits · Compassion fatigue · Emotional costs · Self-compassion · Spiritual care · Palliative care

1 Introduction

Human suffering caused by a chronic illness affects the functioning of a person in all areas of one's life. Suffering from a life-threatening illness demands that the patient be treated with intimacy and dignity, taking into account not only somatic ailments but also emotional, social, and spiritual needs [1]. In their relationship with a healthcare professional, patients want to be treated with compassion, [2] and when interacting with a professional in a white coat, they wish to see a responsive and caring human

M. Fopka-Kowalczyk (✉)
Department of Philosophy and Social Sciences, Nicolaus Copernicus University, Toruń, Poland
e-mail: mfopka-kowalczyk@umk.pl

M. C. Best (ed.), *Spiritual Care in Palliative Care*,
https://doi.org/10.1007/978-3-031-50864-6_16

being rather than a machine doing their job [3]. In addition to advice for such behaviour towards the suffering and the sick, this attitude is also found in recommendations for the soft competencies of healthcare professionals necessary in their relationship with the patient and his relatives, which emphasise the importance of, among other things, adopting an attitude that expresses compassionate care towards the suffering person. These issues are particularly relevant to the situation of a dying patient, when professionals are required to lean on the patient and the entire baggage of his or her experiences, show respect and regard for the individuality of experiences, as well show care and compassion appropriate to the patient's situation.

2 How Do We Define Compassion for Others?

There are many definitions for *compassion* in the reference literature [4] as an interpersonal attitude that involves not only recognising another person's feelings, but also responding in order to relieve the suffering. In general, it can be said that compassion is 'a state of concern for the suffering or unmet need of another person, combined with a desire to alleviate that suffering' [5]. Compassion, then, is an attitude full of warmth and kindness, with the ability to recognise pain and suffering, but in a relationship with another person this suffering does not become the suffering of the helper, but only the experience of caring and wanting to support that person in suffering. It is being truly present for a person who is in a situation that is difficult for them, involving recognising and understanding the suffering of others. In order to be compassionate, one must be characterised by the relevant attributes and skills necessary in practising compassion towards others. Among the most important, according to Gilbert, are:

1. sensitivity—responding to other people's emotions and recognising when they need help, as well as being able to recognise and differentiate between the feelings and needs of the suffering person,
2. sympathy—showing special care when another person is suffering,
3. empathy—putting oneself in the place of the suffering person and being moved by the person's experience and suffering,
4. motivation—being motivated to be patient in responding positively to another's suffering,
5. tolerance of stress and suffering—agreeing to tolerate difficult emotions and experiences rather than avoiding them, fearfully turning away, shutting down or denying them to the healthcare professional,
6. non-judgemental attitude—the ability to accept another person, not condemning or judging them, even if their condition, reaction, or emotion evokes negative feelings in us: frustration, anger, fear, or disgust [6: 202–203].

Compassion is also 'patience, benevolence and non-judgmental understanding, recognising that all people are imperfect and make mistakes. It is an attitude of responding emotionally to the suffering of others, trying to understand cognitively a situation and noticing the suffering experienced, as well as being more focused on the suffering or distress of another' [7, p. 21]. Importantly, it can be directed not only at other people, but also at oneself, where it is assumed to be an attitude of gentleness and kindness towards oneself and treating oneself with patience, especially when something goes wrong or in a personal crisis [8, 9]. The issue of self-compassion is important as a protective factor for people who are compassionate towards others. This will be further discussed below.

3 Compassion and Other Categories of Pro-Social Behaviour

One of the difficulties in understanding compassion comes from confusion with other pro-social attitudes [4, p. 3–4]. The attitude most commonly equated with compassion is *empathy*. Empathy and compassion are two different ways of responding to human suffering: empathy refers to the ability to see another person's perspective, imagine and feel their emotions, while compassion occurs when these feelings and thoughts include the desire to help those who are vulnerable or in danger [10], as well as the ability to understand why this is happening [11]. Empathy, therefore, is an affective state, an emotion, arising as a result of witnessing the experiences of another person, while compassion is an attitude and willingness to take action to remove suffering, together with an understanding of the causes of the suffering experienced.

Another category confused with compassion is *altruism*, understood as pro-social behaviour often triggered by feelings of compassion, although it is possible to feel compassion without acting on it, and altruism is not always motivated by compassion [10]. Kindness and altruism have a much broader meaning than compassion and do not focus on suffering. Arman however claims that empathy and altruism are connected, and are 'a triad of phenomena, with compassion as a basis' [12, p. 6].

Compassion can also be regarded as a form of *pity*. Pity, however, does not require any action or even an inclination to act. Rather, it is evidence of noticing someone's plight or suffering without specifically reacting to the situation. A risk in showing pity is exhibiting a patronising attitude towards the sufferer and treating the person with detachment, with a sense of simple 'arrogance and even fear, and a feeling of "I'm glad it's not me"' [13, p. 52]. This attitude does not occur in compassion, where there is a synchronous partnership relationship, and the assisted person is not treated as inferior or unworthy of help.

Compassion is also regarded as a significant element of human *spirituality* and as one method of communicating or intervening in a relationship with a suffering person, irrespective of stated religion [14]. Every faith includes compassion, which is, in a sense, the test of true spirituality and requires us to focus our attention and care on the person whether friend or foe [15].

4 Compassion Care for Others in Palliative Care in Practice

Compassion for others is an essential component of staff interpersonal competence in palliative care. Acts of compassion involve the ability to focus attention on the suffering person, to show concern for their worries, but also to take action to help them better understand their situation and to encourage them to seek within themselves the strength and resources to find a way out of the difficult situation they are experiencing. Some of the essential methods of showing compassion are techniques known from verbal and non-verbal communication: 'It is necessary to recognise that someone is suffering if one is to intervene to alleviate that suffering. Speech content, vocal cues and facial expressions can individually or collectively inform the observer that someone is suffering' [16, p. 44]. Therefore, it is not only the spoken words that are important, but also the sound of the words, the form of expression and the whole context, the posture and what we communicate with the person who is suffering and looking for compassion. In non-verbal communication, it is especially important to skilfully show benevolence and friendliness as well as interest by means of facial expressions or eye contact, expressing listening, full acceptance, and interest. This involves non-intrusive eye contact that does not make the sufferer uncomfortable, showing interest in the content being said and appropriate gestures (e.g. leaning the body towards the patient, nodding, or encouraging words such as: 'I am listening', 'I would like you to tell me more about this'). Another technique used in compassion can be the use of touch—research shows that touch is a primary source for developing close and constructive bonds and relationships [17]. Touch is the first sign of closeness. In the relationship with the patient, it becomes information to him or her that we, as professionals, do not feel disgusted by the changes taking place in their body, and that they have the right to experience a variety of difficult emotions and behaviours in the situation of progression of the disease or awareness of impending death. Discussions I have had in classes with medical and non-medical students show that they consider that this is a forgotten way of showing compassion to another person in relationships. A kind and non-intrusive touch is a non-verbal message: 'I accept you as you are and respect your opinion on a subject'. Touch is also a forgotten way of showing closeness to the other person, helping to get closer to them, communicating an interest in them and their life as well as focusing on what they are saying [18]. Small acts of kindness such as smiling, companionship, silent presence, and behaviours such as taking a walk together, having tea or being there for the suffering person, but also telling stories and jokes if the patient has the space to do so, are also important [19]. Certainly, the statement 'I am there for you' or 'you are not alone' would be the best act of compassion to offer to another.

Complementary to showing compassion to the other person is verbal communication [20] in addition to active listening techniques (paraphrasing, asking the right questions or giving feedback), it is to show the sufferer your attentiveness and involvement in the story being told, and to communicate your willingness to help and support. In practice, this means asking questions that encourage the person to tell their story (e.g. 'I would like you to tell me more about this'), naming the sick person's feelings (e.g. 'I can see how much you are going through', 'I can hear in your voice that you are suffering') or verbally showing understanding while respecting the individuality of the experience (e.g. 'I cannot even imagine what you are going through', 'I can only imagine how you are suffering').

Julia Wahl [21], for example, points to two essential stages in the practice of compassion:

1. Working with what is difficult and unlearning what is not helpful.
2. Seeking what strengthens, e.g. the search for meaning and significance, the ability to forgive, learning helpful and constructive coping strategies, the ability to ask for help.

Showing a willingness to help is also important. The phrase 'what can I do for you today' or 'what can I do for you as a doctor/nurse/therapist...' strengthens the patient and gives them the courage to go deeper into their story because they know and experience acceptance and hear the declaration of support.

5 Benefits of Compassion for Patients and Healthcare

Paul Gilbert's studies show positive correlations of compassion with various aspects of life, allowing for mutual support and mutual caring in social relationships. Showing and receiving compassion are beneficial and play key roles in emotion regulation, mental health and interpersonal relationships [4]. Compassion takes on particular importance in palliative care, in the relationship with the sick and dying: 'Doctors practising an empathic and compassionate attitude is one of the most important aspects of the therapeutic relationship (...) Among the factors most valued by students and professionals in the development of compassionate care are acting with warmth and empathy, providing patient-centred care and treating others as the professional himself would like to be treated' [2]. Lack of compassion turns healthcare into a mechanical and emotionless performance of work [2, 22], and is also often recognised as a lack of interpersonal skills and a lack of competence in the context of working with a suffering person [2]. Compassion shown towards those who are ill has a strong positive impact on healthcare professionals, reducing their moral suffering, job burnout and occupational stress, while increasing their commitment and work satisfaction [23]. In the relationship with the patient, compassion enhances the quality of that relationship, having a positive impact on treatment planning and patient compliance [24].

Practising compassion in a relationship with a person who is ill or in need of support is not only meaningful for the compassionate person, but also very beneficial for the recipient of this compassion. This also applies to the professional relationship. In the context of chronically ill people, this seems to be a particularly important factor. For example, patients report positively about professionals who use compassion-focused techniques in the treatment process and in therapeutic relationships [25]. As mentioned earlier, a patient experiencing an encounter, not only with a doctor, but also simply with another human being, receives tremendous and positive support during the illness and treatment. As a benefit of compassion, patients highlight, for example, that the compassion shown to them reduces severe physiological symptoms and somatic complaints [26]. Patients surveyed indicate that, thanks to compassion, they also experience significantly less suffering and anxiety [27], which in the relationship with the doctor, increases patients' length of survival [28]. A perceived lack of a compassionate attitude among healthcare professionals intensifies stress. Consequently, dissatisfaction with the established (or not) relationship with the healthcare professional and the care received contributes to and increases patient complaints and medical malpractice lawsuits [2]. Compassion shown also contributes to patient satisfaction [27], influencing the subjectively perceived quality of support and care provided during illness and treatment [29] and the patients' quality of life [24].

Practising and experiencing compassion can also positively influence the patients' ability to cope with the intensification of negative emotions that can accompany a patient at any stage of illness, such as anger, dissatisfaction, or sadness [30]. It also allows patients to feel that they are being treated with dignity and respect by a healthcare professional [31], enhancing patient well-being [29]. It gives the professional helper an opportunity to look at the person in need in a holistic way and gives the sick person the opportunity to meet not only a professional, but also a responsible and concerned human being, prepared to provide help and support according to the needs expressed by the protégé. The results of studies of patients who experienced gestures or small acts of compassion highlighted above show that compassionate care of helpers brought about significant changes in patients' functioning, feelings of relief from suffering, improved well-being, and influenced changes in perceptions and evaluations of the quality of care received from medical professionals [2].

6 Emotional Costs and Compassion Fatigue

Although the provision of compassionate care has wide-ranging benefits for the recipients of the care shown, a compassionate attitude among professional helpers may result in an emotional cost to them [32]. This has a particular dimension in palliative care, where professional workers can be 'let in' to the patient's experiences, establishing often intimate and very deep relationships with the patient while providing care [32, 33]. Among the most highlighted emotional costs are compassion fatigue [34], the deteriorating well-being of helpers resulting in symptoms of professional burnout and loss of interest in helping [35], and the experience of a sense of loss after the death of patients whom they previously cared for with compassion and care/concern [33]. Other negative effects include an increased risk of mental and physical health problems, insomnia [35], and increased use of sedative drugs or drinking alcohol excessively as a way of dealing with it.

Nowadays, employees improving their competence in compassion for others are also provided with information on how to cope when compassion fatigue occurs. A remedy for the difficulties experienced can be, for example, adopting an attitude of self-compassion [36]. Self-compassion means being benevolent and benign towards oneself in situations of experienced anxiety or stress, but also taking a balanced view of one's problems, being attentive to the emotions experienced by oneself and being caring towards oneself. It is also about learning to be patient with oneself, and not adopting an evaluative, critical, or overly demanding attitude towards oneself [8, 9]. It is helpful to practice mindfulness through, for example, breathing practices, visualisations, or meditations as techniques to increase self-awareness, building comfort and a sense of safety at work and with oneself. Nevertheless, Balint groups and supervision seem to be of no less importance, allowing people to look at themselves from a distance, learn about their emotions and learn how to cope. These suggestions can protect healthcare staff and increase compassion for others [37] (see Chap. 29).

Personal working conditions are also a factor in mitigating the risk of compassion fatigue, influencing staff's psychological well-being, and increasing positive emotions about their work and their quality of life and relationships with others. Hence, practitioners emphasise that in the workplace, it is important to nurture compassion both towards and among employees. The effect would be to increase motivation and willingness to work, non-avoidance of work and a sense of being useful [38]. Importantly, employees who experience compassion are less likely to leave their jobs, especially if it is their employer/leader who adopts compassionate attitudes towards their employees. This can be manifested, for example, by not taking criticism '*ad personam*', but talking constructively about the tasks at hand. It is showing understanding and benevolence to an employee who is experiencing difficult situations at work or in their personal life. It is conveying support and acceptance to the employee. It is also agreeing with and taking care to improve the competence of your employees, especially in the aspect of working with the dying.

Compassion towards others has several benefits for the provider. It has been associated with lower blood pressure reactivity, lower cortisol reactivity, and higher HF-HRV (high frequency heart rate variability) reactivity. Higher compassion was also associated with better relationship with and greater liking for the supportive co-workers or supervisors at work. It also suggests that it can serve as a buffer against stress occurring at work [39]. Through this, it also becomes a helpful factor in reducing tension and stress. The use of compassion in workplaces not only increases satisfaction and enjoyment, but also reduces the risk of burnout, facilitates employees' developing emotional resilience [35], increasing trust among employees and willingness to cooperate [40]. Compassion at work makes situations understandable, people feel comfortable and have a greater awareness and sensitivity to what is happening around them. They are able to adapt their behaviour and actions accordingly to the work situation. The trust built up then encourages people to engage in compassionate behaviour, as employees can notice, feel, and respond to their colleagues' pain and problems. In a study of nurses, it was found that a more compassionate attitude on the part of supervisors allows them to feel less stress and has a positive effect on the work they do [41]. The consequence is not only a satisfied employee, but a higher quality of work from them, which translates into a better quality of patient care and improved therapeutic relationships.

7 Conclusion

Compassion for others is a unique expression of caring for others. This kind of care for the other takes on a special significance in palliative care, benefiting patients and their families as well as staff. Awareness of the needs of patients at this stage of life and the intrinsic need and ability to adopt compassionate care towards the suffering person is one of the most important aspects of the relationship with the dying and sick person. Research to date shows that compassion is an innate human trait of which every human being can boast. If this is the case, then perhaps it is worth looking within ourselves and trying to apply this kind of care not only to another person, but also to ourselves. Then the costs of caring for the chronically ill and the dying will not frighten the employee but will become a motivation to develop their skills, while the workplace will become a place where the relationship with the chronically ill and the benefits of applying compassion will outweigh the emotional costs of this relationship.

References

1. Leget C. Art of living, art of dying. Spiritual care for a good death. London/Philadelphia: Jessica Kingsley Publishers; 2017.
2. Davalos-Batallas V, Vargas-Martínez A-M, Bonilla-Sierra P, Leon-Larios F, de las Mercedes Lomas-Campos, M, Vaca-Gallegos S-L, de Diego-Cordero R. Compassionate engagement and action in the education for health care professions: a cross-sectional study at an Ecuadorian university. Int J Environ Res Public Health. 2020;17(15):5425. https://doi.org/10.3390/ijerph17155425.
3. Stepulak M. Problemy etyczno—zawodowe psychologa klinicznego pracującego z chorymi terminalnie. In: Makselon J, editor. Człowiek wobec śmierci. Aspekty psychologiczno – pastoralne. Kraków: Wydawnictwo Naukowe PAT; 2005. p. 77–99.
4. Gilbert P. Creating a compassionate world: addressing the conflicts between sharing and caring versus controlling and holding evolved strategies. Front Psychol. 2021;11:582090. https://doi.org/10.3389/fpsyg.2020.582090.
5. Goetz JL, Keltner D, Simon-Thomas E. Compassion: an evolutionary analysis and empirical review. Psychol Bull. 2010;136(3):351. https://doi.org/10.1348/147608310X526511.
6. Gilbert P. Introducing compassion focused therapy. Adv Psychiatr Treat. 2009;15:202–3. https://doi.org/10.1192/apt.bp.107.005264.
7. Pommier E, Neff KD, Tóth-Király I. The development and validation of the compassion scale. Assessment. 2020;27(1):21–39. https://doi.org/10.1177/1073191119874108.
8. Neff KD. Self-compassion: an alternative conceptualization of a healthy attitude toward oneself. Self Identity. 2003a;2(2):85–101. https://doi.org/10.1080/15298860309032.

9. Neff KD. The development and validation of a scale to measure self-compassion. Self Identity. 2003b;2:223–50. https://doi.org/10.1080/15298860390209035.
10. Gibbs P. Higher education: a compassion business or edifying experience? In: Gibbs WP, editor. The pedagogy of compassion at the heart of higher education. Cham (SUI): Springer International Publishing; 2017. p. 1–16. https://doi.org/10.1007/978-3-319-57783-8_1.
11. Spinrad TL, Eisenberg N. Compassion in children. In: Seppälä EM, Simon-Thomas E, Brown SL, Worline MC, Cameron D, Doty JR, editors. Oxford handbook of compassion science. Oxford University Press; 2017. p. 53–63.
12. Arman M. Empathy, sympathy, and altruism – an evident triad based on compassion. A theoretical model for caring. Scand J Caring Sci. 2023;00:1–10. https://doi.org/10.1111/scs.13163.
13. Schantz ML. Compassion. A concept analysis. Nurs Forum. 2007;42(2):48–55, pp x. https://doi.org/10.1111/j.1744-6198.2007.00067.
14. Halifax J. The precious necessity of compassion. J Pain Symptom Manag. 2011;41(1):146.
15. Amstrong K. As cited in: Head, J. (2018). The spirituality of compassion. 2011; 1–6. Retrieved January 13, 2023, from https://www.rcpsych.ac.uk/docs/default-source/members/sigs/spirituality-spsig/spirituality-special-interest-group-publications-juli-head-thespiritualityofcompassion.pdf?sfvrsn=4a59295b_2
16. Ekman P, Ekman E. Is global compassion achievable? In: Seppälä EM, Simon-Thomas E, Brown SL, Worline MC, Cameron CD, Doty JR, editors. The Oxford handbook of compassion science. New York: Oxford University Press; 2017. p. 41–9.
17. Goetz JL, Simon-Thomas E. The landscape of compassion: definition and scientific. In: Seppälä EM, Simon-Thomas E, Brown SL, Worline MC, Cameron CD, Doty JR, editors. The Oxford handbook of compassion science. New York: Oxford University Press; 2017. p. 3–16.
18. Fopka-Kowalczyk M, Winch B. Wartość dotyku. In: Kowalczyk M, Łącka T, editors. Edukacja terapeutyczna w hospicjum. Toruń: Stowarzyszenie Hospicjum "Światło"; 2011.
19. Larkin P. Compassion as an Interpersonal Skill. An open lecture at NCU Faculty of Pedagogical Sciences. 2018, Dec 6.
20. Fopka-Kowalczyk M. Umiejętności interpersonalne i etyka pomagania chorym przewlekle. In: Fopka-Kowalczyk M, Rębiałkowska-Stankiewicz M, editors. Akademia Walki z Rakiem – wsparcie społeczne. Adam Marszałek: Toruń; 2013.
21. Wahl J. Współczucie. Powrót do wrażliwości i siły. Katowice: Charaktery; 2019.
22. Lesińska-Sawicka M, Grochulska A, Nagórska M, Papadopoulos I. Współczucie w pielęgniarstwie. Czasopismo Pedagogiczne/J Pedagogy. 2016;2(3):111–20.
23. Seppälä EM, Hutcherson CA, Nguyen DT, Doty JR, Gross JJ. Loving-kindness meditation: a tool to improve healthcare provider compassion, resilience, and patient care. J Compassionate Health Care. 2014;1:5. https://doi.org/10.1186/2053-2393-1-5.
24. Bramley L, Matiti M. How does it really feel to be in my shoes? Patients' experiences of compassion within nursing care and their perceptions of developing compassionate nurses. J Clin Nurs. 2014;23(19–20):2790–9. https://doi.org/10.1111/jocn.12537.
25. Lown BA, Rosen J, Marttila J. An agenda for improving compassionate care: a survey shows about half of patients say such care is missing. Health Aff. 2011;30(9):1772–8. https://doi.org/10.1377/hlthaff.2011.0539.
26. Porges SW. Vagal pathways: portals to compassion. In: Seppälä EM, Simon-Thomas E, Brown SL, Worline MC, Cameron CD, Doty JR, editors. The Oxford handbook of compassion science. New York: Oxford University Press; 2017. p. 189–202.
27. Lelorain S, Bredart A, Dolbeault S, Sultan S. A systematic review of the associations between empathy measures and patient outcomes in cancer care. Psycho-Oncology. 2012;21:1255–64. https://doi.org/10.1002/pon.2115.
28. Ironson G, Kremer H, Lucette A. Compassionate love predicts long-term survival among people living with HIV followed for up to 17 years. J Posit Psychol. 2018;13(6):553–62. https://doi.org/10.1080/17439760.2017.1350742.
29. Gilbert P. Compassion. Concepts, research and applications. London-New York: Routledge; 2017.

30. Chapin HL, Darnall BD, Seppala EM, Doty JR, Hah JM, Mackey SC. Pilot study of a compassion meditation intervention in chronic pain. J Compassionate Health Care. 2014;1:4. https://doi.org/10.1186/s40639-014-0004-x.
31. Singh P, King-Shier K, Sinclair S. The colours and contours of compassion: a systematic review of the perspectives of compassion among ethnically diverse patients and healthcare providers. PLoS One. 2018;13(5):e019726. https://doi.org/10.1371/journal.pone.0197261.
32. Fopka-Kowalczyk M. Wypalanie się i koszty emocjonalne pracowników w relacji z osobą przewlekle chorą i umierającą. Wychowanie na co dzień. 2016a;1:39–43.
33. Fopka-Kowalczyk M. Poczucie straty po śmierci pacjenta wśród pracowników opieki paliatywnej. Toruń: NCU Press; 2016b.
34. Palombaro KM, Erdman EA, Duszak McArdle K, Black JD, Steward AR, Jones SA. High civic-mindedness reduce compassion fatigue in the first 3 years of professional physical therapists practice: a pilot study. J Patient Exp. 2020;7(5):771–7. https://doi.org/10.1177/2374373519891346.
35. Kinman G, Grant L. Emotional demands, compassion and mental health in social workers. Occup Med. 2020;70(2):89–94. https://doi.org/10.1093/OCCMEDKQZ144.
36. Delaney MC. Caring for the caregivers: evaluation of the effect of an eight-week pilot mindful self-compassion (MSC) training program on nurses' compassion fatigue and resilience. PLoS One. 2018;13(11):e0207261. https://doi.org/10.1371/journal.pone.0207261.
37. Fopka-Kowalczyk M. Superwizja i grupy Balinta jako formy rozwoju zawodowego i wsparcia osób pomagających profesjonalnie. In: Kustra C, Fopka-Kowalczyk M, Bandura A, editors. Opieka i wsparcie jako zadanie całożyciowe: studia z pedagogiki opiekuńczej. Toruń: Wydawnictwo Edukacyjne "Akapit"; 2017. p. 211–22.
38. Dutton JE, Worline MC, Frost PJ, Lilius J. Explaining compassion organizing. Adm Sci Q. 2006;51(1):59–96.
39. Cosley BJ, McCoy SK, Saslow LR, Epel ES. Is compassion for others stress buffering? Consequences of compassion and social support for physiological reactivity to stress. J Exp Soc Psychol. 2010;46(5):816–23. https://doi.org/10.1016/j.jesp.2010.04.008.
40. Paakkanen M, Martela F, Hakanen J, Uusitalo L, Pessi A. Awakening compassion in managers – a new emotional skills intervention to improve managerial compassion. J Bus Psychol. 2021;36(6):1095–108. https://doi.org/10.1007/s10869-020-09723-2.
41. Lilius JM, Worline MC, Maitlis S, Kanov J, Dutton JE, Frost P. The contours and consequences of compassion at work. J Organ Behav. 2008;29:193–218.

Spiritual Care Therapeutics for the End of Life

Elizabeth Johnston Taylor

Abstract This chapter presents an overview of a variety of approaches to spiritual care that include therapeutics that encourage intrapersonal meaning (i.e. Dignity Therapy, spiritual life review), interpersonal meaning (i.e. forgiveness therapy, altruism), and transpersonal meaning (i.e. religion, prayer, nature). Given there are many approaches to meaning making, these selected therapeutics simply provide a spiritual care sampler. After reviewing some principles of spiritual care, this chapter discusses each of these therapeutics by describing it, presenting empirical evidence about it, and making practical suggestions for implementing it in the context of palliative care.

Keywords Interventions · Therapeutics · Spiritual care · Dignity Therapy Forgiveness · Meaning making · Palliative care · End of life · Spirituality · Religion

1 Introduction

Over 30 years ago, Reed defined spirituality as 'the propensity to make meaning through a sense of relatedness to dimensions that transcend the self in such a way that empowers and does not devalue the individual' [1, p. 350]. This relatedness that is essential to spirituality, Reed asserted, is experienced intra-, inter-, and transpersonally. In concert, these approaches to meaning making transform ordinariness to extraordinariness in people's lives.

E. J. Taylor (✉)
Loma Linda University, School of Nursing, Loma Linda, CA, USA
e-mail: ejtaylor@llu.edu

M. C. Best (ed.), *Spiritual Care in Palliative Care*,
https://doi.org/10.1007/978-3-031-50864-6_17

This chapter, in presenting an overview of a variety of approaches to spiritual care, therefore will include therapeutics that encourage intrapersonal meaning (i.e. Dignity Therapy, spiritual life review), interpersonal meaning (i.e. forgiveness therapy, altruism), and transpersonal meaning (i.e. religion, prayer). Given there are many approaches to meaning making, these selected therapeutics simply provide a spiritual care sampler. While discussing each of these therapeutics, both the evidence informing the use of the therapeutic as well as specific practical suggestions for implementing the therapeutic in palliative care will be offered. First, however, a few general prescriptive principles about providing spiritual care are reviewed.

2 General Principles for Spiritual Care

One might wonder why approaches to spiritual care are termed 'therapeutics' rather than 'interventions'. This intentional word selection is made to avoid inferring that spiritual care is to be used to fix, control, or manipulate a person's spiritual well-being. Rather, spiritual care is about being present, about compassionately and deeply listening, and about honouring the other. It is not assumed that the provider has more knowledge or experience than the patient. Rather, the patient-provider relationship is ideally realised as symmetrical; the spiritual carer is co-journeying though life. Indeed, the ability to be a healer requires self-respect for one's own woundedness [2].

Foundational to honouring the patient is providing spiritual care that is ethical and non-coercive. A simple, yet comprehensive, set of ethical guidelines for spiritual care within the healthcare context was offered by ethicist Winslow and nurse Wehtje-Winslow [3]. These guidelines are as follows:

- seek to know the patient's spiritual needs, resources, and preferences
- follow the patient's expressed wishes
- do not prescribe your own spiritual beliefs or practices or pressure the client to relinquish theirs.

To practice these guidelines, Winslow and Wehtje-Winslow acknowledged the healthcare provider must strive to learn about their own spirituality so that its potential impact on spiritual care can be assessed. They also recognised that spiritual care must be provided with personal integrity, meaning it must be consonant with the provider's own spiritual beliefs or practices [3]. There are common spiritual denominators among all persons, however, that can allow a provider to meet a patient on 'holy ground'. For example, when a Christian patient requests prayer, a Muslim nurse would likely be unable to colloquially verbalise an intercessory prayer to Jesus but could share a ritual prayer to God for peace and wholeness.

Communication is pivotal to spiritual care; whether it is verbal or non-verbal, it can be used like any precision instrument [2, 4]. A few communication principles particularly pertinent to spiritual care include the following:

- Listen not only for facts, but also for the feelings and embodied inner experience. You can learn what the patient is feeling by listening to your own emotional and physical response to the patient. Use this dual listening to inform how you respond.
- Information about the patient's spirituality can be gleaned not only from a spiritual screening or assessment, but from careful listening to the patient's stories and 'chit chat'. Consider: Where does the patient place energy in their story (e.g. talks excitedly, cries, or 'lights up')? What theme undergirds the story (e.g. betrayal, heroism, victimisation)? Respond to these cues to allow the patient to recognise what is occurring deep within them.
- Remember the goal is usually not to instil information; rather, it is to use therapeutic communication skills to allow the patient to hear themselves, gain insight from this, and possibly take action. Given you may only have a few minutes with a patient, your role may be simply to create an environment where spiritual self-awareness is desired and safe to seek.
- When a patient expresses intense emotion, respond empathically by naming the emotions (e.g. some variation on sad, bad, mad, or glad); it is also helpful to verbalise how the feelings might be linked to experience (a 'because'). Notice whether the patient affirms or refines your description of their inner experience and remember that they are the experts of their inner world.
- Avoid responses that will inform the patient that you are disinterested or not safe. For example, do not minimise or deny their negative feelings (e.g. 'Oh, it will all be okay'.), do not interject a distraction or positive remark to alleviate your own discomfort (e.g. 'At least you have....'), and do not imply judgement—positive or negative (e.g. 'It's so good that you pray!').
- When tempted to share your personal experience, first assess for what reason you are self-disclosing. For example, are you uncomfortable and need to fill an awkward silence? Do you have a 'saviour complex'? Only self-disclose when requested or when it is therapeutic.

Indeed, the basic communication skills learned in healthcare training need to be applied in the provision of spiritual care. These skills are essential as a healthcare provider introduces any of the following therapeutics.

Whereas the following therapeutics can be implemented by a solo spiritual care provider, team-provided spiritual care is likely more comprehensive, integrated, and effective [5]. Thus, it is necessary to communicate with colleagues about spiritual care provision (e.g. document therapeutics provided and the patient response to them). Team-provided spiritual care may involve diverse members of the palliative care team (e.g. chaplain, social worker, nurse) as well as the patient's spiritual carers in the community (e.g. clergy, spiritual director, folk healer, family).

3 Promoting Intrapersonal Connectedness

3.1 Dignity Therapy

Research findings support the feasibility and effectiveness of several therapeutics that support intrapersonal connectedness by fostering a sense of meaningfulness. Life review, reminiscence, encouraging patients to tell their stories or spiritual journeying are therapeutics identified as helpful [5]. Likely the most well-researched and widely implemented of these therapeutics among persons at the end of life is Dignity Therapy (DT), a semi-structured therapeutic developed by psychiatrist Chochinov [6].

Much evidence supports the efficacy of DT for persons with advanced disease. Martinez et al.'s systematic review of 28 studies evaluating use of DT with patients living with a life-threatening illness in diverse cultures substantiated that clinicians, patients, and their family carers value DT [7]. In particular, evidence indicated DT reduces anxiety and depression, especially among patients with high distress. Similarly, Zhang et al. conducted a meta-analysis of 14 studies evaluating outcomes of cancer patients receiving DT [8]. They found that DT decreased anxiety, depression, and increased hope. Although these outcomes are the most supported, weaker evidence suggests existential and spiritual well-being are also improved by DT.

DT is a manualised therapeutic that can be implemented by nurses, chaplains, and others trained to provide it [9]. It has also been adapted for use among family caregivers of adults with cancer [10]. DT involves presenting a series of specific open questions to a patient and allowing them to reflect on and integrate the disparate pieces of their life. During these semi-structured interviews, the following questions (slightly truncated here) are posed:

1. Tell me a little about your life history; particularly the parts that you remember most, or think are the most important? When did you feel most alive?
2. Are there specific things that you would want your family to know or remember about you?
3. What are the most important roles you have played in life? Why were they important? What do you think you accomplished?
4. What are your most important accomplishments and what do you feel most proud of?
5. What do you yet want to say (or say again) to your family?
6. What are your hopes and dreams for your loved ones?
7. What have you learned about life that you would want to pass along to others? What advice would you wish to pass along to your children, spouse, others?
8. Are there words or instructions that you would like to offer your family to help prepare them for the future?

The final question asks the patient if there is anything else that they would like in the legacy document that is created from the DT interviews [7]. The interviews are recorded and/or transcribed and made permanent for the patient's family. Along with the recording or transcription, the patient may also wish to add cherished items or pictures. Not only does DT allow a patient to psycho-spiritually process and document their life, but it also leaves a memento for loved ones to treasure and an opportunity for them to make meaning of the decedent's life.

3.2 *Diagrammatic Spiritual Life Histories*

More overt approaches to making meaning of one's spiritual life history were described by social worker Hodge [11]. Although these creative approaches were designed to allow spiritual assessment, they undoubtedly allow reflection and meaning making. After all, given how spirituality inextricably prompts and influences one to make meaning, examining this dimension of one's life story can provide novel insights. These approaches to spiritual life review include:

- Spiritual life maps involve that draw one's spiritual journey. This can include simple pencil sketches or more complex drawings and words to label or accentuate the art. Spiritual life maps may be particularly helpful for those who are challenged to express their deeply inward and private spiritual experiences with words.
- Spiritual genogram or spiritual family tree, like a standard genogram, that allows a patient to depict the intergenerational spiritual issues and influences. Indeed, using a few words or symbols, various people and events that influence spirituality can be notated.
- Spiritual ecomaps that encourage a patient to reflect on current spiritual experience, diagramming how the self (drawn in the centre) relates to the divine or transcendent other/value, other spiritual beings, faith community, or other relationships key to one's spiritual life.
- Spiritual timelines that engage a patient to note sequentially the events that were most influential spiritually.
- Fill-in-the-blank prompts like 'My relation to God…' or 'What I would really like to be…' can also be useful for a patient, perhaps especially if they can respond in a private journal.

These therapeutics for drawing one's spiritual life story can be merged or adapted. Having a variety of approaches, however, gives a clinician a toolbox from which to select what best fits a patient's ability, personality, need, and condition [12].

4 Promoting Interpersonal Connectedness

4.1 *Forgiveness*

In the process of life review or reflection, a patient facing their mortality may become aware of interpersonal disconnection. For example, they may be remorseful about having hurt a co-worker or estranged family member and yearn to restore the relationship before they die. Forgiveness is often conceptualised as a process that involves a deliberate choice to abandon negative responses to an injustice with positive, merciful, pro-social ones [13].

Some evidence about the process and outcomes of forgiveness among patients receiving palliative or end-of-life care exists. Both a scoping review of 23 studies and a systematic review of 39 studies about forgiveness in palliative care identified numerous outcomes of experiencing forgiveness [13, 14]. These included improved quality of life, and psychological and spiritual well-being (e.g. decreased anxiety, depression, anger, increased meaning, hope, inner peace, self-esteem, and self-acceptance). Fascinatingly, a couple of studies have observed physical outcomes: death within 2 days after experiencing a profound forgiveness, and increased ability to have do not resuscitate conversations [13].

While several process models for forgiveness facilitation exist, the Enright 'Forgiveness Therapy' approach may be the most widely known. Hansen et al. delivered this 4-week (about 1 h per week) therapeutic to older patients with cancer in a group setting [15]. These researchers observed significant improvements in psycho-spiritual well-being. The therapeutic involves the following steps:

- Identifying what is anger and differentiating between good and debilitating anger
- Expanding one's perspective about the offender; empathically considering the offender's story and reframing the offence
- Allowing one's heart to be softened; releasing the pain
- Recognising the meaningfulness of this growth and choosing a new way to relate to the offender [15].

While these group meetings were structured to present content, encourage personal application, and nudge completion of assignments between sessions, these components can still be helpful when supporting one patient yearning for forgiveness.

When describing how palliative care clinicians and patients are in the 'same existential boat' and need forgiveness, Breitbart observed that self-forgiveness was essential to forgiving others and experiencing release from existential distress [16]. Requisite to self-forgiveness, Breitbart posited, was knowing one's worthiness to be unconditionally loved. Thus, the 'therapeutic use of self' by palliative care providers may catalyse the process of forgiveness for the patient. Honouring a patient by respecting their struggles, by listening to their distress, by sharing their joy, or by giving a knowing look or caring touch may move the patient, even if incrementally, towards self-worth, and create inner room to give or receive forgiveness.

4.2 Altruism

Decades ago, the existential psychiatrist Yalom recognised how persons create meaning, in part, by dedicating themselves altruistically to a cause or mission [17]. It could be an artistic, scientific, social, or other cause; regardless, the altruism allows the individual to transcend themselves and improve life for others. Thus, it is proposed that this approach to interpersonal connection of fostering altruism may increase spiritual well-being.

Little direct evidence exists about altruism among persons receiving palliative or end-of-life care. Altruism, however, is known to prompt patients with life-threatening illness to participate in research to improve healthcare for others, [18, 19] agree to donate a body organ posthumously, [20] and join an online support group to encourage others [21]. A systematic review of 27 studies of adults who practised kindness interventions indicated that it does significantly improve subjective well-being to a small-moderate degree [22]. This evidence suggests that patients may often already be altruistic and that clinicians can increase patients' spiritual well-being by fostering altruism.

Yet, how can altruism be fostered when a patient is physically debilitated and emotionally distressed? First, a clinician ought to keep in mind that the altruistic activity is one that only the patient can choose. Given that patients may already be practising altruism, but just not recognise it, the clinician can notice and affirm any altruism they hear referenced. Then when a patient identifies that they are struggling to create meaning (e.g. 'I'm useless' or 'I feel like a burden and can't give anything in return'), a clinician can brainstorm about altruism or 'random acts of kindness' with the patient. Indeed, there are many ways to be altruistic even when bedbound. For example: smiling; calling someone who is lonely; writing an encouraging email, text, or card; doing sedentary work or art that helps someone; or praying for others or for the world. Altruistic activities may also be ways to leave a legacy.

5 Promoting Transpersonal Connectedness

5.1 Religion

Religions provide humans with connectedness to Something greater, Absolute, or beyond themselves. Often this Sacred Source, Ultimate Other, or Higher Power is anthropomorphised and labelled God. Most Western definitions for spirituality are careful to distinguish it from religion, which is conceptualised as spiritually oriented beliefs and practices shared by a collective ('faith community') [23, 24]. For a patient who is religious or non-religious, there are inherently spiritual beliefs and practices that guide life: These worldviews typically provide an orientation to the big questions of life (e.g. What created existence? What is the purpose for humans? What happens after death?). When faced with an imminent death, one's religious beliefs often become more comforting—or get re-examined.

Many aspects of receiving healthcare while living at the end of life intersect with religiosity. Chakraborty et al. systematically reviewed literature from the major world religious traditions to summarise how they viewed various end-of-life interventions [25]. Indeed, religious beliefs were observed to impact how believers view advanced directives and when to stop treatment, euthanasia and suicide, artificial hydration and nutrition, pain management, and autopsies. Chakraborty and colleagues noted that these viewpoints about end-of-life interventions were diverse even within one faith tradition. In fact, although religion is an aspect of culture, other aspects of culture also influence how the religion determines end-of-life care.

Ironically, while religions characteristically provide comforting beliefs about an after-life, there is evidence indicating that those who are more religious are more likely to avoid advance care planning, hospice, and prefer more intense end-of-life medical interventions [26]. Balboni et al.'s findings, however, suggested that this trend is explained by a lower understanding of illness among those with higher religiosity [27]. Regardless, it is important to recognise the salient influence of religion on how patients and their families (who may differ in their beliefs from the patient) make healthcare decisions, especially about how to navigate the sacred intersection between life and death [23].

Thus, a few suggestions for how healthcare providers can provide care that respects these religious influences:

- Assess for how religious beliefs and practices shape the patient's response to illness and dying. Many tools exist for spiritual assessment, but most assess the more generic spiritual responses [12]. Of interest is Balboni et al.'s 7-item scale to specifically measure religious beliefs about end-of-life medical care [27]. These include items about miracles (e.g. 'believe God would perform a miracle'), God's sovereignty (e.g. 'belief relieves me of needing to think about…'), the sanctity of life (e.g. 'will accept every possible medical treatment because my faith tells me to…'), and the sanctification of suffering (e.g. 'faith helps me to endure the suffering').
- For patients who are not at home where they can exercise their usual religious practices, negotiate with them how space and time can be allocated to allow uninterrupted quiet 'holy ground' [28]. For example, dedicated quiet spaces like a chapel or garden may be available for those in hospices or hospitals; signage on the patient's room door requesting non-essential workers and visitors stay away during a certain time can also be enforced. Clinicians may also need to respect religious articles at the bedside. They may also provide support by reading or playing a recording of the patient's sacred scripture [24].
- Sometimes a patient may request the presence of a spiritual mentor or leader. Clergy can perform religious rituals that comfort or give hope and provide theological explanations for questions with which the patient is struggling. They may also provide the gift of presence during a difficult time. While patients and their families typically initiate such contact, healthcare providers may need to make the contact if the patient is unable, and family are not involved. Often the chaplain or spiritual care services of the healthcare organisation provide this liaison.

Even if a clinician is not directly providing religious support, it is vital for them to understand the salient influence of religious beliefs and practices in the living and dying of patients and their families.

5.2 *Prayer*

A religious ritual for transcending the self that can be practised in or out of religion is prayer [24]. Prayer is generally thought to be directed to God, spiritual beings, or whatever the person considers to be the divine. Psychoanalyst Ulanov and theologian Ulanov described prayer as 'primary speech' and hypothesised that 'to pray is to listen to and hear this self who is speaking' [29, p. 1]. Indeed, most people pray—especially when in extremis [30].

A mixed-methods study of 70 advanced cancer patients in the USA revealed that 64% agreed that it was appropriate at least occasionally for a clinician to offer to pray with a patient [31]. In general, these respondents believed prayer was supportive, yet they also recognised the circumstances for patient-clinician praying depended on circumstances (e.g. an established relationship). Smith et al. qualitatively studied how 13 women with advanced cancer prayed [32]. They observed how these patients prayed: to make spiritual sense of their illness and move forward through it; to ascertain their priorities; to find strength and courage; and to spiritually grow or grow closer to God. These women prayed in diverse ways: Their prayer experiences were conversational, petitionary, ritual, and of thanksgiving—for themselves and others.

When Taylor et al. interviewed 30 cancer and hospice patients about how they prayed, it was observed that while all reported prayer was beneficial, many also described concurrent spiritual struggle [33]. While talking about how they prayed, these study participants named issues, doubts, and questions. For example: Does God really hear? Does God have the power to cure me? Am I praying in the right way? Should I not ask God for things that are too big? Should I only pray for others and not myself? Maybe I'm not good enough (e.g. not worthy, not good at praying)? Thus, 'unanswered' prayer raised questions of theodicy and the nature of God.

Given the prevalence and salience of prayer for religious and non-religious patients, palliative care clinicians will do well to consider how to ethically incorporate this therapeutic into their practice. Thus, a few suggestions to spur reflection:

- If a patient initiates a request for prayer with a clinician, it is considered ethical to proceed as long as the clinician is comfortable doing so and does not attempt any spiritual coercion in the process [23, 24]. The Winslow & Wehtje-Winslow ethical guidelines for spiritual care presented at the top of this chapter were originally developed to guide clinicians to know when and how to pray with patients [3]. A clinician can apply these guidelines to any inner promptings to offer to pray with a patient.
- Assess for what and how to pray. A non-coercive way to ask is, 'Would a prayer be helpful?' (as opposed to the imposition, 'Do you want me to pray with you?'). If a patient welcomes prayer with the clinician, then follow-up questions that will lead to deeper understanding about the inner life of the patient would include: 'What would you like me to pray for?' and 'Is there a certain way you would like me to pray?'

- Remember that while patients may report that prayer is helpful, there can co-occur spiritual distress related to praying [33]. Using therapeutic communication skills that do not judge positively or negatively a patient's talk about the prayer experience can allow the patient to discuss this and gain insight.
- Remember that there are diverse approaches to prayer. Indeed, any attitude or activity can be laced with prayerfulness. If praying with a patient, a clinician can consider what type of prayer would best align with the patient's personality and circumstances. For example, an introvert may prefer a shared silent prayer. An emergent condition may be best addressed with squeezing the patient's hand and saying, 'God, be with us!'

5.3 Nature

Some posit that while God 'speaks' through sacred scriptures (God's 'word'), God's works are found in the 'book' of nature. Regardless of religiosity, activities that submerge a patient within nature, even if virtually, bring a sense of awe and wonder. Thus, being in nature increases spiritual wellness, as well as mental and physical health [34–36]. One factor contributing to these positive effects is the inhalation of phytoncides, an antimicrobial that plants emit. In addition to improving immune function, being in nature lessens stress and some types of pain.

Supporting a patient to be with nature is an inexpensive and non-religious approach to spiritual care. Taylor [37] suggested the following strategies for clinicians who want to introduce this therapeutic:

- Nature can be brought to the bedside if a patient is unable to go outdoors. (However, might family and/or colleagues be coordinated to help take a patient outside?) Virtual reality, YouTube videos, mobile phones with nature meditation apps, or picture books of nature can be brought to a patient. It is interesting to note that pictures with canopies of trees, bodies of water, and mountains (as opposed to pictures that were close-ups or included unnatural elements) were identified in a study of 40 college students as best representing nature [38]. These researchers observed that such nature pictures are restorative and create awe.
- Ideally, make the nature experience multi-sensory. The more senses employed, the more therapeutic it is [34].
- Recognise nature that is already present (e.g. in a flower or plant at the bedside, the sky out the window). Notice it with the patient and, if they are receptive, encourage them to use it as a visual mantra or focus for meditation. Reflective questions might include: How is this [plant, soil, leaf, cloud] making the body or spirit feel? Is it creating a sense of awe or gratitude? What lessons does this [bud, weed, filtered light] teach? If the patient believes that nature is created by a divine and loving trans-personal being, then a prompt to consider could be, 'What does this say about the character of the Creator?' [37]

Whether through intellectual reflection or subjective experience, nature can be harnessed to nurture the spirit.

6 Conclusion

This sampler of therapeutics can be used to support intra-, inter-, and transpersonal meaning. Many other therapeutics, however, are available. For example, considerable evidence indicates that gratitude can be intentionally cultivated to enhance spiritual well-being [39–41]. Likewise, evidence supports a variety of approaches to meaning-centred therapy for persons with advanced illness [42, 43]. Different approaches to a 5-min mindfulness meditation were also found to bring increased well-being to palliative care patients [44]. Thus, therapeutics for enhancing spiritual well-being abound.

Although a palliative care provider cannot fix a patient's spiritual problems, they can accompany and support a patient's spiritual journeying. Indeed, a clinician's presence can create a safe and sacred space for a patient to begin inner self-exploration. A clinician's precise use of therapeutic communication and wounded healer-ness can provide an environment for a patient to gain spiritual self-awareness. A clinician's support of existing adaptive spiritual and/or religious resources and practices (or support to re-evaluate maladaptive ones) can also aid the patient to experience their end of life more fully. Through spiritual care that increases a sense of meaning, palliative care providers can help patients to move from ordinary to extraordinary [1].

References

1. Reed PG. An emerging paradigm for the investigation of spirituality in nursing. Res Nurs Health. 1992;15(5):349–57.
2. Taylor EJ. What do I say? Talking with patients about spirituality. West Conshohocken, PA: Templeton Press; 2007.
3. Winslow GR, Wehtje-Winslow BJ. Ethical boundaries of spiritual care. Med J Aust. 2007;186(10 Suppl):S63–6.
4. Taylor EJ. Healing communication: a precision instrument for spiritual care. Semin Oncol Nurs. 2021;37(5):151213.
5. Balboni TA, Fitchett G, Handzo GF, Johnson KS, Koenig HG, Pargament KI, et al. State of the science of spirituality and palliative care research part II: screening, assessment, and interventions. J Pain Symptom Manag. 2017;54(3):441–53.
6. Chochinov HM, Hack T, Hassard T, Kristjanson LJ, McClement S, Harlos M. Dignity therapy: a novel psychotherapeutic intervention for patients near the end of life. J Clin Oncol. 2005;23(24):5520–5.
7. Martínez M, Arantzamendi M, Belar A, Carrasco JM, Carvajal A, Rullán M, et al. 'Dignity therapy', a promising intervention in palliative care: a comprehensive systematic literature review. Palliat Med. 2017;31(6):492–509.

8. Zhang Y, Li J, Hu X. The effectiveness of dignity therapy on hope, quality of life, anxiety, and depression in cancer patients: a meta-analysis of randomized controlled trials. Int J Nurs Stud. 2022;132:104273.
9. Schoppee TM, Scarton L, Bluck S, Yao Y, Keenan G, Handzo G, et al. Description of a training protocol to improve research reproducibility for dignity therapy: an interview-based intervention. Palliat Support Care. 2022;20(2):178–88.
10. Xiao J, Chow KM, Choi KC, Ng SNM, Huang C, Ding J, et al. Effects of family-oriented dignity therapy on dignity, depression and spiritual well-being of patients with lung cancer undergoing chemotherapy: a randomised controlled trial. Int J Nurs Stud. 2022;129:104217.
11. Hodge DR. Developing a spiritual assessment toolbox: a discussion of the strengths and limitations of five different assessment methods. Health Soc Work. 2005;30(4):314–23.
12. Taylor EJ. Spiritual screening, history, and assessment. In: Ferrell BRPJ, editor. Textbook of palliative nursing care. 5th ed. New York: Oxford University Press; 2019. p. 432–46.
13. Phoon J, Tan YP, Harding R. A systematic review and narrative synthesis of the evidence underpinning theoretical perspectives and cultural influences on forgiveness in palliative care. J Palliat Med. 2022;25(8):1282–308.
14. Silva RS, Caldeira S, Coelho AN, Apóstolo JLA. Forgiveness facilitation in palliative care: a scoping review. JBI Evid Synth. 2020;18(11):2196–230.
15. Hansen MJ, Enright RD, Baskin TW, Klatt J. A palliative care intervention in forgiveness therapy for elderly terminally ill cancer patients. J Palliat Care. 2009;25(1):51–60.
16. Breitbart W. Forgiveness. Palliat Support Care. 2018;16(3):244–5.
17. Yalom I. Existential psychotherapy. New York: Basic Books; 1980.
18. Godskesen T, Hansson MG, Nygren P, Nordin K, Kihlbom U. Hope for a cure and altruism are the main motives behind participation in phase 3 clinical cancer trials. Eur J Cancer Care (Engl). 2015;24(1):133–41.
19. Gysels M, Shipman C, Higginson IJ. "I will do it if it will help others:" motivations among patients taking part in qualitative studies in palliative care. J Pain Symptom Manag. 2008;35(4):347–55.
20. Nijkamp M, Hollestelle M, Zeegers M, van den Borne B, Reubsaet A. To be(come) or not to be(come) an organ donor, that's the question: a meta-analysis of determinant and intervention studies. Health Psychol Rev. 2008;2(1):20–40.
21. Vilhauer RP. Perceived benefits of online support groups for women with metastatic breast cancer. Women Health. 2009;49(5):381–404.
22. Curry OS, Rowland LA, Van Lissa CJ, Zlotowitz S, McAlaney J, Whitehouse H. Happy to help? A systematic review and meta-analysis of the effects of performing acts of kindness on the well-being of the actor. J Exp Soc Psychol. 2018;76:320–9.
23. Mathew-Geevarughese SE, Corzo O, Figuracion E. Cultural, religious, and spiritual issues in palliative care. Prim Care. 2019;46(3):399–413.
24. Taylor EJ. Religion: a clinical guide for nurses. New York: Springer; 2012.
25. Chakraborty R, El-Jawahri AR, Litzow MR, Syrjala KL, Parnes AD, Hashmi SK. A systematic review of religious beliefs about major end-of-life issues in the five major world religions. Palliat Support Care. 2017;15(5):609–22.
26. Colenda CC, Blazer DG. Review of religious variables in advance care planning for end-of-life care: consideration of faith as a new construct. Am J Geriatr Psychiatry. 2022;30(7):747–58.
27. Balboni TA, Prigerson HG, Balboni MJ, Enzinger AC, VanderWeele TJ, Maciejewski PK. A scale to assess religious beliefs in end-of-life medical care. Cancer. 2019;125(9):1527–35.
28. Anderson D, De Souza J. The importance and meaning of prayer rituals at the end of life. Br J Nurs. 2021;30(1):34–9.
29. Ulanov AB, Ulanov B. Primary speech: the psychology of prayer. Louisville, KY: John Knox Press; 1983.
30. Bentzen JS. In crisis, we pray: religiosity and the COVID-19 pandemic. J Econ Behav Organ. 2021;192:541–83.

31. Balboni MJ, Babar A, Dillinger J, Phelps AC, George E, Block SD, et al. "It Depends": viewpoints of patients, physicians, and nurses on patient-practitioner prayer in the setting of advanced cancer. J Pain Symptom Manag. 2011;41(5):836–47.
32. Smith AR, DeSanto-Madeya S, Pérez JE, Tracey EF, DeCristofaro S, Norris RL, et al. How women with advanced cancer pray: a report from two focus groups. Oncol Nurs Forum. 2012;39(3):E310–6.
33. Taylor EJ, Outlaw FH, Bernardo TR, Roy A. Spiritual conflicts associated with praying about cancer. Psychooncology. 1999;8(5):386–94.
34. Franco LS, Shanahan DF, Fuller RA. A review of the benefits of nature experiences: more than meets the eye. Int J Environ Res Public Health. 2017;14(8):864.
35. Hansen MM, Jones R. The interrelationship of Shinrin-Yoku and spirituality: a scoping review. J Altern Complement Med. 2020;26(12):1093–104.
36. Moeller C, King N, Burr V, Gibbs GR, Gomersall T. Nature-based interventions in institutional and organisational settings: a scoping review. Int J Environ Health Res. 2018;28(3):293–305.
37. Taylor EJ. How can I use nature to nurture the spirit? J Christ Nurs. 2022;39(3):193.
38. Menser T, Baek J, Siahaan J, Kolman JM, Delgado D, Kash B. Validating visual stimuli of nature images and identifying the representative characteristics. Front Psychol. 2021;12:685815.
39. Borelli E, Bigi S, Potenza L, Gilioli F, Artioli F, Porzio G, et al. Gratitude among advanced cancer patients and their caregivers: the role of early palliative care. Front Oncol. 2022;12:991250.
40. McGuire AP, Fogle BM, Tsai J, Southwick SM, Pietrzak RH. Dispositional gratitude and mental health in the U.S. veteran population: results from the National Health and resilience veterans study. J Psychiatr Res. 2021;135:279–88.
41. Mills PJ, Redwine L, Wilson K, Pung MA, Chinh K, Greenberg BH, et al. The role of gratitude in spiritual well-being in asymptomatic heart failure patients. Spiritual Clin Pract (Wash D C). 2015;2(1):5–17.
42. Breitbart W, Rosenfeld B, Pessin H, Applebaum A, Kulikowski J, Lichtenthal WG. Meaning-centered group psychotherapy: an effective intervention for improving psychological well-being in patients with advanced cancer. J Clin Oncol. 2015;33(7):749–54.
43. Breitbart W, Pessin H, Rosenfeld B, Applebaum AJ, Lichtenthal WG, Li Y, et al. Individual meaning-centered psychotherapy for the treatment of psychological and existential distress: a randomized controlled trial in patients with advanced cancer. Cancer. 2018;124(15):3231–9.
44. Yik LL, Ling LM, Ai LM, Ting AB, Capelle DP, Zainuddin SI, et al. The effect of 5-minute mindfulness of peace on suffering and spiritual well-being among palliative care patients: a randomized controlled study. Am J Hosp Palliat Care. 2021;38(9):1083–90.

Struggle and Blessing. Spirituality and Attachment in Palliative Care

Eckhard Frick and Yvonne Petersen

Abstract According to John Bowlby, the attachment system is activated in extreme situations of physical or psychological threats such as separation, bereavement, and absence of an important attachment person. Attachment theory differentiates four attachment styles: secure-autonomous, insecure-avoidant, disorganised (unresolved trauma), insecure-enmeshed. Attachment-to-God theory offers an understanding of transcendent attachment figures such as God, Jesus, Buddha, Mohammed, Mary, etc. and focuses on the individual patient's image of God. Spiritual care in the palliative situation may benefit from an attachment-to-God approach, respecting diverse denominational and religious orientations, and the patient's representations and need of security. This helps nurses, doctors, chaplains, and other accompanying persons provide a secure base for the patient's last departure.

Keywords Attachment theory · Attachment to God · Palliative care · Spiritual care Psychotherapy · God image

1 Introduction

'*Abide with me – fast falls the eventide!*' This poem versified by the dying Anglican priest H.F. Lyte (1793–1847) was made famous by W.H. Monk's (1823–1889) melody, often sung as evensong, at funerals, at military or at sport events, forming for a moment a 'sonic congregation' in otherwise completely secularised contexts [1].

E. Frick (✉)
School of Medicine & Health, Technical University of Munich, Munich, Germany
e-mail: eckhard.frick@tum.de

Y. Petersen
Department of Palliative Medicine, Krankenhaus Barmherzige Brueder, Munich, Germany

M. C. Best (ed.), *Spiritual Care in Palliative Care*,
https://doi.org/10.1007/978-3-031-50864-6_18

Lyte's prayer is inspired by Jesus' walk towards Emmaus together with two disciples. When Jesus makes as though he would go further, '*they constrain him, saying, abide with us: for it is toward evening, and the day is far spent*' (Luke 24). According to Whitehead [2], a sense of permanence is 'dominating the invocation "Abide with Me", and the sense of flux dominating the sequel "Fast Falls the Eventide". [...] In the inescapable flux, there is something that abides; in the overwhelming permanence, there is an element that escapes into flux. Permanence can be snatched only out of flux, and the passing moment can find its adequate intensity only by its submission to permanence'.

Obviously, dying is life's most inescapable flux; however, it is not life's first experience of separation. Attachment theory [3] describes the making and breaking of affectional bonds 'from the cradle to the grave'. Developing a bond to a primary caregiver—mostly to mother or father—in early infancy is crucial from a stable, 'Internal Working Model' (IWM) of interpersonal relationships. These early models will later in life guide the perceptions, emotions, behaviour, and expectations of others. Analogous to childhood inner working models, we can differentiate four adult attachment patterns/styles, developed from the Adult Attachment Interview (see Fig. 1). Individuals with secure-autonomous attachment style are characterised

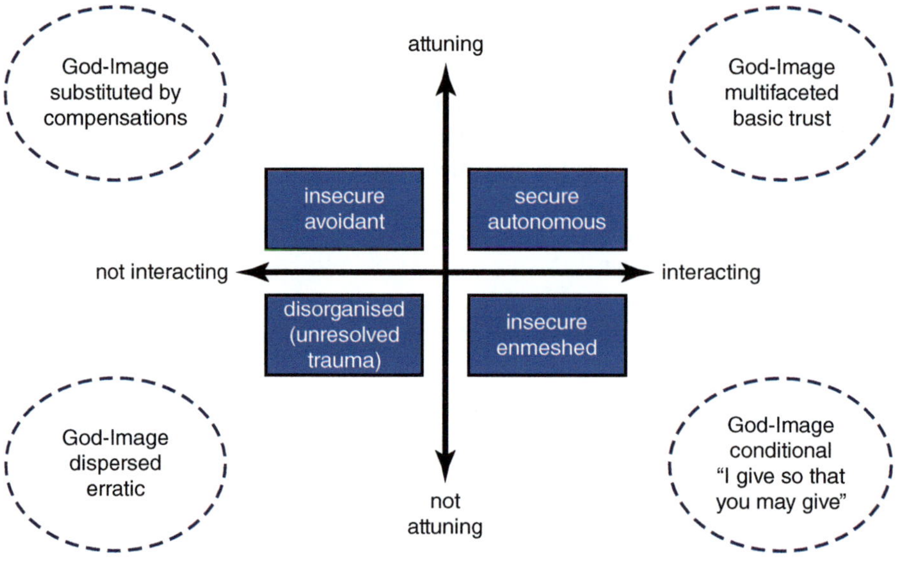

Fig. 1 Attunement and interaction capacities and God image of different attachments styles in dying persons: I: High interacting, high attuning: secure-autonomous. A solid basic trust permits tolerating diverse God image aspects. II: High attuning, not interacting: insecure-avoidant. The person's actions use other persons for one's own needs without committing relatedness. Insecurity is compensated by a manipulated God image. III: Not attuning, not interacting. No clear or rapidly changing patterns: the God image may entail various (esoteric, alternative, fundamentalist...) aspects which provide safety, at least temporarily. IV: Not attuning, high interacting: insecure-enmeshed. Anxious 'clinging' to the other person, incapacity to accept different God image aspects. Negotiating ('*do ut des*') with God

by the capacity to reflect on positive and negative experiences with their caregivers. They are able to show flexible integration and to value their experiences. Respecting God, Buddha, Mohammed, Mary, Jesus, and other transcendent attachment figures, various aspects are tolerated: dark and bright, deceiving, and promising, bad, and good … sides. While Lyte's hymn's first strophe (abide with me, fast falls the eventide…) focuses on proximity seeking [4], the second strophe expresses this capacity to undergo changes and to preserve trust in the other person's or God's permanent presence.

Swift to its close ebbs out life's little day;
Earth's joys grow dim, its glories pass away;
Change and decay in all around I see;
O Thou, who changest not, abide with me.

Previous randomised controlled trials (RCTs) exploring spiritual care in the palliative context addressed the following interventions: reminiscence/life review and group or individual psychotherapy, including Meaning-Centred Behavioural Therapy and Dignity Therapy [5]. With respect to attachment-based interventions, there are RCTs with borderline patients [6] and examining attachment to God among adolescents suffering from conduct disorder [7]. To our knowledge, there are no RCTs exploring attachment-based therapy in palliative care [8, 9].

2 Attachment to God

According to attachment theory, people turn to attachment searching (i) a safe haven (i.e. distress alleviation and comfort) and (ii) a secure base from which to explore, learn, and thrive. Attachment-to-God theory offers an understanding of transcendent attachment figures such as God, Jesus, Buddha, Mohammed, Mary, etc. [10] Now, not all believers have had the experience of secure attachment and they have taken that experience into their lives, as Bowlby puts it, as an IWM that is activated in situations of separation, severe stress, or emotional upheaval. Consequently, a person's IWM will have an impact on her or his dying process.

What is the difference between a concrete, human counterpart, and God as an attachment figure? At first glance, the personal characteristics and qualities of human relationships can be experienced and verified on the basis of concrete experience, while the transcendent God is only a mental construct whose characteristics cannot be verified. However, Rizzuto [11] shows that the image of God arises in the transitional area of parental absence and in this respect includes aspects of bonding experiences with the primary reference person and collective, archetypal contents. The archetypal anchoring of the image of God in the mental inner world has the advantage that concrete interaction experiences cannot shake the image of God, despite all the ambivalences: God remains an unfathomable mystery. More than attachment representations of one's own parents, children, partner, etc., the image of God offers more leeway in dealing with insecurities that affect the otherworldly world. The image of God, as we see with Rizzuto, can be pulled out of the attic like a dreamy and almost forgotten teddy bear from childhood and endowed with a new 'libido', indicating in psychoanalytic terminology new energy and new meaning. This can happen in the course of life whenever the attachment system is activated, e.g. in one of the many goodbye situations that run through our lives and finally in the dying situation.

Attachment theory not only offers a basis for psychotherapeutic interventions in palliative medicine [12]. It also helps us to understand the different manifestations of the image of God and their meaning in the dying situation.

The four attachment types (see Fig. 1) are not pathological categories, although disturbances in experience, behaviour, and relationships can also be understood and treated with the help of attachment theory. Above all, however, the allocation to one of the attachment types can help the palliative care staff to respond sensitively to the needs of the dying person and their relatives. This includes the spiritual orientation, which is condensed in the respective image of God.

3 Attachment Styles and God Image in the Palliative Situation

The following four clinical cases have been chosen from the long clinical experience of one of the authors (Y.P.) as a physician and psychotherapist in palliative care (German originals available) [13].

3.1 Secure Attachment Style in the Dying Process

Ms H. was 87 years old. She was suffering from advanced breast carcinoma and had been admitted because of severe pain and deterioration in her general condition.

According to the information provided by the nurse and the doctor in charge, she seemed to recognise her situation very well and also spoke about her impending death. She was very sad and had a strong wish to die, which was interpreted as a depressive mood.

When I knock, I hear a clear 'Come in'.

The patient is lying in bed, turns her head to me when I enter and smiles: 'Are you the psychotherapist?' I confirm. She makes an inviting gesture and asks me to sit down. She waits until I am seated, then she says, 'I'm glad you came to me'. I sit and look at her.

She begins to speak: 'I have had a good life, experienced good times and difficult times. My childhood was happy. We were four siblings, our parents were very good people, loving and supportive—we liked each other very much. I had to move out early to make money, we were poor'. I ask how she experienced it. The separation was very difficult, but faith always connected her to her family. Her faith carried her through her whole life, even when things were really bad. Here she falls silent and begins to cry. 'I lost my husband and a child at the age of 35. We had an accident, Luischen was seven years old'. She cries, seeks my hand. I hold her hand and caress it gently.

She tells me how the accident happened, and often cannot go on talking; that was too much for her—she felt guilty about the accident and did not want to go on living. It took a long time to find the courage to live. I ask what helped her to overcome this crisis: 'My little son and my faith in God. I knew that I had to go on living for my child. That saved me'. She was active in her church community at the time, received a lot of encouragement and help from there, for which she is grateful to heaven.

Ms H. tells of other incidents from her earlier life and accompanies the experiences with appropriate emotions.

She has lived enough, and now she can go in peace. Her son died 2 years ago—she cries again but smiles at me: she will be happy to see him again. She found the thought reassuring.

She looks very tired now. It was good for her to talk about her life and the pain of life. She takes my hand and looks at me: 'Thanks for listening'.

When I want to visit her again a few days later, I learn that she had asked for the last sacraments and died quietly that night.

3.2 Insecure-Avoidant Attachment Style

Mr S., 65 years old, was admitted to the hospital because of severe pain and poor general condition with a far advanced pancreatic carcinoma. His son had brought him in but left as soon as Mr S. was admitted: he had a lot to do, had to go to the office now, couldn't wait for a doctor who should contact him if there was anything special.

During the initial consultation, the patient lies in bed with his eyes closed. I notice a very tense facial expression, hands clenched on the covers.

I introduce myself as his ward doctor and sit down in a chair next to him on the bed. 'I'm waiting for the chief doctor; I'm a private patient and I'm feeling bad. I'm in pain'. I felt anger, but also despair. 'Is it okay if I treat the pain until he visits you later?' He opens his eyes and looks at me briefly: 'Can you do that too?' I smiled at him: 'Well, I think so'. 'Well, do it then!' he says and closes his eyes without changing his facial expressions.

I check on him often. He needs painkillers several times until the pain noticeably subsides. 'It took quite a while before you managed it', he says, 'but thanks anyway'. I feel a little annoyed, but I think it's not the right moment for a confrontation. 'I'm a doctor and I acted professionally', I reply. He closes his eyes without answering.

In the coming days, he remains pain-free with medication but is difficult to manage. The sisters complain that he wants to do everything independently and is in danger of falling. At night, he does not ring for help and goes to the bathroom alone. He is demanding; it is difficult to please him. He emphasises his status as a very successful, well-known academic. His son only visited him once, left quickly and did not report to the staff.

During visits, he talks a lot about his professional successes, emphasising his difficult career path; he had to work a lot to finance his studies. The parents would have supported him, but according to their own ideas. His father, a strict pastor, preferred a theological education and disapproved of his academic path to becoming an economist. When I ask about the mother, he shrugs his shoulders and makes a dismissive gesture: 'She only prayed and did everything that father wanted'.

He was often 'bad' as a teenager; he also would run away. He repeatedly received 'strict' punishment for his rebelliousness—he certainly deserved it. When asked how often his father punished him, he can't remember exactly, it was so long ago that he didn't mind. He still had a good relationship with his father. He can only vaguely remember other details from his childhood.

When I ask about his current family, he changes the subject. I find out from the nursing staff that his wife has been separated from him for several years. The only son is a successful lawyer. He was extremely proud of him, and it was completely acceptable that he didn't have time for him now either. 'I don't want to be a burden to him'.

He is worse after an acute medical event and would like to speak to me.

He begins hesitantly, unable to continue. He grips my hand, which I had spontaneously placed on his arm, very tightly. He cries, first cautiously, then more and more heavily. I remain still and hold his hand. After a long time, he regains his composure and smiles at me. 'Thank you', he says, 'that was good'. I smile back, stay with him. 'I'm so scared of dying. I was a very religious child; faith often helped me a lot. God was like an anchor for me. Then I forgot about faith during my career, everything else became more important: my success; my money. I only laughed about faith'. The night before, he had had a very touching experience that shook him: A nurse, an Indian nun, had offered to pray with him. She spoke the old words of 'The Lord's Prayer' with him and made a cross on his forehead when he said goodbye. That moved him a lot. Now he feels that he will not live long and is afraid but feels that he is no longer 'entitled' to prayer and religious attention.

I offer him a chaplain, but he refuses; he wanted to talk to me about his fear. He asks me about my own thoughts on faith and my experiences on this topic in my work as a palliative care doctor. I'm happy to provide information. We talk about my experiences and about his fears of 'invalidity'. He listens very carefully and says it helped him. He feels calmer now.

The following night there is acute deterioration. The following morning, he is dying.

When I sit down next to him on the bed, he opens his eyes briefly; he looks relaxed, I think I see a smile. He dies peacefully a few hours later.

The compensating figure, 'God', becomes a stabilising resource that enables the patient to die in peace.

3.3 *Disorganised Style (Unresolved Trauma)*

Ms N. was 41 years old. For 2 years, she had been suffering from a very advanced breast carcinoma, which had previously only been irradiated; the patient had rejected chemotherapy or other reasonable tumour-specific therapies. According to the doctor's report, she had turned to alternative therapies that had not stopped the tumour progression. She was now suffering from severe local pain in the area of the open breast tumour and pain when moving, which was probably caused by bone metastases.

The family doctor had informed us that he had significant problems with the patient: she denied the progression of the cancer and put all her hope in healing objects that she had received from her spiritual master, a healer. He couldn't do anything for the patient and couldn't think of any way to help her. She only agreed to treatment in the palliative care ward if she could walk again after a day.

During the first contact, I see an emaciated, mask-like smiling woman who greets me with the words: 'I'm glad you're coming, I want to go home tomorrow!' She is sitting on a chair; it smells very unpleasant. An unpacked bag is next to her. 'Great', I say, 'it's good that you came to us. We only have one day to help you—so let's start right away!' I smile at her too and sit down next to her. She seems to like the light, open tone. 'Okay,' she says. 'Great', I reply, 'Then please tell me how I can help you'. 'My chest. It's healing very nicely, but the healing process hurts a lot. And my back, I can hardly walk—every movement hurts'. I ask if I can look at her breasts and do a careful physical exam. She looks at me and hesitates. She fixes her eyes searchingly on me. I hold her gaze, smile. 'Well, well', she says.

I help her get up. She tries to lie down, moaning loudly. 'Oh, you poor thing', I say, 'you're in terrible pain. If you want, I'll bring you some painkillers'. She closes her eyes and nods.

After the administration of a strong painkiller, I wait but keep checking on her. She's feeling better. She allows the physical examination. The tumour findings and the physical findings indicate extensive metastasis formation. During the examination, she closes her eyes and holds a grey stone in her hand. It is her 'healing stone', she says when asked. There are more stones in different colours on the bedside table. Interested, I ask about the meaning of the stones. She looks at me again searchingly: 'They help me to get well', she says. 'Then the stones have a very important function', I say.

The night is problematic, the patient is in pain and administering the medication is difficult. She's waiting for my visit. A conversation about the desired release from the clinic develops. I'm not pushing her; she wants to leave the clinic. We agree that she can come back at any time.

The next morning, she is waiting at the door. 'I can't bear the pain any longer'. We admit her to the clinic without comment and are able to take good care of her over the next few days. The stones are with her; she holds the 'healing stone' tightly.

During one of the rounds, she spontaneously talks about herself. Thanks to a healer, she recognised the tumour as a challenge to confront. She is convinced that she will be healed by the blessed stones and then start a new, better life.

When asked, she talks about her biography. She was born as an illegitimate child, her mother was mentally unstable, could not take good care of her, and had been in psychiatric clinics for extended periods of time. As a foster child, she had lived with several families. Here she suddenly breaks off and drifts away. I touch her carefully, say her name. She looks at me, then turns away.

On my next rounds, I learn about her problematic youth. The mother tried again and again to take care of her. As a teenager, she often ran away and repeatedly took drugs. Nevertheless, she completed her apprenticeship as a businesswoman and earned money with it. After several failed relationships, later she met a man and had two children with him.

Her husband was not a nice person and she started to study religion and became a member of a religious sect. 'That's when I got answers for the first time to all my questions. I went to the sect, left my children and my husband'. For the first time I see tears in her eyes, she is crying. 'I've done so many things wrong. My healer says that's why I was given the tumour as a chance to start all over again'. I don't comment but touch her arm comfortingly. She cries, takes her 'healing stone' and holds it tightly to her cheek.

Physically, she gets worse almost every day, but she doesn't seem to notice it. In response to a careful confrontation on my part, she comments: 'Things have to get worse before they get better again'.

Her visitors appear to be members of the sect. Singing and praying can be heard coming from the room. After the visits, she seems exhausted but satisfied. 'This is my family', she says, 'they help me get better'.

Her condition deteriorates acutely and then she is no longer responsive. I sit down next to her. It seems to me that she is restless inside. On impulse, I put the 'healing stone' in her hand and close my fingers around it. She embraces it and instantly becomes calmer. A short time later she dies peacefully.

Up until to the last minute, the healing stone acts as a spiritual helper and helps to achieve a peaceful dying process.

3.4 Insecure-Enmeshed Attachment Style

Ms L. is 65 years old. She has been suffering from a colon carcinoma that has been far advanced for several years. She had visited our palliative care clinic several times and had been unsure how to proceed. Her family, a husband and two daughters aged 26 and 28, were always present at the outpatient clinic meetings. According to the outpatient report, her mood was usually very emotional. Her children and husband had always pushed the patient to continue the chemotherapy. Now a new recurrence had been found and she and her family had decided to come to the palliative care ward for symptom control and a possible change in therapy goals. She suffered from severe nausea.

During the admissions interview, there is an agitated mood in the room: the two daughters are sitting on her bed and stroking her. They are both crying. The husband is standing at the end of the bed and straightening the covers. A young man is standing to one side. The patient has a bowl in front of her and is gagging. 'Please, doctor, quickly! Mama is doing badly! Do something, she's dying!!'

I take a chair and ask one daughter to get up from the bed. She gets up a little reluctantly and with a worried look at her mother: 'Mom, this is the doctor, she'll help you right away!' I ask all family members to sit down, then I look at the patient, introduce myself and ask how I can help her. 'I'm feeling just awful', she says, and retches. I sense that it is important to calm the situation down now and ask the patient if she would like to send the relatives outside during the physical examination. She nods. I politely ask the family, with their mother's permission, to leave the room for a moment so that I can do my job better. I felt a momentary insecurity, the family members look at each other. 'Mom, we're going out for a moment, but then we'll be back'. I say thank you and lead the family to our lounge.

Then I sit down next to the patient, and she holds the bowl in front of her. I get the nurse taking care of her to bring her some medicine and administer it: 'It will do you good and calm you down'.

The patient closes her eyes. 'I can't take it anymore, I'm so scared. My family is so important to me. I want to die'. She sobs. I put my hand comfortingly on her arm, wait a while until she has calmed down a bit, then carry out the examination.

The physical findings are reassuring. I assure her that, first of all, we would help her to alleviate her present ailments; there is no sign that she is near death at the moment. She throws her arms up with folded hands: 'Then all the prayers have helped after all!' When asked, she tells me that the family has started on a pilgrimage for her recovery. 'Now I can believe again', she exclaims. She had always been a believer, but since she became ill, she had lost all trust in God.

I share my findings with the family members who are already waiting impatiently across from the door, and they immediately jump up excitedly. 'Then she won't die right away?' My soothing explanations trigger strong emotional excitement again. The daughters cry and storm into their mother's room. The young man introduces himself as a son, and he would like to speak to me. He tells me that he's trying to keep a clear head amid the chaos—his father is very devoted to his wife, as are his sisters. There is a lot of prayer in the family, which he can't go along with. He has the feeling that there is a deal with God: the family has decided to pay a large sum to pilgrimage to site X if the mother does not die. I thank him and assure him that we would help the mother.

In the coming days, the patient's condition stabilises, and she seems calmer. The family comes for many hours every day and stays with her into the night.

On one of my rounds, Ms L. looks at me openly and wants to know if she still has a chance. It becomes an intense conversation in which we discuss the possible perspectives. The patient thanks me and says: 'My family always decides what I should do—I only live for them!' 'But it's about YOUR life and the time left to YOU', I reply, 'The family will live on'. After a short pause, during which she looks at me, I add that only she can decide about her life, it's her life after all. Thoughtfully, she says that actually, I'm right. She hadn't seen it like that before.

During the next visit, when asked, she tells me her biography. She was a refugee child, her mother fled Poland during the war. She was an only child, her father died in the war. The mother was always worried about her, was always afraid for her. 'I was all she had'. She only married her husband after her mother's death, before which she took care of her. Like her mother, she believes in a God, but she has never had complete trust in him, he is not really reliable. A deep conversation about meaning and faith develops in which I am also asked about my thoughts and experiences.

In a further conversation, we can bring biographically problematic events, which she has seen as stressful, into meaningful causal connections. Thoughtfully, Ms L. says she has discovered something like a 'common thread' in her life. 'I guess I have been guided throughout my life', she says, and, deeply touched, expresses her gratitude for the interview.

The family would like to meet me and now that the mother's condition is more stable, they would like to think about further therapy options. When I asked the patient if she was aware of this, she answered almost indignantly: The family knew best what to do!

I ask for a family discussion, including the patient.

In the family conversation, I realise that the patient has changed—she can express her wishes regarding further treatment. At one point, she even says that it is her life that is at stake. At first, the family reacts almost angrily and irritated, then takes on a harassing tone. There is a lot of crying. Ms L. sticks to her decision to continue the palliative treatment and to forego chemotherapy.

After the conversation, the family wants to speak to me alone again: the daughters are very excited and anxious, they keep questioning the procedure, the course of the tumour and the possible dying process. They decide to be with their mother day and night.

The next day, the patient asks for a priest, she wants a conversation.

Afterwards, she seems relaxed and much calmer.

Her physical condition changes, complications arise. The patient requires more painkillers and palliative, symptom-oriented treatment. The daughters and the husband are very present; the patient accepts it. The patient herself seems increasingly calmer, which also affects her family: the mood is less emotionally charged. At the patient's request, the son now visits frequently; he can better accept the now calmer atmosphere.

After the sacrament of anointing of the sick is performed in the presence of all family members, in a room they have lovingly decorated, her condition deteriorates very quickly, and she dies quietly and peacefully in the family's presence.

It is possible to re-establish the resource of God/faith by recognising a meaningful, 'guided' way of life. This enables the patient to recognise God as a reliable, secure basis for herself and leads to a visible, emotional calm that facilitates the dying process.

4 Discussion

The hymn 'abide with me' quoted at the beginning of this chapter comprises a 'security potency' for the bereaved and terminally sick. 'Abide with me' is a 'therapeutic hymn that guarantees the assurance of God's divine presence in times of tragedy'. [14] The framework of attachment theory, used through this chapter, does not pathologise different interaction styles. It helps, however, find tailored therapeutic responses to the patient's distress by providing resources to the terminal patient, especially respecting the individual God image. Attachment theory permits a structured clinical observation of patients, families, and therapeutic team in the palliative situation, resulting in hypothetical classification of a given attachment style. Questions orienting this clinical observation are: How does the patient interact and utter his or her needs and distress? How does the patient interact with the therapeutic team, with the family? How does the patient express emotions and wishes by gestural, mimic, verbal, and non-verbal signs?

Broadening attachment theory to attachment-to-God theory [15] shows resources and suffering expressed by God images. This approach focuses equally on 'blessing' (inner and outer resources) and 'struggle' (intra and interpersonal conflicts and the patient's wrestling with her or his God). Exline et al. [16] integrate attachment research and other previous research and differentiate four behaviours towards God in the context of spiritual struggle, focusing on two orthogonal dimensions (with opposites at their endpoints: constructive versus destructive; active versus passive):

I. APPROACH (constructive for relationship; move towards partner, corresponding to a secure-autonomous attachment pattern).
II. DISENGAGEMENT (destructive for relationship; create distance or conflict, corresponding to an insecure-avoidant or dismissive attachment pattern).
III. SUPPRESSION (actively suppress or avoid negative emotions, corresponding to an unresolved attachment pattern).
IV. PROTEST (express concerns or questions; assertion, arguing with God, corresponding to an insecure-enmeshed attachment pattern).

Exline et al. [17] describe six domains of spiritual struggle: (I) divine (e.g. feeling angry at God or punished by God), (II) demonic (e.g. feeling tempted or attacked by the devil or evil spirits), (III) ultimate meaning (e.g. questioning whether life has a deeper meaning or purpose), (IV) doubt (e.g. doubts or confusion about beliefs), (V) moral (e.g. struggling to follow moral principles; concern about moral failures), and (VI) interpersonal religious struggles (e.g. conflicts or hurts involving religious people or religious issues; anger at organised religion). In all these domains, spiritual struggle may be associated with emotional distress but also with spiritual growth. It may, for example, clarify one's ideas about God and this life's reality. Exline et al. [17] suggest 'that simply providing a safe, accepting environment can help provide space for clients to explore their struggles without pressuring them (or the therapist) to find quick answers or solutions'. Seen from an attachment orientation, this safe therapeutic space is crucial as a safe haven (i.e. distress alleviation and comfort) [18], especially for patients and families presenting an insecure attachment-style. Struggling with God or spiritual representations does not need catechetical or otherwise normative answers in order to close (or deny) the patient's questions. On the contrary, by providing a secure base (from which to explore, learn, and thrive) and therapeutic interventions tailored to the perceived attachment style, the therapist will foster the patient's capacity of exploration, despite his or her distress and beyond 'darkness, change, and decay'. We interviewed Ken Pargament about his vision of spiritual struggles and he answered the following (Pargament et al., 2014/2018, pp. 216–217) [19]:

So, I think we have to be careful of romanticising struggle, and responding reassuringly to our clients: 'Oh, you're having pain but you'll grow'. Not necessarily! Not everyone does. Part of our obligation, then, is to discern when struggle is in fact problematic and potentially deadly and when people are taking a more constructive, healthy path through their struggle. Now, how do you do that? How do you distinguish whether struggle is leading people to growth or to decline? I think that's a clinical question, but it's also a vital research question that is, as yet, unanswered. I wouldn't say that struggle is inherently destructive. That's why I wasn't really happy with the term 'negative religious coping' because it suggests that it's negative and that there's no benefit to it. I prefer the term 'religious struggle' to 'negative religious coping', and I try to use the language of struggle more myself. So there's positive religious coping where we're speaking about religion as a resource to people in dealing with difficult situations. It's a resource that is generally helpful. And then there are people who are struggling with religious/spiritual issues in their coping. These struggles are not necessarily a problem. Sometimes, they propel us forward in our lives.

Struggling with God may be a consequence of divine entitlement, expressed by the following exemplary convictions: 'God will always give me what I want', 'I deserve more spiritual blessings', 'I expect God to make me happy all the time', 'I expect to be blessed, no matter what I do', and 'God owes me'. [20] Divine entitlement fits particularly well with the conditional, negotiating insecure-enmeshed attachment style. More generally, deserving blessings in divine entitlement may challenge, as in romantic entitlement, academic entitlement, and sexual entitlement, a sort of recompense for experienced deceptions during the lifespan or for suffering in the palliative situation. In the biblical tradition, we find many persons who struggle with God. The most important is Jacob's wrestling with a dark being (Angel? Demon? God?):

'And Jacob was left alone. And a man wrestled with him until the breaking of the day. When the man saw that he did not prevail against Jacob, he touched his hip socket, and Jacob's hip was put out of joint as he wrestled with him. Then he said, 'Let me go, for the day has broken'. Jacob said, 'I will not let you go unless you bless me' (Genesis 32:24–26).

Jacob will be hurt, limping the rest of his life. However, he will be blessed: His wound will be beneficial, a resource. Respecting a dying patient's struggling with

God, angels, demons, or other spiritual representations, the therapist cannot decide whether it is blessing, growth, or mere suffering. All the therapist can do is to provide a safe space and to accompany the patient's exploration.

References

1. Johnson-Williams EG. Sonic congregating: the hymn as national British spectacle. Yale J Music Relig. 2022;8(2):7.
2. Whitehead AN. Process and reality. Macmillan; 1957.
3. Bowlby J. The making and breaking of affectional bonds: I. Aetiology and psychopathology in the light of attachment theory. Br J Psychiatry. 1977;130(3):201–10.
4. Feeney JA, Noller P. Adult attachment, vol. 14. Thousand Oaks: SAGE; 1996. https://doi.org/10.4135/9781452243276.
5. Best MC, Vivat B, Gijsberts M-J. Spiritual care in palliative care. Religions. 2023;14(3):320.
6. Buchheim A, Hörz-Sagstetter S, Doering S, Rentrop M, Schuster P, Buchheim P, Pokorny D, Fischer-Kern M. Change of unresolved attachment in borderline personality disorder: RCT study of transference-focused psychotherapy. Psychother Psychosom. 2017;86(5):314–6. https://doi.org/10.1159/000460257.
7. Salmanian M, Ghobari-Bonab B, Hooshyari Z, Mohammadi M-R. Effectiveness of spiritual psychotherapy on attachment to god among adolescents with conduct disorder: a randomized controlled trial. Psychol Relig Spiritual. 2020;12(3):269–75. https://doi.org/10.1037/rel0000241.
8. Kunsmann-Leutiger E, Loetz C, Frick E, Petersen Y, Müller JJ. Attachment style and spiritual coping in palliative patients. J Hosp Palliat Nurs. 2018;20(4):385–91. https://doi.org/10.1097/NJH.0000000000000455.
9. Petersen Y, Köhler L. Application of attachment theory for psychological support in palliative medicine during the terminal phase. Gerontology. 2006;52(2):111–23. http://www.karger.com/DOI/10.1159/000090957
10. Cherniak AD, Mikulincer M, Shaver PR, Granqvist P. Attachment theory and religion. Curr Opin Psychol. 2021;40:126–30. https://doi.org/10.1016/j.copsyc.2020.08.020.
11. Rizzuto AM. The birth of the living God. A psychoanalytic study. Chicago: University of Chicago Press; 2002.
12. Müller JJ, Petersen Y. Bindungstheorie als Grundlage psychotherapeutischer Interventionen in der Palliativmedizin. In: Anneser J, Frick E, editors. Psychosomatische Medizin und Palliative Care. Perspektiven und Ansätze aus multiprofessioneller Sicht. Stuttgart: Kohlhammer; 2023. p. 105–23.
13. Frick E. Gerufen oder nicht gerufen? Stuttgart: Kohlhammer; 2024.
14. Adenike LA. Analytical discourse on the security potency structure of abide with me. In: Ojukwu EV, Esimone CC, Okeke IN, Ugoo-Okonkwo I, editors. The prodigious musicologist: celebrating Professor Agatha Ijeoma Onwuekwe (Ugonabo). ArchRockCreativesMedia, Umodioka; 2023. p. 416–30.
15. Granqvist P, Mikulincer M, Gewirtz V, Shaver PR. Experimental findings on God as an attachment figure: normative processes and moderating effects of internal working models. J Pers Soc Psychol. 2012;103(5):804–18. https://doi.org/10.1037/a0029344.
16. Exline JJ, Wilt JA, Stauner N, Schutt WA, Pargament KI, Fincham FD, May RW. Supernatural operating rules: how people envision and experience God, the devil, ghosts/spirits, fate/destiny, karma, and luck. Psychol Relig Spiritual. 2021;15:504. https://doi.org/10.1037/rel0000444.
17. Exline JJ, Pargament KI, Wilt JA, Pait KC, Schutt WA. Research on spiritual struggles: a brief snapshot focusing on new horizons. Spiritual Care. 2024;13(2):103–14.

18. Best M, Butow P, Olver I. Creating a safe space: a qualitative inquiry into the way doctors discuss spirituality. Palliat Support Care. 2016;14(5):519–31. https://doi.org/10.1017/S1478951515001236.
19. Pargament KI, Frick E, Roser T. "Struggles are not necessarily destructive or dangerous". The Wasan Island talk with Kenneth I. Pargament. Spiritual Care. 2014/2018;7(2):215–8.
20. Grubbs JB, Exline JJ, Campbell WK, Twenge JM, Pargament KI. God owes me: the role of divine entitlement in predicting struggles with a deity. Psychol Relig Spiritual. 2018;10(4):356–67. https://doi.org/10.1037/rel0000147.

Reaching Spiritual Realms Through Music Therapy and Music in Palliative Care

Clare C. O'Callaghan

Abstract Spiritual care focuses on helping people to connect with what they find sacred or important and brings an overall feeling of health and well-being. Music is a fundamental part of being human and can profoundly support this endeavour. Music can inspire, soothe, transport, and enable transcendence. Some project anthropomorphic properties onto music, describing it as a friend or saviour; it can convey understanding, validate, and give a voice. Music can powerfully elicit memories and accompanying emotions, enable emotional release, and connect people with significant others, places, values, and religious beliefs. Alternatively, music that does not resonate may need avoidance; and music associated with devastating loss may need silencing while it safely holds painful states, available for returning to when ready. The chapter describes music therapy in the care of serious illness, with a focus on contributions to generalist spiritual care. Additionally, the chapter includes suggestions for how specialist and generalist spiritual carers can use music to extend spiritual support. Research findings and case illustrations demonstrate that music therapy and thoughtful music-based applications can extend the multisensorial scope of reaching and supporting spiritual realms in those affected by serious illnesses.

Keywords Music therapy · Music · Spirituality · Religion · Generalist spiritual care · Palliative care · Serious illness · Informal carers

---

C. C. O'Callaghan (✉)
Caritas Christi Palliative Care Unit and Psychosocial Cancer Care, St Vincent's Hospital, Melbourne, VIC, Australia

Department of Medicine, The University of Melbourne, Melbourne, VIC, Australia
e-mail: clare.ocallaghan@svha.org.au

M. C. Best (ed.), *Spiritual Care in Palliative Care*,
https://doi.org/10.1007/978-3-031-50864-6_19

1 Introduction

Spiritual care can refer to secular practices and religious rituals that help people to connect with what they consider sacred or important, attend to spiritual suffering, and bring an overall sense of resilience, hope, peace, and transcendence [1–5]. Patients and informal carers affected by serious and advanced illnesses report wide-ranging spiritual concerns [6], which are associated with patients' reduced quality of life [7], coping [8], and healthcare satisfaction [9]. Spiritual care is a core domain within international palliative care guidelines [10–12], with many turning to spirituality when dealing with advanced illness [8, 13]; however, hospital-based spiritual care remains inadequately offered [6, 14–17] and sparsely described [3, 13, 18]. Specialist spiritual care focuses on those especially challenged by existential issues [1], and its increased presence in serious illness settings remains essential. Generalist spiritual care also warrants attention, which refers to how other health workers help patients and families to feel that what is sacred or important to them is respected [1]. This chapter describes music therapy in the generalist spiritual care of those affected by serious, life threatening, and end-stage illnesses. It will also offer suggestions for how other health workers may use music to support spiritual well-being in this context. Music 'makes sense' in spiritual care as it often reaches and affects significant realms in private and social lives, and deepens transpersonal aspects of spiritual practices, including meditation, worship, and ritual [19].

Spirituality is a complex, multidimensional, culturally laden concept, critiqued for overinclusive meaning, and defined in widely varied ways by health workers, [20–22] patients, and caregivers [6, 23]. In Australia, many patients with advanced illness and their caregivers do not resonate with the term and more relatable terms are postulated as adjuncts, including 'values-based care' and 'hospitality' when communicating about spiritual care [1]. This chapter reflects one music therapist's interpretation of how music therapy, and music in general, can help patients and those significant to them (hereafter called families) connect with their personhood, that is, their values, sense of dignity, self-respect, and self-compassion. Following a definition and description of music therapy, the evidence base for music therapy and music in 'generalist spiritual care' (hereafter called 'spiritual care') of those affected by serious illness is summarised. Illustrative case studies will be outlined, followed by general suggestions for offering music in serious illness care.

2 Music Therapy, Spirituality, and Serious Illness: Definition and Description

The World Federation of Music Therapy (WFMT) defines music therapy as:

> the professional use of music and its elements as an intervention in medical, educational, and everyday environments with individuals, groups, families, or communities who seek to optimize their quality of life and improve their physical, social, communicative, emotional,

> intellectual, and spiritual health and wellbeing. Research, practice, education, and clinical training in music therapy are based on professional standards according to cultural, social, and political contexts [24].

Music therapy emphasises the music therapist–client therapeutic relationship, and clients do not need musical backgrounds to benefit. Music therapists are university educated and accredited by national registration committees. The profession is distinguishable from 'music medicine' wherein music is applied for therapeutic intention without the therapeutic relationship [25], and 'music thanatology', which refers to a compassionate musician offering 'prescriptive music, using harp and voice at bedside' [26, p. 80].

Recognition of the scope and significance of addressing clients' spiritual well-being pervades music therapy practice [27–30]. Spirituality is highlighted in the WFMT definition of music therapy and in the earliest publication on music therapy in palliative care: Susan Munro and Balfour Mount in 1978 discussed how music therapy provided a 'means of expressing spiritual feelings and feeling comforted and reassured (and provided) an avenue for expressing doubts, anger, fear of punishment, and questions on the ultimate meaning of life' [31, p. 1030]. Deborah Salmon, another music therapist who worked with Balfour Mount at the Royal Victoria Hospital Palliative Care Unit, Montreal, wrote:

> The ultimate purpose of a music therapist in palliative care is to provide a safe space in which … connections to the psychospiritual realm may be facilitated, enabling the patient to experience a greater sense of meaning, integrity, and well-being. [27, p. 145]

In an international study examining the relevance of spirituality for music therapists (n = 358), 79% reported that spirituality was connected to their work and 91% believed that music therapy contributes to clients' spiritual well-being [32]. Many added, however, that this was not the primary focus of their therapeutic work.

When working with people affected by serious illness, music therapy programmes vary according to cultural, organisational, and music therapist-related factors. The core that connects all music therapists' work in serious illness care is 'a belief that music can affect the expression of loss' [33, p 6]. The work can occur in home-based and inpatient hospice and palliative care programmes, residential care (nursing homes), palliative rehabilitation, and acute care settings. Music therapists use a holistic care approach, guided by the 'total pain' construct which asserts that pain sensation is a manifestation of physical, social, emotional, and spiritual distress [34]: This means that amelioration of spiritual distress may reduce pain sensation. The broad range of psychosocial, physical, and existential concerns that may be addressed by music therapy include loss, grief, fear, anxiety, communication issues, regret, pain, delirium, insomnia, tension, social disconnection, funeral planning, legacy creation, and need for a music-related aesthetic or religious connection. Further concerns that music therapy can address are extensively detailed elsewhere [35, 36]. Like other creative arts therapists, music therapists importantly offer activities to 'open up possibilities' from the client's illness experience [37, p 17] and accompany patients and families [38]. The welcoming hospitality framework can guide this work wherein patients and family members are each regarded as unique and unrepeatable individuals rather than 'problems' to be solved [39], and caring acts are intended to convey concern for comfort, availability, and 'something of oneself' rather than purely duty [40, 41]. Patients and families are sourced through referrals from interdisciplinary team members and through self-referrals as the therapist offers sessions in inpatient settings. People choose if and the extent to which they engage in music therapy, as with other supportive care modalities. Music therapy methods and brief descriptions of their uses follow:

Replaying the Music from One's Life When the author visits patients, who are sometimes with their families, she takes an electric piano and sheet music of over 5000 songs from varied genres (including religious) and cultures, and classical music pieces that can be immediately played live. Recorded music is also available. Music requests are invited. Patients and families may listen, sing, dance, cry, and laugh. Music-elicited memories and statements about who/what is valued may be shared, and accompanying emotions may be witnessed and acknowledged. 'Re-storying' may follow, as 'fragmented understandings' [37] arising from challenging illnesses or earlier life experiences are spoken, and the therapist listens, validates, and perhaps offers reframing. Music shared with families may validate each other's significance, and memories of these significant moments can sustain the bereaved. Song choices can send strong messages. The song 'I will always love you' [42] may be requested as someone sits with a dying relative; a dying patient may ask for their parent's favourite song in every shared session (in one case it was 'Love Me Tender' [43]); and religious songs may be requested to connect with faith-based values.

In these sessions, music therapy can allow patients and families to move into a therapeutic space in relatively non-confrontational ways. Music therapists are trained to consider when to invite verbal reflection or to be a quiet presence. Music has personal meaning: individuals and families requesting songs do not have to talk about them, but in their minds, memories, imagery, emotions, and thoughts can flow. Meaningful shared secrets may be non-verbally conveyed through timely shared eye contact, nods and touch, and this can be especially powerful in clinical, public institutional settings.

Exploring 'New' Music This includes therapeutic song writing, unfamiliar live or recorded music, music improvisation, and therapeutic music lessons. Music instruments such as tuned *hapi* drums are available for people to play, even if they have never played an instrument before. After one patient played a hapi drum for the first time she said, 'I never thought I would experience anything beautiful ever again'. These instruments can be loaned to patients and such improvisations can also be shared between patients and families.

Music-Based Legacy Work This includes patients' song compositions, created with music therapist support. The songs can include the creation of new lyrics and music, or simply new lyrics for familiar songs. They can be recorded by patients, solo or with therapist support and the recordings given as gifts. One inpatient replaced the lyrics in 'Twinkle Twinkle, Little Star' [44] with lyrics which invited her infant child to find her mother's support in the starlight after her death.

Guided Uses of Music This includes music-based relaxation, sometimes using the iso-principle whereby live musical elements are performed to resonate with the patient's tension, with musical elements shifting to support a more relaxed state over time. It may also include guided imagery and music, after which patients may draw and consider the meaning of imagery experienced. For example, before he died, one inpatient described comforting imagery of returning to a former country home, where native animals came to farewell him.

Environmental Music Therapy This involves live music played in public areas in serious illness setting following permission and possible requests from patients and families. Patients and families sometimes prefer music played outside their rooms in initial or all sessions. The music therapist will occasionally enter rooms to assess responses, and invite further requests, or engage in therapeutic conversation as music-elicited stories are shared. This approach may be helpful for those ambivalent about engaging in music therapy. Patients and families sometimes come and sit near the therapist as she plays in public ward areas and verbal exchanges are shared. Occasionally, patients and families play the piano, an available guitar, or percussion instruments. The space is also open for staff to engage with patients and families: they may discuss music-related themes, sing, or even dance. The focus is on sensitively offering opportunities to enable the palliative care unit's (or hospital ward's) transient community involvement [45], and enhance the quality of life of all members.

3 Music Therapy, Spirituality, and Serious Illness: Illustrations

The following scenarios illustrate in further detail how music therapy can help patients to reach spiritual realms through music therapy. The first scenario describes how music therapy helped a patient to revisit and integrate traumatic personal hardship and to experience more comfort and self-worth before his death. The second describes how music therapy helped a patient to deal with grief related to her expected death.

3.1 Atith

Atith was aged in his late 50s, born in Laos, lived alone, and described as having 'some English' and a long-standing addiction problem. He was hospitalised and diagnosed with end stage metastatic cancer, dying several weeks later. His issues included fluctuating respiratory distress and anxiety due to dyspnoea. Through an interpreter, Atith had conveyed to medical staff that he feared that he would die through breathlessness. On hearing me play classical music for another patient, the music therapist overheard Atith repeat the phrase, 'music beautiful'. Before leaving the ward area, the therapist offered to play an Asian folk song (by showing Atith the song's textual name), which Atith recognised. He smiled widely and nodded 'yes' as it was played. In following days, Atith asked a staff member for help to die, and he regularly expressed suicidal ideation. When the music therapist visited Atith for his first individual music therapy session, Atith used fragmented sentences and hand gestures to request a song about a boat being hit by a big wave. He smiled and nodded 'yes' when the melody of 'The Morning After" [46] was played on the electric piano. After finishing the song, Atith looked downcast and said 'tough'. 'Tough memories?' the therapist said, and he nodded 'yes'. On being invited to talk about these memories, Atith used short phrases and gestures to describe how he had previously led a boat with many refugees from Cambodia to Indonesia when it was attacked by thieves and the boat's motor stolen. Although frightened, Atith told the refugees to pull wood panels from the boat's cabin and use them to row. They reached the shore days later, where many dead bodies lay on the beach. Atith fell silent and nodded gently as the music therapist acknowledged his trauma and added that he sounded like a hero. The following day, Atith's shortness of breath improved, and the medical team reported that he was 'happy'. In the next music therapy session, Atith and the therapist shared a piano and drum musical improvisation, and Atith then pretended to play a mouth organ. On being lent a mouth organ, he played some melodic fragments, and smiled with delight when others nearby recognised the songs he played. Over following days, Atith deteriorated and died, recognising that he was now known by palliative care staff as a hero and musician, with unfathomable trauma acknowledged, and not just as an end-stage cancer patient who had a drug addiction.

Comment Atith's story demonstrates how music therapy provided generalist spiritual care related to two of the five spiritual need areas in The Standards for Hospice & Palliative Care Chaplaincy [47]. These are: (a) exploring a person's sense of meaning and purpose in life; and (b) affirming life and worth by encouraging reminiscence.

Atith's story demonstrates how music therapy may support story evocation and telling in less threatening ways than traditional medical history-taking, and how music therapy can powerfully help people to 'restore some coherence to the story of their lives, … (and be reminded) of their previous capabilities to transcend' [37, p. 15]. Atith's request for a song from a film about a sinking cruise liner, The Poseidon Adventure [48], indicated he wanted to revisit an earlier traumatic memory. This arguably illustrated Stein's depiction of music potentially being an internal 'sacred conservatory' associated with internal emotions and images, available to return to, if and when ready. Atith's traumatic experience as an asylum seeker 'boat person' was relived, reworked, and integrated with therapist support, empowering him to live more peacefully in his final days. Atith's story is also testament to the power of music therapy in supporting patients' 'double awareness' at the end of mortal life, that is, their connection with quality life possibilities while preparing for death [49]. Atith's story also reminds us of the importance of cultural sensitivity in music therapy and spiritual care practice. When working with people from culturally and linguistically diverse backgrounds, it is especially important to check people's responses to music as varied barriers, norms, and values towards music are evident across cultures [50]. Offering to play a nationalist song for a refugee with traumatic memories from their country of origin, for example, needs to be avoided.

3.2 Angela

For 28 months, Angela, in her mid-50s, rotated between palliative and nursing home care, spending a total of 39 weeks in the inpatient palliative care unit before her death. Her metastatic disease was causing increasing quadriplegia, pain, anxiety, and other issues. Angela's response to anxiolytics was poor due to sedating and confusion effects. Angela worked as a schoolteacher until not long before her first palliative care admission and had two very supportive young adult daughters.

Angela experienced 16 music therapy sessions during her palliative care unit admissions. In sessions, Angela sang favourite songs on her own or with her daughters, occasionally improvised on instruments, and composed songs with music therapist support. In one session, Angela added a prayerful verse to the song, 'One Day at a Time' [51], asking for God's support: *'How'd I be feeling; Walking again? Lord I need you to hold onto me; And be my guide; Please support me; and hold me up; Give me the strength to be positive; And to succeed'.*

Angela later wrote an original song, with music therapy assistance, about dealing with her illness. The song was sung and recorded by Angela, her daughters, and about six medical and nursing staff (who the family invited to join in), which brought much joy. The song's chorus was:

> It's not for a reason, it is what it is,
> Not what you'd hope for, we've had to adjust
> We've come a long way, confident and strong
> Determined women, together life moves on

Some of the other lyrics in the song were:

> No words will take the pain away
> The essence is time, it helps to process …
> People do their bit; it gives me hope
> Helping hands, prayers of faith
> St Anthony, Mary McKillop, and other saints
> Each little miracle goes a long way

After recording the song with staff, one daughter commented: '*We will cherish this moment singing with staff forever'.* Angela's daughters also recorded the song, which was played at Angela's funeral.

In another admission, Angela and her daughters together composed and recorded a play song, with many expressive horn sounds, for a loved 2-year-old relative. The daughters later recorded the child singing it and brought it into the hospital for Angela to listen to who was delighted. Angela also later composed another song for her daughters, which included the following chorus lyrics:

> The time has come, you are adults
> You've taken on responsibilities
> You've stepped up when required
> Live life normally, remember family
> Seeing that makes me happy and proud

Comment Arguably, Angela's story demonstrates how music therapy provides generalist spiritual care related to three of the five spiritual need areas in The Standards for Hospice & Palliative Care Chaplaincy [47]. These are: (a) exploring attitudes, beliefs, ideas, values, and concerns about life and death issues; (b) exploring the individual's hopes and fears for themselves and their families/carers; and (c) exploring the 'why' questions in relation to life, suffering, and death.

Music therapy supports patient and families to navigate devastating, distressing, and sad conditions in visually confronting, and sometimes noisy and smelly hospital environments. In music therapy, patients' and families' choice of music reflects the feelings, memories, and spiritual realms they want and are ready to connect with. The oscillation between lighter and sombre states echoes the dual process model of bereavement [52] whereby one processes loss through oscillating between confronting and retreating from grief tasks. Angela demonstrated this throughout her time in the palliative care unit. At times, she declined music therapy sessions because she was too distressed or disinterested; at other times she used music therapy to express and process grief and distress; engage with religious beliefs and her mortality; connect with and communicate important messages and hopes to people close to her; and express joy. Music can help people to feel held in a safe place to mourn [53] or bring joyful relief. Joy is also described as a 'key to spirituality' through its personal associations with self-expansion, self-transcendence, other embracing, and power to connect people with each other [54].

4 Spiritual-Based Research: Music Therapy and Music in Serious Illness Care

4.1 Music Therapy

Over the past three decades extensive, heterogeneous research has examined the role of music therapy in serious illness care [55], with many studies including its impact on patients' and families' spirituality and spiritual well-being. Brief descriptions of these spiritual-related findings follow:

Quantitative and Mixed Methods Findings

A systematic review of experimental or quasi-experimental studies on the effects of music interventions on patients' spirituality found seven studies which met the inclusion criteria, five of which included patients with cancer or receiving palliative care. Of those five U.S. studies, all included music therapists, most used participants' music preferences or choices in the interventions, and most examined individual sessions. Participant numbers ranged from 9 to 90, and session numbers conducted ranged from 3 to 6. Measures included the Functional Assessment of Chronic Illness Therapy-Spiritual Well-Being (FACIT-Sp) [56, 57], Reed Spiritual Perspective Scale [58, 59], and the Inspirit Scale (adapted from the Spiritual Well-Being Scale) [60]. Music interventions were compared to standard care or treatment [56, 57, 60] or another audio-stimulus [58, 59]. Two studies reported statistical pre-post improvements in the music therapy group compared to the control group (Cook et al. [57]: meaning $p = 0.677$, peace $p = 0.018$, faith $p = 0.001$, and full scale $p = 0.089$; Wlodarczyk [60]: $d = 1$, $p = 0.01$). The other three studies reported no differences. While the benefit of music therapy on spirituality was unclear, review authors stated that the non-significant results did not demonstrate ineffective treatment and that further studies were needed, including studies which used measurement instruments that did not imply religious beliefs, such as the FACIT-Sp [61], and qualitative studies. Notably, the randomised controlled trial by Cook and colleagues included interviews with four participants in a mixed methods study, wherein all reported that music therapy addressed patients' spiritual needs, including positive effects on their peace, faith, and meaning in life. Some participants also reported that music therapy helped them to feel closer to God and that provision of music therapy would improve the hospital's spiritual care [57].

A more recent randomised controlled trial in Germany, which used the FACIT-Sp, provided further support for music therapy in the spiritual care of those receiving palliative care. The study examined the 'song of life' (SOL) music therapy 3-session intervention wherein: the palliative care inpatient ($n = 104$) identified a biographically meaningful song, the song was transformed into lullaby style, and the patient reflected on elicited feelings and memories while responding to pre-defined questions, with the final two sessions audio-recorded. The comparison was a relaxation intervention. FACIT-Sp 12 scores were measured on the first baseline music therapy visit and the third (final) visit two days later. Patients receiving SOL reported significantly higher spiritual well-being ($F = 5.53$, $p = 0.04$; [$d = 0.52$]) and ego integrity ($F = 16.03$, $p < 0.01$) following SOL when compared to the relaxation intervention [62].

Other evidence to support music therapy for spiritual care in serious illness contexts is found in two retrospective studies. In a retrospective cross-sectional analysis of electronic medical records studies, cancer patients ($n = 10{,}534$) who received hospice care and music therapy in the USA reported that their spiritual support was adequate (OR = 1.59, $p = 0.06$) and that they had been involved in discussions about spirituality (odds ratio [OR] =1.59, $p = 0.01$) [63]. In another retrospective programme evaluation of cancer patients' ($n = 358$) involvement in music therapy sessions, a subgroup of Black patients were closely examined ($n = 75$). The study found that Black U.S. patients discussed spirituality more commonly than White patients during sessions (Blacks 39.4%; Whites: 3.1%), whereas White patients focussed more on family bonds (Blacks 18.2%; Whites: 40.6%). Authors discussed findings in relation to music's key role in Black churches, and historical role in black communities for helping self-expression, hope for ultimate justice, and stoicism. They suggested that music was therefore a culturally relevant approach for helping Black patients to process and work through pain experiences [64].

Qualitative Findings

Heterogeneous qualitative studies demonstrate further support for music therapy in the spiritual care of those with serious illness. A qualitative content analysis of listening logs recorded by eight participants with breast cancer in the U.S. indicated that specific songs could inspire spiritual thoughts, which could calm and help with coping with cancer treatment. The songs were on a CD created by a music therapist after individual sessions. Patients received up to five sessions and were asked to listen to the CD daily [65]. In a 5-day retreat which included a one-off music therapy session at a U.K. cancer centre, participants with cancer ($n = 23$) expressed thoughts which indicated experiences of transcendence, connectedness, and meaning making in the session. The sessions included music improvisation, relaxation to classical music, and verbal discussion [66].

In a U.S. naturalistic inquiry, open-ended interviews were conducted with seven bereaved caregivers of home hospice care patients, who reflected on their memories of music therapy experiences shared with the now deceased patients. Caregivers remembered spiritual experiences of: joy (both personally and seeing joy in the loved one); empowerment (happiness to be able to help the loved one); connectedness (with the loved one and the greater scheme of life); remembrance (gratitude for the loved one); and hope (peace in music and looking forward to doing desired things). An overall thematic finding from this study was that caregivers experienced 'meaning through transcendence' [67].

A 'coping through spirituality' theme was found in a study examining U.S. parents' ($n = 11$) lived experience of their children's heartbeat recordings (HBR) when the children were receiving palliative care for progressive neurodegenerative illnesses. In this intervention, music therapists synchronised the child's heartbeat rhythm with one of the child's or parent's favourite songs. One parent stated that s/he felt that the song was spiritual because the:

> heartbeat is what gives you life (and) to hear your loved one's heart beat on a song that has deep meaning to it really hits on so many levels, spiritually on so many chambers of your heart, in your mind, in your thought process and things. [68, p. 1026]

Finally, song lyrics that patients with serious illness composed in music therapy regularly included spiritual themes, leading authors to extrapolate that therapeutic song writing can therefore spiritually affirm and support these song writer patients. In an analysis of 64 songs' lyrics written by 39 Australian palliative care patients, seven songs (11%) included prayers to God, and 10 (16%) included expressions of gratitude to family members, staff, and God [69]. In another analysis of 36 songs written by 27 parents with cancer for their children, category (sub-theme) findings included: (a) 'Parents reflect directly and metaphorically on existential and metaphysical matters through references to hope, faith, blessings, God, prayer, and to being present now and after life'; (b) 'Parents reflect on the beauty, "miracle" and wonder of life'; and (c) 'Messages and requests depicting comfort, support, encouragement, existential beliefs, and coping strategies, including parents immortally remaining a part of their children's lives' [70, p 1153]. The final statement of findings also included the message that: While some parents apologise or request their children's optimism and forgiveness, many convey their personal reflections to them, including their existential and metaphysical beliefs, making direct or metaphorical reference to hope, faith, blessings, God, prayer, and to being present, now and after life [70, p 1154].

4.2 *Musicians and Music for Self-Care*

Studies on the role of musicians, and the relevance of music for people affected by serious illness, have also generated important information about how music can maintain spiritual well-being. A U.S. study examined the effect of a live flautist playing patients' preferred music when they received hospice or palliative care consults ($n = 46$). Spirituality was one of the thematic findings with some patients reporting that the music made them feel closer to God and that it brought 'strength, peace, and hope' [71]. In a similar French study ($n = 10$), however, the spirituality theme was 'less developed' which authors ascribed to 'cultural reasons'. This study included two musicians playing varied musical instruments in a palliative care unit's hallway. While the majority of patients experienced pleasant emotions, including relaxation, well-being, and joy, some reflected on the difficulty of choosing songs and fatigue affecting the experience.

My own constructivist (qualitative) research on the relevance of music in the lives of people affected by serious illness demonstrated substantial evidence for the importance of music in spiritual self-care in many people's lives. Five studies examined music's relevance (what music does for them and whether it helps) in the lives of children with cancer ($n = 26$), parents of children with cancer ($n = 28$) [72], adolescents and young adults with cancer ($n = 12$) [73], adults with cancer ($n = 52$) [74], caregivers of adults with cancer ($n = 12$) [75], and bereaved cancer carers ($n = 8$) [76]. The synthesis of the five studies' findings concluded that: 'Music can be a lifeline; support biopsychosocial well-being and/or spiritual life; remain an incidental presence; be avoided; or become elusive, whereby it is difficult to experience' [77, p 410]. Music could inspire, soothe, connect, transport, and enable transcendence. Some people projected anthropomorphic properties onto music, describing it as a friend or saviour; it could convey understanding, validate, and give a voice. Alternatively, music that elicited discomfort may have needed avoidance; and music associated with devastating loss may have needed to be silenced, while it safely (metaphorically) held painful states and remained available for returning to when ready. While many found music spiritually supportive, some did not connect music with spirituality at all, and one Catholic patient avoided hymns because they were associated with a punishing God. Further, one participant who spoke of sacred music being 'an expression of God in the universe', said that sacred music did not offer solace because it was too emotional [75]. Illustrative quotes demonstrating music's spiritual, including religious, elicitations when affected by cancer included:

> Mother to 12-year-old girl (G)
>
> *(Music therapist) recorded you playing the clarinet...there was a school performance, and you were supposed to be playing the clarinet...you were neutropenic, but they actually played your CD at the school, and they said all the class stood up and held hands on the stage... G (patient): [giggled].* [72, p 785]
>
> *Feeling of moving to a higher plane or being in a different kind of situation to where you are ... only when I hear particularly good music.* (23-year-old male patient) [73, p 691]
>
> *Ave Maria which I listened to over and over again during my first chemo. ...Now it instantly takes me back to that... I was petrified...I was just bawling, and I had this song blaring in my ears and I just kind of shut out the world and got lost in Ave Maria. ... I listen to it now.... I still kind of feel ... the beauty ... it helped me kind of make peace.* (37-year-old, female patient) [74, p 5]
>
> *(Music) is like transformation into another world. It's relaxation. It's a spiritual connection. It's an emotional broadening, emotions at times that's hard to express or communicate ... it leaves a lovely feeling, ... it's just like something's touching my heart and I need to get it out somehow.* (Mother of young adult cancer patient) [75, p 50]
>
> *For the first 9 or 10 months I would listen over and over and over again to the songs that were played at [son's] funeral ... I couldn't listen to them without flood, flood of tears .... It's almost like putting on a relief valve ... all this grief and sadness ... I'd cry and cry and then I'd feel a bit better, sad but a bit better .... You almost know you're going to be in pain, so in a way you try not to (listen to son's music) but then there's some days when you can't help it, because it's just a comfort.* (Mother) [76, p 115]

5 Generalist Music-Based Care

Music can amplify and intensify spiritual experiences, potentiating new and transcendent ways of being in the world [28]. Offering music to patients in palliative care therefore expands opportunities for palliative care patients and families to connect with important spiritual realms. Health workers caring for those affected by serious illness are encouraged to ask them about the role of music in their lives, for example, their music preferences, first album bought, favourite musicians, and genres. Many patients feel recognised as a person, not just a patient, when staff inquire about their life interests such as music. Talking about music and its significance can be as profoundly emotionally evocative as experiencing it.

Many patients now bring personal devices with favourite playlists into healthcare settings; however, with the hard work of managing life-threatening and advanced illnesses, many lose connection with their music. In these instances, staff caregivers may gently inquire about whether music is something patients and their families may like to use again, mindful that some may not be ready to return to the intense emotional states that music can elicit. An extensive list of suggestions for staff caregivers offering music in palliative care is found elsewhere and some follow [78].

- Develop diverse music libraries with CDs and CD players as many still like to borrow and listen to CDs in palliative care settings. Availability of music devices with music streaming services are excellent when funds allow.
- Offer to play inpatients' familiar and liked music when they cannot work their devices, keeping in mind that music choice is imperative, including type, volume, when/where, and length of time it is heard. Research has implied that familiar songs with particular significance may be important with the experience of sacred moments [79], and preferred music is also most associated with relaxation [80] and pain reduction [81]. Religious music or TV programmes which include music, such as Songs of Praise [82], can also help those unable to attend religious community gatherings to remain connected to specific faith traditions [28].
- When music-lover patients have cognitive impairment (e.g. adynamic, memory loss) affecting their initiation of music listening, regularly offer to put on their favourite music. Patients with significant memory loss often find listening to their favourite music repeatedly very enjoyable.
- Invite patient and family music-based interactions, for example, enable a space where musical instruments can be borrowed or brought into an inpatient unit and played; suggest to family members that they can bring patients' favourite CDs into the ward.
- Consider inviting people to listen to birdsong in outside areas (where possible) or birdsong playlists on music streaming services.
- When helping patients with autobiographies, consider inviting reflections on music and including audios within the final products.
- When involving live musicians in inpatient services, try to ensure that patients and families can either 'tune in' or not listen. Presenting music in places that patients and families can easily move towards and away from is helpful. Avoid songs with obvious death-related themes in public settings, unless checking with those nearby. It is important to inquire about people's views about music heard in public settings as much as possible. Anonymous feedback can be simply gathered, for example, through placing strategically located feedback boxes, and providing pens and paper so that people can leave anonymous comments. This kind of information was collected to examine the impact of a staff choir, which had been singing Christmas carols for 52 years on patient wards at Peter MacCallum Cancer Centre, Melbourne, Australia. The straight-forward study was conducted after several staff complained that the music might offend non-Christian patients.

Findings from the 175 patients, visitors [83], and staff members [84], mostly anonymous responses confirmed that people from varied religious and cultural backgrounds valued the choir, resulting in its continuance to this day.
- Indiscriminate or 'piped' recorded music in palliative care settings needs caution or avoidance: what one person finds helpful may aggravate another.
- Towards the end of a patient's life, consider inviting family members to play soft music that they believe that the patient would like, or softly hum or sing one of their favourite songs or hymns, for example, a song they remembered the patient singing to them as a child.

6 Coda

> It (music) gives you the confidence and tools to go to that dark place … to mould that emotion…construct something musically and then express that … (you) get to the light by going down there (41-year-old, male with cancer). [74, p 1042]

Music experiences offer opportunities for people to feel heard and known at deep, felt, and multisensorial levels [77], and to feel transported to realms beyond ordinary awareness [27]. Many patients and families affected by serious illness already recognise and use music in soothing and revelatory ways and for religious support. Many also use music therapy to support their venture into deeper awareness, and to bring helpful insights gained back into ordinary consciousness. Such insights may be explored verbally or evident non-verbally through a smile or the touch of another's hand [27]. They may also be apparent in a musical epiphany, such as when a patient stridently sang out the lyrics, 'I did it my way', after requesting 'My Way' [85] hours before his death. In sum, music therapy and generalist music-based care, offered by all health workers, can profoundly extend the multisensorial scope of reaching and supporting spiritual realms. Both should ideally exist in any context holistically caring for those affected by serious illnesses.

References

1. O'Callaghan C, Brooker J, de Silva W, Glenister D, Melia A, Symons X, et al. Patients' and caregivers' contested perspectives on spiritual care for those affected by advanced illnesses: a qualitative descriptive study. J Pain Symptom Manag. 2019;58:977–88. https://www.ncbi.nlm.nih.gov/pubmed/31404641.
2. Balboni T, Balboni M, Paulk ME, Phelps A, Wright A, Peteet J, al. Support of cancer patients' spiritual needs and associations with medical care costs at the end of life. Cancer. 2011;117:5383–91. https://www.ncbi.nlm.nih.gov/pubmed/21563177.
3. Puchalski CM. Restorative medicine. In: Cobb M, Puchalski CM, Rumbold B, editors. Oxford book of spirituality in healthcare. Oxford: Oxford Universiity Press; 2012. p. 197–210.
4. Hanson LC, Dobbs D, Usher BM, Williams S, Rawlings J, Daaleman TP. Providers and types of spiritual care during serious illness. J Palliat Med. 2008;11:907–14. https://www.ncbi.nlm.nih.gov/pubmed/18715183.

5. Handzo G, Puchalski C. The role of the chaplain in palliative care. In: Cherny NT, Fallon M, Kaasa SK, Portneboy RK, Currow DC, editors. Oxford textbook of palliative medicine. Oxford: Oxford University Press; 2015. p. 170–6.
6. Selman LE, Brighton LJ, Sinclair S, Karvinen I, Egan R, Speck P, et al. Patients' and caregivers' needs, experiences, preferences and research priorities in spiritual care: a focus group study across nine countries. Palliat Med. 2018;32:216–30. https://doi.org/10.1177/0269216317734954.
7. Perez-Cruz PE, Langer P, Carrasco C, Bonati P, Batic B, Tupper Satt L, et al. Spiritual pain is associated with decreased quality of life in advanced cancer patients in palliative care: an exploratory study. J Palliat Med. 2019;22:663–9. https://www.ncbi.nlm.nih.gov/pubmed/30649985.
8. Vallurupalli M, Lauderdale K, Balboni MJ, Phelps AC, Block SD, Ng AK, et al. The role of spirituality and religious coping in the quality of life of patients with advanced cancer receiving palliative radiation therapy. J Support Oncol. 2012;10:81–7. https://www.ncbi.nlm.nih.gov/pubmed/22088828.
9. Astrow AB, Kwok G, Sharma RK, Fromer N, Sulmasy DP. Spiritual needs and perception of quality of care and satisfaction with care in hematology/medical oncology patients: a multicultural assessment. J Pain Symptom Manag. 2018;55:56–64. https://www.ncbi.nlm.nih.gov/pubmed/28842220.
10. Puchalski C, Ferrell B, Virani R, Otis-Green S, Baird P, Bull J, et al. Improving the quality of spiritual care as a dimension of palliative care: the report of the Consensus Conference. J Palliat Med. 2009;12:885–904. http://www.ncbi.nlm.nih.gov/pubmed/19807235.
11. Australian Health Ministers. Supporting Australians to live well at the end of life: national palliative care strategy 2010. Commonwealth of Australia; 2010. http://www.health.gov.au/internet/main/publishing.nsf/Content/EF57056BDB047E2FCA257BF000206168/$File/NationalPalliativeCareStrategy.pdf. Accessed 1 Oct 2018.
12. World Health Organization. World Health Organisation definition of palliative care. 2015. http://www.who.int/cancer/palliative/definition/en/. Accessed 18 July 2015.
13. Piderman KM, Kung S, Jenkins SM, Eurele TT, Yoder TJ, Kwete GM, et al. Respecting the spiritual side of advanced cancer care: a systematic review. Curr Oncol Rep. 2015;17:6. https://doi.org/10.1007/s11912-014-0429-6.
14. Pearce MJ, Coan AD, Herndon JE 2nd, Koenig HG, Abernethy AP. Unmet spiritual care needs impact emotional and spiritual well-being in advanced cancer patients. Support Care Cancer. 2012;20:2269–76. https://doi.org/10.1007/s00520-011-1335-1.
15. Epstein-Peterson ZD, Sullivan AJ, Enzinger AC, Trevino KM, Zollfrank AA, Balboni MJ, et al. Examining forms of spiritual care provided in the advanced cancer setting. Am J Hosp Palliat Care. 2015;32:750–7. https://www.ncbi.nlm.nih.gov/pubmed/25005589.
16. Balboni TA, Vanderwerker LC, Block SD, Paulk ME, Lathan CS, Peteet JR, et al. Religiousness and spiritual support among advanced cancer patients and associations with end-of-life treatment preferences and quality of life. J Clin Oncol. 2007;25:555–60. http://www.ncbi.nlm.nih.gov/pubmed/17290065.
17. Hegarty MM, Abernethy AP, Olver I, Currow DC. Former palliative caregivers who identify that additional spiritual support would have been helpful in a population survey. Palliat Med. 2011;25:266–77. https://doi.org/10.1177/0269216310389225.
18. Massey K, Barnes MJ, Villines D, Goldstein JD, Pierson AL, Scherer C, et al. What do I do? Developing a taxonomy of chaplaincy activities and interventions for spiritual care in intensive care unit palliative care. BMC Palliat Care. 2015;14:10. http://www.ncbi.nlm.nih.gov/pubmed/25878558.
19. Potvin. Music and spirituality at the end of life. OUPblog, September 24, 2019. https://blog.oup.com/2019/09/music-and-spirituality-at-the-end-of-life/. Accessed 14 Aug 2023.
20. Egan R, Maclead R, Jaye C, McGee R, Baxter R, Baxter J, et al. What is spirituality? Evidence from a New Zealand hospice study. Mortality. 2011;16:307–24. https://doi.org/10.1080/13576275.2011.613267.
21. Wynne L. Spiritual care at the end of life. Nurs Stand. 2013;28:41–5. https://www.ncbi.nlm.nih.gov/pubmed/24020576.

22. Walker A, Breitsameter C. The provision of spiritual care in hospices: a study in four hospices in North Rhine-Westphalia. J Relig Health. 2017;56:2237–50. https://www.ncbi.nlm.nih.gov/pubmed/28444607.
23. Stein EM, Kolidas E, Moadel A. Do spiritual patients want spiritual interventions? A qualitative exploration of underserved cancer patients' perspectives on religion and spirituality. Palliat Support Care. 2015;13:19–25. https://doi.org/10.1017/S1478951513000217.
24. World Federation of Music Therapy. Announcing WFMT's NEW definition of music therapy. https://www.wfmt.info/about. Accessed 14 Aug 2023.
25. Bradt J, Potvin N, Kesslick A, Shim M, Radl D, Schriver E, et al. The impact of music therapy versus music medicine on psychological outcomes and pain in cancer patients: a mixed methods study. Support Care Cancer. 2015;23:1261–71. http://www.ncbi.nlm.nih.gov/pubmed/25322972.
26. Cox H, Roberts P. From music to silence: an exploration of music-thanatology vigils at end of life. Spiritual Health Int. 2007;8:80–91. https://doi.org/10.1002/shi.288.
27. Salmon D. Music therapy as psychospiritual process in palliative care. J Palliat Care. 2001;17:142–6.
28. Potvin N, Argue J. Theoretical considerations of spirit and spirituality in music therapy. Music Ther Perspect. 2014;32:118–28. https://doi.org/10.1093/mtp/miu022.
29. O'Callaghan C. Musc therapy and spiritual care. In: Carey LB, Mathisen BA, editors. Spiritual care for allied health practice. Jessica Kingsley Publications: London; 2018. p. 162–82.
30. Magill L. Music therapy: enhancing spirituality at the end-of-life. In: Dileo C, Loewy J, editors. Music therapy at the end of life. Cherry Hill: Jeffrey Books; 2005. p. 3–15.
31. Munro S, Mount BM. Music therapy in palliative care. Can Med Assoc J. 1978;119:1029–34.
32. Tsiris G. Music therapy and spirituality: an international survey of music therapists' perceptions. Nord J Music Ther. 2017;26:293–319. https://doi.org/10.1080/08098131.2016.1239647.
33. Lee CA. Introduction: music and dying. In: Lee CA, editor. Lonely waters: proceedings of the international conference, music therapy in palliative care. London: Sobell Publications; 1995. p. 3–10.
34. Saunders C, Baines M, Dunlop R. Living with dying: a guide to palliative care. 3rd ed. Oxford: Oxford University Press; 1995.
35. Clements-Cortés A, O'Callaghan C. Music therapy at the end of life. In: Viega M, Dos Santos A, Wheeler B. Music therapy handbook. 3rd ed. New York: Guildford Press; in press.
36. Dileo C, Loewy J, editors. Music therapy at the end of life. Cherry Hill: Jeffrey Books; 2005.
37. Rumbold B. Introduction: spiritual care for allied health practice. In: Carey LB, Mathisen BA, editors. Spiritual care for allied health practice. London: Jessica Kingsley Publishers; 2018. p. 11–21.
38. Aldridge D. Music therapy and the creative act. In: Aldridge D, editor. Music therapy in palliative care: new voices. London: Jessica Kingsley Publications; 1999. p. 15–28.
39. Gula RM. The good life: where morality and spirituality converge. Mahwah: Paulist Press; 1999.
40. Telfer E. The philosophy of hospitableness. In: Lashley C, editor. The Routledge handbook of hospitality studies. New York: Routledge; 2016.
41. Marcel G. Creative fidelity, trs., Robert Rosthal. New York: Fordham University Press; 2002.
42. Parton D. I will always love you [song]. 1973.
43. Poulton GR, Darby K. Love me tender [song]. RCA Victor; 1956.
44. Taylor J. Twinkle, twinkle, little star [song]. In: Taylor J, Taylor A, editors. Rhymes for the nursery; 1806.
45. O'Callaghan C. Music therapy inspired transient ward communities in oncology. In: Edwards J, editor. Music in health care: international perspectives to inform theory and practice. Cambridge: Cambridge Scholars Press; 2007. p. 1–18.
46. Kasha A, Hirschhorn J. The morning after. 20th Century; 1973.
47. Association of Hospice & Palliative Care Chaplains, editor. Standards for hospice & palliative care chaplaincy. 2nd ed. Association of Hospice & Palliative Care Chaplains; 2006.

48. Neame R. The poseidon adventure [film]. 20th Century Fox; 1972.
49. Colosimo K, Nissim R, Psos AE, Hales S, Zimmermann C, Rodin G. "Double awareness" in psychotherapy for patients living with advanced cancer. J Psychother Integr. 2017;28:125–40. https://doi.org/10.1037/int0000078.
50. Bahcivan O. Possible cross-cultural role in effectiveness of music therapy in palliative and hospice care. Support Care Cancer. 2017;25:2373. https://www.ncbi.nlm.nih.gov/pubmed/28536885.
51. Wilkin M, Kristofferson K. One day at a time. 1974. https://secondhandsongs.com/work/94280/all.
52. Stroebe M, Schut H. The dual process model of coping with bereavement: rationale and description. Death Stud. 1999;23:197–224. https://doi.org/10.1080/074811899201046.
53. Saresma T. "Art as a way to life": bereavement and the healing power of arts and writing. Qual Inq. 2003;9:603–20. https://doi.org/10.1177/1077800403254226.
54. van der Merwe L, Morelli J. Explaining how community music engagement facilitates social cohesion through ritualised belonging. Religions. 2022;13:1170. https://doi.org/10.3390/rel13121170.
55. O'Callaghan C. Research on hospice music therapy. In: Dileo C, Baroni M, editors. Music therapy at the end of life. 2nd ed. Cherry Hill: Jeffrey Books. in press.
56. Hanser SB, Bauer-Wu S, Kubicek L, Healy M, Manola J, Hernandez M, et al. Effects of a music therapy intervention on quality of life and distress in women with metastatic breast cancer. J Soc Integr Oncol. 2006;4:116–24. https://doi.org/10.2310/7200.2006.014.
57. Cook E, Silverman MJ. Effects of music therapy on spirituality with patients on a medical oncology/hematology unit: a mixed-methods approach. Arts Psychother. 2013;40:239–44. https://doi.org/10.1016/j.aip.2013.02.004.
58. Burns DS, Robb SL, Haase JE. Exploring the feasibility of a therapeutic music video intervention in adolescents and young adults during stem-cell transplantation. Cancer Nurs. 2009;32:E8–E16. https://doi.org/10.1097/NCC.0b013e3181a4802c.
59. Robb SL, Burns DS, Stegenga KA, Haut PR, Monahan PO, Meza J, et al. Randomized clinical trial of therapeutic music video intervention for resilience outcomes in adolescents/young adults undergoing hematopoietic stem cell transplant: a report from the Children's Oncology Group. Cancer. 2014;120:909–17. http://www.ncbi.nlm.nih.gov/pubmed/24469862.
60. Wlodarczyk N. The effect of music therapy on the spirituality of persons in an in-patient hospice unit as measured by self-report. J Music Ther. 2007;44:113–22. https://doi.org/10.1093/jmt/44.2.113.
61. Alvarenga WA, Leite A, Oliveira MS, Nascimento LC, Silva-Rodrigues FM, Nunes MDR, et al. The effect of music on the spirituality of patients: a systematic review. J Holist Nurs. 2018;36:192–204. https://www.ncbi.nlm.nih.gov/pubmed/28589782.
62. Warth M, Koehler F, Brehmen M, Weber M, Bardenheuer HJ, Ditzen B, et al. "Song of life": results of a multicenter randomized trial on the effects of biographical music therapy in palliative care. Palliat Med. 2021;35:1126–36. https://www.ncbi.nlm.nih.gov/pubmed/33876660.
63. Burns DS, Perkins SM, Tong Y, Hilliard RE, Cripe LD. Music therapy is associated with family perception of more spiritual support and decreased breathing problems in cancer patients receiving hospice care. J Pain Symptom Manag. 2015;50(2):225–31. http://www.ncbi.nlm.nih.gov/pubmed/25839735.
64. Lichtl A, Casaw C, Edwards J, Popkin K, Yu J, Li QS, et al. Music therapy for pain in black and white cancer patients: a retrospective study. J Pain Symptom Manag. 2022;64:478–85. https://www.ncbi.nlm.nih.gov/pubmed/35870654
65. Elwafi PR, Wheeler BL. Listening to music as part of treatment for breast cancer: a qualitative content analysis of patients' listening logs. Arts Psychother. 2016;48:38–45. https://doi.org/10.1016/j.aip.2015.12.004.
66. McClean S, Bunt L, Daykin N. The healing and spiritual properties of music therapy at a cancer care center. J Altern Complement Med. 2012;18:402–7. https://www.ncbi.nlm.nih.gov/pubmed/22384974.

67. Magill L. The spiritual meaning of pre-loss music therapy to bereaved caregivers of advanced cancer patients. J Palliat Support Care. 2009;7:97–108. https://doi.org/10.1017/S1478951509000121.
68. Walden M, Charley Elliott E, Ghrayeb A, Lovenstein A, Ramick A, Adams G, et al. And the beat goes on: heartbeat recordings through music therapy for parents of children with progressive neurodegenerative illnesses. J Palliat Med. 2021;24:1023–9. https://www.ncbi.nlm.nih.gov/pubmed/33305998.
69. O'Callaghan C. Lyrical themes in songs written by palliative care patients. J Music Ther. 1996;33:74–92. https://doi.org/10.1093/jmt/33.2.74.
70. O'Callaghan C, O'Brien E, Magill L, Ballinger E. Resounding attachment: cancer inpatients' song lyrics for their children in music therapy. Support Care Cancer. 2009;17:1149–57. https://doi.org/10.1007/s00520-008-0555-5.
71. Peng CS, Baxter K, Lally KM. Music intervention as a tool in improving patient experience in palliative care. Am J Hosp Palliat Care. 2019;36:45–9. https://www.ncbi.nlm.nih.gov/pubmed/30045627.
72. O'Callaghan C, Baron A, Barry P, Dun B. Music's relevance for pediatric cancer patients: a constructivist and mosaic research approach. Support Care Cancer. 2011;19:779–88. http://www.ncbi.nlm.nih.gov/pubmed/20422229.
73. O'Callaghan C, Barry P, Thompson K. Music's relevance for adolescents and young adults with cancer: a constructivist research approach. Support Care Cancer. 2012;20:687–97. http://www.ncbi.nlm.nih.gov/pubmed/21311914.
74. O'Callaghan C, McDermott F, Michael N, Daveson BA, Hudson PL, Zalcberg JR. "A quiet still voice that just touches": music's relevance for adults living with life-threatening cancer diagnoses. Support Care Cancer. 2014;22:1037–47. http://www.ncbi.nlm.nih.gov/pubmed/24287507.
75. O'Callaghan C, Hudson P, McDermott F, Zalcberg JR. Music among family carers of people with life-threatening cancer. Music Med. 2011;3:47–55. https://doi.org/10.47513/mmd.v3i1.257.
76. O'Callaghan C, McDermott F, Hudson P, Zalcberg JR. Sound continuing bonds with the deceased: the relevance of music, including preloss music therapy, for eight bereaved caregivers. Death Stud. 2013;37:101–25. http://www.ncbi.nlm.nih.gov/pubmed/24520844.
77. O'Callaghan CC, McDermott F, Reid P, Michael N, Hudson J, Zalcberg J, et al. Music's relevance for people affected by cancer: a meta-ethnography and implications for music therapists. J Music Ther. 2016;53(4):398–429. http://www.ncbi.nlm.nih.gov/pubmed/27980035.
78. O'Callaghan C. Music therapy in palliative medicine. In: Cherny N, Fallon M, Kaasa S, Portnoy R, Currow D, Morita J, editors. Oxford textbook of palliative medicine. 5th ed. London: Oxford University Press; 2015. p. 184–90.
79. Griffith FJ, Wong ST, Dietrich KM, Exline JJ, Pargament KI. 'The music was speaking to me': using narrative inquiry to describe sacred moments with music. Arts Psychother. 2022;79:101911. https://doi.org/10.1016/j.aip.2022.101911.
80. Stratton V, Zalanowski A. The relationship between music, degree of liking and self-reported relaxation. J Music Ther. 1984;21:184–92. https://doi.org/10.1093/jmt/21.4.184.
81. Mitchell LA, MacDonald RA. An experimental investigation of the effects of preferred and relaxing music listening on pain perception. J Music Ther. 2006;43:295–316. https://doi.org/10.1093/jmt/43.4.295.
82. British Broadcasting Commission. Songs of praise [Television series]. https://www.bbc.co.uk/programmes/b006ttc5. Accessed 14 Aug 2023.
83. O'Callaghan CC, Hornby CJ, Pearson EJ, Ball DL. "The moment is all we have": patients and visitors reflect on a staff Christmas choir. Med J Aust. 2009;191:684–7. https://www.ncbi.nlm.nih.gov/pubmed/20028308.
84. O'Callaghan CC, Hornby CJ, Pearson EJ, Ball DL. Oncology staff reflections about a 52-year-old staff Christmas choir: constructivist research. J Palliat Med. 2010;13:1421–5. http://www.ncbi.nlm.nih.gov/pubmed/21117947.
85. Anka P. My way [song]: Reprise; 1969.

Ritual in Palliative Care

Denise Hess

Abstract Spirituality refers to the human predilection to find meaning, purpose, connection, and transcendence through an endless variety of beliefs, values, traditions, and practices that span cultures, religions, and eras. Spirituality includes religious beliefs and practices, and yet as religious belief and engagement decline in some parts of the globe, spirituality has also come to include beliefs and practices that are not tied to any particular religious tradition. Rituals, or actions that have been imbued with symbolic meaning and significance, are no longer only religious rites, ceremonies, traditions, or sacraments. Rituals are now a part of organisational and wellness cultures as well. People living with a serious illness and the people who care for them have spiritual needs, and palliative care best practice includes attention to the spiritual needs of patients, family members, and the professionals who work in palliative care. One spiritual intervention provided by spiritual care professionals is ritual facilitation. This chapter explores ritual facilitation in palliative care clinical practice. Ritual facilitation includes the individual, communal, formal, informal, repeated, occasional, literal, and metaphorical actions that help patients, family members, individual clinicians, and interdisciplinary teams find meaning, purpose, and transcendence in the midst of challenging circumstances.

Keywords Ritual · Palliative care · Ritualisation · Spirituality · Spiritual care

---

D. Hess (✉)
School of Pharmacy, University of Maryland, Baltimore, MD, USA
e-mail: Denise.hess@rx.umaryland.edu

M. C. Best (ed.), *Spiritual Care in Palliative Care*,
https://doi.org/10.1007/978-3-031-50864-6_20

1 The Need for Ritual

If there is a meaning in life at all, then there must be a meaning in suffering.
Victor Frankl: Man's Search for Meaning [1]

People living with a serious illness and those who care for them are faced with life's biggest questions. Who am I? Why am I here? What is the purpose of my life? What will happen when I die? How will I be remembered? What legacy will I leave?

These questions arise not just for the person living with a life-limiting diagnosis, but also for those in their immediate family, circle of friends, as well as the collection of health care professionals who are involved in the patient and family's lives.

In the face of life's existential questions, humans seek to make sense of the non-sensical.

'She was so healthy, she did everything right, how can she have cancer?'
'Children should never die before their parents'.
'I guess this lung cancer is God's punishment for my sin of smoking'.
'God needed another angel'.
'This suffering purifies my soul for the life to come'.
'They are in a better place'.
'At least their suffering is over'.

Human attempts to make sense of the painful, chaotic, unpredictable, and uncertain aspects of life can be undergirded by communal and individual beliefs, values, and frameworks. For some, a specific religious or spiritual tradition provides meaning in the face of suffering. For others, a personal world view offers a way forward amid struggles. For still others, a combination of communal and individual beliefs affords a way to make meaning out of distress.

Spiritual care professionals or SCPs (also known as chaplains, pastoral care professionals or spiritual counsellors), and specifically SCPs working within palliative care team settings, provide specialist level assessment and interventions to address patient and family spiritual distress. SCPs also attend to the spiritual distress of the palliative care team members and other professional colleagues to promote professional well-being and resilience [2].

One of the many tools in the palliative care SCP's toolkit is ritual support or facilitation [3]. When an SCP is not available, ritual support can be provided by other members of the interdisciplinary team [4]. In most contexts, ritual support almost exclusively includes religious or cultural rituals, either facilitated by the SCP themselves, or coordinated with the appropriate religious or cultural leader on behalf of the patient, family, or professional colleague who has requested the ritual.

Examples of religious or cultural ritual support can include specific prayers, sacraments, rites, ceremonies, observances, traditions, celebrations, solemnities, and rite of passage practices to name a few. For more information on these types of religious, faith-based, or cultural rituals, see Chaps. 5, 6, 7, 8, 9, 10 and 11.

2 The Shape of Ritual

Rituals are a popular topic among the 'nones', or the growing segment of western populations that identifies as 'none' on survey questions about religious preference [5–8]. Religiously inspired chanting, prayers, sacraments, body blessings, and culturally minded rituals around body placement, body washing, and body contact with the earth are replete in hospice and end of life care [9–14].

Many palliative care teams engage in regular services of remembrance or memorialisation of patients who have died. Some hospital-based services partner with community-based hospices to provide bereavement ritual support [15–17]. For example, one cancer centre team created two rituals of remembrance where friends and family of the deceased participated in a co-created art piece centred around a traditional Jewish litany 'We Remember Them'. Similarly, and separately, the cancer centre staff were invited to participate in a bereavement ritual centred around the creation of a mandala [18].

Ideally, palliative care team support is accessed close to diagnosis and is uninterrupted until death [19–21]. Ritual needs will change across the disease trajectory according to the acuity of the symptom burden. As suggested above in the memorialisation work at a cancer centre, patients, family members, and the teams of professionals who care for seriously ill people will have differing ritual needs. Family needs will centre on grieving and integrating the loss. Clinical staff needs will centre on cumulative grief.

The field of ritual studies was pioneered by Van Gennep in the 1960s and further developed as an academic discipline by Grimes and others in the mid-1970s [22, 23]. Building on Van Gennep and Grimes, van der Weegen and colleagues provide this definition of ritual in palliative care:

> Ritual is a more or less repeatable sequence of action units which take on a symbolic dimension through formalisation, stylisation, and their situation in place and time. On the one hand, individuals and groups express their ideas and ideals, their mentalities and identities through these rituals, on the other hand the ritual actions shape, foster, and transform these ideas, mentalities and identities [4].

A ritual is an action. Yet, implicit in this definition is the assertion that actions in and of themselves do not carry intrinsic meaning. Thus, any ordinary act can become extraordinary. Human actors can assign meaning and significance to actions by infusing them with symbolic elements that create meaning and significance. A ritual can be routine, but not mere habit. A ritual can take place once in a lifetime or every day. And, most importantly, rituals are bi-directional: they shape humans while simultaneously being shaped by them. A study examining rituals in a Dutch Hospice setting found that everyday practices, such as washing a patient, could be enriched with elements that have a strong symbolic meaning, thereby creating a ritual which promoted a good death for patients [24].

In addition, rituals are often created in liminal spaces, or spaces of being 'in between'. Rituals provide a form or container to create, express, and connect with the spiritual dimension of life. Similarly, rituals are one expression of human spirituality. Like spirituality, rituals help people find ultimate meaning, purpose, and transcendence by experiencing relationship to self, family, others, community, society, nature, and the significant or sacred. As such they take on numerous forms that enact significant functions.

Within the various forms and functions, rituals serve to enact what cannot be fully expressed with words, to integrate head knowledge with heart sensing, and to sacralise time by making the invisible visible.

3 The Impact of Ritual in Palliative Care

There has not been much investigation of the impact of ritual in the palliative care setting. One study has shown that the use of ritual can benefit patients, family members and staff in the end-of-life setting. Montross Thomas and colleagues found that hospice staff and volunteers who used personally meaningful rituals to help them cope after the death of their patients had significantly higher compassion satisfaction and significantly lower burnout as measured by the Professional Quality of Life scale [12]. Qualitative research on the *Code Lavender* intervention found that it created space for staff to make sense of particularly impactful losses and lessen the negative effects of staff moral distress. This intervention was a group ritual practice for staff in the aftermath of a stressful event in their unit and included an opening prayer followed by a 'listening round' and a facilitated dialogue [25]. Palliative care team 'remembrance rounds' promote team resiliency and sustainability through the monthly reading of names of patients who have died. This ritual includes a team discussion about the family's potential bereavement needs and risks [26]. Similarly, family rituals were found to provide important outlets for the bereavement needs of children whose siblings died in the Neonatal Intensive Care Unit [27].

4 The Practice of Ritual

Following Tables 1 and 2 above, the remainder of this chapter will explore the various forms and functions of rituals that are likely to arise in palliative care practice through case examples derived from the author's own practice. In the day-to-day life of a palliative care team, what rituals are present, what forms do they take, and what functions are they intended to achieve?

Table 1 Ritual forms

Individual	Communal
Formal	Informal
Repeated	Occasional
Literal	Metaphorical

Table 2 Ritual functions

Meaning
Purpose
Transcendence
Relationship

4.1 Case Example 1: Ventilator Removal Litany

Background: A hospital-based palliative care team is frequently consulted by the intensive care unit (ICU) team for assistance with patients who are nearing the end of life. The palliative care team facilitates goals of care-focused family meetings to help the family decision-makers align the intensity of care with the patient's values, beliefs, and goals. The physicians and advanced practice clinicians also assist with symptom management. While some of these palliative care patients will be discharged from the hospital to receive hospice care in another setting, a large proportion of the patients will be transitioned to a more palliative-focused type of inpatient care. This can include cessation of active therapies such as vasopressors, dialysis, nasogastric or intravenous nutrition and hydration, or ventilator support and introduction of comfort care such as opioids, benzodiazepines, antipsychotics, and other medications to decrease symptoms that may arise when other treatments are stopped.

Over time, the ICU team has come to rely on and prefer that the palliative care team provide patient and family support from the time of the goals of care family meeting until death or discharge. As a result, the palliative care team is usually involved when a family decides to de-escalate an ICU patient's care and focus exclusively on the patient's comfort.

Ritualisation: When this transition occurs, the team SCP and social worker provide spiritual and psychoeducational support, respectively. The social worker will prepare the family for what to expect when certain medical treatments are stopped, and the dying process begins. The SCP will meet with the family to assess their spiritual and ritual needs, and where appropriate facilitate the following ritual prior to the removal of a medical treatment where death is expected imminently.

The family members and others present encircle the patient's bed, holding hands when desired, as the SCP guides those present through the following litany.

SCP: Let us join together in this prayer of release
Acknowledging the unique gift of your life,
Those present are invited to speak aloud one word that captures the uniqueness of the patient.
SCP: We all say, we release you.
All: We release you.
SCP: In knowing that you have touched each one here and many who are not here,
Those present are invited to speak their names and the names of family members not present.
SCP: We all say, we release you.
All: We release you.
One: In knowing we are grateful for the time we shared with you,

Those present are invited to name a place, event, or shared memory with the patient.
SCP: We all say, we release you.
All: We release you.
One: In knowing that all is forgiven between us,
Those present hold a moment of silence together where they are invited to give and receive any forgiveness that they need between themselves and the patient.
SCP: We all say, we release you.
All: We release you.
One: In knowing that our love for you continues,
Those present are invited to say goodbye to the patient.
SCP: We all say, we release you.
All: We release you.

Following Tables 1 and 2, this ritual is communal, formal, occasional, and both literal and metaphorical. With the addition of family chosen, faith-based prayers or sacred texts the ritual can connect families to their beliefs about life after death, the meaning of a life, and deepen their connections to each other and the patient. More specifically,

- What could be a solely medical treatment-focused moment in the patient's care becomes a *communal* ritual and often the last time the family will be together in the patient's living presence before death occurs. The ritual mediates the liminal spaces not only between living and dying, but also between what some family's experience as 'doing everything' to 'doing nothing'. This ritual communicates to the patient's family that even as the type of medical care changes, care never ceases, care is never 'withdrawn'.
- The ritual includes both *formal*, call and response style spoken prayer and *informal*, spontaneous sharing about the patient. This allows for the emotional safety that comes with structure while also providing opportunities to express personal feelings of love, grief, appreciation, gratitude, and loss.
- The ritual is *specific to the occasion* of anticipated death after stopping a medical treatment. As such it is *not usually repeated.* It is specific to a singular and poignant moment in the patient and family's life together. It marks a significant milestone in the family's shared life.
- The repeated phrase, 'we release you', has both *literal and metaphorical* meanings. In a very real sense, those gathered are saying goodbye and releasing the patient. In another sense, the patient is dying and not being 'released'. Yet, the intersection of the literal and metaphorical meanings of 'releasing' provides consolation to the newly grieving. Death is not in our control, yet we can participate in witnessing its arrival.
- If the SCP determines that the family is connected to a specific, shared faith tradition, the SCP can add in readings from sacred texts and familiar prayers to preface and close the ritual. This can elucidate the *meaning and purpose* of life and death and deepen the *transcendent* dimension of the ritual.
- As the family encircles the patient's bed, including the patient in the circle, possibly for the last time, the family *relationships* are embodied and enacted. Their encircling represents their continued care and love for the patient.

4.2 Case Example 2: The Clean Sweep

Background: An outpatient palliative care team in the United States of America (USA) serves a rural patient population with high rates of poverty, lack of access to resources and social supports. In addition to living with a serious illness, their typical patient may be challenged to find adequate housing, health services, and employment. Many of their patients live alone and do not have family or friends in the immediate area. Many of their patients are living with multiple serious illnesses, both physical and psychological. Since they are the only outpatient palliative care programme in the region, they also see paediatric patients. While paediatric patients have family support, the systemic effects of poverty often add to the experienced suffering for these children and their families.

The palliative care team is well established, fully staffed, and specialty trained, yet, even for this mature team, the repeated exposure to the suffering experienced by their patients takes a toll on each team member's emotional and psychological well-being. To address this, the team has educated themselves on countertransference [28], emotional exhaustion [29], professional boundaries, and team well-being [30]. While this knowledge has been helpful, the team felt the need for some way to enact their commitment to caring for their patients while also caring for themselves.

The team was caring for a 7-year-old patient who was dying of advanced leukaemia. The child lived with her parents and five siblings in a garage near the farm where the parents worked as farm labourers. The family did not have electricity or running water. They relied on donations from local church food banks for most of their food. And, because of they had not yet secured visas to live and work in the U.S.A, none of the family members had access to basic medical care until the emergency room visit that led to their child's diagnosis.

After a visit to the patient and her mother at their home, the team nurse and social worker found themselves overcome by the enormity of this family's suffering. As they completed the visit and began driving to their next visit of the day, they both began to weep. They together realised that they were not ready to go to their next patient visit. They needed a way to acknowledge their emotions, tend to them, and then set them to the side to be present to their next patient.

Drawing on her hospice experience, the nurse suggested they try a practice she learned from a SCP colleague. She called it her 'clean sweep'.

Ritualisation: After being profoundly affected by a patient and her family's suffering, the nurse and social worker return to their car and drive a short distance away from the patient's home. They begin with a pause to pay attention to their breath. They scan their body from head to toe and breathe into any tension or discomfort. They allow their breathing to naturally deepen and slow down. After a minute or so, silently, on an inhale, they say, 'I see…' and name the emotional, physical, relational, and cognitive suffering they notice in themselves and in the situation. Silently, on each exhale, they say, 'and I set this to the side….' After a few minutes, they end the ritual by brushing their hovering hands over their bodies from head to toe. When they are done, they pause again and return their attention to their breath, closing their eyes if helpful. They eventually share this practice with their team, and it becomes a part of their monthly remembrance ritual for patients who have died or have been discharged from their service.

Returning to Tables 1 and 2, what ritual forms and functions are present?

- An *individual* ritual became a *communal* act as the nurse and the social worker practised the clean sweep together and later shared this practice with the whole team. However, the ritual can be practised both individually and communally.
- A *formal* ritual from the nurse's previous clinical experience in hospice was further formalised by sharing it with her clinical dyad partner and the team.
- The ritual remained both *occasional*, used on an as-needed basis by individual team members, and *repeated*, as it was incorporated into the team's regular remembrance ritual.
- A *literal* action was used for its *metaphorical* meaning. Even though the team had a deep understanding of countertransference, empathic exhaustion, and professional boundaries, the symbol-infused actions of breathing and brushing served to connect the team members with the deeper meaning of these concepts.
- This ritual helped the team clarify the *meaning and purpose* of being present to suffering. Specifically, the ritual led to the team coalescing around the idea of caring versus carrying. They found that 'exquisite empathy' [30] for the suffering of others includes engaging with others in their suffering while not being overtaken by it. The team redefined their sense of their posture towards their work as having a 'soft front, and strong back'. The team found renewed agreement that their *purpose* is not to fix, or cure, or take away all suffering, but to instead create the conditions where patients and their family members can find their own healing amid their suffering.
- Some team members found that this ritual aligned with their spiritual beliefs and practices. One team member changed the 'I see…' and 'I set aside…' to 'let go, and let God', as that fit better with his spiritual tradition. Another team member used the breath and body scan to silently recite a passage from the sacred text of his religion. Some, but not all, team members found *transcendence* in this ritual.
- Paradoxically, over time, this ritual helped several team members discover that they needed to leave clinical practice. Their greater attention to the cumulative impact of being present to suffering was harmful to their *personal* well-being. Other team members reported a greater feeling of connection to the patients and families that they had previously dreaded seeing. Somehow the ritual created more space inside for them to connect to *others*. Practising this ritual as a *team* reminded each team member that they did not carry this suffering alone.

4.3 Case Example 3: The Body Blessing

Background: An outpatient palliative care SCP serves a patient population that is predominantly 'spiritual but not religious'. During the first year at the oncology clinic where she spends most of her time, she found that when Admissions staff asked, 'would you like to see the SCP?' as part of their initial visit screening, the refusal rate hovered around 70%. After conducting a quality improvement project designed to analyse and decrease the number of spiritual care refusals, the SCP discovered that both the patients and staff had a limited understanding of the breadth and depth of spiritual care. The SCP provided staff education in spiritual care and trained the Admissions staff to use a spiritual distress screening tool [31]. Additionally, to give the staff an experiential sense of spiritual care, she introduced and facilitated a ritual called a 'body blessing'. The ritual was designed for patients in the infusion clinic but was also warmly received by the staff. After these interventions, the admission staff reported greater confidence in screening patients for spiritual distress and a fuller understanding of spiritual care in patient care.

Ritualisation: The SCP created two versions of this ritual. Only the one for patients in treatment in the infusion clinic is included here.

Prior to beginning the ritual, the SCP shares a description of the ritual and provides time for the patient to consider and give consent. Patients are informed that this blessing can be repeated as often as they like. The blessing of the abdomen includes an acknowledgment of the patient's children when applicable. The ritual begins with 'For a Friend on the Arrival of an Illness' from 'To Bless the Space Between Us', by John O'Donohue [32].

Now is the time of dark invitation
Beyond a frontier you did not expect;
Abruptly, your old life seems distant.
You barely noticed how each day opened
A path through fields never questioned,
Yet expected, deep down, to hold treasure.
Now your time on earth becomes full of threat;
Before your eyes your future shrinks.
You lived absorbed in the day-to-day,
So continuous with everything around you,
That you could forget you were separate;
Now this dark companion has come between you.
Distances have opened in your eyes.
You feel that against your will
A stranger has married your heart.
Nothing before has made you
Feel so isolated and lost.
When the reverberations of shock subside in you,
May grace come to restore you to balance.
May it shape a new space in your heart
To embrace this illness as a teacher
Who has come to open your life to new worlds.
May you find in yourself
A courageous hospitality
Toward what is difficult,
Painful, and unknown.
May you learn to use this illness
As a lantern to illuminate
The new qualities that will emerge in you.
May the fragile harvesting of this slow light
Help to release whatever has become false in you.

May you trust this light to clear a path
Through all the fog of old unease and anxiety
Until you feel arising within you a tranquillity
Profound enough to call the storm to stillness.
May you find the wisdom to listen to your illness:
Ask it why it came.
Why it chose your friendship.
Where it wants to take you.
What it wants you to know.
What quality of space it wants to create in you.
What you need to learn to become more fully yourself
That your presence may shine in the world.
May you keep faith with your body,
Learning to see it as a holy sanctuary
Which can bring this night-wound gradually
Toward the healing and freedom of dawn.
May you be granted the courage and vision
To work through passivity and self-pity,
To see the beauty you can harvest
From the riches of this dark invitation.
May you learn to receive it graciously,
And promise to learn swiftly
That it may leave you newborn,
Willing to dedicate your time to birth.

The ritual continues with a body blessing modelled on Joyce Rupp's work [33].

SCP: (Name), we pause to bless you as you receive treatment today.

The SCP invites those present to place a hand on the patient's shoulder or upper back.

SCP: (Name), we are going to bless your whole body. It houses a wonderful life and is a gift to many people. Thank you for the privilege of blessing you.

Blessing of the head—the SCP touches the forehead with a dot of oil.

All: We bless your head, (Name). Thank you for the ways that you have influenced many by your beliefs, attitudes, and values. Thank you for sharing your hopes and dreams.

Blessing of the eyes—the SCP touches the closed eyes with a dot of oil.

All: We bless your eyes, (Name). We are grateful for what these eyes have seen to bring you joy and happiness. We are thankful for the times when these eyes have looked on others with love.

Blessing of the ears—the SCP touches the ears with a dot of oil.

All: We bless your ears, (Name). Thank you for the ways they have been attuned to both the outer and inner world. Thank you for the times you have listened. Thank you for the times you have heard.

Blessing of the mouth—the SCP touches the chin with a dot of oil.

All: We bless your mouth, (Name). This mouth is the carrier of your wisdom. Thank you for words of courage and kindness that you have spoken. Thank you for the truths you share.

Blessing of the hands—the SCP touches the hands with a dot of oil.

All: We bless your hands, (Name). Your hands are a source of welcome and of help in countless ways. We are grateful for all the good that these hands have done.

Blessing of the abdomen—the SCP touches the abdomen with a dot of oil.

For a woman with biological children

All: We bless your abdomen recalling how it was filled with new life. We thank you for the children you carried, nurtured, and brought forth.

For a man with biological children

All: We bless the children you brought forth. We give thanks for the gift of life you gave, nurtured, and sent forth into the world.

For someone who has adopted children

All: We bless the children you nurtured and raised. We thank you for your welcoming heart that gave birth to a loving family that is a blessing to the world.

For someone who do not have children

All: We bless your passions, your desires, your joy in life. We thank you for your longings to make the world a better place.

Blessing of the feet—the SCP touches each foot with a dot of oil.

All: We bless your feet. You have stood and walked on these feet since your youth. These feet have carried you through many of your life's joys and sorrows.

Blessing of the heart—the SCP touches the sternum with a dot of oil.

All: We bless your heart. This heart pulses with life. It has given and received love. It contains bonds with many people both near and far. It gives you energy to live.

Final blessing

All: As we lay our hands upon you may our love surround you, embrace you, bear you up, bring you peace, take you by the hand and lead you through.

Using Tables 1 and 2, the body blessing ritual exemplifies,

- An *individual* blessing done by a *community* of colleagues, friends, family, and clinic staff.
- The ritual is *formal* and scripted so that all those present can participate.
- While the ritual is *repeatable,* the SCP found that patients were most likely to receive the blessing near the beginning or end of treatment.
- The ritual is *literal* in its focus on the function and blessing of each body part, yet it also carries deep *symbolic* significance for clinicians and patients. The body is blessed both physically and spiritually for what is has literally done, held, spoken, walked, seen and what it has metaphorically done, imparted wisdom, endured trials, embraced joy, offered companionship.
- The ritual reminded them of the miracle of the body, the ways they have healed in the past, and the gift of being alive in the moment. This perspective helped them remember the 'why', or *meaning and purpose*, of seeking treatment which for most patients was to extend the quality of their lives.
- The ritual straddles the *transcendent* and the immanent frames. The body is an immanent, physical reality, yet the ritual connects the physical body to its larger transcendent function, namely, to mediate care and love.
- The ritual allows all those present to participate at the level with which they are comfortable. Oftentimes, all persons present, whether family members, friends, or clinic staff would join the blessing ritual creating connections to *self* and to *others*.

5 Conclusion

Rituals are individual and communal, repeatable actions that are infused with meaning and purpose through connection to the self, others, and the transcendent. The ritualisation of everyday actions can be of benefit to palliative care clinicians, teams, patients, and families. People shape rituals and are shaped by them. They may provide a way to incorporate the spiritual dimension of life in places where the need for meaning and transcendence are heightened. Approaching rituals from the broad lens of spirituality and spiritual practices opens wide the gates of individual and group creativity and expression. Attention to repeated acts such as washing or sanitising one's hands in between patient visits, fluffing a patient's pillow, playing a certain song on the drive home from work each day, lighting a candle, keeping a gratitude list, attending a service of remembrance, and even sharing a meal can, with intention, creates a ritual. As the body of research on the benefits of rituals grows, the positive impact on patients, family members, and the professionals who work in palliative care will increase our commitment to incorporate this dimension into the practice of whole person care.

References

1. Frankl VE. Man's search for meaning. Gift ed. Boston: Beacon Press; 2014, p. 63.
2. Jeuland J, Fitchett G, Schulman-Green D, Kapo J. Chaplains working in palliative care: who they are and what they do. J Palliat Med [Internet]. 2017 [cited 2023 Jun 22];20(5):502–8. Available from: https://search-ebscohost-com.proxy-hs.researchport.umd.edu/login.aspx?direct=true&db=rzh&AN=122811492&site=eds-live
3. Massey K, Barnes MJD, Villines D, Goldstein JD, Hisey Pierson AL, Scherer C, et al. What do I do? Developing a taxonomy of chaplaincy activities and interventions for spiritual care in intensive care unit palliative care. BMC Palliat Care [Internet]. 2015 [cited 2023 Jun 22];14(1):1–8. Available from: https://search-ebscohost-com.proxy-hs.researchport.umd.edu/login.aspx?direct=true&db=asn&AN=103221010&site=eds-live
4. van der Weegen K, Hoondert M, Timmermann M, van der Heide A. Ritualization as alternative approach to the spiritual dimension of palliative care: a concept analysis. J ReligHealth [Internet]. 2019 [cited 2023 Jun 22];58(6):2036–46. Available from: https://search-ebscohost-com.proxy-hs.researchport.umd.edu/login.aspx?direct=true&db=rzh&AN=139585812&site=ehost-live
5. Pew Research Center. About three-in-ten U.S. adults are now religiously unaffiliated. 2021 Dec 14. Available from: https://www.pewresearch.org/religion/2021/12/14/about-three-in-ten-u-s-adults-are-now-religiously-unaffiliated/
6. Bowles N. God is dead. So is the office. These people want to save both. The New York Times [Internet]. 2020 Aug 28. Available from: https://www.nytimes.com/2020/08/28/business/remote-work-spiritual-consultants.html
7. Ter Kuile C, Thurston A. How we gather. 2015. Available from: https://caspertk.files.wordpress.com/2015/04/how-we-gather.pdf
8. Ter Kuile C. The Power of Ritual: Turning Everyday Activities into Soulful Practices. New York: Harper One; 2020.
9. Reid JC, Dennis B, Hoad N, Clarke F, Hanmiah R, Vegas DB, et al. Enhancing end of life care on general internal medical wards: the 3 wishes project. BMC Palliat Care [Internet]. 2023 [cited 2023 Jun 22];22(1):1–10. Available from: https://search-ebscohost-com.proxy-hs.researchport.umd.edu/login.aspx?direct=true&db=rzh&AN=161883763&site=ehost-live
10. Kaur R, Harmon E, Joseph A, Dhliwayo NL, Kramer N, Chen E. Palliative ventilator withdrawal practices in an inpatient Hospice unit. Am J Hosp Palliat Med [Internet]. 2023 [cited 2023 Jun 22];40(7):720–6. Available from: https://search-ebscohost-com.proxy-hs.researchport.umd.edu/login.aspx?direct=true&db=rzh&AN=164077697&site=ehost-live

11. Orloff MA, Hosley BB. Initiating a ceremony at the time of death in a medical facility. Int J Hum Caring [Internet]. 2022 Oct [cited 2023 Jun 22];26(4):209–14. Available from: https://search-ebscohost-com.proxy-hs.researchport.umd.edu/login.aspx?direct=true&db=rzh&AN=162939346&site=ehost-live
12. Montross-Thomas LP, Scheiber C, Meier EA, Irwin SA. Personally meaningful rituals: a way to increase compassion and decrease burnout among HOSPICE staff and volunteers. J Palliat Med [Internet]. 2016 [cited 2023 Jun 22];19(10):1043–50. Available from: https://search-ebscohost-com.proxy-hs.researchport.umd.edu/login.aspx?direct=true&db=rzh&AN=120830328&site=ehost-live
13. Rutenberg M. Casting the spirit: a handmade legacy. Art Ther [Internet]. 2008 [cited 2023];25(3):108–14. Available from: https://search-ebscohost-com.proxy-hs.researchport.umd.edu/login.aspx?direct=true&db=rzh&AN=105710233&site=ehost-live
14. Søfting GH, Dyregrov A, Dyregrov K. Because I'm also part of the family. Children's participation in rituals after the loss of a parent or sibling. Omega J Death Dying [Internet]. 2016 [cited 2023 Jun 22];73(2):141–58. Available from: https://search-ebscohost-com.proxy-hs.researchport.umd.edu/login.aspx?direct=true&db=rzh&AN=114896053&site=ehost-live
15. Vale-Taylor P. "We will remember them": a mixed-method study to explore which post-funeral remembrance activities are most significant and important to bereaved people living with loss, and why those particular activities are chosen. Palliat Med [Internet]. 2009 [cited 2023 Aug 7];23(6):537–44. Available from: https://search.ebscohost.com/login.aspx?direct=true&db=pbh&AN=105411532&site=eds-live
16. Silloway CJ, Glover TL, Coleman BJ, Kittelson S. Filling the void: hospital palliative care and community hospice: a collaborative approach to providing hospital bereavement support. J Soc Work End Life Palliat Care [Internet]. 2018 [cited 2023 Aug 7];14(2/3):153–61. Available from: https://search.ebscohost.com/login.aspx?direct=true&db=sih&AN=133743711&site=eds-live
17. Rawlings D, Glynn T. The development of a palliative care-led memorial service in an acute hospital setting. Int J Palliat Nurs [Internet]. 2002 [cited 2023 Aug 7];8(1):40. Available from: https://search.ebscohost.com/login.aspx?direct=true&db=asn&AN=6435358&site=eds-live, 40
18. Knight L, Cooper R, Hypki C. Service of remembrance: a comprehensive cancer center's response to Bereaved family members. J Soc Work End Life Palliat Care [Internet]. 2012 [cited 2023 Aug 7];8(2):182–98. Available from: https://search.ebscohost.com/login.aspx?direct=true&db=sih&AN=76446176&site=eds-live
19. https://www.who.int/news-room/fact-sheets/detail/palliative-care
20. https://hospicecare.com/what-we-do/projects/consensus-based-definition-of-palliative-care/definition/
21. https://www.capc.org/about/palliative-care/
22. Romanoff BD, Thompson BE. Meaning construction in palliative care: the use of narrative ritual, and the expressive arts. Am J Hosp Palliat Med [Internet]. 2006 [cited 2023 Jun 22];23(4):309–16. Available from: https://search-ebscohost-com.proxy-hs.researchport.umd.edu/login.aspx?direct=true&db=rzh&AN=106355181&site=ehost-live
23. Grimes RL. Chapter five. Ritual, performance, and the sequestering sacred space. In: Discourse in ritual studies. Leiden; 2007. https://doi.org/10.1163/ej.9789004158009.i-305.34.
24. van der Weegen K, Hoondert M, van der Heide A, Timmermann M. Practices of ritualization in a Dutch hospice setting. Religions [Internet]. 2020 [cited 2023 Sep 13];11(571):571. Available from: https://search-ebscohost-com.proxy-hs.researchport.umd.edu/login.aspx?direct=true&db=edsdoj&AN=edsdoj.012a1b8c85f6459da7cb79ca7bcacaa3&site=eds-live
25. Stone RSB. Code Lavender: a tool for staff support. Nursing [Internet]. 2018 [cited 2023 Sep 13];48(4):15–7. Available from: https://search.ebscohost.com/login.aspx?direct=true&db=cmedm&AN=29561364&site=eds-live
26. Morris SE, Kearns JP, Moment A, Lee KA, deLima TJ. "Remembrance": a self-care tool for clinicians. J Palliat Med [Internet]. 2019 [cited 2023 Sep 13];22(3):316–8. Available from:

https://search.ebscohost.com/login.aspx?direct=true&db=cmedm&AN=30556757&site=eds-live
27. Fanos JH, Little GA, Edwards WH. Candles in the snow: ritual and memory for siblings of infants who died in the intensive care nursery. J Pediatr [Internet]. 2009 [cited 2023 Sep 13];154(6):849–53. Available from: https://search-ebscohost-com.proxy-hs.researchport.umd.edu/login.aspx?direct=true&db=edselp&AN=S0022347608010585&site=eds-live
28. Rosenberg LB, Brenner KO, Jackson VA, Jacobsen JC, Shalev D, Byrne-Martelli S, et al. The meaning of together: exploring transference and countertransference in palliative care settings. J Palliat Med [Internet]. 2021 [cited 2023 Jul 18];24(11):1598–602. Available from: https://search.ebscohost.com/login.aspx?direct=true&db=cmedm&AN=34491110&site=eds-live
29. Back AL, Rushton CH, Kaszniak AW, Halifax JS. "Why are we doing this?": clinician helplessness in the face of suffering. J Palliat Med [Internet]. 2015 [cited 2023 Jul 18];18(1):26–30. Available from: https://search.ebscohost.com/login.aspx?direct=true&db=cmedm&AN=25555085&site=eds-live
30. Kearney MK, Weininger RB, Vachon MLS, Harrison RL, Mount BM. Self-care of physicians caring for patients at the end of life: "Being connected… a key to my survival." JAMA [Internet]. 2009 [cited 2023 Jul 18];301(11):1155. Available from: https://search.ebscohost.com/login.aspx?direct=true&db=cmedm&AN=19293416&site=eds-live
31. Kestenbaum A, Fitchett G, Galchutt P, Labuschagne D, Varner-Perez SE, Torke AM, et al. Top Ten tips palliative care clinicians should know about spirituality in serious illness. J Palliat Med [Internet]. 2022 [cited 2023 Jun 22];25(2):312–8. Available from: https://search-ebscohost-com.proxy-hs.researchport.umd.edu/login.aspx?direct=true&db=rzh&AN=155086081&site=ehost-live
32. O'Donohue J. To bless the space between us: a book of blessings. Kindle ed. The Crown Publishing Group; 2008. pp. 142–143. Used with permission.
33. Excerpted from *Out of the Ordinary.* Copyright © 2000, 2010 by Joyce Rupp. Used with permission of the publisher, Ave Maria Press®, Inc., P.O. Box 428, Notre Dame, IN 46556. www.avemariapress.com

Barriers to Spiritual Care in Palliative Care

Paul Galchutt and Edward Peñate

Abstract The majority of palliative care patients and their loved ones desire for their spiritual care needs and preferences to be assessed and addressed. Most clinicians also desire to provide some form of spiritual care to patients and those within the patient's inner circle of support. Barriers persist, however, to the delivery of this spiritual care. This chapter will examine the evidence base concerning professional, personal, and institutional barriers as well as explore ways of overcoming these barriers. The professional barriers discussed include confusion regarding whose job it is to provide spiritual care, communication concerns about spiritual care within the interdisciplinary team, the need for spiritual care training, and existing structural challenges. From a clinician's stated discomfort to the possible fear of offending patients, personal barriers are also considered. The institutional barriers of time and money are also explored from the lens of both the chaplain and non-chaplains. This chapter concludes with suggestions for overcoming spiritual care barriers. Three possible solutions include expanding the knowledge and evidence base for spiritual

Prefacing Note
As the authors of this chapter, we are chaplains (also known as spiritual care providers) based in the United States. As a result, many of the clinical examples provided and evidence cited come from this context. While we incorporate international sources within this text, our unintentional bias towards United States-based literature could be perceived. Our intent throughout this chapter is to discuss the persistent barriers evident in many settings.

P. Galchutt (✉)
Transforming Chaplaincy, Rush University, Chicago, IL, USA
e-mail: paul_galchutt@rush.edu

E. Peñate
Section of Palliative Medicine and Spiritual Care & Education, Northwestern Memorial Hospital, Chicago, IL, USA
e-mail: epenate@nm.org

M. C. Best (ed.), *Spiritual Care in Palliative Care*,
https://doi.org/10.1007/978-3-031-50864-6_21

care, optimising the use of telehealth, and promoting professional development. As spiritual barriers are overcome, the healing benefits received will strengthen whole person care for those living with serious illness.

Keywords Chaplain · Communication · Generalist-specialist · Prayer · Preferences · Time · Training · Spiritual care · Palliative care

1 Introduction

During any person's experience of serious illness, aspects of who they are as a person and what is important to them can become heightened due to the rigours of increased symptom burden, the existential stressors related to complicated decision-making, and the possibility of imminent death. One of those aspects is a person's spirituality. Spirituality, a challenging, dynamic concept to define [1, 2] can involve religion or a faith-based community, but it also involves a person's identity and what specifically is of meaning, connection, purpose, and transcendence to them [3, 4]. Adding to this complexity is that spirituality can conceptually overlap with identified existential components such as meaning, connection, and purpose [5, 6]. Any patient's spirituality can be rich in depth. It deserves attention from all members of the palliative care team. To begin to address barriers to spiritual care in patients receiving palliative care, it is important to first identify that spiritual care needs exist as well as to discuss the supporting evidence regarding these needs and associated benefits when needs are addressed [7].

A systematic review of the literature found that a majority of patients believe it is relevant for their physician to ask about their spirituality in some instances [8], especially for patients living with advanced cancer (78%) [9]. Among advanced cancer clinicians, oncologists (72%) and oncology nurses (85%) believe that regular spiritual care would have a positive influence on patients [9]. Despite these preferences from patients and the attitudes of their professional caregivers, evidence suggests that this is not happening as often as desired [1]. For instance, in a large study conducted in the United States, 249 intensive care unit (ICU) care conferences were audio recorded and then analysed, revealing that patients' family members agreed religion or spirituality to be important (78%), but that religion or spirituality were only discussed in 16% of these care conferences [10]. This significant gap between what is desired by ICU care recipients (78%) and what is received (16%) is a crude but powerful measure towards the work that is necessary to close this gap for addressing possible religious struggle or spiritual distress.

Another large investigation [11] helps show the need for screening within an outpatient cancer population from several United States cities for those aged 55 years or older also receiving palliative care ($n = 331$). Damen and her team [11] examined the prevalence of religious and spiritual struggle [12]. These investigators reported that while two out of three in this outpatient sample indicated having some religious and spiritual struggle, one in five experienced this struggle in a moderate to high range [11]. These kinds of data serve as a guiding reminder for how common these struggles can be and how critical it is to address them.

When patients and their loved ones receive spiritual care, beneficial outcomes can occur. Seriously ill patients' perceptions of spiritual care from treatment teams is associated with decisions to transition from the ICU and enrol in hospice, with the accompanying reduction in hospital costs for patients pursuing a less curative care trajectory [13]. Another example comes from a U.S. randomised trial comparing usual chaplaincy care with chaplains offering early intervention for family members in the ICU. Family members who received the early involvement of chaplaincy care relative to usual chaplaincy care were more likely to experience significant anxiety reduction as well as increased spiritual well-being [14]. Family members of patients assigned to the usual chaplaincy care control group had access to a chaplain assigned to the ICU. Chaplaincy care with this group occurred either through other clinicians making a referral or through chaplain discretion. All the ICUs were staffed by a full-time board-certified staff chaplain who also covered two to three other non-ICU clinical areas. Chaplain students (interns, residents, and fellows) also provided coverage on the ICUs during the off-shifts and would occasionally assist with care as part of a clinical rotation. Chaplaincy care within the intervention group was similar relative to the control group apart from two aspects, proactive contact with the ICU patient's family member and that the chaplain continued to support the family member after discharge from the ICU. These data offer evidence of what can be possible when working towards reducing spiritual care barriers.

By recognising patient spiritual care preferences, needs, and outcomes, the next section of this chapter will explore the pertinent data concerning professional, personal, and institutional barriers that can obstruct the way towards practising spiritual care as well as ways to overcome them.

2 Professional Barriers

Early on in the COVID-19 pandemic, nursing professor and researcher, Betty Ferrell, along with an interprofessional team of palliative care experts, reflected, '...spiritual care is not a luxury, it is a necessity for any system that claims to care for people' [15]. Pandemic or otherwise, spiritual care needs to be available to each person with serious illness delivered by professional members of the palliative care team such as physicians, advanced practice registered nurses, physician assistants, nurses, social workers, chaplains, and pharmacists [16, 17]. This section discusses the evidence base pointing to professional barriers preventing the delivery of spiritual care through four areas: (1) the Generalist-Specialist Approach; (2) Communicating with the Chaplain; (3) Training; and (4) Structural Challenges.

2.1 The Generalist-Specialist Approach

Some clinicians believe that spiritual care is not their job [18], and that spiritual care is, rather, the responsibility of the chaplain or spiritual care provider [19]. As a field, though, palliative care systemically contends that spiritual care is the role of everyone on the interdisciplinary team [16]. One recommended way to conceptualise how spiritual care is conducted by each palliative team member is through the generalist-specialist model [20, 21]. This model proposes that the chaplain serves as the spiritual care specialist and the other non-chaplain team members serve as the generalists [20]. The way this model works is that generalists conduct a spiritual history as well as regular spiritual screening and the chaplain, when warranted and referral is made, conducts a full spiritual assessment and addresses spiritual distress [16]. The spiritual history helps the clinician to get to know the patient with a brief interview concerning the patient's values, hopes, and resources [3, 4, 7]. The spiritual screen triages for spiritual need and for determining whether a chaplain referral is necessary [3, 4, 7]. Although chaplains fulfil this specialised spiritual care role in many countries, there are some contexts throughout the world where a recognised specialised spiritual care role such as a chaplain does not exist [4]. In those settings without chaplains, spiritual care needs are either not assessed by other staff or they are evaluated and addressed by non-chaplain clinicians. Beyond chaplains and clinician partners, United States patients may indicate family members or friends to be their primary providers of spiritual care [22].

Conducting a spiritual history can be a complex task involving possible barriers such as the clinician not recognising their own spiritual self [23]. If a palliative clinician is not self-aware of their own spiritual needs for connection, meaning, purpose, and transcendence, it is not likely that these needs will be facilitated for those within their care. Paal and team discuss additional spiritual history taking barriers such as an inability to cultivate a relationship with the patient, a lack of reading nonverbal cues, and only seeing this duty as the mere completion of a checklist [23]. One barrier complicating the spiritual screening process is that among the many tools available within the peer-reviewed literature, the majority have not been psychometrically validated. One tool, however, has undergone sensitivity and specificity testing with an adult population in a U.S. outpatient cancer setting [24]. This research team [24] recommend the following two questions as the most sensitive to being able to capture whether a person is experiencing spiritual distress within an outpatient cancer setting:

1. Do you struggle with the loss of meaning and joy in your life?
2. Do you currently have what you would describe as religious or spiritual struggles?

While these cancer outpatient data [24] are an important step forward, more studies are needed, especially in other clinical environments such as those experiencing an acute hospitalisation, or for people enrolling in hospice in the United States and internationally.

When spiritual generalists discover spiritual information through conducting a spiritual history or attend to more urgent needs identified through a spiritual screen, this aspect of whole person care is strengthened. While the data are limited concerning how often spiritual history or screening occurs in clinical care or what can happen as a result, one investigation using a structured chart review analysis from the United States discovered that among a serious illness inpatient population, 55% of patients received spiritual screening by non-chaplain team members, and of these, 91% desired chaplaincy care [25]. While it is not explored why nine out of ten screened patients wanted chaplaincy care, it is an example of the significant impact made with collaboratively oriented spiritual care among non-chaplain interprofessional palliative team members. Conducting this screening resulted in staff communicating with the chaplain about patient spiritual care needs or concerns. These data further indicate that 97% of those nine out ten patients desiring chaplaincy care were seen by a chaplain demonstrating how this spiritual generalist-specialist approach can be effectively administered [25].

2.2 Communication with the Chaplain

After being equipped with spiritual history and screening information from a non-chaplain team member shared through interdisciplinary rounds or perhaps in a consultation note, a chaplain collects and integrates these vital details to shape their clinical care. While this is the ideal scenario, some data, however, indicate that communication can at times be hindered with poor cooperation between chaplains and other healthcare providers [18, 26]. One example of this low amount of cooperation occurred in a nationwide survey of Dutch general practitioners (GPs) concerning their involvement with palliative care at home identifying that GPs involve chaplains considerably less compared to nurses, other physicians, or pharmacists [26]. Borgsteede and team [26] interpret that this is due to a few reasons including that GPs do not see this as their role or that relatively few patients have spiritual concerns. In a mixed-methods study, other examples of this poor cooperation were discussed including Dutch GPs and nurses not referring to chaplains because, like Borgsteede and team's [26] cross-sectional survey, they do not perceive that it was their responsibility to do so [18]. Furthermore, these Dutch GPs and nurses expressed their sense that it was solely the patient's responsibility to seek spiritual care if a need was present [18].

Another barrier for communication between chaplains and team members is the lack of shared understanding concerning the chaplains' scope of practice. For instance, chaplains indicate that a significant component of their role involves assisting patients and family members with their decision-making [27, 28]. However, in one study, this understanding was not shared among non-chaplain team members with less than 10% having an awareness that chaplains can be involved in this role [29]. Palliative care clinicians, however, have expressed a desire for chaplains to address decision-making within their scope of practice [30].

This gap in understanding aspects of the palliative care chaplain's role is unsurprising when considering the known communication challenges in having the chaplain's progress note in a patient's chart as the most common means of communicating [31] with the palliative care team. There is a lack of documentation standardisation in training [32] for professional chaplains generally [33] and specifically for palliative care specialists [34]. The literature also shows that many chaplain progress notes communicate minimal content [35] and in two small U.S.-based ICU studies, these notes are, first, written in a profession-specific language unhelpful to a non-chaplain reader [36] and second, they are read infrequently [37]. There are also problems related to content, with palliative care non-chaplain team members reporting that in chaplain progress notes '…the things that are missing are the things that are helpful' [30, p. 186] and that information about chaplaincy impact on patient outcomes is not clearly shared in chaplaincy documentation [36].

2.3 Training

Lack of training has been identified as the strongest predictor for spiritual care provision [38]. Important for inclusion within this training is to address the identified lack of knowledge and uncertainty for opening a conversation concerning religious or spiritual matters [8]. Because 'language is the medium in which substantive understanding and agreement take place between two people' [39, p. 386], learning the language of religious and spiritual literacy is another area where non-chaplain team members have requested guidance concerning their self-reported lack of vocabulary [1]. Based on the interpretation of their findings, McGee and team, however, contend that 'gaining knowledge about diverse patient belief systems' [40, p. 307] will not increase spiritual care provision without also cultivating self-reflection and self-awareness.

Also, among the interprofessional palliative care team members, physicians affirm a lack of confidence in spiritual care skills [1, 8, 19, 38, 41, 42]. Other barriers include physicians reporting that it is challenging for them to address spiritual needs due to prioritising biomedical needs [19]. These biomedical and spiritual needs, however, are interrelated as Delgado Guay and team [43] demonstrated within a U.S.-based advanced cancer population (n = 100). Their evidence showed that for people reporting the experience of spiritual pain, there was an increase in physical and emotional symptoms, except for shortness of breath [43].

Discussing the evidence base concerning spiritual care is important and is a part of comprehensive spiritual care training for generalists discussed in Chap. 27. Along with these data, this training encourages clinician spiritual self-awareness [40]. In other words, a participant leaves with more than a few new acronyms and a handful of novel evidence-based references. Each participant is also invited to integrate spiritual care throughout their other aspects of care and not separate it as an item for a checklist [44]. Finally, clinicians and chaplains leave this training collaboratively equipped for addressing the spiritual care needs with each patient in their local setting.

2.4 *Structural Challenges*

The demanding realities for any palliative care interprofessional team member are essential to recognise as are structural or organisational hurdles that could unintentionally create barriers for spiritual care to be assessed and addressed. Concerning these competing demands, time is the structural challenge most often cited [7, 18, 19, 38, 41]. Another organisational barrier named is the lack of private space for clinician and patient consultation [38]. Additionally, in a qualitative interview study with ICU physicians, they indicated that there are insufficient electronic health record reminders concerning addressing spiritual care and that it would be helpful to include these reminders among other care needs to be addressed [19]. There was also uncertainty related to how best to contact a chaplain when specialised spiritual care was warranted [19].

3 Personal Barriers

Non-chaplain medical team members, unrelated to palliative care specialisation, have also reported personal reasons to account for why they do not assess spiritual needs or concerns. Two common reasons were feeling uncomfortable to address a patient's spirituality [19, 40] and fear of offending the patient with spiritual inquiry [41, 45]. Perhaps connected with the fear of offending the patient is the perceived and unfounded barrier held by some clinicians that their religion, faith, or worldview needs to be concordant or aligned with the patient's [8, 19]. Specifically related to physicians, many prefer to directly refer to a chaplain rather than cultivate a discussion concerning religion or spirituality [1]. In a large cross-sectional survey with seriously ill patients in the United States, physicians, and other care providers (nurses, social workers, chaplains, and hospice volunteers), Steinhauser and team [46] sought to determine the factors considered important at the end of life for each of these groups. With the patients and their bereaved family members, both ranked 'to be at peace with God' second on a list of nine pre-selected attributes important at the end of life [46]. 'Freedom from pain' was narrowly ranked first [46]. These findings are significant to note for any clinician considering transcending personal barriers towards addressing what is most important to patients.

One other possible personal barrier meriting special consideration is when a clinician is requested to pray with a patient. In the United States, a clinician need not wonder if this will occur, only when it will happen. Recognising how often this occurs for clinicians, Balboni and colleagues [47] conducted a cross-sectional mixed-method investigation with people living with advanced cancer ($n = 70$) as well as with their physicians ($n = 206$) and nurses ($n = 115$). Generally, most participants, that is both the clinicians and patients, viewed prayer to be occasionally appropriate. Specifically, patients reported that to offer prayer would be spiritually supportive of them [47]. Among the six themes generated through the qualitative interviews, the authors discuss the (1) conditions, (2) benefits, (3) critical attitudes, and (4) positive attitudes as well as (5) possible negative consequences towards patient–clinician prayer [47]. These five themes and supportive subthemes are discussed in more detail below:

1. Conditions: Patients wondered if a physician knew their spiritual background, was it concordant with the practitioner, and what was the depth of their relationship. Practitioners also highlighted the nature of the relationship with the patient, a consideration for the practitioner's comfort level, and was there a shared religion or spirituality.
2. Benefits: The expressed benefits of sharing prayer are that it could be perceived as a source of support and perhaps lead to a better relationship between a patient and their clinician.
3. Critical attitudes: Patients were concerned that prayer could violate professional boundaries. Staff also mentioned a desire to keep their religion private and a perception that addressing spirituality was not the scope of non-chaplain staff.
4. Positive attitudes: Prayer was also discussed by staff as being intrinsically good as well as being beyond religion when framed within a lens towards whole person care.
5. Possible negative consequences towards patient–clinician prayer: Various concerns were identified by physicians about transgressing personal boundaries or fostering relational misunderstandings with patients by creating a sense that a medically scientific approach was forsaken. Patients also identified not wanting to feel pressured by a physician's religion.

The sixth theme concerned alternatives to sharing prayer together [47], which is also explored through a brief *Fast Facts and Concepts* article [48]. Both sources [47, 48] suggest the middle ground possibility for clinicians and patients to stay in the same physical space while a patient prays as the clinician respectfully and silently bears witness. Clinicians also, of course, have the option to either decline to participate or to actively join in the prayer.

4 Institutional Barriers

Beyond the professional and personal barriers already described, sometimes the employing organisations, payor sources such as health insurance companies, or government systems can serve as barriers to spiritual care being available and delivered in a suitable way. Among these organisations and systems, these barriers are usually due to financial concerns.

With competing institutional demands on nursing for patient care at the end of life, time constraints are a barrier for offering spiritual care with the time required to develop spiritual care relationships as discussed by Batsone and colleagues in their systematic review [49]. In a study with nurses in South Africa, Chandramohan and Bhagwan also affirmed that it requires extra time to deliver spiritual care [50]. A snapshot example of how long discipline-specific spiritual care training could take comes from the nursing staff of a Danish hospice [51]. Following their eight-hour training, the authors discuss the growth in knowledge, confidence, and skills [51].

Ellis and team [52] discuss how physicians are reluctant to invest the time to conduct a form of spiritual assessment, unless there was a clear source of remuneration connected. Within the necessary monetising considerations configured into any healthcare system are the accompanying considerations of how long a service will take and what it is going to cost. Unlike physicians, nurses, or other allied health professionals, the majority of chaplains as the spiritual specialists are not tied to third-party reimbursement requirements with the exception of U.S. hospice chaplains [53]. As a result, many chaplains are not bound by strict considerations on time. This can have a positive effect. For instance, in a United Kingdom project involving outpatient clinic primary chaplaincy care, it was observed that 'The single most important contribution offered by the chaplain was the gift of time' [54, p. 168]. Each patient experiencing the disruptive challenges of serious illness deserves a palliative care professional's attention and time towards addressing spiritual needs. Ideally, each palliative team member, including a chaplain, is institutionally supported in this duty.

While it is recommended that there is a chaplain as the spiritual specialist on each palliative care team [16], there are no data indicating how often and to what extent this happens in most settings. While Spetz and colleagues [55] offer data that within the United States, almost two out of five (38%) inpatient palliative care teams have a funded chaplain, it is unknown how many and to what degree palliative teams rely on spiritual or pastoral care department staff chaplains or chaplain students. Standardising chaplaincy staffing, in general, has been a historical challenge [56]. There are even more limited data concerning outpatient palliative chaplaincy care, apart from one study from the State of California noting that among ten safety net healthcare system's palliative care clinics, five had a chaplaincy team member [57]. Additionally, when these palliative teams were asked which team member would be added next to their staff, three of the ten indicated a chaplain [57].

It is essential to recognise professional, personal, and institutional barriers towards conducting spiritual care. It is also imperative to examine that data while simultaneously offering windows of possibility into where spiritual care needs are most needed and what desirable outcomes are achievable when spiritual care is addressed. Overcoming the barriers towards the work of spiritual care is the necessary next step.

5 Overcoming Barriers

Healthcare systems must confront and overcome several barriers so patients and their caregivers can receive quality and equitable care. To that end, we suggest that barriers to spiritual care are a multidimensional construct and context dependent. It is essential that one considers the barrier types highlighted in this chapter, which may include the presence of multiple barriers at many levels (e.g. personal, professional, and/or institutional barriers).

From leading evidence-based decisions and strategies to the latest educational and professional development resources, we describe three possible solutions highlighted by international colleagues.

1. Improving the evidence base related to overcoming barriers [58]: There is still much to understand about the barriers previously described, including how these barriers differ in various settings globally. Moreover, there is more to understanding how to overcome such barriers in various settings—researching to get a better understanding of what is working or not working in spiritual care in the setting of palliative care and then using the findings to improve the quality and results in various realms such as clinical, education, leadership, policy. This matters across the entire continuum of care. Healthcare professionals must quickly identify values and needs, conduct assessments, offer interventions, and improve outcomes.
2. Optimising Telehealth and Virtual Care [59, 60]: One of the most promising solutions to mitigate access and the provision of spiritual care is the utilisation of telehealth technology such as the example discussed in this chapter's case study. The COVID-19 pandemic increased the use of telehealth (see Chap. 22). This approach to care has significant power as chaplains take advantage of telehealth technology and request flexible care models to meet spiritual needs [61].
3. More Training for Healthcare Staff: Healthcare professionals may have limited knowledge and understanding of the importance of spiritual care and how to provide it. Two studies found that healthcare professionals often felt unprepared and lacked confidence in addressing spiritual needs due to inadequate training and education [38, 41]. Moreover, two studies found that the strongest predictor for providing spiritual care is training [41, 62]. Healthcare information is dynamic and ever-changing. From emerging evidence to changing policies, guidelines, industry standards, technologies, and trends, there's always something new to learn about spiritual care for healthcare professionals. However, it's not just about content—the delivery matters too.

6 Case Study

This case description explores the barriers to spiritual care based on one of the author's (PG) previous clinical experience as the chaplain for an outpatient cancer infusion clinic. This narrative offers a detailed overview of the duties for both the in-person as well as telehealth aspects of spiritual care.

6.1 In-Person

One aspect of my chaplaincy role was to offer emotional and spiritual care while people received their cancer infusion therapies. These treatments could range in length from two to six hours. The first barrier I professionally encountered was that my availability for chaplaincy care in this setting was limited to only eight to ten hours per week. As a result, I was not able to sustain a consistent presence so staff could know when I would be there. My capacity to provide care there was determined by balancing other clinical inpatient assignments. Additionally, with patients and their caregivers, I was unable to reliably provide follow up care when it was requested due to not having more hours allocated for expanded or scheduled coverage.

Another challenge encountered was the professional barrier of knowing who needed or desired chaplaincy care. Nurses or other staff were not required to inquire about spiritual concerns during these scheduled infusion clinic therapies. As a result, I relied on their real time personal and professional discernment about any person's specific needs when I was visible on the unit. As described above, confounding these possible staff referrals was factoring in co-workers not knowing when I would be there or missing me when I was there. It is difficult for staff to offer chaplaincy care if it is not readily and reliably available.

From the chaplaincy perspective, my approach towards specialised patient spiritual care involved consideration that something was better than nothing. I repeatedly encountered the institutional barrier of funding. Although it had been repeatedly requested to increase chaplaincy care availability for this environment, it had not been fulfilled. Bearing the barriers in mind, my professional practice for determining who would receive chaplaincy care was guided by a combination of nursing referrals and a review of the electronic health record to discover if someone, for instance, had previously received chaplaincy care during a hospitalisation.

6.2 Telehealth

Another aspect of my outpatient cancer infusion clinic chaplain role occurred through telehealth. The process began when I would receive a referral through the electronic health record. These referrals were generated when rooming nursing assistant staff would ask patients a battery of required questions once a month involving such matters as nutritional concerns and psychosocial needs prior to their encounter with their physician and/or advanced practice provider (nurse practitioner or physician assistant). Also included within this bank of questions were two related to spiritual distress recommended by King and team [24] for the outpatient cancer clinic setting:

1. Do you struggle with the loss of meaning and joy in your life?
2. Do you currently have what you would describe as religious or spiritual struggles?

The ordinal responses available for each of these questions are: (1) Not at all; (2) somewhat; (3) quite a bit; (4) a great deal. Any self-reported response at the level 'somewhat' to 'a great dea'l triggered a response to a chaplain. Before describing my process for responding to these referrals, it is worth considering possible localised professional barriers to these questions.

First, based on the best evidence [24] available, these two spiritual distress questions and their possible responses (above) were incorporated into my healthcare system's holistic questionnaire for screening. These questions were not, however, locally tested for feasibility with the staff nor for acceptability with patients. Second, real world implementation considerations warrant discussion because reports from my local context began to emerge that rooming staff reported the personal barrier of not feeling comfortable asking these questions. Specifically, anecdotal reports revealed that my nursing assistant co-workers' discomfort stemmed from patient responses. Specifically, patients refused to not only not answer these two spiritual distress screening questions, but some patients also requested that these questions no longer be asked in the future.

With the referrals I did receive, I was expected to contact patients by phone within 48 h. I encountered professional barriers with the competing demands of my role such as needing to arrange coverage with other chaplains if on vacation. Another professional barrier was the timing of my call in relationship to when the patient was asked the spiritual distress screening questions. I, for example, came to expect the possible patient response that spiritual distress was being experienced when the questions were asked in clinic but that that distress was no longer present at the time of our phone conversation. Sometimes patients stated they were expecting results from their diagnostic scans and could have used support at that time. A third professional barrier experienced was that that a phone call was not expected from a chaplain, sometimes requiring me to quell fears that I was not calling to share unwelcome news about disease advancement. To address this fear and accompanying anxiety, I segued into a well-rehearsed explanation that the intent of my call was to offer support related to the spiritual distress questions that were asked in clinic and were occasionally not remembered by the patient.

In summary, this case description highlights institutional and professional barriers encountered as well as practical workarounds for addressing spiritual needs amid the day-to-day work of an outpatient cancer infusion therapy clinic and related chaplaincy care provision. The personal barrier I encountered through this outpatient cancer work concerned telehealth aspects. I quickly recognised that the process of making the phone calls was less fulfilling in comparison to the in-person interactions that have become meaningfully fulfilling throughout my 20 years of chaplaincy care. This barrier was immediately transcended, however, when a cancer patient amid spiritual distress welcomed the call and opportunity to receive care. In those moments that become thick in time and consume our attention, the healing available through compassion and skilled care nurtures both the caregiver and care receiver.

7 Conclusion

Spiritual care disparities exist across a spectrum of financial, geographic, cultural, and social challenges. Disparities and barriers to spiritual care exist on the micro and macro levels. At times, barriers stand out clearly, but they are often concealed in the cracks and crevices at personal, professional, and institutional levels, making them harder to observe and address.

In this chapter, we introduced a body of evidence on these barriers. We listed them under three categories (personal, professional, and institutional), hoping that they will contribute to our ability to understand and address these complex problems. We offer recommendations, including highlighting the need for additional work to validate barrier types and solutions, and investigations that examine the relationship between these barrier types and other types we have not described, such as limited availability of healthcare resources that may reduce access to healthcare services and increase the risk of poor health outcomes. Another example is reducing unwarranted variations in spiritual care. Following guidelines helps avoid unnecessary variation in clinical practice.

References

1. Best M, Butow P, Olver I. Doctors discussing religion and spirituality: a systematic literature review. Palliat Med. 2016;30(4):327–37.
2. Rushton L. What are the barriers to spiritual care in a hospital setting? Br J Nurs. 2014;23(7):370–4.
3. Puchalski C, Ferrell B, Virani R, Otis-Green S, Baird P, Bull J, et al. Improving the quality of spiritual care as a dimension of palliative care: the report of the consensus conference. J Palliat Med. 2009;12(10):885–904.
4. Puchalski CM, Vitillo R, Hull SK, Reller N. Improving the spiritual dimension of whole person care: reaching national and international consensus. J Palliat Med. 2014;17(6):642–56.
5. Boston P, Bruce A, Schreiber R. Existential suffering in the palliative care setting: an integrated literature review. J Pain Symptom Manag. 2011;41(3):604–18.
6. Tarbi EC, Meghani SH. A concept analysis of the existential experience of adults with advanced cancer. Nurs Outlook. 2019;67(5):540–57.
7. Best M, Leget C, Goodhead A, Paal P. An EAPC white paper on multi-disciplinary education for spiritual care in palliative care. BMC Palliat Care. 2020;19(1):9.
8. Best M, Butow P, Olver I. Do patients want doctors to talk about spirituality? A systematic literature review. Patient Educ Couns. 2015;98(11):1320–8.
9. Phelps AC, Lauderdale KE, Alcorn S, Dillinger J, Balboni MT, Van Wert M, et al. Addressing spirituality within the care of patients at the end of life: perspectives of patients with advanced cancer, oncologists, and oncology nurses. J Clin Oncol. 2012;30(20):2538–44.
10. Ernecoff NC, Curlin FA, Buddadhumaruk P, White DB. Health care professionals' responses to religious or spiritual statements by surrogate decision makers during goals-of-care discussions. JAMA Intern Med. 2015;175(10):1662–9.
11. Damen A, Exline J, Pargament K, Yao Y, Chochinov H, Emanuel L, et al. Prevalence, predictors and correlates of religious and spiritual struggles in palliative cancer patients. J Pain Symptom Manag. 2021;62(3):e139–e47.

12. Exline JJ, Pargament KI, Wilt JA, Grubbs JB, Yali AM. The RSS-14: development and preliminary validation of a 14-item form of the religious and spiritual struggles scale. Psychol Relig Spiritual. 2023;15(4):592–604.
13. Balboni T, Balboni M, Paulk ME, Phelps A, Wright A, Peteet J, et al. Support of cancer patients' spiritual needs and associations with medical care costs at the end of life. Cancer. 2011;117(23):5383–91.
14. Torke AM, Varner-Perez SE, Burke ES, Taylor TA, Slaven JE, Kozinski KL, et al. Effects of spiritual care on well-being of intensive care family surrogates: a clinical trial. J Pain Symptom Manag. 2023;65(4):296–307.
15. Ferrell BR, Handzo G, Picchi T, Puchalski C, Rosa WE. The urgency of spiritual care: COVID-19 and the critical need for whole-person palliation. J Pain Symptom Manag. 2020;60(3):e7–e11.
16. Ferrell BR, Twaddle ML, Melnick A, Meier DE. National Consensus Project Clinical Practice Guidelines for quality palliative care guidelines, 4th Edition. J Palliat Med. 2018;21:1684.
17. Geiger J, Enck G, Luciani L, Fudin J, McPherson ML. Evolving roles of palliative care pharmacists. J Pain Symptom Manag. 2022;64(6):e357–61.
18. Koper I, Pasman HRW, Onwuteaka-Philipsen BD. Experiences of Dutch general practitioners and district nurses with involving care services and facilities in palliative care: a mixed methods study. BMC Health Serv Res. 2018;18(1):841.
19. Alch CK, Wright CL, Collier KM, Choi PJ. Barriers to addressing the spiritual and religious needs of patients and families in the intensive care unit: a qualitative study of critical care physicians. Am J Hosp Palliat Med. 2020;38:104990912097090.
20. Robinson MR, Thiel MM, Meyer EC. On being a spiritual care generalist. Am J Bioeth. 2007;7(7):24–6.
21. Beaussant Y, Tulsky J, Guerin B, Schwarz-Plaschg C, Sanders JJ. Radcliffe institute for advanced study working group on psychedelic research in serious I. Mapping an agenda for psychedelic-assisted therapy research in patients with serious illness. J Palliat Med. 2021;24:1657.
22. Hanson LC, Dobbs D, Usher BM, Williams S, Rawlings J, Daaleman TP. Providers and types of spiritual care during serious illness. J Palliat Med. 2008;11(6):907–14.
23. Paal P, Frick E, Roser T, Jobin G. Expert discussion on taking a spiritual history. J Palliat Care. 2017;32(1):19–25.
24. King SD, Fitchett G, Murphy PE, Pargament KI, Harrison DA, Loggers ET. Determining best methods to screen for religious/spiritual distress. Support Care Cancer. 2017;25(2):471–9.
25. Ernecoff NC, Wessell KL, Hanson LC, Dusetzina SB, Shea CM, Weinberger M, Bennett AV. Elements of palliative care in the last 6 months of life: frequency, predictors, and timing. J Gen Intern Med. 2020;35(3):753–61.
26. Borgsteede SD, Deliens L, van der Wal G, Francke AL, Stalman WA, van Eijk JT. Interdisciplinary cooperation of GPs in palliative care at home: a nationwide survey in The Netherlands. Scand J Prim Health Care. 2007;25(4):226–31.
27. Jeuland J, Fitchett G, Schulman-Green D, Kapo J. Chaplains working in palliative care: who they are and what they do. J Palliat Med. 2017;20(5):502–8.
28. Wirpsa JM, Johnson ER, Bieler J, Boyken L, Pugliese K, Rosencrans E, Murphy P. Interprofessional models for shared decision making: the role of the health care chaplain. J Health Care Chaplain. 2019;25(1):20–44.
29. Damen A, Labuschagne D, Fosler L, O'Mahony S, Levine S, Fitchett G. What do chaplains do: the views of palliative care physicians, nurses, and social workers. Am J Hosp Palliat Care. 2019;36(5):396–401.
30. Galchutt P, Connolly J. Palliative chaplain spiritual assessment progress notes. In: Peng-Keller S, Neuhold D, editors. Charting spiritual care: the emerging role of chaplaincy records in global health care. Cham: Springer; 2020. p. 181–98.
31. Hultman GM, Marquard JL, Lindemann E, Arsoniadis E, Pakhomov S, Melton GB. Challenges and opportunities to improve the clinician experience reviewing electronic progress notes. Appl Clin Inform. 2019;10(3):446–53.

32. Tartaglia A, Dodd-McCue D, Ford T, Demm C, Hassell A. Chaplain documentation and the electronic medical record: a survey of ACPE residency programs. J Health Care Chaplain. 2016;22(2):41–53.
33. O'Connor TC, O'Neill K, Van Staalduinen G, Meakes E, Penner C, Davis K. Not well know, used little and needed: Canadian chaplain's experiences of published spiritual assessment tools. J Pastoral Care Counsel. 2005;59(1–2):97–107.
34. Handzo G, Buhuro RDJ, Kidd R, Saks RNT, Ferrell B. A statement on the role and qualifications of health care chaplains for research and quality. J Pain Symptom Manag. 2023;65(6):e745–e55.
35. Cadge W. Paging god: religion in the halls of medicine. Chicago: University of Chicago Press; 2012.
36. Lee BM, Curlin FA, Choi PJ. Documenting presence: a descriptive study of chaplain notes in the intensive care unit. Palliat Support Care. 2017;15(2):190–6.
37. Choi PJ, Chow V, Curlin FA, Cox CE. Intensive care clinicians' views on the role of chaplains. J Health Care Chaplain. 2019;25(3):89–98.
38. Balboni MJ, Sullivan A, Enzinger AC, Epstein-Peterson ZD, Tseng YD, Mitchell C, et al. Nurse and physician barriers to spiritual care provision at the end of life. J Pain Symptom Manag. 2014;48(3):400–10.
39. Gadamer HG. Truth and method. 2nd rev. ed. (Weinsheimer J, Marshall DG, Trans.). New York: Continuum; 2004. (Original work published 1960).
40. McGee J, Palmer Kelly E, Kelly-Brown J, Stevens E, Waterman BL, Pawlik TM. Assessing the impact of provider training and perceived barriers on the provision of spiritual care: a mixed methods study. J Cancer Educ. 2023;38(1):301–8.
41. Balboni MJ, Sullivan A, Amobi A, Phelps AC, Gorman DP, Zollfrank A, et al. Why is spiritual care infrequent at the end of life? Spiritual care perceptions among patients, nurses, and physicians and the role of training. J Clin Oncol. 2013;31(4):461–7.
42. Ledford CJ, Canzona MR, Seehusen DA, Cafferty LA, Schmidt ME, Huang JC, Villagran MM. Differences in physician communication when patients ask versus tell about religion/spirituality: a pilot study. Fam Med. 2015;47(2):138–42.
43. Delgado-Guay MO, Hui D, Parsons HA, Govan K, De la Cruz M, Thorney S, Bruera E. Spirituality, religiosity, and spiritual pain in advanced cancer patients. J Pain Symptom Manag. 2011;41(6):986–94.
44. Tarbi EC, Gramling R, Bradway C, Meghani SH. "If it's the time, it's the time": existential communication in naturally occurring palliative care conversations with individuals with advanced cancer, their families, and clinicians. Patient Educ Couns. 2021;104(12):2963–8.
45. Sinclair S, Booker R, Fung T, Raffin-Bouchal S, Enns B, Beamer K, Ager N. Factors associated with post-traumatic growth, quality of life, and spiritual well-being in outpatients undergoing bone marrow transplantation: a pilot study. Oncol Nurs Forum. 2016;43(6):772–80.
46. Steinhauser KE, Christakis NA, Clipp EC, McNeilly M, McIntyre L, Tulsky JA. Factors considered important at the end of life by patients, family, physicians, and other care providers. JAMA. 2000;284(19):2476–82.
47. Balboni MJ, Babar A, Dillinger J, Phelps AC, George E, Block SD, et al. "It depends": viewpoints of patients, physicians, and nurses on patient-practitioner prayer in the setting of advanced cancer. J Pain Symptom Manag. 2011;41(5):836–47.
48. Kwiatkowski K, Arnold RM, Barnard D. Physicians and prayer requests #120. J Palliat Med. 2011;14(11):1259–60.
49. Batstone E, Bailey C, Hallett N. Spiritual care provision to end-of-life patients: a systematic literature review. J Clin Nurs. 2020;29(19–20):3609–24.
50. Chandramohan S, Bhagwan R. Utilization of spirituality and spiritual care in nursing practice in public hospitals in KwaZulu-Natal, South Africa. Religions. 2016;7(3):23.
51. Viftrup DT, Rosenbaek F, Damgaard HH, Hemdrup M, Nielsen M, Nissen RD. Caring spiritually: a study on spiritual care training in a hospice setting. J Hosp Palliat Nurs. 2023;25(3):156–64.

52. Ellis MR, Vinson DC, Ewigman B. Addressing spiritual concerns of patients: family physicians' attitudes and practices. J Fam Pract. 1999;48(2):105–9.
53. Centers for Medicare & Medicaid Services. Hospice [Internet]. CMS.gov; 2023. [updated 2023; cited 2023 Sept 28]. https://www.cms.gov/Medicare/Medicare-Fee-for-Service-Payment/Hospice
54. McSherry W, Boughey A, Kevern P. "Chaplains for wellbeing" in primary care: a qualitative investigation of their perceived impact for patients' health and wellbeing. J Health Care Chaplain. 2016;22(4):151–70.
55. Spetz J, Dudley N, Trupin L, Rogers M, Meier DE, Dumanovsky T. Few hospitals palliative care programs meet national staffing recommendations. Health Aff (Millwood). 2016;35(9):1690–7.
56. Tartaglia A, White KB, Corson T, Charlescraft A, Johnson T, Jackson-Jordan E, Fitchett G. Supporting staff: The role of health care chaplains. J Health Care Chaplain. 2022;30:1–14.
57. Rabow MW, Parrish M, Kinderman A, Freedman J, Harris H, Cox D, et al. Staffing in California public hospital palliative care clinics: a report from the California Health Care Foundation Palliative Care in Public Hospitals Learning Community. J Palliat Med. 2021;24(7):1045–50.
58. Nolan S, Saltmarsh P, Leget C. Spiritual Care in Palliative Care: working towards an EAPC task force. European. J Palliat Care. 2011;18:86–9.
59. Ogunseitan AB, Smith MM. Telehealth: an avenue for expanding access to specialist palliative care. Jt Comm J Qual Patient Saf. 2022;48(12):625–6.
60. Xu X, Ho MH, Lin CC. Telehealth in palliative care during the COVID-19 pandemic: a systematic mixed studies review. Worldviews Evid-Based Nurs. 2023;20(5):476–91.
61. Sprik PJ, Janssen Keenan A, Boselli D, Grossoehme DH. Chaplains and telechaplaincy: best practices, strengths, weaknesses-a national study. J Health Care Chaplain. 2022;29:1–23.
62. Gijsberts M-JHE, Liefbroer AI, Otten R, Olsman E. Spiritual Care in Palliative Care: a systematic review of the recent European literature. Med Sci. 2019;7(2):25.

Spiritual Care During a Pandemic

George F. Handzo

Abstract The COVID-19 pandemic impacted every aspect of how we live, work, and lead our lives including the delivery of spiritual care in health care. It amplified many aspects of spiritual care both positive and negative. It came on swiftly and dramatically and, in spiritual care, caused the loss of in-person ritual, loss of touch and presence which are central and sacred to chaplaincy, and role confusion for chaplains. Many chaplains were considered non-essential and excluded from patient rooms or even from the institutions. Spiritual care and education had to pivot to virtual techniques which many did well. However, international research found that many chaplains were marginalised during this time. At the same time, others became more visible, and their contributions much better understood. The distinction seems to be largely due to whether the chaplains understood their role and were integrated into their institutions before the pandemic. Those who were well integrated pre-pandemic were much more likely to thrive during this time. Chaplains need to learn how to advocate for spiritual care and for what they contribute to care.

Keywords Chaplaincy · Spiritual Care · COVID-19 · Palliative Care · Pandemic

1 Introduction

While much of what is discussed in this chapter is true for the whole world, the author lives and works in the United States of America (USA). Thus, the content is written within the context of that system. When research or commentary exists from

---

G. F. Handzo (✉)
Health Services Research & Quality, HealthCare Chaplaincy Network, New York, NY, USA
e-mail: ghandzo@healthcarechaplaincy.org

M. C. Best (ed.), *Spiritual Care in Palliative Care*,
https://doi.org/10.1007/978-3-031-50864-6_22

other counties, that was included. The major international survey referenced repeatedly here was conducted in North America, Europe, Australia, and New Zealand.

The COVID-19 pandemic was arguably one of the major health events to occur in the world in modern times. It certainly impacted every aspect of how we live, work, and lead our lives. It also had major impacts on how we die and how we grieve for those who have died. Many of those changes appear to be permanent—for better or for worse. None of those impacts was more dramatic and visible that the impact on how we care for the sick and dying. Health delivery systems were unprepared for the swiftness of the spread of the disease, the resources needed to protect others including health care providers from contagion, and the emotional as well as physical toll the disease would take on providers and the general population. Health care providers of all disciplines were not fully trained for the technical or medical knowledge they needed or for how to care for themselves and others emotionally and spiritually. Religious and spiritual communities were unprepared for the impact on their communities, both individually and corporately. In all these domains, the pandemic called for ways of taking care of others, some of which were previously thought to be either undoable or at least not optimal.

One of the hallmarks of this pandemic was that it impacted virtually every country in the world. Even countries that knew it was coming were unable to prevent it. The experience across these countries had many similarities despite the differences in culture and medical resources including the impact on the elderly and the difficulties in providing for end-of-life care. An upside was that countries were motivated to work together to standardise treatment protocols and speed the development of vaccines. At one time when intensive care units in northern Italy were overwhelmed, some of their physicians appeared on a webinar open to physicians from all over the world discussing some of the treatment protocols they found that helped and some that did not.

Another hallmark was that the pandemic amplified the strengths and weaknesses of health care delivery systems everywhere including the delivery of spiritual care. As an example, there was already a worsening workforce shortage in palliative care in the United States before the pandemic [1]. The pandemic increased the workforce needs while simultaneously speeding up the number of providers leaving the workforce early. Many hospitals were already under financial stress. The pandemic added significantly to that stress even in the face of special government supports. All these stresses put increasing burdens on the systems and the people who work in them. The situation also morphed over time as many caregivers went from being seen as heroes in their communities to being seen as villains who were not telling the truth about the disease.

In many of these situations, chaplains did or could have acted as the supports for staff, families, and caregivers [2]. Staff support particularly has been recognised as part of the health care chaplain's role for many years as has support for families in crisis. For instance, chaplains are often delegated to be with families in trauma centres and emergency departments as they wait for news of loved ones. Unfortunately, too many times, the chaplains, like other team members, lacked the training or the amount of staffing needed to meet these needs.

Before discussing the particulars of these issues in depth, it is important to define some terms. While this is a book written for an international audience, some essential terms are used differently in different parts of the world. The definitions used in this chapter are those that have come to be generally used in the United States. No representation is made that these should be the preferred terms everywhere. The definitions are given only so that readers will know exactly what the author is referring to with each.

'Chaplain' as used here should be assumed to refer to a professional health care chaplain who serves patients, family members and staff without regard to their belief system or culture. A recently developed consensus definition written for the United States is summarised as:

> The chaplain is the spiritual care specialist on the health care team. They support patients, families, their caregivers, and staff to draw on their spiritual, religious, emotional, and cultural resources, as well as their personal values to cope with their experiences in the health care context. They are unique and essential members of the interdisciplinary team with the goal of providing person-centered care. [3]

Palliative care 'focuses on expert assessment and management of pain and other symptoms, assessment and support of caregiver needs, and coordination of care. Palliative care attends to the physical, functional, psychological, practical, and spiritual consequences of a serious illness. It is a person- and family-centred approach to care, providing people living with serious illness relief from the symptoms and stress of an illness'. [4]

Health care chaplaincy for decades has functioned according to the values and behaviours of palliative care. It starts with determining the beliefs and values of the patient and family and using those as the basis for a care plan. It is about relieving suffering—in this case spiritual suffering. Thus, no distinction will be made here between health care chaplaincy in general and palliative care chaplaincy.

2 Health Care Chaplaincy Before COVID-19

Even before the pandemic, health care, certainly in the developed world, was changing and the role of the chaplain along with it. Palliative care had grown significantly and with it the attention to the spiritual dimension of care [6]. Chaplains started to become more a part of a team than a solo practitioner. These changes were codified in the United States in 2018 by the 4th edition of the National Consensus Project Clinical Practice Guidelines for Quality Palliative Care in which chaplains were named one of the four required members of the palliative care team [4]. Nonetheless, in the United States, only a small percentage of teams have a dedicated chaplain—far fewer than social work, for example. In the United States, it is possible to get specialty certification in palliative care chaplaincy. However, the total number of chaplains so certified as of 2023 is only slightly over 100. The likely cause is that many palliative team chiefs do not appreciate the value added by a fully trained and professional chaplain. Others have been served by chaplains who did not understand palliative care or what it meant to be a member of a palliative care team. Many chaplains do not know how to attend to helping the institutions understand what chaplains do, or they simply think that it will be evident to others. They often do not know how to succinctly state who they are and what their role is. This became clear during the pandemic when those who could not be clear about what they contributed were often marginalised [7]. Chaplains are often not very good at limiting their stress and so are subject to burnout. This characteristic was evident in New York City post-9/11 when many chaplains routinely far exceeded the guidelines for how much time they should spend at the World Trade Center site working with the first responders.

On the positive side, chaplains were often designated as participants in the institution's disaster plan. They also tended to spend time providing care for institutional staff whether or not this was officially part of their job description [8].

3 Rapid Onset

Even after the initial appearance of COVID-19, locations were often not prepared for how fast the onset would be both for individuals and for systems. Even for systems and providers who knew it was coming, the onset was a shock [9]. The onset was often called a 'wave' or even a 'tsunami'. Once it hit, there was often little or no time to adjust [9–11]. There were times when there was not enough Personal Protective Equipment (PPE) to go around which made chaplains particularly vulnerable to marginalisation. There certainly was not enough time for the chaplain to establish a leadership role in the institution if they did not already have one.

One seemingly universal administrative response to the pandemic's onset was to pare down those who were allowed patient contact or even allowed in the institution. 'Essential' employees were often only those deemed necessary for the physical dimension of care and the physical running of the institution which sometimes did not include chaplains. Volunteers were routinely excluded. Many of those volunteers, including representatives of local faith communities, were delivering spiritual care [12–14]. Chaplaincy students were also often part of this excluded group. Certainly, in the United States, students and volunteers deliver most of the spiritual care in many institutions so this change often reduced the spiritual care delivered to a very low level at a time when it was most needed [2].

This juncture in the process was critical for the delivery of spiritual care since, once the chaplains were excluded, they had little ability to make the case for their inclusion. Vandenhoeck, Snowdon, and colleagues conducted a very important survey of health care chaplains in North America, Europe, New Zealand, and Australia in which they asked about various aspects of what the chaplains had done during the pandemic [7]. A critical finding was that many chaplains were unsure of their role, both before the pandemic and during it. Additionally, many chaplains reported that their institutions were not clear about the chaplain's role. It seems logical that if the chaplains cannot articulate their role, the institution will not understand it. Many chaplains blamed lack of chaplaincy leadership for this situation. They believed they were often not properly deployed because chaplains were not in the meetings where the responses of the institution to the pandemic were discussed. While there is no reason to believe that this conclusion is in error, the root cause is likely deeper. Chaplains have long been resistant to standardisation of any kind and, often, chaplain training has encouraged chaplains to develop their own way of operating. The problem in the pandemic was that, once the first wave had set it, it was too late to change the situation. In the meantime, some chaplaincy services did very well. They were even able to expand their services during the pandemic. Anecdotal evidence suggests that this achievement was related to the clarity with which they articulated their role and their degree of integration before the pandemic.

4 Changes in Patient Care

Perhaps the major intervention central to all trained health care chaplains is called *presence*. This implies more than just physical presence. It indicates that the chaplain is with the patient on a spiritual/existential level as well as a physical and social one. To be present in this way does not require speaking but does require the chaplain to be giving their undivided attention to the patient. The assumption in chaplaincy has been that this presence can only be effectively delivered face to face. Further, touch has long been central to communicating this presence.

In general, all over the world, an immediate and dramatic change in patient care occurred with the onset of COVID-19. There was a sudden reduction in the contact COVID-19 patients had with other people, including the patient's family and other visitors as well as many staff including chaplains [10, 12]. In Scotland where many chaplains work in outpatient settings and do home visits, both of those options were stopped [15]. This change was a significant loss for patients, families, and for the chaplains who often felt that they could no longer deliver effective spiritual care [14]. Patients were faced with loneliness as well as increased anxiety. Even chaplains who were allowed to visit patients had to deal with the barriers of gloves and particularly masks. In an interaction like chaplaincy where non-verbal communication is an important element in the relationship, masks turned out to be a significant barrier [12]. This was widely recognised for all staff and, eventually for this reason, many institutions purchased masks with the part over the mouth replaced with transparent plastic.

A population that was particularly impacted by these changes were the institutionalised elderly. Previously many families spent a lot of time with them and provided a significant amount of their care [9]. Many of these patients had some form of dementia, making it additionally difficult for them to understand what was going on during the pandemic, and why visitors were not coming.

To their credit, chaplains generally responded promptly and used the avenues that remained available to them to deliver the care patients and families needed. They went through the work of putting on PPE where that was allowed and communicated despite it [10]. Where in-person visiting was no longer possible, chaplains quickly switched to the telephone even though it was hard for them to get used to and seemed less effective [9, 15]. They often endured being labelled as non-essential and rejoiced that they were able to provide some care for those who were so sick [14].

Family visiting, or the prohibition of it, was a major issue during the pandemic. While medical safety was understandably paramount, the psychologic consequences for families were sometimes significant to the point of causing security issues when families demanded to see their sick loved ones [16]. Communication with families became a significant task for many chaplains especially since it could be done remotely from the chaplain's office or from home. Not being able to come into the hospital posed a barrier to keeping families informed and chaplains could often be the bridge to communicating the need for information to medical staff and facilitating calls [17].

For many patients, prayer and religious ritual are still very important and still a desired part of their regular lives despite hospitalisation. While prayer and some of the rituals can be done without touching the patient or even being in the same room, some require the presence of the person administering the ritual, or recipients expect the sacrament to be administered in person. Eucharist for some Christian patients is an example. The communion wafer is normally placed in the recipient's mouth or in their hand by the priest. In the AIDS pandemic, this was not a problem once if was understood that AIDS is not transmitted by air. COVID-19, however, is mainly airborne so a chaplain coming near to an unmasked patient can be problematic. The Sacrament of the Sick (formerly known as Last Rites) in which holy oil is applied to the patient's forehead is also problematic because of the physical proximity required. As the pandemic progressed, health care institutions and religious communities structured ways to satisfy these important needs without violating safety protocols. Many religious bodies legitimised forms of sacraments that were safe and let their adherents know about them. Prayers and reading of sacred texts were done through various technologies including telephone, Zoom, and iPAD.

End-of-life rituals and funerals posed significant issues on many levels in several faith groups. At the beginning of the pandemic, families were not allowed to visit at all. Thus, patients often died alone. This process caused significant distress for the family and, presumably, for the patient as well, especially in religious and cultural communities in which family is supposed to be with the patient at the time of death. Nurses often had to be the family surrogates which put an extra physical and psychological burden on them.

In several religious traditions, the corpse is required to be moved quickly and buried by the community in a very short time after death. However, for a long time, it was not clear how long the COVID-19 virus lived on in the human body, and thus, it was unclear how soon the body could be transferred to funeral directors or those in faith communities. In some faith communities, the funeral homes that served that community were overwhelmed and unable to keep up with the demand. It often fell to the chaplains to support the families through these difficult periods. In the African American Muslim community in New York City, the local Muslim chaplain often had to explain to families that the *Janazah* prayer required at Muslim funerals to make sure the deceased went to Paradise could be said without a body present. In New York City, this had already been done all too often after 9/11 [18].

In more recent times, protocols have been worked out to allow at least a small number of close family to visit a patient immediately before death. The issue still is that, in some diseases such as dementia, predicting the time of death with any precision is very difficult. Thus, patients still die unattended by loved ones. Virtual funerals became the norm and provided the benefit of allowing people who could not attend a funeral for any reason to now attend. Providing virtual worship services became commonplace, which again, provide benefits for those who previously had not been able to go to worship in person.

5 Emergence of Spiritual/Existential Needs

A critical feature of this pandemic was that the spiritual/existential needs it generated seem to have been similar world-wide. Bahramnezhad and Asgari, writing from Iran, point out the need for attention to the dying patient and the anxiety caused for patient, family, and care staff by not having family present at the time of death [19]. Ferrell and colleagues writing from the United States point out the need for care for the 'wounded' caregivers who have their own spiritual needs [2]. Roman and colleagues, writing from South Africa raise the need for listening to hopes and fears and the promotion of compassionate care [20]. The fact that these issues seem to cover such a diversity of geographies and cultures suggests that something quite basic is being touched. Part of the issue may be that no one was, or is, immune to this disease and, if contracted, it can be swiftly fatal. Everyone was disconnected, isolated, and dealing with loneliness. Thus, everyone, including the medical caregivers and the chaplains, is prone to the same fear and anxiety as their patients. In answer to these intense feeling, chaplains provided 'calm presence, being available, holding out hope, and introducing creative ways to provide spiritual care'. [12] However, this was often done at some psychological and spiritual cost to the chaplains.

5.1 Virtual Spiritual Care

Maybe no change in spiritual care delivery and education was more dramatic than the emergence and acceptance of technology and virtual delivery of spiritual care. As mentioned previously, nothing is more sacred to chaplaincy than the idea that it had to be done in person. It was widely considered impossible to be present virtually in the way chaplains claimed was central to their practice. That said, contacting patients and families by telephone had been practised for years for various reasons including calling pre-operative patients before their admission, following up with families after a death, and reaching out to patients and families in rural areas. Doing chaplaincy clinical training by Zoom was beginning in the United States but was assumed to be far inferior to in-person training [13]. This was due in part to the inexperience of educators with this modality. There was one association using Zoom as part of their chaplaincy certification process. These changes did make clinical services and education much more widely available.

As in health care, the change to more virtual care was dramatic and seemingly instantaneous. To their credit, chaplains generally did not resist since often this was their only way to continue care, but it was clearly hard work and not nearly as professionally satisfying [15]. The change was especially dramatic for those in the outpatient setting where clinics were closed. Many chaplains who were no longer permitted to go into patient rooms adopted telephonic visits as the only way available to interact with patients. Chaplains were known to call patients on the chaplains' cell phones from outside the room where they could see the patient from a distance. This strategy enabled them to talk to the patient safely and see them without a mask on. As chaplains began to be allowed back into patient rooms, many chaplains were given iPADs. These were used mainly to allow communication in the room between the patient and loved ones. Over time, more and more communication migrated from telephone to Zoom. A 2019 United States survey found that about half of United States health care chaplains did some part of their work virtually [21]. Today, certainly, in the United States, being able to visit by Zoom is considered to be a standard part of a health care chaplain's toolkit. A survey of best practices did find that telehealth improved health care [22]. However, this change did highlight how many people in the United States do not have access to this technology or still live in areas without internet reception.

6 Staff Care

As mentioned above, one of the unique aspects of this pandemic was that staff were as susceptible to the disease as patients and therefore were subject to the same fears. Many were afraid of bringing COVID-19 home to their families to the point that they cut themselves off from physical contact with them thus adding to their overall stress [12]. It was quickly realised that there was a need for spiritual care of staff [23]. Staff were also surrounded by sudden death often without the time in between deaths to process their grief. These were often staff who were already burdened by workforce shortages, and pressures to deliver more care without extra staff. Thus, at a point when they needed more time for self-care, they had less time. In many places, the chaplains were central to providing the staff care. As with the other staff, chaplains had their own stresses and grief to deal with and now were being asked to share the grief of other staff usually with no additional staffing. There were exceptions where chaplains were already well integrated and already seen as central to staff support. In some of these institutions, chaplaincy staff were added during the pandemic. Chaplains helped set up quiet rooms to which staff could retreat when they felt overwhelmed. There were attempts at group interventions. However, these often failed because staff clearly preferred to go home rather than stay to attend a group. Anecdotally, the stress on small or single person chaplaincy services was especially severe and under-appreciated since these chaplains were the least likely to take the time to respond to surveys.

During all the stresses, many chaplains reported increased attention to staff care and use of creative strategies to reach out to staff even in situations where they were not allowed in the institution [8]. There are several staff support strategies that have been well validated and found to be effective. *Resilience in Stressful Events* (RISE) was originally developed several years ago at Johns Hopkins Medical Center in Baltimore, Maryland (United States), as a staff support and resilience building programme. It is not a programme that is normally led by chaplains but does involve chaplains in the implementation. It has been quite successful and is now used in several medical centres in the United States. One of its most successful features is that it relies on peer support and peer support leaders. Thus, after it is up and running, it is self-sustaining and very low cost. However, it did rely on in person interactions. To deal with the need for social isolation during COVID-19, the RISE team implemented some virtual encounters and rounded on certain units [24].

Three Good Things is another intervention that has been in use for some years and is based in positive psychology. The intervention consists of each day naming three good things that happened that day. It requires no training and can be used by people of almost any age. In a trial with health care workers, it demonstrated benefits including improvements in emotional exhaustion, symptoms of depression and happiness [25].

7 Education

As in all other aspects of spiritual care during the pandemic, weaknesses were exposed in spiritual care training that impeded the work of chaplains and other spiritual care providers [26]. Chief among these was the insistence on in-person training. The use of Zoom and other technologies was beginning to be used pre-pandemic but was not favoured by many educators. However, virtual *clinical pastoral education* (CPE, the basic training for professional health care chaplains) quickly became central to both education and practice although some educators adapted more readily than others [13]. Virtual supervision became fully acceptable and has remained so post-pandemic.

The concept of specialist and generalist spiritual care providers had been introduced some years ago and was increasingly integrated in the United States and other countries [27]. In this model, the professional chaplain is the spiritual care specialist who is the authority on all aspects of spiritual care such as spiritual distress and beliefs of different faith groups. Other clinical members of the team such as nurses are the spiritual generalists. The chaplains are expected to provide generalist training [28]. In the pandemic, the role of the nurse as spiritual generalist often came to the fore as the chaplain was not as available and chaplaincy volunteers who previously delivered a great deal of generalist care were no longer in the hospital. For example, spiritual/religious interventions such as reading prayers which were rarely delegated to nurses pre-pandemic were now often expected from them because no one else was in the room to do it. In general, nurses recognised this as part of their role and were willing to provide the services but needed training [29, 30]. This task fell to the chaplains as the spiritual care specialists. Serving people of all faiths, integrating with other disciplines, and working in a crisis setting had long been standard training for some such as military chaplains but was usually not part of the training of health care chaplains. They now became standard practice in health care and needed to be incorporated into training.

The foundational modality for training professional health care chaplains, CPE, is widely available in North America and less so elsewhere. The training is based on the action-reflection-action model in which the action is providing direct spiritual care and the reflection is group and individual supervision. With the onset of COVID-19, all these processes had to pivot to virtual formats which had previously been considered at least inferior and at worst incapable of producing the expected CPE outcomes. Some programmes were even shut down until this pivot could happen. It took a while in some places to find ways for students to connect with patients and families virtually. It is still unclear how well this pivot did work. What is known is that it did happen quite quickly in many places and not quickly or successfully in others. The results suggest that some educators and programmes adapted very well, and some did not. The reasons for this are not yet clear [13].

8 Self-Care

Self-care for chaplains and religious/spiritual professionals generally is a topic that every practitioner thinks is a good idea, but which many are not diligent to follow up. Often the ethos in this profession is one of selfless giving which does not include taking care of oneself. Like many health care professionals, chaplains were often cut off from their normal social and professional supports especially if they were working virtually. Religious, spiritual, and social communities were not gathering. One study found that those chaplains who belonged to a professional association received more supervision and, in turn, gave more staff support [31]. Another study found that chaplains being well integrated in their institutional structure and having good leadership and supervision was critical to their self-care [32]. Like others, they were often understaffed and working long hours. On the positive side, many chaplains were able to take advantage of private pre-existing spiritual and religious practices which provided support. Thus, professional connections seem to have a positive impact on the chaplain's self-care and thus presumably on the quality and quantity of care they were able to deliver.

9 Going Forward

Clearly, COVID-19 is here to stay at some level. Along with that reality is the general realisation in health care that another pandemic is almost a certainty at some time in the future and continued vigilance is in order. It also seems a reality that virtual health care is here to stay at some level. Patients like it. It not only provides good quality care in many circumstances but enables outreach that would be otherwise difficult [21]. Additionally, care is moving into the outpatient and community settings often with palliative care in the lead. The palliative model is also a team-based model.

To be included in this new reality, spiritual care will have to adapt. This includes provision of virtual spiritual care as part of what health care chaplains do, the ability to work in various care settings, skills in supporting staff as well as patients, and the ability to work as a member of an interdisciplinary team. The international survey done during COVID-19 found that the chaplain skill that was most effective during the pandemic was the ability and willingness to be flexible and creative [31].

This pandemic has raised the visibility and value of spiritual care in health care. It has demonstrated much of the breadth and depth of what spiritual care can do for patients, families, and staff [14]. Yet, spiritual care is not fully integrated in many places and chaplains are not always at the tables where their voices can be heard. A consequence of this situation is that policy is made, and programmes are set up without chaplains included to their full potential or not included at all.

This issue seems rooted in the finding of Snowden that many chaplains cannot articulate their role [7]. If this is true, it seems only logical that the administrators would not and could not know what the role is either. Further, many chaplains still operate by the religion-based model. Professional health care chaplaincy worldwide needs to adopt standards for the role of the health care chaplain just as consistency in the definition of spirituality was established [5]. These standards will likely not be identical across all cultures and geographies, but they should give evidence of some common roots. Hopefully, a recent attempt in the United States will spur similar efforts worldwide [3]. Snowden and colleagues also found that chaplains who belonged to professional associations felt much more supported and were much more likely to be well integrated [7].

Perhaps most damaging to the cause of inclusion of chaplaincy in health care is the inability, and sometimes unwillingness, of many chaplains to advocate for themselves. This is partly a fault of the chaplaincy education system which does not promote the importance of advocacy or indeed teach it. There is now much evidence for the inclusion of chaplaincy [33–35]. However, chaplains need to be familiar with that evidence, able to articulate it, and, most importantly, know how to use it to their advantage [36]. Until this happens, Snowdon warns, chaplains will not be considered of value to the system or fully integrated [7].

In COVID-19, many health care chaplains served heroically and provided tremendous benefit for patients, loved ones, and staff while showcasing the value-added care that professional chaplains can provide. However, many did not even get the opportunity to do this often because they were not well integrated into their institution's structure or because they did not advocate for their inclusion [7].

Permissions Permissions from the *J of Pain and Symptom Management* and the *J of Palliative Medicine* are automatically granted by journal policy because the author of this chapter is also an author on the paper quoted.

The National Consensus Project Clinical Practice Guidelines are in the public domain.

The policy of Sage Publications, publisher of the *J of Pastoral Care and Counselling*, is that permissions are automatically granted if the quotation is under 200 words or under 10% of the total article whichever is smaller. All quotations from that journal fall within this policy.

References

1. Kamal AH, Wolf SP, Troy J, Leff V, Dahlin C, Rotella JD, Handzo G, Rodgers PE, Myers ER. Policy changes key to promoting sustainability and growth of the specialty palliative care workforce. Health Aff. 2019;38(6):910–8.
2. Ferrell BR, Handzo G, Picchi T, Puchalski C, Rosa WE. The urgency of spiritual care: COVID-19 and the critical need for whole-person palliation. J Pain Symptom Manag. 2020;60(3):e7–11.
3. Handzo G, Buhuro RD, Kidd R, Saks RN, Ferrell B. A statement on the role and qualifications of health care chaplains for research and quality. J Pain Symptom Manag. 2023;65(6):e745–55.
4. National Consensus Project for Quality Palliative Care (NCP). Clinical practice guidelines quality palliative care. 4th ed. Richmond: National Coalition for Hospice and Palliative Care; 2018. https://www.nationalcoalitionhpc.org/ncp. Accessed 26 July 2023
5. Puchalski C, Ferrell B, Virani R, Otis-Green S, Baird P, Bull J, Chochinov H, Handzo G, Nelson-Becker H, Prince-Paul M, Pugliese K. Improving the quality of spiritual care as a dimension of palliative care: the report of the Consensus Conference. J Palliat Med. 2009;12(10):885–904.
6. Dumanovsky T, Augustin R, Rogers M, Lettang K, Meier DE, Morrison RS. The growth of palliative care in US hospitals: a status report. J Palliat Med. 2016;19(1):8–15.
7. Snowden A. What did chaplains do during the Covid pandemic? An international survey. J Pastoral Care Counsel. 2021;75(1_suppl):6–16.
8. Tata B, Nuzum D, Murphy K, Karimi L, Cadge W. Staff-care by chaplains during COVID-19. J Pastoral Care Counsel. 2021;75(1_suppl):24–9.
9. Drummond DA, Carey LB. Chaplaincy and spiritual care response to COVID-19: an Australian case study–the McKellar Centre. Health Soc Care Chaplain. 2020;8(2):165–79.
10. Busfield L. Listening on the outside–screaming on the inside: reflections from an acute hospital chaplain during the first weeks of COVID-19. Health Soc Care Chaplain. 2020;8(2):218–22.
11. Muehlhausen BL, Desjardins CM, Chappelle C, Schwartzman G, Tata-Mbeng B, Fitchett G. Managing spiritual care departments during the COVID-19 pandemic: a qualitative study. J Pastoral Care Counsel. 2022;76(4):294–303.
12. Jones KF, Washington J, Kearney M, Best MC. Responding to the "unknown assailant": a qualitative exploration with Australian health and aged care chaplains on the impact of COVID-19. J Health Care Chaplain. 2022;28(3):295–309.
13. Szilagyi C, Tartaglia A, Palmer PK, Fleenor DW, Jackson-Jordan E, Knoll Sweeney S, Slaven JE. Delivering Clinical Pastoral Education (CPE) remotely: educators' views and perspectives during the COVID-19 pandemic and beyond. J Pastoral Care Counsel. 2022;76(3):189–209.
14. Domaradzki J. Hospital chaplains facing the pandemic. A qualitative study. J Health Care Chaplain. 2023;29(1):145–60.

15. Giffen S, Macdonald G. Report for the association of chaplaincy in general practice on spiritual care during the COVID-19 pandemic. Health Soc Care Chaplain. 2020;8(2):265–76.
16. Downar J, Kekewich M. Improving family access to dying patients during the COVID-19 pandemic. Lancet Respir Med. 2021;9(4):335–7.
17. Singh N, Giannitrapani K, Gamboa R, Walling A, Lindvall C, Lorenz K. "Shoot from the hip": what patients with cancer want from communication about serious illness during COVID-19 (S526). J Pain Symptom Manag. 2022;63(5):919–20.
18. Al-Hajii Imam Yusuf Hasan. Personal communication, July 15, 2023.
19. Bahramnezhad F, Asgari P. Spiritual care for COVID-19 patients: a neglected necessity. Infect Dis Clin Pract. 2021;29(1):e63.
20. Roman NV, Mthembu TG, Hoosen M. Spiritual care–'a deeper immunity'–a response to Covid-19 pandemic. Afr J Prim Health Care Fam Med. 2020;12(1):1–3.
21. Sprik PJ, Janssen Keenan A, Boselli D, Grossoehme DH. Chaplains and telechaplaincy: best practices, strengths, weaknesses – a national study. J Health Care Chaplain. 2023;29(1):41–63.
22. Monaghesh E, Hajizadeh A. The role of telehealth during COVID-19 outbreak: a systematic review based on current evidence. BMC Public Health. 2020;20:1–9.
23. Sarmiento PJ. Wounded healers: a call for spiritual care towards healthcare professionals in time of COVID-19 pandemic. J Public Health. 2021;43(2):e273–4.
24. Wu AW, Connors CA, Norvell M. Adapting RISE: meeting the needs of healthcare workers during the COVID-19 pandemic. Int Rev Psychiatry. 2021;33(8):711–7.
25. Sexton JB, Adair KC. Forty-five good things: a prospective pilot study of the Three Good Things well-being intervention in the USA for healthcare worker emotional exhaustion, depression, work–life balance and happiness. BMJ Open. 2019;9(3):e022695.
26. Flynn E, Tan H, Vandenhoeck A. "We need to learn from what we have learned!": the possible impact of covid-19 on the education and training of chaplains. J Pastoral Care Counsel. 2021;75(1_suppl):37–40.
27. Handzo G, Koenig H. Spiritual care: whose job is it anyway? South Med J. 2004;97(12):1242–5.
28. Jones KF, Washington J, Kearney M, Best MC. What is the role of spiritual care specialists in teaching generalist spiritual care? The perspectives of pastoral care staff in a large Catholic health and aged care organisation. J Health Care Chaplain. 2022;29:368–80.
29. de Diego-Cordero R, López-Gómez L, Lucchetti G, Badanta B. Spiritual care in critically ill patients during COVID-19 pandemic. Nurs Outlook. 2022;70(1):64–77.
30. Timmins F, Connolly M, Palmisano S, Burgos D, Juárez LM, Gusman A, Soriano V, Jewdokimow M, Sadłoń W, Serrano AL, Caballero DC. Providing spiritual care to in-hospital patients during COVID-19: a preliminary European fact-finding study. J Relig Health. 2022;61(3):2212–32.
31. Tan H, Holmes C, Flynn E, Karimi L. "Essential not optional": spiritual care in Australia during a pandemic. J Pastoral Care Counsel. 2021;75(1_suppl):41–5.
32. Desjardins CM, Bovo A, Cagna M, Steegen M, Vandenhoeck A. Scared but powerful: healthcare chaplains' emotional responses and self-care modes during the SARS-Cov-19 pandemic. J Pastoral Care Counsel. 2021;75(1_suppl):30–6.
33. Balboni TA, VanderWeele TJ, Doan-Soares SD, et al. Spirituality in serious illness and health. JAMA. 2022;328(2):184–97.
34. Marin DB, Sharma V, Sosunov E, Egorova N, Goldstein R, Handzo GF. Relationship between chaplain visits and patient satisfaction. J Health Care Chaplain. 2015;21(1):14–24.
35. Schultz M, Baziliansky S, Mitnik I, Ulitzur N, Campisi-Pinto S, Givoli S, Bar-Sela G, Zalman D. Some differences between social work, spiritual care, and psychology: content variance in end-of-life conversations. Palliat Support Care. 2023;22:306–13.
36. Best M, Washington J, Condello M, Kearney M. 'This ward has no ears': role of the pastoral care practitioner in the hospital ward. J Health Care Chaplain. 2022;28(2):179–93. https://doi.org/10.1080/08854726.2020.1814089. Epub 2020 Sep 13.

Part V
Suffering

Existential Distress at the End of Life

Betty Ferrell and Tami Borneman

Abstract Existential distress at the end of life is a common experience for patients with a serious illness and those caring for them. Of paramount importance is the interdisciplinary team's response to issues of faith, spirituality, and existential concerns, with compassion, intentional listening, and complete presence. This chapter will examine the multidimensional nature of distress at the end of life, the challenges of diagnosing and treating existential distress, suffering, and opportunities for spiritual growth.

Keywords Existential distress · Spirituality · End of life · Meaning · Spiritual care Palliative care

1 Introduction

Facing the end of life pushes one on a spiritual journey that often was not planned for. Many patients experience existential or spiritual distress necessitating sensitive and effective palliative care services.

There are many definitions for terms such as existential distress, suffering, spiritual distress, and spiritual pain, which are provided by various sources and are helpful in highlighting differing and overlapping components. Many times, these terms are used interchangeably in research literature, incorporated into definitions of general distress, or identified as an element of psychological distress. The North

B. Ferrell (✉) · T. Borneman
Division of Nursing Research and Education, City of Hope National Medical Center, Duarte, CA, USA
e-mail: bferrell@coh.org; tborneman@coh.org

M. C. Best (ed.), *Spiritual Care in Palliative Care*,
https://doi.org/10.1007/978-3-031-50864-6_23

American Nursing Diagnosis Association-International (NANDA-I) defines spiritual distress as 'a state in which one's sense of relationship to the sacred or transcendent has been frayed; that is, inner resources and connection to the divine, higher power or beliefs about life and death have been compromised and/or challenged'. [1]

The United States' (U.S.) National Comprehensive Cancer Network (NCCN) incorporates spiritual distress into their general distress definition of a '…multifactorial, unpleasant experience of a psychological (i.e., cognitive, behavioural, emotional), social, spiritual, and/or physical nature that may interfere with one's ability to cope effectively with cancer, its physical symptoms, and its treatment…to problems that can become disabling, such as depression, anxiety, panic, social isolation, and existential and spiritual crisis'. [2]

The Diagnostic and Statistical Manual of Mental Disorders, Fifth Edition (DSM-5), and the International Classification of Diseases, 10th revision (ICD-10) provide a code for a Religious or Spiritual Problem under the section 'Problems Related to Other Psychosocial, Personal, and Environmental Circumstances' which are considered non-mental disorders. Examples include 'distressing experiences that involve loss or questioning of faith, problems associated with conversion to a new faith, or questioning of spiritual values that may not necessarily be related to an organised church or religious institution'. [3]

Vehling and Kissane [4] place existential distress in the psychological realm that includes, but is not limited to, hopelessness, death anxiety, and desire for hastened death. Using two case studies, Tang and colleagues [5] demonstrate the multiplicity of existential suffering experienced by each patient, including the expression of existential suffering in the four domains of mortality, freedom, meaninglessness, and isolation, as put forth by Strang et al. [6] For Grech and Marks [7], spiritual/religious distress is a type of existential suffering. Although spirituality is a part of the aforementioned domains, Grech and Marks state that 'all spiritual suffering is existential suffering, but not all existential suffering is spiritual suffering' (p. 2) (see Box 1 for an example of existential suffering that is not spiritual suffering). According to Yeh and Chernicoff [8], existential distress can be manifested via physical symptoms such as pain, or psychologically as depression or anxiety. Spiritual pain is defined by Illueca et al. [9] as a 'self-identified experience of personal discomfort, or actual or potential harm, triggered by a threat to a person's relationship with God or a higher power' (p. 1920). As evident from the literature, defining these terms is not clear cut, and spiritual distress and its associated terms are often intertwined with physical and psychological dimensions. What is clearly expressed in the literature is the reality of the patient's experience and that spiritual distress greatly impacts the patient facing serious illness. One definition of spirituality that helps to encapsulate its various aspects is provided by a Consensus Report on Spirituality [10, p. 3]: 'Spirituality is the aspect of humanity that refers to the way individuals seek and express meaning and purpose and the way they experience their connectedness to the moment, to self, to others, to nature, and to the significant or sacred'.

Box 1
Dr. Brad Thorton is a 72-year-old English Professor who is dying of heart failure. His disease has progressed more quickly than anticipated and he is now aware that he likely has only a few months of life remaining. Dr. Thorton has no religious affiliation, is a 'lifelong agnostic', has no immediate family but has been very devoted to his work and mentoring students. Since hearing the news of his worsened prognosis Dr. Thorton has been very distressed and shares that he had hoped to have at least another year to complete his writing, complete mentorship of doctoral students and accept an award from his university scheduled for the end of the year. He feels he 'has been cheated' and that each day now is 'meaningless and torture' as he struggles with limited function and worsened breathing.

Family caregivers may also experience existential or spiritual distress as they co-journey the serious illness with the patient and anticipate the death of their loved one. Palliative care is a service designed to improve the quality of life for both patients and their families facing a life-threatening illness by preventing or mitigating suffering, whether that is physically, psychosocially, or spiritually [11]. Family caregiver existential and spiritual distress is not unlike the patient's in that they too search for meaning and ask 'why?' Selman and colleagues [12] conducted focus groups at 11 sites across nine countries with patients and caregivers (n = 71). Family caregiver spiritual concerns included existential ('why me?' searching for meaning), psychological (guilt, feeling overwhelmed, isolation and loneliness, doubting their ability to cope), religious (anger at God or questioning God), and social and relational concerns (changes in relationships in general and with the patient).

The prevalence of spiritual distress and spiritual needs in family members of patients with advanced disease has often been neglected. Family caregivers often report spiritual distress as well as unmet needs when caring for a loved one approaching end of life [13]. Family members often look for meaning in caring for their loved one, in relationships with others and the environment, and in their own lives. Similar themes were found among family caregivers of patients in the Intensive Care Unit: loss of meaning, purpose, connection with others, questioning core beliefs, and feeling vulnerable [14]. Wikert [15] conducted a secondary analysis of 29 family caregiver interviews to determine how spirituality was manifested in their lives as they cared for a loved one with terminal cancer. All 29 narratives included themes of spirituality and four themes emerged as to what was important to them: connectedness, religious faith, transcendence, or hope with a fifth central theme of 'ongoing integration of spiritual experience'(p. 45). The importance of addressing spiritual distress as part of palliative care for the family caregiver cannot be overstated (see Chap. 37 for further discussion of this topic).

2 Aspects/Examples of Existential/Spiritual Distress in Facing End of Life

2.1 *Loss of Meaning*

Meaning is defined as 'something which gives one a sense of purpose, value…the perceived purpose of existence or of a person's life'. [16] Meaning doesn't happen in a vacuum, it requires relationships, connectedness and spirituality, and facing the end of life often leads to a reappraisal of those very things [17, 18]. According to Antonovsky, a sense of coherence involves three components: comprehensibility, manageability, and meaningfulness. It reveals one's perception of life and internal capacity to deal with stressful stimuli [19, 20]. Patients who struggle with a loss of meaning or purpose experience a disrupted sense of coherence; very little makes sense anymore. Pinho et al. [21] reported 'lack of meaning and purpose in life' as the most prevalent defining characteristic for spiritual distress in patients with HIV/AIDS. Finding meaning in life is important for terminally ill patients experiencing new aspects of loss every day in their decline.

2.2 *Connection to Others*

Research has shown that a loss of connection to others whether by social isolation or a sense of loneliness without isolation is a negative risk factor for health decline and increases mortality [22–24]. Connection to others is a basic innate human need and does not stop because of serious illness. Patients grieve the loss of ordinary daily life. Every day is controlled by illness and its related symptoms, reducing involvement in relationships and activities. Energy is lacking and at some point, the disease progresses, and the patient is confined to bed. Seventeen patients with incurable oesophageal cancer were interviewed about their everyday experiences including life before and with their cancer, social relationships, symptoms, and other aspects of late-stage disease [25]. The first of the four themes reported was a sense of isolation, feeling relegated to a 'table in the corner', followed by 'being in a zombie-like state', 'one day at a time', and 'at sea' (p. 1). The need for social (family and others') connections was also found in studies with older hospitalised patients [26], as well as patients with other types of cancer [27] and Alzheimer's disease [24], and frequently cited in systematic reviews across disease groups [28]. A quote from *Tuesdays with Morrie* [29] is an apropos summary, '*In the beginning of life, when we are infants, we need others to survive, right? And at the end of life, when you get like me, you need others to survive, right?…But here's the secret: in between, we need others as well*'(p. 157).

2.3 *Connection to God/Spiritual Longing*

Patients who previously have not had a strong faith affiliation may experience the need for spiritual support when facing serious illness or the end of life. In a sample of 68 patients with advanced illness, one of the most commonly reported items by approximately half the patients was 'seeking a closer connection with God or one's faith'. [30] Patients may feel the need for transcendence by strengthening their spiritual beliefs, communicating with God and by prayer [27]. Two systematic reviews report 'sense of spiritual connection to God (or Higher Power or Divine) or to the transcendent' as important spiritual needs [26, 28]. All 100 patients in a study by Ramezani [31] reported at least one spiritual need with 'requesting help from God' rated as the highest need.

2.4 *Despair/Randomness/Hopelessness*

The word 'random' comes from *randon* (Old French), meaning speed and violence. It implies lacking a careful choice, an impetuous and haphazard movement [32]. Being diagnosed with a terminal illness can feel like a violent blow, leaving one feeling very vulnerable, sometimes angry and spiritually abandoned [17]. Feeling hopeless was found to be a major indicator of spiritual distress as well as reinforcing feelings of depression and suffering [33]. A sense of hopelessness was one of the defining characteristics of spiritual distress in a systematic review by Eshghi [34]. Despair may also be felt by those facing the end of life. One aspect of despair is when one turns to an inward solitude and withdraws from the world, thus abandoning relationships and focusing only on the impending death [35]. Patients can also feel despair facing the loss of a future life, and goals that will never be achieved [36].

2.5 *Guilt/Shame/Regret*

When faced with the end of life, patients often undergo a life review which may lead to difficult feelings including spiritual distress. Some patients feel guilt over burdening family members with their care and others feel regret over missed opportunities or troubled relationships [18, 21]. Ohnsorge [37, 38] interviewed 62 patients (cancer $n = 30$, neurological disease $n = 10$, organ failure $n = 11$, frailty $n = 11$) about their wishes to die and the most common themes were guilt and shame over being a burden to family. That burden included not only physical care but the emotional and financial burdens as well.

2.6 Forgiveness

The need to forgive and be forgiven is important for maintaining dignity, completing unfinished business, overall spiritual health, and provides an opportunity for spiritual and moral growth [18, 26, 31, 39, 40]. Forgiving oneself is just as important and may present as an acknowledgement of regret or personal failure [41]. One area of self-forgiveness that is less often thought of, but equally important, is moral injury, a wound to the core of one's being. Moral injury involves the violation of moral beliefs, either by oneself or others, that has resulted in a myriad of negative feelings (e.g. anger, moral guilt), destruction of meaning and purpose in life, broken relationships with the Sacred and others, and for some, suicide [42, 43]. Patient expressions of a need for forgiveness are often symptoms of deep spiritual distress and suffering. Deep concerns such as the need for forgiveness may be shared in the clinical setting and illustrate the critical need for collaboration between clinicians and chaplains to respond to this distress.

3 Interventions to Address Existential/Spiritual Distress

3.1 Presence and Therapeutic Listening

One way to address existential distress is by presence and therapeutic listening. This involves more than an acknowledging nod of the head; it involves complete presence of body, mind, and spirit. The word 'presence' comes from the Latin word *praesentia*, 'being at hand' and the verb *praeesse* (present), 'fully focused on or involved in what one is doing or experiencing'. [44] It is bearing witness to the patient's existential/spiritual distress. 'Being at hand' means offering to be present to the patient and opens the door for the clinician to journey alongside and be allowed to see, to share, to touch, and to hear the brokenness, vulnerability, and suffering of another [45, p. 505, 46].

Therapeutic listening is more than just hearing and involves all the senses, incorporates being present, recognises metaphors and repeated spiritual themes, and provides pause and space for the patient's story to unfold [17, 47–49]. In her earlier work, Taylor [50] provided four dimensions of listening: intellectual (ability to reiterate facts back to the patient in a way understood by the patient); emotional (identifying the patient's feelings or importance of what was said and reflecting it back to the patient); physical (being aware of both the patient's and one's own nonverbal and postural messages); and spiritual (listening for the holy or divine). Presence and therapeutic listening are important interventions that allow space for the patient to express their existential/spiritual distress.

3.2 Referral to a Spiritual Care Specialist

Two main themes emerged from a focus group with nine spiritual care providers regarding lack of referrals to their services: [1] a lack of knowledge by healthcare providers; and [2] not knowing who the spiritual care providers are or how to find them [51]. Suggestions given by the focus group included better training for healthcare providers to recognise spiritual care needs and knowing when to make the referral. Additionally, spiritual care providers need to make themselves and their services known to healthcare providers. These suggestions are key because according to The National Consensus Project Clinical Practice Guidelines for Quality Palliative Care for the United States [52], all clinicians are to provide spiritual care and collaborate with chaplains. Clinicians provide generalist level spiritual care through screening and history, and chaplains provide specialist-spiritual care based on an in-depth assessment and contributing to spiritual care (Domain 5).

Patients experiencing existential/spiritual distress require care by a spiritual care specialist, specifically a chaplain, who can help them at a level beyond the scope of practice for the general healthcare provider. An interesting study by Poncin and colleagues [53] involved 12 healthcare providers (six nurses, two nursing auxiliaries, three doctors, and one physical therapist) to learn what motivated them to refer to a chaplain. Actual referral requests were submitted by each participant, followed by an interview that sought to clarify the intention of the healthcare provider in making the referral, the aim of the referral, and the benefit to the patient by receiving a chaplain visit. Three themes emerged from the referral requests responding to difficult patients, supporting patients, and understanding patients (e.g. experiences and feelings). The most common themes from the interviews for referring to a chaplain were the patient's need for support followed by acquiring a better understanding of the patient (e.g. their psychological suffering, questions about life, and need to express suffering and distress). The third theme, spiritual care, pertained to the meaning given by patients to their life and experiences. Overall, while healthcare providers in this study were motivated to refer to chaplaincy for various reasons, the study findings point to the need for more education regarding the need for spiritual care and validates the role of the chaplain [53]. Chaplains can provide much needed specialised spiritual care for patients at the end of life as well as providing an invaluable service to the clinician.

3.3 Meaning-Centred Approaches

Frankl [54] reminded us that man's search for meaning is not merely an instinctual drive but rather the primary basic drive that is unique to each individual, that when fulfilled, will satisfy the need for meaning. A terminal illness invites the question of meaning. Meaning making is a process whereby the patient tries to reconcile their global beliefs (others, self, world) to their understanding of a stressful life event and in this case a terminal disease [55]. Patients may also interpret the life event in a way that is compatible with their global beliefs or conversely change their global beliefs to match the life event [55, 56]. To help patients in this process, some practical suggestions are offered.

Leaving a legacy can have a profound effect on both the patient and the recipient. Some of the ways patients leave a legacy is by planning their own memorial service and/or funeral. Others have created scrap books for each member of the family, written letters to each child, created videos (home and professional), painted pictures, or participated in videotaped interviews. Dignity therapy as well as life review and legacy documents are other options for patients [57–59]. Blogging and vlogging are ways to record experiences that others can read and watch [60–62]. Reframing hope is also a helpful intervention [63, 64].

3.4 *Mind/Body Interventions*

Mindfulness is an acute awareness of one's thoughts, feelings and surroundings and the connection between them [65, 66]. Given the mind/body connection it is not surprising that Mind/Body Interventions (MBIs) have been shown to help various mental and physical health conditions such as depression, pain, anxiety, and symptoms from cancer [66]. Mindfulness interventions can be formal, such as breathing or walking, and requires a concerted effort to maintain an 'in the moment' experience [67]. Informal mindfulness exercises can simply involve an awareness of everyday moments [66]. Types of MBIs include mindfulness-based stress reduction [68], mindfulness-based cognitive therapy [69], mindfulness-based retreats [70], internet/smartphone applications [71, 72], and mindfulness-related interventions that seek to enhance mindfulness [67]. Yik and colleagues [73] conducted a five minute mindfulness of peace exercise with 40 patients receiving palliative care with moderate to severe levels of suffering. Patients in the control arm received active listening for five minutes. The *Suffering Pictogram* and *Functional Assessment of Chronic Illness Therapy-Spiritual Wellbeing* (FACIT-Sp-12) measured pre- and post-intervention suffering and spiritual well-being. Results showed the efficacy of the intervention to provide immediate relief from suffering as well as to improve spiritual well-being.

3.5 *The Importance of Relationships*

Part of what gives meaning in life is relationships with family, friends, and the community. Social (broader social network) and especially emotional (intimate friend/partner) loneliness was reported by cancer patients who were persistently fatigued and cognitively impaired [74]. Twenty palliative patients with a terminal disease and their family caregivers were interviewed about their feelings and perceptions and experiences of existential isolation [75]. The primary reason for experiencing existential isolation was the patient's impending death. A common experience was feeling alone. The illness limited social interactions which also affected a sense of community.

The supportive relationships of friends that provide meaning to life was described by one patient as 'cream that comes to the top' while the superficial friends fall away, and supportive spouses were seen as 'champions' [76]. In the same study by Maiko et al. [76], other patients who considered themselves spiritual felt their relationship with God was deepened and He became a stronger source of support. Faith community was also important as patients felt cared for, through their prayers, gifts, comfort, and encouragement. Contacting the patient's spiritual care provider in the community may be one way of facilitating connection.

3.6 Reappraisal

Patients facing serious illness or death may recognise that perhaps something positive can come from a terminal diagnosis. In its own way, this fosters a hope that is not contingent on physical healing but is able to focus on whatever time is left reconciling relationships and finding meaning. Valuing the time left once death was accepted for some patients may reduce suffering and create a sense of peace [17].

4 Assessment of Existential Distress

Several instruments have been developed for clinical practice or research purposes to assess existential distress. These tools include items assessing lack of meaning or purpose, despair, hopelessness, religious struggle, loss of dignity, grief, abandonment, and numerous other aspects of patient experience. Johnston-Taylor [49] has provided a useful summary of these instruments. These tools range from single items to assessment of multiple aspects of distress.

These tools can be useful for clinical assessment to identify specific aspects of distress which can facilitate identification of potentially useful therapies. These quantitative measures should be used in conjunction with interviews to elicit each patient's personal experiences since active listening and presence by clinicians is at the core of both assessment and response to suffering.

5 Case Examples

The following case examples are provided to illustrate common themes of existential suffering.

5.1 Case 1—Meaning/Purpose

Mr. Conrad was a 77-year-old man from Guatemala who had resided most of his adult life in California. He was recently admitted to home-based hospice for end-stage heart failure. His heart failure rapidly declined after having COVID-19. On admission to hospice, the nurse and social worker noted that Mr. Conrad was very depressed and anxious, and when asked about spiritual needs, he became very tearful.

Mr. Conrad shared that he was raised as Catholic, moved to the United States and was able to start a family and to have a successful gardening business. For the next 20 years, his life was good; however, he then became an alcoholic and lost his business and became estranged from his family. At age 60 years, he became sober and was reunited with his wife and was able to support her through breast cancer. However, his absence of over 20 years left the family with great financial distress, and his adult children and grandchildren remained distant. Mr. Conrad was seen by the hospice Chaplain who shared her assessment with the team. The Chaplain confirmed his spiritual distress and feeling of having 'wasted most of my life'. He shared that as a Catholic he 'failed God' by abandoning the most important thing in life 'to be a good husband and father'. The team is also aware that his extreme spiritual distress is impacting his dyspnoea, depression, anxiety, and insomnia. After a team discussion, the chaplain contacted Mr. Conrad to see if he would like to talk about his feelings and concerns with his parish priest. He consented and a date and time was then planned for the priest to visit.

5.2 Case 2—Spiritual Longing/Connection

Elizabeth Levy is a 58-year-old woman diagnosed 1 year ago with Amyotrophic Lateral Sclerosis (ALS, also known as Motor Neurone Disease). Her disease is now progressing, and she is well aware of the difficult decisions she faces ahead related to her ALS symptoms and eventual death. Elizabeth is single, has been an accountant, and is now residing with her younger sister who agreed to be her caretaker.

Elizabeth describes herself as a 'cultural Jew' and states that she and her sister Kerry have not been involved in their Jewish religion since childhood. Elizabeth shares with the hospice nurse that as she faces the end of her life, she is longing to be reconnected to her Jewish faith. Kerry has no desire to participate in religious services, and Elizabeth is reluctant to share her desire with Kerry as she doesn't want to add any further burden. Elizabeth also says she hopes to attend a temple service while she is still able and while she has her voice to participate in prayer. The hospice nurse meets with the Chaplain and has also involved a Social Worker, Ben, who is Jewish. The team discusses Elizabeth's care and her spiritual longing as they plan for her months ahead. With Elizabeth's permission, Ben arranged a ride to the local temple so Elizabeth could attend a service as well as have her name included prior to the saying of the *Mi Shebeirach.*

5.3 Case 3—Forgiveness

Sargent Michael Moley is being seen in the oncology clinic of a Veterans Affairs hospital for newly diagnosed head and neck cancer. His cancer is suspected to be related to chemical exposure he experienced in war in Afghanistan. Michael is accompanied by his wife, JoAnn, a strong source of support. Michael and JoAnn are Catholic and have met with the hospital Chaplain.

Over the next several weeks Michael comes to the outpatient radiation therapy centre for six weeks of daily radiation. He becomes very close to Sam, the radiology technical assistant, as he is also a war Veteran and Catholic. As Michael's suffering increases from several oral side effects of treatment, he confides in Sam that he believes his cancer and suffering are punishment from 'bad things' he did in the war. Sam expresses that he understands. Michael also shares that he has never shared with JoAnn the 'real story' of the war and that he can't speak of the 'nightmare'. He asks Sam to pray for him and that he will be forgiven. Sam willingly prays for Michael and then asks him if he would feel comfortable sharing more with the hospital chaplain he has met, or perhaps a priest. Michael is unsure and states he will think about it. Sam shared that he understood.

5.4 Case 4—Family Caregiver Despair

Monica Brightman is a 45-year-old single mother of Bryan, a 23-year-old patient with relapsed leukaemia. Monica and Bryan immigrated from Ukraine to the United States five years ago, and Monica was able to work as a chemist and support Bryan through college. Their dream of their new life was shattered with Bryan's leukaemia diagnosis, and they now await stem cell transplant for his recurrent disease.

The transplant team meets with Monica to discuss how they can best support her in the weeks ahead during Bryan's transplant. Monica shares that she 'used to believe in God' and that they were previously very devout Orthodox Christians. They saw their successful immigration, her employment and Bryan's college completion as signs of God's love but that 'all is gone now. God abandoned us. I don't know why we are being punished'. Monica does not want to meet with a Chaplain, is very worried about the transplant and fears that God's ultimate betrayal may be Bryan's death. She says she needs no support, and that everyone should just concentrate on Bryan as he must survive. Given that Monica stated she 'needs no support', the team decides to rotate who connects with her each day and to keep the chaplain informed so that he can help guide them in their interactions with her.

5.5 *Case 5—Support of Spirituality in Illness*

Mr. Carlson was an 87-year-old man who had devoted the last 20 years to caring for his wife Jane with dementia who recently died. Mr. Carlson is proud to have cared for her at home. He was recently diagnosed with late stage prostate cancer and has had a difficult time with symptom control, depression, and diminished function. He has declined his family's invitations to move across the country to be near them as he likes to visit Jane's grave and talk to her. Mr. Carlson is visited by the chaplain during his hospitalisation for surgery and he shares that he and Jane were 'very faithful church goers' for many years but stopped attending church 15 years ago when Jane's dementia worsened. He says he hasn't had any contact with the church in years. The chaplain contacts the church, arranges a visit from the minister and follows up once Mr. Carlson returns home. The church has arranged for members of the men's group to visit weekly and to drive him to church when he is able. He is added to the church prayer list.

Mr. Carlson tells the chaplain he is so grateful to have been reconnected to the church. The men's group visitors read scripture and pray with him and also talk with him about his wife. They also volunteer to go to the cemetery if he isn't able. The chaplain also has been in contact with the church minister to offer assistance in arranging for home hospice care as his physician feels his disease is likely progressing.

6 Conclusion

Existential distress is inevitable in serious illness and for those facing the end of life. This distress involves all aspects of faith, spirituality, and existential concerns. Responding to this distress is greatly facilitated by deep listening and presence by compassionate clinicians and by interdisciplinary collaboration by all members of the care team.

References

1. North American Nursing Diagnosis Association. Spiritual distress. NANDA. https://nanda-diagnoses.com/spiritual-distress/#NANDA_Nursing_Diagnosis_Definition. Published 2023. Accessed 10 May 2023.
2. National Comprehensive Cancer Network. Distress management (Version 2.2023). https://www.nccn.org/guidelines/guidelines-detail?category=3&id=1431. Published 2023. Accessed 16 May 2023.
3. American Psychiatric Association. Other conditions that may be a focus of clinical attention. In: American Psychiatric Association: diagnostic and statistical manual of mental disorders. 5th ed. Arlington: American Psychiatric Association; 2013. p. 725.
4. Vehling S, Kissane DW. Existential distress in cancer: alleviating suffering from fundamental loss and change. Psychooncology. 2018;27:2525.

5. Tang M, Nguyen N-N, Bruera E, Tanco K, Delgado-Guay M. Expression of existential suffering in two patients with advanced cancer in an acute palliative care unit. Palliat Support Care. 2020;18(6):748–50.
6. Strang P, Strang S, Hultborn R, Arner S. Existential pain – an entity, a provocation, or a challenge? J Pain Symptom Manag. 2004;27(3):241–50.
7. Grech A, Marks A. Existential suffering part 1: definition and diagnosis #319. J Palliat Med. 2017;20(1):93–4.
8. Yeh A, Chernicoff H. Existential distress: identification and management by hospice and palliative medicine fellows. BMJ Support Palliat Care. 2023;13:e765.
9. Illueca M, Bradshaw YS, Carr DB. Spiritual pain: a symptom in search of a clinical definition. J Relig Health. 2023;62(3):1920–32.
10. Puchalski C, Ferrell B, Virani R, et al. Improving the quality of spiritual care as a dimension of palliative care: the report of the Consensus Conference. J Palliat Med. 2009;12(10):885–904.
11. Worldwide Hospice PCA. Global atlas of palliative care. 2nd ed. London: Worldwide Palliative Care Alliance; 2020. http://www.thewhpca.org
12. Selman LE, Brighton LJ, Sinclair S, et al. Patients' and caregivers' needs, experiences, preferences and research priorities in spiritual care: a focus group study across nine countries. Palliat Med. 2018;32(1):216–30.
13. Goncalves F, Teixeira MI, Magalhaes B. The role of spirituality in people with amyotrophic lateral sclerosis and their caregivers: scoping review. Palliat Support Care. 2022;21:1–11.
14. Roze des Ordons AL, Stelfox HT, Sinuff T, Grindrod-Millar K, Smiechowski J, Sinclair S. Spiritual distress in family members of critically ill patients: perceptions and experiences. J Palliat Med. 2020;23(2):198–210.
15. Wikert J, Treutlein M, Theochari M, Bokemeyer C, Oechsle K, Ullrich A. How does spirituality manifest in family caregivers of terminally ill cancer patients? A qualitative secondary analysis. Palliat Support Care. 2022;20(1):45–54.
16. Wiktionary Contributers. Meaning. https://en.wiktionary.org/w/index.php?title=meaning&oldid=73503252. Published 2023. Accessed 6 June 2023.
17. Borneman T, Brown-Saltzman K. Meaning in illness. In: Ferrell BR, Paice JA, editors. Oxford textbook of palliative nursing. 5th ed. New York: Oxford University Press; 2019. p. 456–66.
18. Ellington L, Billitteri J, Reblin M, Clayton MF. Spiritual care communication in cancer patients. Paper presented at: seminars in oncology nursing. 2017.
19. Antonovsky A. The structure and properties of the sense of coherence scale. Soc Sci Med. 1993;36(6):725–33.
20. Eriksson M. The sense of coherence: the concept and its relationship to health. In: Mittelmark MB, Bauer GF, Vaandrager L, et al., editors. The handbook of salutogenesis. Cham: Springer International Publishing; 2022. p. 61–8.
21. Pinho CM, Gomes ET, Trajano MFC, Cavalcanti A, Andrade MS, Valenca MP. Impaired religiosity and spiritual distress in people living with HIV/AIDS. Rev Gaucha Enferm. 2017;38(2):e67712.
22. Golaszewski NM, LaCroix AZ, Godino JG, et al. Evaluation of social isolation, loneliness, and cardiovascular disease among older women in the US. JAMA Netw Open. 2022;5(2):e2146461.
23. Holt-Lunstad J. Loneliness and social isolation as risk factors: the power of social connection in prevention. Am J Lifestyle Med. 2021;15(5):567–73.
24. Ren Y, Savadlou A, Park S, Siska P, Epp JR, Sargin D. The impact of loneliness and social isolation on the development of cognitive decline and Alzheimer's disease. Front Neuroendocrinol. 2023;69:101061.
25. Laursen L, Schønau MN, Bergenholtz HM, Siemsen M, Christensen M, Missel M. Table in the corner: a qualitative study of life situation and perspectives of the everyday lives of oesophageal cancer patients in palliative care. BMC Palliat Care. 2019;18(1):60.
26. Desmet L, Dezutter J, Vandenhoeck A, Dillen A. Spiritual needs of older adults during hospitalization: an integrative review. Religions. 2020;11(10):529.
27. Hatamipour K, Rassouli M, Yaghmaie F, Zendedel K, Majd HA. Spiritual needs of cancer patients: a qualitative study. Indian J Palliat Care. 2015;21(1):61–7.

28. de Brito Sena MA, Damiano RF, Lucchetti G, Peres MFP. Defining spirituality in healthcare: a systematic review and conceptual framework. Front Psychol. 2021;12:756080.
29. Albom M. Tuesdays with Morrie. New York: Doubleday; 1997.
30. Balboni TA, Balboni MJ. The spiritual event of serious illness. J Pain Symptom Manag. 2018;56:816.
31. Ramezani T, Karimi Z. Exploring spiritual needs and its relation with anxiety and depression in the elderly patients with chronic diseases. Health Spiritual Med Ethics. 2019;6(2):10–6.
32. Etymology of random. https://www.etymonline.com/word/random#:~:text=random%20(adj.),1300). Accessed 12 July 2023.
33. Caldeira S, Timmins F, de Carvalho EC, Vieira M. Clinical validation of the nursing diagnosis spiritual distress in cancer patients undergoing chemotherapy. Int J Nurs Knowl. 2017;28(1):44–52.
34. Eshghi F, Nikfarid L, Zareiyan A. An integrative review of defining characteristic of the nursing diagnosis "spiritual distress". Nurs Open. 2023;10(5):2831–41.
35. Wrigley A. Hope, dying and solidarity. Ethical Theory Moral Pract. 2019;22(1):187–204.
36. Olsman E, Leget C, Duggleby W, Willems D. A singing choir: understanding the dynamics of hope, hopelessness, and despair in palliative care patients. A longitudinal qualitative study. Palliat Support Care. 2015;13:1643–50.
37. Ohnsorge K, Gudat H, Rehmann-Sutter C. What a wish to die can mean: reasons, meanings and functions of wishes to die, reported from 30 qualitative case studies of terminally ill cancer patients in palliative care. BMC Palliat Care. 2014;13:38.
38. Ohnsorge K, Rehmann-Sutter C, Streeck N, Gudat H. Wishes to die at the end of life and subjective experience of four different typical dying trajectories. A qualitative interview study. PLoS One. 2019;14(1):e0210784.
39. Glenn CT, Pieper B. Forgiveness and spiritual distress: implications for nursing. J Christ Nurs. 2019;36(3):185–9.
40. Worthington EL Jr, Witvliet CV, Pietrini P, Miller AJ. Forgiveness, health, and well-being: a review of evidence for emotional versus decisional forgiveness, dispositional forgivingness, and reduced unforgiveness. J Behav Med. 2007;30(4):291–302.
41. Mullen LM, Bistany BR, Kim JJ, et al. Facilitation of forgiveness: impact on health and well-being. Holist Nurs Pract. 2023;37(1):15–23.
42. Brémault-Phillips S, Cherwick T, Smith-MacDonald LA, Huh J, Vermetten E. Forgiveness: a key component of healing from moral injury? Front Psych. 2022;13:906945.
43. Purcell N, Griffin BJ, Burkman K, Maguen S. "Opening a door to a new life": the role of forgiveness in healing from moral injury. Front Psych. 2018;9:498.
44. Wiktionary Contributers. Presence. https://en.wiktionary.org/w/index.php?title=presence&oldid=72932557. Published 2023. Accessed 6 June 2023.
45. Pettigrew J. Intensive nursing care. The ministry of presence. Crit Care Nurs Clin North Am. 1990;2(3):503–8.
46. Fredriksson L. Modes of relating in a caring conversation: a research synthesis on presence, touch and listening. J Adv Nurs. 1999;30(5):1167–76.
47. Bullington J, Söderlund M, Sparén EB, Kneck Å, Omérov P, Cronqvist A. Communication skills in nursing: a phenomenologically-based communication training approach. Nurse Educ Pract. 2019;39:136–41.
48. Ellison DL, Meyer CK. Presence and therapeutic listening. Nurs Clin. 2020;55(4):457–65.
49. Taylor EJ. Spiritual screening, history, and assessment. In: Ferrell B, Paice J, editors. Oxford textbook of palliative nursing. New York: Oxford University Press; 2019. p. 432–46.
50. Taylor EJ. What do I say? Talking with patients about spirituality. West Conshohocken: Templeton Foundation Press; 2007.
51. Koper I, Pasman HRW, Schweitzer BPM, Kuin A, Onwuteaka-Philipsen BD. Spiritual care at the end of life in the primary care setting: experiences from spiritual caregivers – a mixed methods study. BMC Palliat Care. 2019;18(1):98.
52. National Consensus Project for Quality Palliative Care. Clinical practice guidelines for quality palliative care. Richmond: National Coalition for Hospice and Palliative Care; 2018.

53. Poncin E, Niquille B, Jobin G, Benaim C, Rochat E. What motivates healthcare professionals' referrals to chaplains, and how to help them formulate referrals that accurately reflect patients' spiritual needs? J Health Care Chaplain. 2020;26(1):1–15.
54. Frankl VE. Man's search for meaning: an introduction to logotherapy. Boston: Beacon; 1959.
55. Kopacz MS, Lockman J, Lusk J, et al. How meaningful is meaning-making? New Ideas Psychol. 2019;54:76–81.
56. Sloan DH, BrintzenhofeSzoc K, Mistretta E, Cheng MJ, Berger A. The influence of relationships on the meaning making process: patients' perspectives. Ann Palliat Med. 2017;6(3):220–6.
57. Cuevas PE, Davidson P, Mejilla J, Rodney T. Dignity therapy for end-of-life care patients: a literature review. J Patient Exp. 2021;8:2374373521996951.
58. Martinez M, Arantzamendi M, Belar A, et al. 'Dignity therapy', a promising intervention in palliative care: a comprehensive systematic literature review. Palliat Med. 2017;31(6):492–509.
59. Vuksanovic D, Green HJ, Dyck M, Morrissey SA. Dignity therapy and life review for palliative care patients: a randomized controlled trial. J Pain Symptom Manag. 2017;53(2):162–170 e161.
60. Lagerkvist A, Andersson Y. The grand interruption: death online and mediated lifelines of shared vulnerability. Fem Media Stud. 2017;17(4):550–64.
61. Lee JL, Frey M, Frey P, Hollin IL, Wu AW. Seeing is engaging: vlogs as a tool for patient engagement. Patient. 2017;10(3):267–70.
62. Taylor J, Pagliari C. #Deathbedlive: the end-of-life trajectory, reflected in a cancer patient's tweets. BMC Palliat Care. 2018;17(1):17.
63. Grossman M. Psychosocial processes of resilience. In: Promoting healing and resilience in people with cancer: a nursing perspective. Cham: Springer; 2022. p. 65–92.
64. Rosenfeld B, Saracino R, Tobias K, et al. Adapting meaning-centered psychotherapy for the palliative care setting: results of a pilot study. Palliat Med. 2017;31(2):140–6.
65. Cooper Z. Spirituality in primary care settings: addressing the whole person through Christian mindfulness. Religions. 2022;13(4):346. https://doi.org/10.3390/rel13040346.
66. Zhang D, Lee EKP, Mak ECW, Ho CY, Wong SYS. Mindfulness-based interventions: an overall review. Br Med Bull. 2021;138(1):41–57.
67. Creswell JD. Mindfulness interventions. Annu Rev Psychol. 2017;68(1):491–516.
68. Kabat-Zinn J. An outpatient program in behavioral medicine for chronic pain patients based on the practice of mindfulness meditation: theoretical considerations and preliminary results. Gen Hosp Psychiatry. 1982;4(1):33–47.
69. Teasdale JD, Segal ZV, Williams JM, Ridgeway VA, Soulsby JM, Lau MA. Prevention of relapse/recurrence in major depression by mindfulness-based cognitive therapy. J Consult Clin Psychol. 2000;68(4):615–23.
70. Creswell JD, Taren AA, Lindsay EK, et al. Alterations in resting-state functional connectivity link mindfulness meditation with reduced Interleukin-6: a randomized controlled trial. Biol Psychiatry. 2016;80(1):53–61.
71. Boettcher J, Astrom V, Pahlsson D, Schenstrom O, Andersson G, Carlbring P. Internet-based mindfulness treatment for anxiety disorders: a randomized controlled trial. Behav Ther. 2014;45(2):241–53.
72. Lim D, Condon P, DeSteno D. Mindfulness and compassion: an examination of mechanism and scalability. PLoS One. 2015;10(2):e0118221.
73. Yik LL, Ling LM, Ai LM, et al. The effect of 5-minute mindfulness of peace on suffering and spiritual Well-being among palliative care patients: a randomized controlled study. Am J Hosp Palliat Med. 2021;38(9):1083–90.
74. Deckx L, van den Akker M, van Driel M, et al. Loneliness in patients with cancer: the first year after cancer diagnosis. Psychooncology. 2015;24(11):1521–8.
75. Sand L, Strang P. Existential loneliness in a palliative home care setting. J Palliat Med. 2006;9(6):1376–87.
76. Maiko S, Johns SA, Helft PR, Slaven JE, Cottingham AH, Torke AM. Spiritual experiences of adults with advanced cancer in outpatient clinical settings. J Pain Symptom Manag. 2019;57(3):576–586.e571.

Demoralisation

Ana Cláudia Mesquita Garcia

Abstract This chapter discusses the relationship between demoralisation and spirituality in the clinical context of palliative care. Demoralisation involves the loss of hope, purpose, and meaning in life when faced with stressful situations, and can be aggravated by the imminence of death and need for coping with an illness over time, affecting patients' quality of life. Addressing demoralisation clinically requires sensitive identification, assessment, and empathic communication. Furthermore, the inverse relationship between demoralisation and spirituality is highlighted, according to the available evidence, with spirituality acting as a preventative measure against the emergence of demoralisation. This finding emphasises the possibility that spiritual care could play a significant role in the management of demoralisation. The importance of spiritual care for patients affected by a severe illness and their caregivers is well known, providing an outlet to seek meaning and connection to something greater. Understanding and addressing demoralisation and spirituality in palliative care are key to providing comprehensive support and meeting the emotional, existential, and spiritual needs of patients.

Keywords Demoralisation · Palliative care · Hospice · Spirituality · Spiritual care

1 Introduction

Frank [1] introduced the term 'demoralisation' to identify a persistent state of feelings of subjective incompetence, such as the loss of a sense of agency, the failure to meet expectations, and the inability to cope with and solve problems [1, 2].

A. C. M. Garcia (✉)
School of Nursing, Federal University of Alfenas, Alfenas, Brazil
e-mail: ana.mesquita@unifal-mg.edu.br

M. C. Best (ed.), *Spiritual Care in Palliative Care*,
https://doi.org/10.1007/978-3-031-50864-6_24

Demoralisation has been proposed as an important diagnosis that can direct the management of complex situations [3], such as when an individual is faced with death, perceiving themselves as worthless or living an empty and meaningless life, which can result in a profound sense of hopelessness [4]. Demoralisation, most commonly reported in oncology and palliative care settings, is also commonly present in other chronic illnesses, mental disorders, refugees, substance users, adolescents, in the postnatal period, and in adjusting to stressors, such as a relationship breakup [4–7].

There is evidence that demoralisation is associated with increased death anxiety [8], increased existential distress [9], worsened psychological well-being [10, 11], depression [12], suicidal ideation [13], and lower quality of life [12, 14]. Although demoralisation is among one of the most debilitating conditions in people affected with a severe illness, it is still a neglected theme in the palliative care context due to factors such as the limited number of documented interventions for the treatment of this condition [15]. In this regard, it is worth noting that recent studies suggest an inverse association between spirituality and demoralisation, where the higher the levels of spirituality, the lower the level of demoralisation [12, 14, 16, 17].

Spirituality encompasses connection, whether religious or otherwise, with a non-physical reality perceived by an individual [18]. In a study exploring the relationship between spirituality/religiousness and physical and mental quality of life among cancer survivors, the mental quality of life of those with high spirituality was significantly higher than those with low spirituality [19]. Balboni et al. [20] suggest that addressing spirituality in the treatment of people with a serious illness is part of a person-centred care that is sensible to their values.

In summary, the available literature suggests the intertwining of demoralisation and spirituality in healthcare. An understanding of the concept of demoralisation is key to exploring this field further.

2 Demoralisation: Concept

The discussion regarding the definition of demoralisation is not new, with questions being raised as to whether this condition is a disorder or just a normal reaction to a state of overwhelming circumstances [21]. Slavney reasons that demoralisation is not a psychiatric disorder, but a normal response to adversity, such as grief, which is a non-pathological reaction to stress, but can be the focus of clinical attention in which the patient requires understanding, encouragement, and greater engagement [22]. On the other hand, given the severe impact that demoralisation can have on function [23], de Figueiredo considers demoralisation to always be abnormal [24]. Conceptually, this debate may be best resolved through a dimensional approach, wherein mild disheartenment is not considered maladaptive, while at the other end of the spectrum, severe demoralisation or despair impairs functionality and represents pathological coping.

As proposed by Irvin Yalom, existential psychotherapy is a dynamic therapy focused on suffering that is rooted in one's existence. For Yalom, conflict emerges when the reality of existence is faced. Thus, demoralisation can be understood as a result of this existential conflict, when an individual lacks the resources to address it [25, 26]. Demoralisation, which is a syndrome consisting of distress associated with subjective incompetence [27], is clinically characterised by hopelessness, loss of meaning/significance, dysphoria (a state of intense distress, discomfort, or dissatisfaction), discouragement, helplessness, and a sense of failure—usually associated with stressful conditions, as in the case of a severe illness [28]. Distress is manifested through symptoms such as anxiety, sadness, discouragement, anger, and resentment [27].

Subjective incompetence is defined as a state of perceived inability to cope or perform at some minimal level according to an internalised standard in a stressful situation [27]. It occurs in people who perceive themselves as being unable to perform their tasks and express the feelings they consider appropriate in a stressful situation. They often seek several solutions to address this situation—eventually exhausting all possibilities—however, all of them are ultimately unsuccessful. Unable to cope with the situation, they fear that the circumstances will become worse [27]. The stressful situation reveals to these people that things they took for granted, whether about themselves or about other people, are no longer certain, leading to doubts regarding the future they had previously imagined [27]. As the stressful situation increases in duration or intensity, some people with subjective incompetence experience helplessness and may become desperate and sometimes suicidal [5, 27].

In summary, the dominant conceptualisation of demoralisation is that it is a form of psychological distress stemming from a state of impaired coping ability, characterised by symptoms of low morale, hopelessness, a sense of entrapment, helplessness, and loss of meaning and purpose in life, and may be strongly associated with suicidal ideation [3, 7]. The experience imposed by a disease (treatment, disease progression, prognosis, bothersome symptoms) challenges the patient's coping capacity, leading to suffering and possibly lowering their morale [7]. Demoralisation syndrome has been commonly found in patients at the end of life, when existential concerns come into focus [29].

From a clinical perspective, the main question is whether demoralisation can be reliably distinguished from depression or adjustment disorder (AD) [21].

2.1 Demoralisation and Adjustment Disorder

AD is a diagnosis recognised in psychiatric nosological systems as a stress response syndrome, that is, a maladaptive reaction to an identifiable stressor. As such, it pinpoints an impaired coping [7]. As a failure to adapt to and cope satisfactorily with the situation, demoralisation is consistent with AD [4]. The categories of AD in the

Diagnostic and Statistical Manual of Mental Disorders, Fifth Edition (DSM-5), and of the International Classification of Diseases, 10th revision (ICD)-10 have been criticised for using broad and subjective criteria [30]. Studies on AD for ICD-11 have pointed to their own distinct phenomena, which are separate from those that define depressive or anxiety disorders, rather than being hierarchically considered a subliminal disorder when the diagnostic requirements for depression or anxiety have not been met [30, 31]. The one-dimensional concept of AD proposed by Glaesmer and colleagues demonstrated that it was characterised by maladaptive concern with a stressor, failure to adapt with significant functional impairment, and additional symptoms, including depression, anxiety, avoidance, and impulsivity [31]. This definition of inability to cope with stress, with functional impairment and distress, overlaps the concept of demoralisation [32].

The suggestion that distress is relieved by removing the stressor in AD, as opposed to demoralisation, is underwhelming for distinguishing these conditions in the setting of a chronic or life-threatening illness [21]. In a study that explored latent class structure to evaluate the contribution of demoralisation symptoms to anhedonic depression, anxiety, adjustment, and somatic disorders in a cohort of 1527 cancer patients, moderate demoralisation was grouped with AD symptoms, characterising a clinical picture consistent with a unidimensional model of AD [32]. In a study on demoralisation, mental disorders, and suicidal ideation in the context of a severe illness, demoralisation was present in tandem with mood/anxiety disorder in 7% of patients, and 14% were demoralised without any mood/anxiety disorder [33]. Demoralisation and adjustment disorders were present in 2% of those studied. Demoralisation, but not depression, was associated with a significantly higher risk of suicidal ideation after controlling for mental disorders. The authors concluded that clinically relevant demoralisation is often present independently of a mental disorder in cancer patients and has a unique contribution to suicidal ideation [33].

2.2 *Demoralisation and Depression*

Demoralisation is often conflated with depression as some of its symptoms overlap. de Figueiredo noted that patients experiencing demoralisation do not exhibit symptoms that are typical of depression, especially those involving sleep, appetite, and motivation [34]. However, this may be difficult to assess clinically, as most hospitalised patients suffering from a severe physical illness suffer disturbances in physiological functions, such as appetite and/or sleep [21]. Other symptoms that characterise demoralisation include feelings of hopelessness and helplessness, confusion, loss of meaning, isolation, subjective incompetence, distress, and concern, most of which are shared with other depressive disorders [21]. However, as there are mixed states between anxiety and depression, for example, demoralisation can also develop as a comorbidity along with other psychological disorders [32].

There are significant clinical differences between demoralisation and Major Depressive Disorder (MDD) [32]. Through techniques such as binary factor analysis and latent class analysis, discrete groupings show a distinction between anhedonia (loss of pleasure), demoralisation (loss of hope and meaning), anxiety (concern and fear), somatic symptoms (pain and fatigue), and grief (emotions of loss) in hospitalised patients [35–37].

Anhedonia, the loss of pleasure in pleasant activities, has been suggested as a defining trait, being present only in depression, whereas demoralisation is marked by the absence of anticipated but unconsummated pleasure [21]. Unlike a patient suffering from depression, a patient experiencing demoralisation usually does not present with a full set of neurovegetative symptoms—specifically, anhedonia [23]. The main symptom of MDD is anhedonia (general loss of interest) in the present moment. A person experiencing demoralisation may not present with anhedonia, but feels uncertain about the future, and there is an anticipated loss of hope and meaning in life [23].

The literature points to a distinction between demoralisation and depression in the context of psychopathology among physically ill patients [7, 38]. Researchers have found that anhedonic depression symptoms are different from demoralisation symptoms, and suicidal thoughts are more strongly associated with demoralisation symptoms [38]. These studies suggest that identifying symptom groupings related to entrapment and helplessness could help characterise depressed and demoralised patients. While demoralisation and depression are related, they should be considered as separate conditions, as not all demoralised patients exhibit depression, and vice versa [33, 39–42].

Mood reactivity is usually preserved in demoralised patients [34], such that in contrast to a depressed individual, a demoralised patient may experience hope and pleasure when an adversity is overcome. For instance, a patient who is suffering from demoralisation may experience an improvement in mood in response to a vacation, successful pain management, or a visit from someone important, in contrast to a depressed patient who is unable to break free from the dysphoric state [23]. However, Belvederi Murri et al. suggest that the defining traits of depression and demoralisation are independent, with the exception of low mood and self-censorship [38]. In addition, both demoralisation and depression are followed by a loss of motivation that leads to an interruption in their actions, i.e. in both, people lose the will and/or the energy to carry out their daily activities [43]. However, the distinction between demoralisation and depression can be found in the relative intensity of the collapse of the two measurable aspects of motivation, namely: magnitude and direction [5]. Demoralisation is characterised by uncertainty and a lack of direction in motivation, leading to inhibited action. Demoralised individuals want to end their distress but lack a clear plan for future action. Depressed individuals, on the other hand, struggle with insufficient motivation, even though they know what to do to improve their situation [34].

2.3 *Demoralisation and Spiritual Distress*

Frankl [44], a Holocaust survivor and psychiatrist, asserts that what makes humans unique is the search for meaning, which he called the will to meaning. Frankl argued that society has medicalised the spiritual aspect of the human being and pathologised the innate quest for purpose [44]. Robinson et al. draw attention to studies indicating that at least one spiritual need is reported by up to 79% of cancer patients, and between 23% and 44% report spiritual distress [45]. Moderate evidence was found for a relationship between demoralisation and spiritual needs or lack of a clear spiritual dimension in life, and psychological factors such as distress, hope, purpose, and sense of coherence regarding the value of life [46].

Spiritual distress is conceptualised as deficiency in seven constructs of a person's sense of spirituality: connection, faith and religious belief system, value system, meaning and purpose in life, self-esteem and transcendence, inner peace and harmony, and inner strength and energy [47]. A validation study of the nursing diagnosis of spiritual distress proposed the following definition for this condition: 'a state of suffering associated with the meaning of one's life, related to a connection with oneself, with others, with the world, or with a Higher Power' [48].

Spiritual and religious beliefs can be listed as important resilience resources—supporting the ability to recover from or cope with adverse situations. According to a systematic review that investigated the relationship between spirituality/religiosity and resilience, a moderate positive correlation was identified between these variables ($r = 0.40$ (IC 95%, 0.32–0.48], $p < 0.01$) [49]. According to the authors, although the mechanisms of this relationship are unknown, it can be explained, at least in part, by the existence of common factors underlying both resilience and religious/spiritual qualities, such as optimism, positive emotions, social support, and the pursuit of meaning and purpose [49]. Individual Meaning-Centred Psychotherapy (IMCP), an intervention designed to address the need for brief interventions aimed at spiritual well-being and a sense of meaning for patients with advanced cancer, has shown clear short-term benefits for controlling spiritual suffering and improving the quality of life [50, 51].

3 Demoralisation in the Hospice and Palliative Care Context

The number of demoralisation studies has increased significantly since 2000 [6]. Clinically relevant demoralisation is found in 21% of patients with severe illnesses [33]. Among cancer patients, its prevalence is 24–36%, higher than non-oncological populations (24–32%) [52]. In Hong Kong palliative care patients, it is 64.8% [39], and among Italian end-of-life cancer patients, severe demoralisation reaches almost 52% [53]. In various populations, demoralisation exists in 27.4% of elderly people with chronic diseases, 43.5% in palliative care, 29–52.5% in terminally ill patients, and up to 64% in end-of-life cancer patients [54].

The experience of suffering encompasses physical, psychological, social, spiritual, and existential components [55]. Palliative care patients, especially those at the end of life, often face considerable physical and psychological suffering [39]. In the existential dimension, patients may lose the will to live and wish for death due to a lack of meaning in life [56]. Existential concerns revolve around questions about human limitations, mortality, attachment, and freedom, with the search for meaning approached from both religious and secular perspectives [57]. Spirituality involves a connection with what is considered sacred, and may or may not be related to religion [58].

According to the literature, demoralisation is more common in cancer patients, especially those in the advanced stages of the disease, which is why research on demoralisation in this population is currently growing [43]. The diagnosis of metastatic cancer and subsequent disease progression signals proximity to the end of life. This can challenge the coping and adaptation processes, resulting in the development of AD and demoralisation [7]. Regarding cancer specifically, during cancer diagnosis, treatment, and rehabilitation, psychological distress can occur on a continuum that ranges from normal fear, worry, or sadness, to severe anxiety, depression, and existential despair [59, 60]. Two distinct approaches have been used to understand the patterns of cancer-related distress, namely: mental disorders and demoralisation [60]. At the most severe end, a diagnosis of a mental disorder identifies a clearly defined pattern of morbidity. In the middle of the spectrum, ADs represent a category of impaired coping that is rather nonspecific, but dominant in psycho-oncological practice [61]. At the lower end of the distress spectrum, subthreshold symptoms may not qualify as disorders, but remain clinically relevant for treatment [60], considering that they can have a negative impact on the patient's well-being.

Demoralisation tends to increase as cancer patients approach the end of life, so that lower performance status, reduced functionality and greater frailty are all linked to greater demoralisation [17]. Suffering at the end of life can be mentally distressing, leading to a loss of what is valuable including the imminent end of life [62]. Among the main ways to alleviate suffering at the end of life is spiritual counselling, through which the patient can be assisted in seeing their existence as meaningful [62].

Demoralisation can affect not only patients with serious illnesses, but also their overburdened caregivers, with a stronger link to spiritual and psychological suffering than to care tasks [17, 63]. Complex interactions between patients and caregivers, including projective identification (a defence mechanism in which the person who is the target of the projection starts to behave, think, and feel according to what has been projected onto them), also play an important role [4].

Demoralisation is a contributing factor to the deterioration of health-related quality of life for end-of-life cancer patients [53]. Considering that dignity and respect for life are core values, demoralisation in the context of palliative care represents a harsh reality that cannot be ignored. To truly honour the experience of those facing the end of life, it is imperative for palliative care to be rooted in empathy, compassion, and understanding, ensuring that each person is treated as a whole human being, worthy of respect, including support for their spiritual or religious traditions. Therefore, it is necessary to identify interventions that, whenever possible, focus on preventing demoralisation [53].

4 Clinical Approach to Demoralisation

Demoralisation is included in the expressions of existential distress, among other aspects, such as fear of cancer recurrence and death anxiety [3, 64]. These aspects focus, with varying emphasis, on fear of death, concerns regarding autonomy, suffering, or being a burden to others; a sense of profound loneliness, worthlessness, or hopelessness; spiritual distress or loss of faith; lament, regret, or bitterness about what has been lost in life; and shame if dignity is lost or if expectations regarding coping are not met [64].

In order to establish a therapeutic plan adequate to patients' needs, healthcare professionals must know how to correctly identify cases of demoralisation, based on an appropriate assessment and diagnosis.

4.1 Assessment and Diagnosis

A 74-year-old widower and retired gardener, "Joe" was afflicted with multiple squamous cell carcinomas on his head and neck, which were the result of prolonged sun exposure throughout his lifetime. He had lost most of his nose and both ears entirely. He had enlarged neck nodes with facial palsy. Although provided with a facial prosthesis to cover his wounds, he was often too bothered to wear it. Feeling highly embarrassed by his disfigurement, he withdrew socially, only finding enjoyment when spending time with his family. Life had become boring otherwise. He stated, "What's the point of going on? My life is meaningless now. I want to die". [65]

The case presented above is an example of a typical case of demoralisation in the hospice and palliative care setting. The main core of demoralisation is the loss of meaning and purpose. Kissane proposed a set of **criteria for diagnosing** Demoralisation Syndrome, which include [66]:

- the experience of emotional distress, such as hopelessness and loss of meaning and purpose in life;
- a sense of powerlessness, failure, pessimism, and the lack of a worthwhile future;
- reduced capacity to react differently;
- social isolation and deficiencies in social support;
- persistence of the aforementioned phenomena for 2 or more weeks; and
- traits of major depression have not superseded as the primary disorder.

Rates of severe demoralisation have been associated with factors such as younger age, being female, physical symptom burden, depression, and anxiety [46], which is

Table 1 Diagnostic criteria for the identification of demoralisation versus AD [7]

Demoralisation	Adjustment disorder
• Low morale, discouragement, or demotivation • A feeling that one is coping poorly with a given situation, that one is unable to cope with this situation, or that one feels like a failure • Feeling trapped, stuck, or unable to change the situation • Being hopeless and pessimistic about the future • A feeling of worthlessness, with a loss of meaning, value, and purpose in life • Resulting excessive distress or impairment in normal life functions • Potential for suicidal thoughts or plans	• The illness as a stressor that challenges coping • The presence of distressing symptoms out of proportion to what is expected from the predicament • A timeline linking the symptoms to the stressor/illness • Maladaptive coping resulting in impairment in personal, family, social, educational, occupational, or other important areas of functioning

in line with the previous hypotheses posed by Frank and de Figueiredo [2, 34]. Risk factors for demoralisation also include expensive treatments, prolonged or recurrent hospitalisations, lower education and health literacy, lower income and socioeconomic deprivation, and lack of social support [7].

Kissane et al. point out that being single (in addition to being separated, divorced, or widowed) is also a risk factor for demoralisation [7]. However, Chan et al. in a study carried out with demoralised patients in palliative care found that participants with partners (married), with more depressive symptoms and less family support had a significantly higher level of demoralisation compared to the others [39].

Given the strong association between demoralisation and AD, Tables 1 and 2 present, respectively, the **diagnostic criteria for the identification of Demoralisation versus AD** and **the common symptoms and signs of AD and Demoralisation** [7].

Demoralisation Measurement

The Demoralisation Scale (DS) was developed in populations representative of psycho-oncology and palliative care settings, with the objective of creating a measurement tool that could reliably assess the various dimensions of demoralisation, in addition to allowing the monitoring of this variable over time [28]. This 24-item self-report scale (scored from 0 to 96), is divided into five factors (loss of meaning and purpose, dysphoria, disheartenment, helplessness, and a sense of failure) [28]. The DS-II also exists, which is a short version (16-item) of the DS [67]. The DS has been validated in a range of languages, such as: Italian [14, 53, 63, 68, 69], Chinese [12, 16], Mandarin [13, 70], and German [71].

In general, the DS has adequate psychometric properties, although confirmatory factor analysis has been recommended, and test-retest reliability has not yet been assessed [67]. Establishing divergent validity also remains a problem, as there is a high level of convergence between depression and demoralisation [67]. The DS

Table 2 The common symptoms and signs of AD and demoralisation [7]

Symptoms	Signs
• Distress, upset, grief, and sadness • Low morale, feeling disheartened, discouraged, losing confidence in the treatment • A sense of poor coping, feeling a failure, struggling to cope with the illness • Feeling trapped by the illness, stuck, with growing helplessness • Hopelessness, feeling pessimistic about the future • Pointlessness and meaninglessness, with the loss of the value of life • Purposelessness, with the loss of direction and goals • Feeling alone, isolated, or alienated from others • The loss of roles, creativity, ways of achieving fulfilment, including relationships • The loss of self-worth, dignity, feelings of embarrassment, or shame • The loss of control, not feeling choices are yours to make • Other dysphoric emotions, including irritability and anger • Resulting impairment in life functions and social withdrawal • Ruminating thoughts about everything and feeling in despair • A readiness to give up on life, a desire for death, or wish to hasten death • Suicidal plans • Spiritual concerns (guilt, regret, shame, loss of faith, etc.)	• Waves of tearfulness, but yet with the ability to rally again • Reactivity of affects is retained, being able to smile freely • A sense of humour that persists, with spontaneous laughter being evident • The ability to enjoy visits, reading, or to be entertained • Having interest in activities and being able to enjoy pleasant experiences • Cognitive function remains intact, fully oriented, with a reasonable memory and sound judgement • Health literacy may not be great, with limited understanding of the prognosis • Insight into the loss of morale and hope is generally present

assesses a specific type of existential psychological distress related to end of life and physical suffering that is present in terminal and life-threatening illnesses; in fact, this instrument has been primarily used to assess samples of cancer patients [54].

4.2 General Measurements for Interventions in Demoralisation Frameworks

According to a systematic review on the clinical utility of demoralisation, several interventions have been identified as being promising for the management of this condition [54]. A sequential combination of cognitive-behavioural therapy (CBT) and well-being therapy (WBT) reduced depressive symptoms compared to clinical control in patients with acute coronary syndromes affected by demoralisation and/or depression [72]. Acceptance and commitment-based therapy led to a significant reduction in demoralisation in breast cancer patients and survivors compared to non-treated controls [73]. A randomised feasibility trial was carried out to compare the Individual Meaning-Centred Psychotherapy-Palliative Care (IMCP-PC) with the counselling-based psychotherapy in patients receiving palliative care at home [74]. The results showed that IMCP-PC was more effective than counselling in the reduction of all variables (anxiety, depression, and emotional distress), except for demoralisation. Participants who received counselling-based psychotherapy (three psychotherapeutic sessions aiming to help patients cope with advanced cancer by encouraging them to share their concerns about the disease and/or treatment) presented a reduction in demoralisation, compared to those who received IMCP-PC [74]. The psilocybin-assisted group therapy demonstrated viability, relative safety, and potential effectiveness for demoralisation in older long-term AIDS survivors [75]. The psilocybin-assisted psychotherapy (PAP) led to a reduction in cancer-related demoralisation and hopelessness [76, 77], with results suggesting that PAP may be an effective anti-suicidal intervention following a cancer diagnosis due to its positive impact on hopelessness and demoralisation and its effects on meaning making [76]. End-of-life patients presented a significant reduction in demoralisation following Dignity Therapy associated with the palliative care approach compared to palliative care alone [78], in contrast to what was found in terminally ill patients [79].

In addition to the interventions presented above, it is worth mentioning that being present and listening to the patient's suffering with compassion are also essential interventions in the search for the relief of human suffering [80]. Consoling existential and spiritual distress is a deeply personal and relational practice, involving a high degree of sensitivity and the courage to be there solely as wounded healers, willing and ready to share the fear of death and the finitude of life with patients and their loved ones [81]. In a study on the meaning of the lived experience of palliative care nurses with the relief of the spiritual and existential suffering of terminally ill patients, the investigators indicate that nurses have the capacity to lessen existential and spiritual suffering through the force of their comforting presence [81]. Nurses have the chance to support patients' strength and enable their bravery to live a meaningful life and die with dignity by developing close relationships with patients and their families [81].

With regard to the suffering caused by demoralisation, it is important to note that these are protective factors [7]:

- Resilient character strengths with strong education, maturity, and wisdom;
- Coherent narrative of a fulfilling and creative life;
- Strong religious belief and availability of a faith community;
- Supportive network of family and friends;
- Open communication, openness to new experiences, adaptability, and flexibility.

4.3 Spiritual Care

All individuals may experience moments of disorientation in their lives and seek spiritual care to find their bearings [82]. Evidence suggests that spirituality is inversely related to demoralisation, with higher spirituality linked to lower levels of demoralisation, serving as a *protective* fator [17]. On the contrary, unmet spiritual needs are associated with increased demoralisation in cancer patients, and even caregivers of these patients can experience demoralisation, often linked to spiritual distress [17].

Demoralisation signifies the loss of meaning, hope, and purpose, often associated with suffering from a stressful event like advanced illness [4]. Spirituality, on the other hand, involves seeking meaning, purpose, and transcendence [83]. Demoralisation results from a lack of meaning, while spirituality helps (re)discover meaning in life and the experience of illness. Loss of meaning precedes a loss of morale, leading to potential despair and demoralisation [4]. Coping based on finding meaning is an important way to address stressful situations [84]. Religious and spiritual beliefs can influence how patients cope with illness by providing a sense of meaning, purpose, and hope [85–87].

Spiritual concerns can include: existential concerns, abandonment by God or others, anger at God or others, concerns about relationship with deity, conflicted or challenged belief systems, despair/hopelessness, grief/loss, guilt/shame, reconciliation, isolation, religious/spiritual struggle [88]. In this context, Puchalski et al. suggest three major groups of spiritual interventions [88]:

- Therapeutic communication techniques: Compassionate presence; Reflective listening, query about important life events; Support patient's sources of spiritual strength; Open-ended questions to illicit feelings; Inquiry about spiritual beliefs, values, and practices; Life review, listening to the patient's story; Continued presence and follow-up;
- Therapy: Guided visualisation for 'meaningless pain'; Progressive relaxation; Breathing practice or contemplation; Meaning-oriented therapy; Referral to spiritual care provider as indicated; Use of storytelling; Dignity-conserving therapy;
- Self-care: Massage; Reconciliation with self or others; Spiritual support groups; Meditation; Sacred/spiritual readings or rituals; Yoga, tai chi; Exercise; Art therapy (music, art, dance); Journaling.

The incorporation of pastoral care providers into the interdisciplinary team is also an important source of spiritual care for patients who wish to have their religious/spiritual needs integrated into their care [85, 89]. Pastoral care providers (also known as chaplains or spiritual care specialists) are trained to recognise and respond to the patient's spiritual suffering, often manifested by an inability to find hope and a sense of meaning and purpose [85, 88].

5 Concluding Remarks

In this chapter, we have explored demoralisation and spirituality in the palliative care setting. Demoralisation, characterised by the loss of hope and purpose, can negatively affect patients with terminal illnesses. However, spirituality provides a powerful resource for coping with demoralisation, bringing comfort and meaning to patients. Palliative care recognises the importance of spirituality by providing a space for the patients' spiritual expression. Multidisciplinary collaboration and continued research are needed to further the knowledge in this field.

Ultimately, demoralisation is related to patients' life stories; thus, Frank states that it is possible to learn how to recognise and alleviate patients' demoralisation by learning their life stories [5]. The enduring human need for dignity and meaning in life transcends cultures and highlights the importance of meaning making and relationships for human well-being [7].

References

1. Frank JD. Persuasion and healing. Baltimore: Johns Hopkins University Press; 1961.
2. Frank JD, Frank JB. Persuasion and healing: a comparative study of psychotherapy. Baltimore: JHU Press; 1991.
3. Kissane DW, Clarke DM, Street AF. Demoralization syndrome: a relevant psychiatric diagnosis for palliative care. J Palliat Care. 2001;17(1):12–21.
4. Kissane DW. Demoralization: a life-preserving diagnosis to make for the severely medically ill. J Palliat Care. 2014;30(4):255–8.
5. de Figueiredo JM. Advances in the study of demoralization: an overview. Eur J Psychiat. 2013;27(1):5–6.
6. Zheng Q, Xiong L, Li H, et al. Demoralization: where it stands-and where we can take it: a bibliometric analysis. Front Psychol. 2022;13:1016601. https://doi.org/10.3389/fpsyg.2022.1016601.
7. Kissane DW, Grassi L, Fang CK. Adjustment disorder and demoralization. In: Kissane DW, Watson M, Breitbart WS, editors. Psycho-oncology in palliative and end of life care. New York: Oxford University Press; 2023. p. 48–69.
8. Eggen AC, Reyners AKL, Shen G, et al. Death anxiety in patients with metastatic non-small cell lung cancer with and without brain metastases. J Pain Symptom Manage. 2020;60(2):422–429.e1. https://doi.org/10.1016/j.jpainsymman.2020.02.023.
9. Bovero A, Sedghi NA, Opezzo M, et al. Dignity-related existential distress in end-of-life cancer patients: prevalence, underlying factors, and associated coping strategies. Psychooncology. 2018;27(11):2631–7. https://doi.org/10.1002/pon.4884.
10. Peng HL, Hsueh HW, Chang YH, et al. The mediation and suppression effect of demoralization in breast cancer patients after primary therapy: a structural equation model. J Nurs Res. 2021;29(2):e144. https://doi.org/10.1097/JNR.0000000000000421.
11. Kouhpas N, Karimi Z, Rahmani B, et al. The relationship between existential anxiety and demoralization syndrome in predicting psychological well-being of patient with cancer. Pract Clin Psychol. 2020;8:175–82.

12. Lin F, Hong Y, Lin X, et al. Demoralization profiles and their association with depression and quality of life in Chinese patients with cancer: a latent class analysis. Support Care Cancer. 2022;30(12):10019–30. https://doi.org/10.1007/s00520-022-07412-9.
13. Chang TG, Huang PC, Hsu CY, et al. Demoralization in oral cancer inpatients and its association with spiritual needs, quality of life, and suicidal ideation: a cross-sectional study. Health Qual Life Outcomes. 2022a;20(1):60. https://doi.org/10.1186/s12955-022-01962-6.
14. Ghiggia A, Pierotti V, Tesio V, et al. Personality matters: relationship between personality characteristics, spirituality, demoralization, and perceived quality of life in a sample of end-of-life cancer patients. Support Care Cancer. 2021;29(12):7775–83. https://doi.org/10.1007/s00520-021-06363-x.
15. Boston P, Bruce A, Schreiber R. Existential suffering in the palliative care setting: an integrated literature review. J Pain Symptom Manage. 2011;41(3):604–18. https://doi.org/10.1016/j.jpainsymman.2010.05.010.
16. Liu ML, Hsiao YC. The impact of demoralization on spiritual well-being in terminally ill patients. Hu Li Za Zhi. 2019;66:48–59. https://doi.org/10.6224/JN.201902_66(1).07.
17. Garcia ACM, Schneiders M, da Mota KS, et al. Demoralization and spirituality in oncology: an integrative systematic review. Support Care Cancer. 2023;31(5):259. https://doi.org/10.1007/s00520-023-07722-6.
18. Rosmarin DH, Pargament KI, Koenig HG. Spirituality and mental health: challenges and opportunities. Lancet Psychiatry. 2021;8(2):92–3.
19. Cannon AJ, Dokucu ME, Loberiza FR Jr. Interplay between spirituality and religiosity on the physical and mental well-being of cancer survivors. Support Care Cancer. 2022;30(2):1407–17. https://doi.org/10.1007/s00520-021-06534-w.
20. Balboni TA, VanderWeele TJ, Doan-Soares SD, et al. Spirituality in serious illness and health [published correction appears in JAMA 2022 Aug 23;328(8):780]. JAMA. 2022;328(2):184–97. https://doi.org/10.1001/jama.2022.11086.
21. O'Keeffe N, Ranjith G. Depression, demoralisation or adjustment disorder? Understanding emotional distress in the severely medically ill. Clin Med (Lond). 2007;7(5):478–81. https://doi.org/10.7861/clinmedicine.7-5-478.
22. Slavney PR. Diagnosing demoralization in consultation psychiatry. Psychosomatics. 1999;40:325–9.
23. Jacobsen J, Vanderwerker L, Block S, et al. Depression and demoralization as distinct syndromes: preliminary data from a cohort of advanced cancer patients. Indian J Palliat Care. 2006;12(1):8–15.
24. de Figueiredo J. Diagnosing demoralization in consultation psychiatry [letter]. Psychosomatics. 2000;41:449–50.
25. Yalom ID. Existential psychotherapy. New York: Yalom Family Trust; 1980.
26. Yalom ID. The Yalom reader: selections from the work of a master therapist and storyteller. New York: Basic Books; 1998.
27. de Figueiredo JM, Frank JD. Subjective incompetence, the clinical hallmark of demoralization. Compr Psychiatry. 1982;23(4):353–63.
28. Kissane DW, Wein S, Love A, et al. The demoralization scale: a report of its development and preliminary validation. J Palliat Care. 2004;20(4):269–76.
29. Clarke DM, Kissane DW. Demoralization: its phenomenology and importance. Aust N Z J Psychiatry. 2002;36(6):733–42. https://doi.org/10.1046/j.1440-1614.2002.01086.x.
30. Bachem R, Casey P. Adjustment disorder: a diagnosis whose time has come. J Affect Disord. 2018;227:243–53. https://doi.org/10.1016/j.jad.2017.10.034.
31. Glaesmer H, Romppel M, Brähler E, et al. Adjustment disorder as proposed for ICD-11: dimensionality and symptom differentiation. Psychiatry Res. 2015;229(3):940–8.
32. Bobevski I, Kissane DW, Vehling S, et al. Latent class analysis differentiation of adjustment disorder and demoralization, more severe depressive and anxiety disorders, and somatic symptoms in patients with cancer. Psychooncology. 2018;27(11):2623–30. https://doi.org/10.1002/pon.4761.

33. Vehling S, Kissane DW, Lo C, et al. The association of demoralization with mental disorders and suicidal ideation in patients with cancer. Cancer. 2017a;123(17):3394–401. https://doi.org/10.1002/cncr.30749.
34. de Figueiredo JM. Depression and demoralization: phenomenological differences and research perspectives. Compr Psychiatry. 1993;34(5):308–11.
35. Clarke DM, Mackinnon AJ, Smith GC, et al. Dimensions of psychopathology in the medically ill: a latent trait analysis. Psychosomatics. 2000;41(5):418–25. https://doi.org/10.1176/appi.psy.41.5.418.
36. Clarke DM, Smith GC, Dowe DL, et al. An empirically derived taxonomy of common distress syndromes in the medically ill. J Psychosom Res. 2003;54(4):323–30.
37. McKenzie DP, Clarke DM, Forbes AB, et al. Pessimism, worthlessness, anhedonia, and thoughts of death identify DSM-IV major depression in hospitalized, medically ill patients. Psychosomatics. 2010;51(4):302–11.
38. Belvederi Murri M, Caruso R, Ounalli H, et al. The relationship between demoralization and depressive symptoms among patients from the general hospital: network and exploratory graph analysis. J Affect Disord. 2020;276:137–46. https://doi.org/10.1016/j.jad.2020.06.074.
39. Chan WCH, Yu CTK, Kwok DKS, et al. Prevalence and factors associated with demoralization in palliative care patients: a cross-sectional study from Hong Kong [published online ahead of print, 2022 Sep 2]. Palliat Support Care. 2022:1–9. https://doi.org/10.1017/S1478951522001171.
40. Fang CK, Chang MC, Chen PJ, et al. A correlational study of suicidal ideation with psychological distress, depression, and demoralization in patients with cancer. Support Care Cancer. 2014;22(12):3165–74. https://doi.org/10.1007/s00520-014-2290-4.
41. Nanni MG, Caruso R, Travado L, et al. Relationship of demoralization with anxiety, depression, and quality of life: a southern European study of Italian and Portuguese cancer patients. Psychooncology. 2018;27(11):2616–22. https://doi.org/10.1002/pon.4824.
42. Ignatius J, De La Garza IIR. Frequency of demoralization and depression in cancer patients. Gen Hosp Psychiatry. 2019;60(Sep–Oct):137–40.
43. Wang Y, Sun H, Ji Q, et al. Prevalence, associated factors and adverse outcomes of demoralization in cancer patients: a decade of systematic review [published online ahead of print, 2023 Jan 31]. Am J Hosp Palliat Care. 2023;40(11):1216–30. https://doi.org/10.1177/10499091231154887.
44. Frankl VE. Man's search for meaning. New York: Simon and Schuster; 1985.
45. Robinson KL, Connelly CD, Georges JM. Pain and spiritual distress at end of life: a correlational study. J Palliat Care. 2022;37(4):526–34. https://doi.org/10.1177/08258597221090482.
46. Robinson S, Kissane DW, Brooker J, et al. A systematic review of the demoralization syndrome in individuals with progressive disease and cancer: a decade of research. J Pain Symptom Manage. 2015;49(3):595–610.
47. Villagomeza LR. Spiritual distress in adult cancer patients: toward conceptual clarity. Holist Nurs Pract. 2005;19(6):285–94. https://doi.org/10.1097/00004650-200511000-00010.
48. Caldeira S, Carvalho EC, Vieira M. Spiritual distress-proposing a new definition and defining characteristics. Int J Nurs Knowl. 2013;24(2):77–84. https://doi.org/10.1111/j.2047-3095.2013.01234.x.
49. Schwalm FD, Zandavalli RB, de Castro Filho ED, et al. Is there a relationship between spirituality/religiosity and resilience? A systematic review and meta-analysis of observational studies. J Health Psychol. 2022;27(5):1218–32. https://doi.org/10.1177/1359105320984537.
50. Breitbart W, Pessin H, Rosenfeld B, et al. Individual meaning-centered psychotherapy for the treatment of psychological and existential distress: a randomized controlled trial in patients with advanced cancer. Cancer. 2018;124(15):3231–9. https://doi.org/10.1002/cncr.31539.
51. Breitbart W, Poppito S, Rosenfeld B, et al. Pilot randomized controlled trial of individual meaning-centered psychotherapy for patients with advanced cancer. J Clin Oncol. 2012;30(12):1304–9. https://doi.org/10.1200/JCO.2011.36.2517.

52. Gan LL, Gong S, Kissane DW. Mental state of demoralisation across diverse clinical settings: a systematic review, meta-analysis and proposal for its use as a 'specifier' in mental illness. Aust N Z J Psychiatry. 2022;56(9):1104–29. https://doi.org/10.1177/00048674211060746.
53. Bovero A, Opezzo M, Tesio V. Relationship between demoralization and quality of life in end-of-life cancer patients. Psychooncology. 2023;32(3):429–37. https://doi.org/10.1002/pon.6095.
54. Woźniewicz A, Cosci F. Clinical utility of demoralization: a systematic review of the literature. Clin Psychol Rev. 2023;99:102227. https://doi.org/10.1016/j.cpr.2022.102227.
55. Hartogh GD. Suffering and dying well: on the proper aim of palliative care. Med Health Care Philos. 2017;20(3):413–24. https://doi.org/10.1007/s11019-017-9764-3.
56. Chen W, Chen Y, Xiao H. Existential distress in cancer patients: a concept analysis. Cancer Nurs. 2022;45(2):E471–86. https://doi.org/10.1097/NCC.0000000000000925.
57. Sullivan D, Palitsky R. An existential psychological perspective on the human essence. In: The Oxford handbook of the human essence. Oxford: Oxford University Press; 2018. p. 21–34.
58. Palitsky R, Kaplan DM, Peacock C, et al. Importance of integrating spiritual, existential, religious, and theological components in psychedelic-assisted therapies. JAMA Psychiatry. 2023;80(7):743–9. https://doi.org/10.1001/jamapsychiatry.2023.1554.
59. Holland JC, editor. Psycho-oncology. 3rd ed. Oxford: Oxford University Press; 2015.
60. Vehling S, Mehnert A. The 1-year longitudinal association of demoralization and depression. In: Psycho-oncology world congress. Hoboken: Wiley; 2017b.
61. Li M, Hales S, Rodin G. Adjustment disorders. In: Holland JC, editor. Psycho-oncology. 3rd ed. Oxford: Oxford University Press; 2015. p. 274–80.
62. Varelius J. Suffering at the end of life. Bioethics. 2019;33(1):195–200. https://doi.org/10.1111/bioe.12513.
63. Bovero A, Vitiello LP, Botto R, et al. Demoralization in end-of-life cancer patients' family caregivers: a cross-sectional study. Am J Hosp Palliat Care. 2022;39(3):332–9. https://doi.org/10.1177/10499091211023482.
64. Vehling S, Kissane DW. Existential distress in cancer: alleviating suffering from fundamental loss and change. Psychooncology. 2018;27(11):2525–30. https://doi.org/10.1002/pon.4872.
65. Robinson S, Kissane DW, Brooker J, et al. A review of the construct of demoralization: history, definitions, and future directions for palliative care. Am J Hosp Palliat Care. 2016a;33(1):93–101. https://doi.org/10.1177/1049909114553461.
66. Kissane DW. Distress, demoralisation and depression in palliative care. Curr Ther (Seaforth). 2000;41(6):14–9.
67. Robinson S, Kissane DW, Brooker J, et al. Refinement and revalidation of the demoralization scale: the DS-II—internal validity. Cancer. 2016b;122(14):2251–9. https://doi.org/10.1002/cncr.30015.
68. Bovero A, Opezzo M, Botto R, et al. Hope in end-of-life cancer patients: a cross-sectional analysis. Palliat Support Care. 2021;19(5):563–9. https://doi.org/10.1017/S1478951520001388.
69. Bovero A, Botto R, Adriano B, et al. Exploring demoralization in end-of-life cancer patients: prevalence, latent dimensions, and associations with other psychosocial variables. Palliat Support Care. 2019;17(5):596–603. https://doi.org/10.1017/S1478951519000191.
70. Chang TG, Hung CC, Huang PC, et al. Demoralization and its association with quality of life, sleep quality, spiritual interests, and suicide risk in breast cancer inpatients: a cross-sectional study. Int J Environ Res Public Health. 2022b;19(19):12815. https://doi.org/10.3390/ijerph191912815.
71. Mehnert A, Vehling S, Höcker A, et al. Demoralization and depression in patients with advanced cancer: validation of the German version of the demoralization scale. J Pain Symptom Manag. 2011;42(5):768–76. https://doi.org/10.1016/j.jpainsymman.2011.02.013.
72. Rafanelli C, Gostoli S, Buzzichelli S, et al. Sequential combination of cognitive-behavioral treatment and well-being therapy in depressed patients with acute coronary syndromes: a randomized controlled trial (TREATED-ACS study). Psychother Psychosom. 2020;89(6):345–56.

73. Sarizadeh MS, Boogar IR, Talepasand S, et al. Acceptance and commitment therapy for demoralization syndrome and cancer-related trauma: a randomized clinical trial study. Int J Cancer Manag. 2021;4(11):e114637.
74. Fraguell-Hernando C, Limonero J, Gil F. Psychological intervention in patients with advanced cancer at home through individual meaning-centered psychotherapy-palliative care: a pilot study. Support Care Cancer. 2020;28(10):4803–11.
75. Agin-Liebes GI, Malone T, Yalch MM, et al. Long-term follow-up of psilocybin-assisted psychotherapy for psychiatric and existential distress in patients with life-threatening cancer. J Psychopharmacol. 2020;34(2):155–66. https://doi.org/10.1177/0269881119897615.
76. Ross S, Agin-Liebes G, Lo S, et al. Acute and sustained reductions in loss of meaning and suicidal ideation following psilocybin-assisted psychotherapy for psychiatric and existential distress in life-threatening cancer. ACS Pharmacol Transl Sci. 2021;4(2):553–62.
77. Ross S, Bossis A, Guss J, et al. Rapid and sustained symptom reduction following psilocybin treatment for anxiety and depression in patients with life-threatening cancer: a randomized controlled trial. J Psychopharmacol. 2016;30(12):1165–80. https://doi.org/10.1177/0269881116675512.
78. Juliao M, Oliveira F, Nunes B, et al. Effect of dignity therapy on end-of-life psychological distress in terminally ill Portuguese patients: a randomized controlled trial. Palliat Support Care. 2017;15(6):628–37.
79. Iani L, De Vincenzo F, Maruelli A, et al. Dignity therapy helps terminally ill patients maintain a sense of peace: early results of a randomized controlled trial. Front Psychol. 2020;11:1468. https://doi.org/10.3389/fpsyg.2020.01468.
80. Silva LHP, Garcia ACM. A′meeting with the world's suffering. J Pain Symptom Manag. 2023. Published: July 01, 2023. https://doi.org/10.1016/j.jpainsymman.2023.06.031.
81. Tornøe KA, Danbolt LJ, Kvigne K, et al. The power of consoling presence – hospice nurses' lived experience with spiritual and existential care for the dying. BMC Nurs. 2014;13:25. https://doi.org/10.1186/1472-6955-13-25.
82. Schuhmann C, Damen A. Representing the good: pastoral care in a secular age. Pastoral Psychol. 2018;67(4):405–17. https://doi.org/10.1007/s11089-018-0826-0.
83. Puchalski CM, Vitillo R, Hull SK, et al. Improving the spiritual dimension of whole person care: reaching national and international consensus. J Palliat Med. 2014;17(6):642–56.
84. Folkman S. Positive psychological states and coping with severe stress. Soc Sci Med. 1997;45(8):1207–21. https://doi.org/10.1016/s0277-9536(97)00040-3.
85. Puchalski CM. Spirituality in the cancer trajectory. Ann Oncol. 2012;23:49–55. https://doi.org/10.1093/annonc/mds088.
86. Delgado-Guay MO. Spirituality and religiosity in supportive and palliative care. Curr Opin Support Palliat Care. 2014;8(3):308–13. https://doi.org/10.1097/SPC.0000000000000079.
87. Garssen B, Visser A, de Jager ME. Examining whether spirituality predicts subjective well-being: how to avoid tautology. Psychol Relig Spiritual. 2016;8:141–8.
88. Puchalski CM, Ferrell B, Virani R, et al. Improving the quality of spiritual care as a dimension of palliative care: the report of the Consensus Conference. J Palliat Med. 2009;12(10):885–904. https://doi.org/10.1089/jpm.2009.0142.
89. Puchalski CM, Lunsford B, Harris MH, et al. Interdisciplinary spiritual care for seriously ill and dying patients: a collaborative model. Cancer J. 2006;12(5):398–416.

The Existential Dimension of Loss and Grief

Carlo Leget and Mai-Britt Guldin

Abstract This chapter discusses integrating grief support and spiritual care in palliative care. It explores the existential dimension of grieving and focuses on the process of loss both patients and families are going through. First, the state of the art of grief research is sketched, and some reasons are given why until now the existential dimension of loss and grief has not had sufficient attention. From there, we will develop a multi-dimensional understanding of loss and grief, connected with the four ultimate concerns identified by Irvin Yalom in his existential therapy. Following the total pain approach in palliative care, we will develop an understanding of loss and grief that brings together the physical, emotional, cognitive, social, and spiritual dimension of the phenomena. We will conclude the chapter by introducing a case of a palliative care patient and his wife, illustrating how an integrative understanding of loss and grief in palliative care may lead to a deeper and more comprehensive approach to loss as a universal human experience.

Keywords Loss · Grief · Bereavement · Existential · Spiritual · Spiritual care Palliative care

C. Leget (✉)
Care Ethics, University of Humanistic Studies, Utrecht, The Netherlands
e-mail: c.leget@uvh.nl

M.-B. Guldin
Research Unit for General Practice, Aarhus University, Aarhus, Denmark
e-mail: m.guldin@ph.au.dk

M. C. Best (ed.), *Spiritual Care in Palliative Care*,
https://doi.org/10.1007/978-3-031-50864-6_25

1 Loss and Grief: State of the Art

Loss and grief are intrinsically intertwined with palliative care. From the diagnosis of an incurable disease, both patient and family are confronted with a process of loss and grief. Even before the diagnosis, in many cases forms of loss have been experienced relating to well-being, energy, and functional capacity. The process of losing one's life is impactful for the patient and continues for the family long after the dying process. In a world café at the conference of the European Association for Palliative Care, 32 healthcare professionals from 16 countries identified a range of different losses experienced in palliative care, such as a planned future, hope, stability, certainty, control, flexibility, normality, connectedness, social relations, sense of self, identity, social life, health social roles, love life, trust, communication, faith, dreams, and body security [1].

Although palliative care as an approach is built around the idea of total pain—suffering is understood as being multi-dimensional and care is understood as an interdisciplinary approach involving different healthcare professionals—in general loss and grief are not approached from an interdisciplinary perspective [2]. Both loss and grief are typically understood as relevant for family and friends after the death of the patient and most of the research in this dimension is about post-death bereavement. Grief support for patients and family is described as opportunities for family members to take part in bereavement groups after the funeral more than being accompanied during the process of losing a loved one [3].

This narrowed attention to loss and grief after death is accompanied by another reduction of the phenomenon: loss and grief are seen as mainly psychological issues. Historically, there is a long tradition of consolation literature both in philosophy and theology, yet since the beginning of the twentieth century, the focus of understanding loss and grief has shifted towards the discipline of psychology. Since Sigmund Freud published his influential text *Mourning and Melancholia* in 1917, theories about loss and grief have been mainly developed within the disciplines of psychiatry and psychology, including the Five Phases Model, the Four Tasks model, the Continuing Bonds theory, and the Dual Process Model [4–8].

Looking at the current state of the art, there seem to be some developments that are working against an integrative approach of loss and grief in palliative care. Firstly, the focus on loss and grief as predominantly relevant after death does not recognise the processes both patient and families are going through. During the process of receiving palliative care, patients and families are faced with many losses as health and function decline, roles are changed, and social life and relations are affected. Often old losses are even re-grieved as they resonate with the situation of loss the patient and family find themselves in. From this perspective, the term 'anticipatory grief' (defined as the state of grief that occurs before an impending loss) is unfortunate since it undervalues these losses by suggesting that the only loss is death.

Secondly, most of the scientific research that has been done in the past years on grief support is focused on the 10% of 'high grievers', people who experience mental health problems in their grieving process, or pathological forms of grief such as prolonged grief disorder, with core symptoms including intense, persistent yearning, preoccupation with the deceased, extending the period of acute grief, and impaired functioning [9]. However important this research is, it has left the majority of grieving persons under-researched.

Thirdly, there seems to be a tendency of introducing a growing number of distinctions and labels for specific forms of loss such as delayed grief, inhibited grief, absent grief, secondary grief, waiting grief and many more, suggesting that loss and grief are a complicated field of subspecialties. Although this trend is understandable from the perspective of people who are suffering and need support, it is not helpful for becoming aware of the omnipresence of loss and grief in palliative care. Finally, most psychological studies on bereavement fail to recognise the existential dimension of loss and grief: the grief over a loss is not only a form of suffering, it also has the potential of becoming more aware of what is existentially meaningful to us, who we are, and what our central values as human beings are [10]. In other words: the shift from the religious to the psychological approach is not compensated by integrating the existential dimension of grief in research and therapy.

In this chapter, we aim to present an integrative approach to loss and grief in palliative care, inspired by the total pain model as it was introduced in the work of Cicely Saunders [2]. We provide an explanation for why it is important to acknowledge the existential dimension of loss and grief by arguing that it is connected with the four ultimate concerns that are distinguished in existential therapy: death, freedom, isolation, and meaninglessness. These ultimate concerns can become very confronting in palliative care for both patients and families. Subsequently, a five-dimensional understanding of loss and grief is introduced that enables palliative care teams to help patients and family members navigate different existential tensions that are related to the ultimate concerns. Finally, the implications to the palliative care approach are presented.

2 The Existential Dimension of Loss and Grief

Being alive unavoidably means being in processes of growth and decline, development and degeneration, growth, and loss. A loss is usually felt and can become a problem when it is not wanted and concerns something that really matters to us. How much it matters can only be determined by the grieving person. 'Where there is sorrow, there is holy ground', Oscar Wilde wrote in a long letter from prison that was later published as *De profundis*. From an existential perspective, one could say that all grief is sacred ground [11]. Only the griever can tell how much a particular loss has meant. The importance of any loss is deeply personal since it is our unique biography during which certain people and things have become more valuable than others. One could say that there are as many forms of grief as there are people (although according to zoologists, animals also grieve).

At the same time, loss and grief are universal phenomena, connected to our human existence. One way of understanding the universal existential dimension of loss and grief is to consider these phenomena against the background of the ultimate concerns that are used in existential therapy [12]. According to Yalom, every individual is confronted with four ultimate concerns in life that ask for a personal and authentic answer: death, freedom, isolation, and meaninglessness. Being aware that existential thinkers differ in the number and distinction of ultimate concerns in life, we will use the four ultimate concerns that have been used by the most influential writer in existential therapy, Irvin Yalom [13]. What is the relation of these ultimate concerns to loss and grief, and how can they help to increase our awareness of the existential dimension of these two phenomena?

When Yalom speaks of ultimate concerns, he follows a tradition of existentialist thinking that starts from the idea that humans differ from other animals in the way they are fundamentally open to the world. A cow does not need to figure out what it means to be a cow. Human beings, however, do need to figure out what it means to be human, since there is no predefined divine master plan or meaning of life that can be followed or adopted. Human life and what it means to be human are principally open to definition and the world in which we find ourselves is completely contingent, meaning that it could have been different or not have been at all. Living a human life demands that we must find our personal answer to the big question of what the meaning of our life is. Each one of the ultimate concerns deals with the totality of human life, and each one of them is connected to a fundamental anxiety.

The ultimate concern of death is connected to our mortality as human beings. When we realise that any moment in time, we may lose all that matters to us, or any person that is intensely loved by us, we are confronted with the vulnerability of human life. The reality of death can hardly be grasped and Yalom quotes the French thinker La Rochefoucauld in stating that '*neither the sun nor death can be looked at steadily*' [14]. Because the naked truth about our vulnerability is hardly bearable, we have found innumerable ways of diverting from this truth. The grief that relates to a big loss, brings us back to the realisation that all of us will ultimately lose our life and everything that is dear to us. Becoming aware that my existence is threatened raises fundamental questions about the meaning of my life and what my personal way of dying looks like.

The ultimate concern of freedom is related to our potential as human beings to make choices. Although, from its beginning, every human life is determined by many cultural, biological, and genetic factors, there is always the possibility to respond personally to what happens to us as described by one of the founders of existential therapy, Victor Frankl [15]. This freedom makes it possible for us to take responsibility for our lives. It also confronts us with the existential question of how to live a life worth living, how to use our freedom even when we are suffering. The fact that for every direction taken, there are many directions not taken, may result in regret or fear of making mistakes or missing out. When we begin to realise that the whole world might have been different, this may result in a fundamental anxiety about how to live with the freedom that we have. When we are subjected to loss and grief, it is understandable to try and escape the pain or want to avoid it. However, in an existential understanding, we all will face loss and grief and therefore can choose to increase our awareness of how to meet and take responsibility for our responses.

The ultimate concern of isolation is rooted in the social dimension of human nature. Human beings are essentially social beings who can only survive and thrive in connectedness with other humans. Isolation is the loss of connectedness and the fear of losing this connectedness with those who are dear to us plays a big role in the choices and decisions that are made at the end of life. When facing loss and grief, most people report challenges with connecting to other people and declare how painful the lack of connectedness is. Loss and grief can change the personal sense of vulnerability and place different demands on communication and social relations resulting in painful experiences of isolation.

Finally, the ultimate concern of meaninglessness is a big challenge for every human being. As humans, we orient ourselves in the world by making sense of it. This gives a sense of security and direction in our life. The situational meaning of everyday experiences is embedded in global meaning structures that give an answer to the bigger questions in life [16]. Once we experience a big loss, this global meaning structure can be challenged or even collapse. We fall into an existential void and realise that it is impossible to face the cold and indifference of a life without meaning. This can be very painful and anxiety provoking.

All four ultimate concerns confront us with the question of how I respond to the call of life, what my personal answer is to the situation I find myself in, and how to deal with the suffering that can be connected to it. This means that loss and grief can be a window to existential awareness. It is evident that in the case of being diagnosed with a terminal illness or losing someone we love, all four ultimate concerns resonate. How could palliative care respond to this existential dimension of loss and grief? How does the four-dimensional total pain approach work out when applied to the existential dimension of loss and grief?

3 An Integrative Approach to Loss and Grief

The total pain approach that is central to palliative care distinguishes between physical, psychological, social, and spiritual dimensions [2]. Although one could easily connect each dimension with one or more disciplines or professions, the idea that suffering is four dimensional urges us to reflect on the temptation to simplify a complex phenomenon like suffering by assigning different aspects to different domains or disciplines. The challenge and the strength of total pain are to develop an interdisciplinary or interprofessional approach to pain and suffering. Since the existential dimension of loss and grief has a similar structure—resonating with all dimensions of our being—we propose to follow this interdisciplinary perspective and connect each dimension with an ultimate concern: the physical (death), psychological (freedom), social (isolation), and spiritual (meaninglessness).

As described above, most of the research on loss and grief has been done from the disciplinary perspective of psychology. The vast amount of psychological research that was done in the last decades has given some important building blocks that can be integrated into an interprofessional approach that aligns with the palliative care approach. One building block is the finding that processes can be understood in terms of moving between polarities. In the currently most used understanding of grief, the Dual Process Model, the grieving process depicted as an oscillation between two poles: loss-oriented and restoration-oriented activities [17].

A similar approach in polarities is found in spiritual literature around the end of life, from the late medieval art-of-dying tradition to its contemporary adaptation in the Diamond model [18, 19]. In the medieval art-of-dying tradition, the dying person was oscillating between faith and loss of faith, hope and despair, love and avarice, impatience and patience, humility, and complacency. In the Diamond model, the oscillation is between connectedness to myself and others, doing and undergoing, holding on and letting go, remembering and forgetting, and knowing and believing. When the suffering of loss is understood from the ultimate concerns and the polarities, existential tensions emerge that we all know. It is then possible to integrate wisdom from spiritual traditions with knowledge from recent psychological research. To show how such an interprofessional model might help understanding the different dimensions of loss and grief, we now present each dimension and the orientations that can be connected to them when grievers are accompanied in navigating their sorrow (see Fig. 1) [20, 21].

The physical dimension of grief can hardly be overlooked as the grieving body is destabilised and affected by biochemical and neuro-physiological processes [22]. Acute grief is often accompanied by symptoms like loss of appetite, energy loss, sleep disturbances, fatigue, and a many more somatic complaints. The destabilising experience of acute grief calls us to find ground again, connecting to our self and our vulnerability. From an existential perspective, this situation demands that we acknowledge human beings as vulnerable and mortal among all other beings that are alive and thus destined to die one day. Thus, the physical dimension, connected to the ultimate concern of death, is characterised by an existential tension and struggle between embracing life and accepting death.

The psychological dimension of grief, connected to the ultimate concern of freedom, can be divided into two parts to better understand the processes related to navigating the existential dimension of loss and grief. In real life, these dimensions are very much intertwined as we go about our daily business. The emotional dimension of the grief process is connected to freedom since emotions can overwhelm us to such a degree that we are completely swept away or dictated by them. In psychological studies, this relates to the task of emotion regulation [23, 24]. Emotion regulation means to be in contact with one's grief, but also being mindful to withdraw when the impact becomes overwhelming and destructive. Emotion regulation can be characterised by the ability to be connected to one's emotions and simultaneously having the ability to either focus or minimise emotions and thereby regulate the degree to which one is exposed. It is an important form of care for the self to not get emotionally overwhelmed by grief and risk the development of mental health problems. From an existential perspective, we can speak of a polarity of undergoing

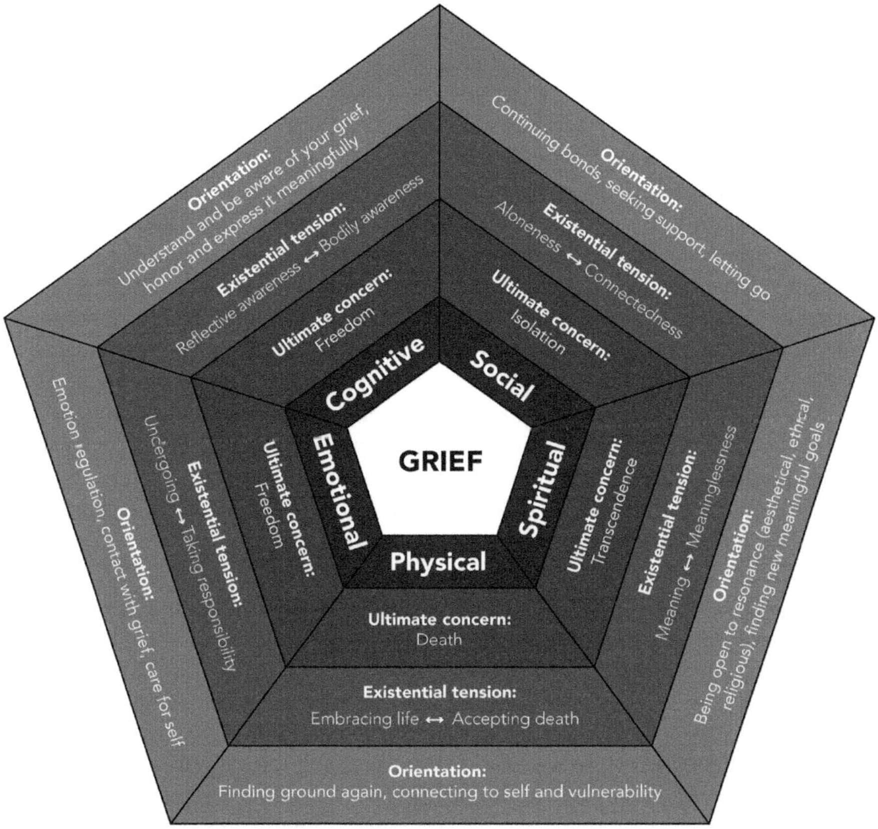

Fig. 1 The Integrative Process Model with all dimensions, ultimate concerns, existential tensions, and orientations

and taking responsibility, by which we focus on or minimise emotions, practice self-care, ask for help, etc. while we navigate the emotional dimension of grief.

The second aspect of the psychological dimension of grief is the cognitive dimension. The cognitive dimension is also connected to the ultimate concern of freedom, since it concerns the schemata that are upholding our understanding of the world. Knowledge is not exclusively connected to our rational capacities. Our body is also full of tacit and unarticulated knowledge about how we are connected to and situated in the world [25]. A striking example of this is the experience that people with dementia who are hardly capable of rational coherent conversation are still able to play the piano as if they have no mental problems at all. As in any mental struggle, the cognitive dimension of grief stretches from reflective awareness to an bodily awareness. Many people ruminate about their loss, maybe even try to deny it, or engage in a type of magical thinking to avoid looking at reality [26, 27]. Navigating this dimension centres around supporting patients and families acknowledging their loss, getting to know their grief, and becoming more aware of the psychological schemata that shape their grief. Existentially this dimension is about the freedom to understand and be aware of our grief, and honour and express it in a meaningful way. In the palliative care setting, transcending old schemata can be helpful to achieve inner freedom and relieve suffering.

The social dimension of grief, connected to the ultimate concern of isolation, possesses many aspects. On an individual level, this dimension confronts us on one side with the question of how to honour the loss and on the other side, the meaningful connectedness to the lost (or dying) of which we become so painfully aware. The continuing bonds theory, showing that people across different cultures continue their relationship with the deceased in different fulfilling and meaningful ways after a loss, has put this insight at the centre of attention [7]. On an interpersonal level, this dimension affirms our social nature as human beings since both being ill and dying are also by nature social processes. Communities and rituals can be a great support, helping to deal with grief and deepening meaningful connections while saying goodbye. Thus, at both levels, the social dimension is characterised by the existential poles of aloneness and connectedness. The existential dimension of this tension is connected to our search for meaningful connections with other human beings who are co-constitutive to our identity.

Lastly, the spiritual dimension of grief refers to the way we find meaning and transcendence while going through the dying process or after a loss that has affected the global meaning structure that helps us make sense of the world [28]. But how to make sense of the world when one's global meaning structure, either religious or non-religious, has collapsed? What can we build on? And will we ever be able to have trust in life again? Here we enter the existential tension between meaning and meaningfulness. To some people it is (medical or scientific) knowledge that brings security and a foothold. Others look for grounding in believing and surrendering to what cannot be completely known or understood. Being open to resonance (aesthetical, ethical, religious) and finding new meaningful goals are central orientations in this dimension [29].

Following this interdisciplinary and interprofessional approach to the existential dimension of grief, it becomes apparent how an integrative approach to loss and grief has the potential of merging knowledge from different disciplines. Spiritual processes are largely dependent on and shaped by psychological processes, rooted in physiological processes, and situated in a social context. Loss and grief are as multi-dimensional and complex as any experiences that affect our existence as a whole.

In the context of palliative care, this comprehensive understanding of loss and grief is also reflected in the best possible relief and outcome for the family, who are in the process of losing or have lost a dear one. In psychological research, this has been coined as post-traumatic growth, the theory which holds that following a struggle and adversity, people can experience positive growth [30]. In our integrative process model, we would understand this growth as the alignment of all five dimensions we discussed. However, existentially, only the person themselves can define what this growth or new insight is about. Per definition this cannot be pre-defined as a goal by others. As pain often starts with an imbalance in one or more dimensions resulting in a reductionist view of the world by the griever, the more balanced the processes are, and the more aligned they develop, they may reinforce each other into more coherence and life energy resulting in the person being able to deal with the struggles the way they would want to.

Having sketched the outline of an integrative process model of grief, let us now see how such an approach would work out in palliative care. How would this model be helpful in understanding the multi-dimensional phenomenon of grief in a palliative care situation?

4 Working with Loss and Grief in Palliative Care

Flora and Robert, both in their mid-fifties, had just been to see the oncologist after Robert had received immune therapy for his bladder cancer for several months. The oncologist recommended stopping treatment and referring Robert to palliative care. The immune therapy had not helped, Robert was in a lot of pain, and he had experienced some complications from earlier treatments. Even though Flora and Robert had been confined to their home, seeing no friends and family for several weeks, the message took them by surprise. On the way home in the car, they were both very quiet. Having met each other only five years ago, Flora had already lost a husband to cancer earlier in her life. Now she kept thinking: 'When will I lose Robert?'

Robert was very quiet, struggling to comprehend the message and feeling overwhelmed by worry. When they came home Flora made a cup of coffee for them and suggested they have a talk. However, Robert excused himself and said he needed to lie down.

In palliative care, loss and grief are present from the moment of breaking bad news, both for the patient and the family. The awareness that Robert cannot be cured from his bladder cancer has great impact on both Robert and Flora. Although both have a different experience of the situation, given their position and life history, each one of them is existentially affected by what happens. How can the integrative process model be of help here to create awareness of the comprehensiveness of what is at stake and how both partners can navigate the existential tensions that they find themselves in?

Being confronted with the ultimate concern of death, Robert is completely overwhelmed. His many worries seem to be confirmed all at once. It leaves him speechless and takes him down. As he loses all hope of being cured, the hope that had kept him and Flora going for several weeks, he must face the loss of his life, his future, his wife, all the plans they had together in a life that was still in a phase of building up a relationship. Being so massively confronted with his vulnerability and mortality, Robert is not able to find or connect to himself. Emotionally, Robert is so overwhelmed that he has a hard time regulating his emotions and feeling any space for a free choice or decisions. His reflective awareness is hardly functioning either. He asks for a time out, excusing himself and in need of a lie down. Robert withdraws to find himself again. It is too early for any social or spiritual support or talk.

Palliative care aims at supporting both the patient and the family. Flora, like Robert, is heavily affected by the bad news. In her case, however, the first thing that happens is an existential activation of a previous loss. The news that Robert cannot be cured brings back the process she had gone through with her first husband. It colours her experience of the here and now so strongly that she too needs time to find herself again and become aware of the space there is to shape the final weeks or months with Robert in the best possible way. Being overwhelmed by the ultimate concern of isolation, she is inclined to hold on tighter to Robert, but she also knows from her earlier experience that eventually she will have to find a way to let go of him. For now, however, the orientation might be to deepen her connectedness with Robert in the time they share. As she also feels the loss of the dream of building a life together, losing the future that she had imagined of growing old together with Robert, she realises that at one point in the future, she will have to face looking for new meaningful goals once again.

The example of Robert and Flora makes clear how in some phases of the process of loss and grief, one or more dimensions are foregrounded, and other dimensions remain in the background. The Integrative Process Model illustrates how the experience of loss and grief as an existential process can be unpacked in the described five dimensions. Each one of these dimensions is present all the time, and although the dimensions can be discerned from each other, they cannot be separated from each other. Nor is one of these five dimensions the whole story of the person's grief. The Integrative Process Model may help patients, significant others, and professionals to understand the comprehensiveness of the existential dimension of loss and grief, so they can navigate in the tensions that ask for an authentic answer to the ultimate concerns in life (see Table 1).

Table 1 Questions that can be used in a conversation for existential reflection on loss and grief

Physical dimension	- How can I stabilise my body? - How can I live with the reality of the loss? - How will I get acquainted with loss and death?
Emotional dimension	- How can I practice self-care? - How/when do I connect to my grief? - How can I honour my grief?
Cognitive dimension	- What is my grief about? - How can I get acquainted with my grief? - How can I grief this loss meaningfully?
Social dimension	- How can I continue the bond? - How can I let go of/change the bond? - How can I reach out to others and connect?
Spiritual dimension	- How is this loss changing my understanding of life? - How can I find meaning again? - What are my revised goals in life?

5 Conclusion

In this chapter, we have introduced an interprofessional and interdisciplinary model to work with existential dimension of loss and grief in palliative care: the Integrative Process Model. The model integrates different mainstream theories of loss and grief around an understanding of loss and grief as an existential and comprehensive experience. The idea behind the model is not to replace existing theories of loss and grief, but to connect them in a meaningful way. Different approaches, models, theoretical understandings, and therapeutic interventions that have been developed are still useful and important. They may even be more helpful when placed in the broader perspective of the Integrative Process Model. In the coming years, the model will be further researched and tested so that the theoretical strength is underpinned with empirical evidence. In this way, palliative care may improve and develop in the spirit of the original total pain approach developed more than half a century ago.

References

1. Guldin MB, Leget C. Integrating existential and psychosocial palliative care: insights from a world café. 2024, forthcoming.
2. Brant J. Holistic total pain management in palliative care: cultural and global considerations. Palliat Med Hosp Care Open J. 2017;1:S32–8.
3. Tam M. Medereiziger, steun voor de partner van een ongeneeslijk zieke. Utrecht: Stili novi; 2014.
4. Freud S. Mourning and melancholia (J. Strachey, trans.). In: Strachey J, editor. The standard edition of the complete psychological works of Sigmund Freud, vol. 14. Hogarth Press & Institute of psychoanalysis (1917); 1957. p. 239–60.
5. Kübler-Ross E. On death and dying. New York: Macmillan; 1969.
6. Worden JW. Grief counseling and grief therapy: a handbook for the mental health practitioner. New York: Springer; 1991.
7. Klass D, Silverman PR, Nickman S. Continuing bonds: new understandings of grief. Washington, DC: Taylor & Francis; 2014.
8. Stroebe M, Schut H. The dual process model of coping with bereavement: rationale and description. Death Stud. 1999;23(3):197–224. https://doi.org/10.1080/074811899201046.
9. Nielsen MK, Carlsen AH, Neergaard MA, Bidstrup PE, Guldin MB. Looking beyond the mean in grief trajectories: a prospective, population-based cohort study. Soc Sci Med. 2019;232:460–9.
10. Cholbi M. Grief. A philosophical guide. Princeton University Press, Princeton; 2021.
11. Guldin MB. Tab og sorg. En gundbog for professionelle [Loss and grief. A handbook for professionals]. 2nd ed. Copenhagen: Hans Reitzels Forlag; 2019.
12. Yalom ID. Existential psychotherapy. New York: Basic Books; 1980.
13. Cooper M. Existential therapies. 2nd ed. London: Sage Publications Ltd; 2003.
14. Yalom ID. Staring at the sun: overcoming the terror of death. Humanist Psychol. 2008;36(3–4):283–97.
15. Frankl V. Man's search for meaning. Boston: Beacon Press; 2006.
16. Park CL. The meaning making model: a framework for understanding meaning, spirituality, and stress-related growth in health psychology. Eur Health Psychol. 2013;15(2):40–7.

17. Stroebe M, Schut H. The dual process model of coping with bereavement: a decade on. Omega (Westport). 2010;61(4):273–89. https://doi.org/10.2190/OM.61.4.b.
18. Girard-Augry P. Ars moriendi (1492) ou L'art de bien mourir. Paris: Dervy; 1986.
19. Leget C. Art of living, art of dying. Spiritual care for a good death. London: Jessica Kingsley Publishers; 2017.
20. Guldin MB, Leget C. The integrated process model of loss and grief – an interprofessional understanding. Death Stud. 2023;48:738. https://doi.org/10.1080/07481187.2023.2272960.
21. Guldin MB, Leget C. Loss, grief and existential awareness. An Integrative Approach. London: Routledge; 2024.
22. O'Connor MF. Grief: a brief history of research on how body, mind, and brain adapt. Psychosom Med. 2019;81(8):731–8. https://doi.org/10.1097/psy.0000000000000717.
23. Bonanno GA, Westphal M, Mancin AD. Resilience to loss and potential trauma. Annu Rev Clin Psychol. 2011;7:511–35. https://doi.org/10.1146/annurev-clinpsy-032210-104526.
24. Gross JJ. Emotion regulation: conceptual and empirical foundations. In: Gross JJ, editor. Handbook of emotion regulation. The Guilford Press; 2014. p. 3–20.
25. Merleau-Ponty M. Phenomenology of perception. Translated by Colin Smith. London: Routledge; 1965.
26. Brennan F, Dash M. The year of magical thinking: Joan Didion and the dialectic of grief. Med Humanit. 2008;34(1):35–9.
27. Neimeyer RA, Pitcho-Prelorentzos S, Mahat-Shamir M. "If Only…": counterfactual thinking in bereavement. Death Stud. 2021;45(9):692–701. https://doi.org/10.1080/07481187.2019.1679959.
28. Nolan S, Saltmarsh P, Leget C. Spiritual care in palliative care: working towards an EAPC task force. EJPC. 2011;18(2):86–9.
29. Rosa H. Resonance: a sociology of our relationship to the world. Cambridge: Polity Press; 2019.
30. Tedeschi RG, Calhoun LG. Posttraumatic growth: conceptual foundations and empirical evidence. Psychol Inq. 2004;15(1):1–18.

Prevention and Treatment of Suffering Through Mindfulness

Tan Seng Beng

Abstract This chapter delves into the realm of preventing and treating psychoexistential suffering within the context of palliative care, taking into account the intricate interplay between suffering and holistic well-being among patients, family caregivers, and healthcare providers. It introduces *The Fractals of Quality of Life* framework, underscoring the significance of integrating mindfulness practices in two distinct phases to effectively address suffering. The initial phase entails the cultivation of mindfulness during patient care, while the subsequent phase centres on guiding individuals through concise mindfulness exercises. By acknowledging the profound interconnectedness of suffering and well-being, and by incorporating mindfulness into practice, healthcare providers can actively engage in the prevention and treatment of suffering and the promotion of overall well-being, thereby fostering a comprehensive and holistic approach to palliative care.

Keywords Suffering · Well-being · Quality of life · Palliative care · Mindfulness Spiritual Care

1 The Triangle of Suffering: Patients, Caregivers, and Healthcare Providers

The triangle of suffering in palliative care acknowledges the interconnectedness of psychoexistential suffering among patients, family caregivers, and healthcare providers [1]. The perceived suffering of any individual within the triangle can impact

T. S. Beng (✉)
Department of Palliative Medicine, Subang Jaya Medical Centre, Subang Jaya, Malaysia
e-mail: tan.seng.beng@rsdhealth.com

M. C. Best (ed.), *Spiritual Care in Palliative Care*,
https://doi.org/10.1007/978-3-031-50864-6_26

the others [2, 3]. To prevent suffering, a comprehensive approach is needed. This involves addressing the suffering of patients through effective symptom management and psychosocial support, supporting family caregivers with resources and education, and promoting the well-being of healthcare providers through self-care programmes and professional development [4, 5]. By recognising and addressing the interrelation of suffering, palliative care teams can create a compassionate environment that promotes healing and dignity for all involved in end-of-life care.

1.1 The First Vertex: Patients

The first vertex within the triangle of suffering pertains to the suffering experienced by palliative care patients. One valuable framework for understanding their suffering is the *existential-experiential model,* which provides insights into the complex nature of suffering from both an events and experiences perspective [6].

Existential suffering, when viewed through the lens of events, encompasses the losses and changes that patients encounter throughout their illness trajectory. These can include physical abilities, independence, social roles, and familiar routines that are disrupted by the disease [7, 8]. Patients may struggle with dependency on others for their basic needs, witnessing the suffering of loved ones, confronting their own disease and mortality, and enduring unpleasant healthcare encounters or hospital stays [9–14].

Experiential suffering involves understanding suffering from the standpoint of patients' subjective experiences. It encompasses sensory, emotional, cognitive, and spiritual dimensions. Sensory suffering involves physical pain, discomfort, and other bodily sensations [7, 15–17]. Emotional suffering encompasses the range of intense emotions such as fear, sadness, anxiety, or anger [18]. Cognitive suffering refers to mental distress arising from thoughts, beliefs, or concerns related to their illness and prognosis [19]. Lastly, spiritual suffering explores the distress patients may encounter when grappling with questions of meaning, purpose, faith, or the uncertainty surrounding their spiritual beliefs [20, 21].

1.2 The Second Vertex: Family Caregivers

The model of *compassion suffering* in family caregivers delves into the complex dynamics of suffering experienced by caregivers as they provide care to their loved ones [22]. Compassion suffering can be understood through the lens of perceptions, intentions, and actions, shedding light on the multifaceted nature of caregivers' experiences and offering insights into the prevention of suffering.

Perceptions of patients' suffering play a crucial role in compassion suffering. Caregivers may undergo empathic suffering as they witness, hear about, and worry about the pain and distress endured by their loved ones [23]. Anticipatory grief may arise from the perceived impending death of patients and the anticipation of their eventual absence [24].

Intentions to relieve patients' suffering can also contribute to compassion suffering. Caregivers may become obsessed with providing the best care. They may also feel compelled to keep the patient alive at all costs, even if it means pursuing futile interventions [25]. The sense of helplessness and powerlessness can emerge when caregivers lack vital information and support, leaving them feeling overwhelmed and incapable of effectively addressing the patient's needs [26].

The actions taken to alleviate the patient's suffering can give rise to further compassion suffering. Caregivers may experience the burden of companionship, shouldering the responsibility of providing emotional support and being present for the patient [27]. Functional assistance, such as attending to daily tasks and medical needs, may also contribute to the caregiver's suffering. Financial burdens and maintaining a cheerful attitude in the face of adversity can also become sources of distress.

Numerous challenges can amplify the experience of compassion suffering during the execution of actions aimed at alleviating the suffering of patients. Patient-related challenges, such as complex physical and psychological issues, disparities in preferences, and the family dynamics and differing opinions regarding the patient's care, can significantly impact the caregiver's well-being [28]. Healthcare-related obstacles, including challenges in obtaining necessary information, navigating interactions with healthcare professionals, and addressing institutional issues, can also add to the caregiver's suffering [29]. Moreover, the caregiver's personal and social life can be profoundly affected, leading to repercussions such as strained relationships, social isolation, and an overall impact on their quality of life [30].

1.3 The Third Vertex: Healthcare Providers

Healthcare providers involved in palliative care often face significant stress and suffering as they face the challenges inherent in their roles. The suffering can emerge from a range of factors, spanning from challenges related to caring for others to challenges related to self-care, with interpersonal issues falling in between [31].

Challenges related to caring for others include organisational issues and care overload. Organisational issues can contribute to the stress experienced by palliative care providers. Team dysfunction and staffing issues, such as inadequate staffing levels or a lack of cohesion within the team, can create additional burdens and hinder the delivery of high-quality care [32]. Limited resources, including financial constraints and limited access to specialised equipment or medications, can further compound the challenges faced by providers [33].

Care overload, both quantitative and qualitative, can be a significant source of stress. Palliative care providers often find themselves faced with a high volume of patients requiring complex care, which can lead to a sense of overwhelming responsibility [34]. Additionally, the qualitative aspects of care, such as managing patients' pain and symptoms effectively, addressing their emotional and spiritual needs, and supporting their families, can place a substantial emotional and psychological burden on providers [35].

Communication challenges can also contribute to stress and suffering. Palliative care providers must navigate difficult conversations with patients and their families, discussing sensitive topics such as prognosis, treatment options, and end-of-life decisions [36]. Differences in opinions among healthcare professionals and patients or families can lead to conflict and additional stress [37]. Misperceptions and misconceptions about palliative care and opioids can further complicate communication, requiring providers to invest additional effort in educating and addressing concerns [38, 39].

Personal expectations can significantly impact the well-being of palliative care providers. They may perceive that they are not doing enough for their patients or feel a sense of failure if they are unable to alleviate suffering completely. The perceived helplessness in the face of patients' uncontrolled symptoms or psychosocial distress can further contribute to feelings of stress and suffering [40].

Emotional involvement is an inherent aspect of palliative care, as providers develop close relationships with patients and their families. This emotional connection can amplify the stress experienced by providers, as they witness the suffering of their patients and share in their grief [41]. The constant exposure to death and dying can also lead to intrusive thoughts and preoccupations further impacting the emotional well-being of providers [42].

2 The Triangle of Well-Being

While the triangular model of suffering elucidates the interconnectedness of distress experienced by patients, family caregivers, and healthcare providers, conversely, an alternative triangular model of well-being exists. This model recognises that the well-being of each element is intricately linked to the well-being of the others. For example, patients' well-being is enhanced by the support and understanding of their families, while healthcare professionals draw strength and fulfilment from witnessing positive patient and family outcomes. Thus, the triangle of well-being in palliative care highlights the holistic nature of care, emphasising the interconnectedness of well-being among patients, families, and healthcare professionals as well as the interconnectedness between the dimensions of well-being.

2.1 The First Vertex: Patients

Merely addressing the presence of suffering in palliative care is insufficient; it is equally imperative to direct attention towards promotion of well-being. The *Seeds Model*, a metaphorical framework, conceptualises the mind as a fertile field wherein various seeds are sown. These seeds encompass our perceptions, thoughts, emotions, actions, and interactions, and they germinate and grow based on how they are nurtured [43]. In the context of preventing suffering, the model highlights six fundamental aspects, each representing a distinct type of seed that, when appropriately watered, can contribute to enhancing the well-being of palliative care patients. These seeds include positive attitudes, cognitions, emotions, engagement, relationships, and circumstances.

Cultivating a positive attitude through acceptance, kindness, and resilience helps patients find peace and navigate challenges [44]. Nurturing positive cognitions, such as hope, optimism, faith, and wisdom, fosters a sense of possibility, optimism, comfort, and purpose [45]. Promoting positive emotions, like calmness and happiness, reduces stress and uplifts spirits [46, 47]. Encouraging positive engagement through routine and leisure activities maintains structure and brings joy [48]. Developing positive relationships provides practical and psychological support, addressing patients' needs and fostering emotional well-being [49]. Creating positive circumstances involves effective symptom management and maximising functional abilities [50]. (See case study in Box 1.)

Box 1 Case Study

Madam B, a woman diagnosed with stage IV pancreatic cancer that has spread to her lungs, exemplifies the Seeds Model approach to enhancing her quality of life. Despite her prognosis, she cultivates a positive attitude through acceptance of her situation, being kind to herself and others, and resilience, engaging in self-care routines and maintaining her determination to cherish each day. Nurturing hope, optimism, and faith, Madam B draws strength from her Buddhist beliefs and remains optimistic about her chemotherapy treatment. Through calming practices like Qigong and her passion for dancing, she fosters positive emotions, managing anxiety and finding moments of happiness. With a structured daily routine encompassing gentle exercises, family time, and leisure activities like dancing, she encourages positive engagement. Madam B's strong support networks provide both practical and psychological support, allowing her to share her feelings openly and maintain a sense of purpose. In fact, at the beginning of the diagnosis of her terminal illness, her children took 6 months unpaid leave to take care of her. As her healthcare team, we focus on managing her cough with opioid, and maximising her functional abilities using oxygen supplement. In Madam B's journey, the convergence of positive attitude, cognitions, emotions, engagement, relationships, and holistic care creates a narrative of dignity and grace amid the challenges of her advanced cancer.

2.2 The Second Vertex: Family Caregivers

Enhancing the well-being of family caregivers in the context of palliative care involves several key factors, including acceptance, gratitude, hope, happiness, and support [51]. Firstly, acceptance plays a vital role. Acknowledging and accepting their caregiver roles, as well as the imminent death of their loved ones, helps them navigate the challenges they face [52]. Acceptance allows caregivers to adapt to their changing circumstances and provide the necessary support to patients during this sensitive phase.

Acceptance is a process that cannot be rushed and is subject to fluctuations. For many, this dynamic acceptance process often oscillates between acceptance and avoidance. To foster acceptance, healthcare providers can play a vital role by engaging in effective communication, providing presence, offering explanations, education, and preparing families for the inevitable outcome. Applying principles from *Acceptance and Commitment Therapy* (ACT), such as focusing on the present moment, cultivating self-awareness, managing thoughts without being controlled by them, embracing difficult thoughts, recognising values, and taking purposeful actions, can significantly aid family caregivers [53]. While not all healthcare providers may be trained in ACT, those who possess the training can effectively apply its techniques to support distressed family caregivers.

Secondly, gratitude is an important aspect of caregiver well-being [54]. Expressing gratitude towards family members, healthcare providers, and their faith can help caregivers find solace and meaning amidst their caregiving journey. Recognising the support received and feeling grateful for it can foster a sense of appreciation and positivity.

Thirdly, maintaining hope is crucial. Family caregivers often hold hope for their loved ones, as well as hope for themselves and their own resilience [55]. Cultivating hope allows caregivers to envision a better future, cope with challenges, and maintain a sense of purpose and motivation. Strategies to nurture hope in caregivers involve building connections, respecting their roles, acknowledging their strengths and bravery, maintaining a light-hearted atmosphere during interactions, assisting them in setting achievable short-term goals, helping them recall positive memories, and acknowledging their spiritual beliefs and practices.

Furthermore, happiness can be nurtured through spending quality time with patients and engaging in activities that bring joy and fulfilment [56]. Recognising the importance of self-care and allocating time for activities they enjoy can help caregivers replenish their energy and experience moments of happiness, contributing to their overall well-being.

Lastly, support from various sources is essential for caregiver well-being [57]. Receiving support from family members, friends, healthcare providers, and having faith-based support can alleviate the emotional and physical burden on caregivers. Social connections and networks provide opportunities for sharing experiences, seeking advice, and finding comfort in knowing they are not alone in their caregiving journey.

2.3 The Third Vertex: Healthcare Providers

The *resilience-reward model* offers insights into the well-being of palliative care providers, focusing on resilience and reward as key components [58]. Resilience is nurtured through values and strengths, coping and work–life balance, as well as social support and spirituality. The reward aspect involves experiencing passion and satisfaction, as well as learning, growth, and transformation.

Resilience is fortified by recognising and cultivating essential values and strengths within palliative care providers [59]. These include love, compassion, empathy, respect, gratitude, competence, and self-awareness. Emphasising these qualities allows providers to draw upon their inner resources, enabling them to navigate the emotional challenges inherent in palliative care. For example, when practising mindfulness during patient interactions, healthcare providers can display genuine care and kindness, actively empathising with patients, treating them with dignity and respect, embracing gratitude while maintaining professional competence, and fostering self-awareness to prevent burnout.

Effective coping strategies and maintaining a healthy work–life balance are also crucial for resilience [60, 61]. Providers can employ techniques such as effective communication, setting professional boundaries, empathy-based cognitive restructuring, calming down strategies, acceptance of reality, and active participation in social and recreational activities. These approaches help manage stress, promote emotional well-being, and prevent burnout.

Social support, both from the professional team and personal networks including family and friends, play a pivotal role in bolstering resilience [62]. Engaging in spiritual practices and drawing strength from one's faith can provide solace and guidance, serving as a source of support in the face of emotional demands [63].

Moving to the reward aspect, passion and satisfaction are essential rewards for palliative care providers [64]. They find passion in caring for patients and derive satisfaction from the impact they make in their patients' lives. Feeling appreciated for their work further reinforces their sense of reward.

Additionally, the model highlights the potential for learning, growth, and transformation. Providers gain insights into human resilience, the intricacies of humanity, the profound dimensions of love, patience, and caring, as well as the limits of caring. They develop awareness of the inevitability and unpredictability of death, becoming less afraid and more accepting of their reality. Through these experiences, providers develop a sense of completeness and purpose, discovering the meaning in life. They strengthen their faith, become more self-aware, and emphasise self-care as they understand the importance of their own well-being [65].

3 The Fractals of Quality of Life

The *Fractals of Quality of Life* is a conceptual framework for assessing and understanding the multidimensional nature of quality of life in palliative care, as shown in Fig. 1. Building upon the triangular model of suffering, which elucidates the interconnectedness of suffering among patients, family caregivers, and healthcare providers, and overlaying it with the triangle of well-being, which highlights the interconnection of well-being among these same groups, the framework forms a hexagon as its foundational structure. This hexagon serves as the base from which the fractal unfolds.

Within the Fractals of Quality of Life, the vertices of the hexagon represent patients, family caregivers, and healthcare providers, forming the core elements of the framework. From these vertices, various experiences of suffering and well-being

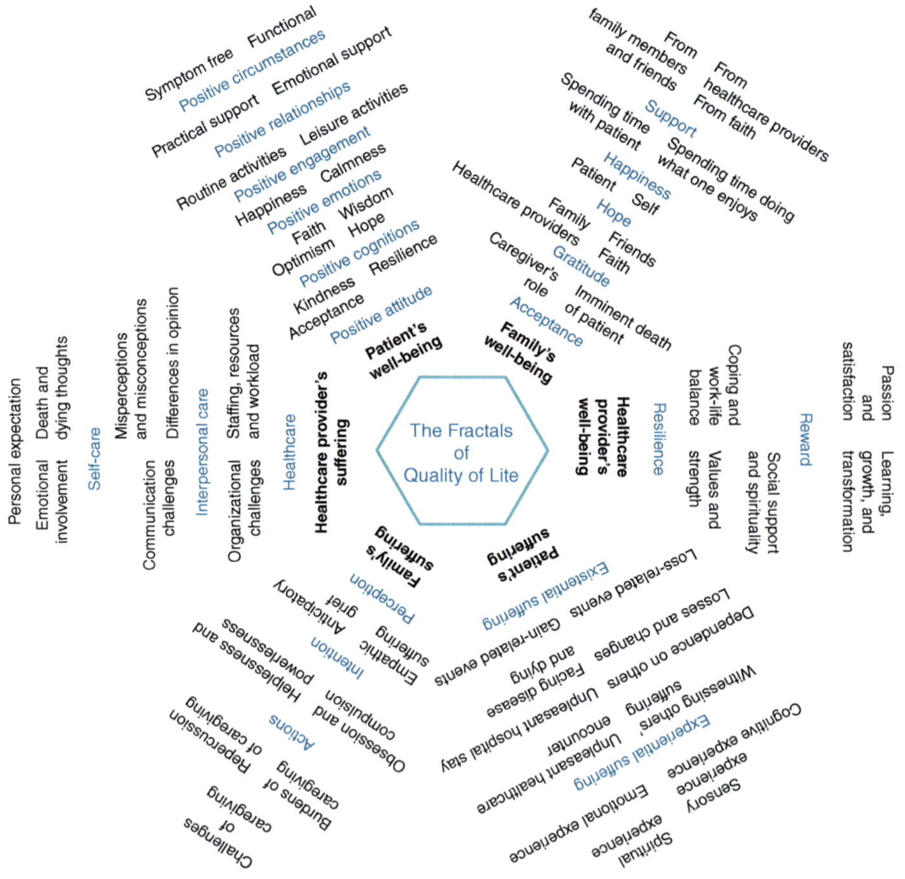

Fig. 1 The fractals of quality of life

emanate, branching out and expanding in a fractal pattern. The fractal nature of the framework implies that the experiences of suffering and well-being occur at multiple levels, encompassing diverse dimensions and intricacies.

The fractal branches symbolise the multifaceted aspects of suffering and well-being within palliative care. They encompass physical, psychological, social, and spiritual dimensions, capturing the complexity of the human experience in the context of illness, caregiving, and healthcare provision. These branches extend beyond the surface level, delving into deeper layers of meaning and significance.

3.1 Strategies to Address Suffering in Palliative Care

Within the framework of The Fractals of Quality of Life, the uniqueness of suffering becomes evident for each patient, family caregiver, and healthcare provider. This fractal recognises that suffering is not a one-size-fits-all experience, but rather a deeply personal and individualised journey. Each person involved in the palliative care process brings their own set of circumstances, and challenges, resulting in a distinct manifestation of suffering.

Understanding this uniqueness is crucial in preventing suffering effectively. By examining the individual Fractal of Quality of Life, we gain insight into the specific areas where suffering may arise. This allows us to tailor interventions and support to address the unique needs and experiences of each person. It reminds us that a comprehensive approach to care goes beyond simply alleviating physical symptoms but also encompasses emotional, psychological, and spiritual aspects.

By acknowledging and addressing the individual Fractal of Quality of Life, we can proactively prevent and minimise suffering. This involves recognising the interconnection between suffering and well-being, and focusing on cultivating positive elements such as compassion, empathy, and resilience. Through this approach, we empower patients, family caregivers, and healthcare providers to navigate their journey with greater support, understanding, and improved quality of life. The individual Fractal serves as a roadmap for personalised care, ensuring that suffering is not only alleviated but prevented wherever possible, fostering a holistic approach to well-being in palliative care. In this context, mindfulness, with its capacity to promote psychological flexibility, could be the key to creating a paradigm shift that has the potential to change the landscape of how we address suffering.

3.2 Mindfulness in the Prevention and Treatment of Suffering

Mindfulness is a practice of intentionally paying attention to the present moment, non-judgementally, and with an attitude of acceptance [66]. It involves bringing awareness to one's thoughts, feelings, bodily sensations, and the surrounding environment. By cultivating mindfulness, individuals develop a deeper understanding of themselves, their experiences, and the interconnectedness of their thoughts, emotions, and actions.

In the context of The Fractals of Quality of Life, mindfulness can be integrated in two phases to address suffering and enhance well-being. The first phase involves the application of mindfulness-based supportive therapy (MBST), a psychotherapy approach tailored for palliative care [67, 68]. In the second phase, brief guided mindfulness exercises can be used to target individual suffering and transform inner experiences [69–72].

4 Mindfulness-Based Supportive Therapy (First Phase)

Mindfulness-based supportive therapy (MBST) represents a pioneering psychotherapeutic approach specifically tailored to address psychoexistential suffering within the context of palliative care [67, 68]. This innovative therapy comprises five integral components, namely mindful presence, mindful listening, mindful empathy, mindful compassion, and mindfulness of boundaries, distinguished from conventional mindfulness-based interventions by its emphasis on fostering the therapist's own mindfulness during patient care.

MBST is a flexible approach that doesn't have specific limits on time or the number of sessions. It can be used by various healthcare providers to help patients, caregivers, or both concurrently. It's useful in different settings like hospitals, homes, or hospices, and can be stopped whenever needed. It can also be a bridge to subsequent psychotherapies based on the specific needs identified from the sessions.

The training regimen encompasses two sessions. The initial session introduces the fundamental underpinnings, framework, and practical application of MBST. Subsequently, the second session concentrates on the active practice of MBST, guided by a palliative care physician well-versed in MBST methodology. In conjunction with these instructional sessions, MBST therapists are encouraged to partake in daily mindfulness exercises conducted at their residence. These exercises comprise a series of brief mindfulness exercises from the four foundations of mindfulness. To facilitate consistent practice, therapists also download a mindfulness bell application as their regular reminders to come back to the present moment during their daily engagements and MBST sessions.

By cultivating the therapist's unhurried presence, non-interruptive listening, objective understanding of the individual Fractal of Quality of Life, compassionate communication and action, and clear awareness of personal and professional boundaries, MBST engenders a transformative framework for alleviating suffering and enhancing the overall therapeutic experience.

4.1 Development of MBST

The conceptualisation of mindfulness-based supportive therapy (MBST) was a result of a systematic process integrating findings from qualitative research. Initially, a comprehensive theory of suffering was developed by merging models of suffering derived from in-depth thematic analysis [6, 22]. This synthesis allowed for a more comprehensive understanding of the multifaceted nature of suffering in the palliative care context.

Building upon this foundation, a secondary thematic analysis was conducted to explore the specific experiences of suffering caused by healthcare interactions [73]. The results of this analysis were then incorporated into the conceptual framework of psychotherapy, adding a nuanced perspective on the impact of healthcare interactions on suffering.

Then, principles of mindfulness were integrated. Mindfulness, with its emphasis on present-moment awareness, non-judgemental acceptance, and compassionate understanding, was recognised as a valuable tool in addressing and alleviating suffering. By incorporating mindfulness into the conceptualisation, MBST was created as a mindfulness-based psychotherapy tailored to the unique needs of individuals in palliative care, aiming to provide support and relief from suffering within a compassionate and holistic therapeutic approach.

4.2 Evidence for MBST

A randomised controlled trial (RCT) conducted at the University of Malaya Medical Centre in Malaysia provided evidence supporting the efficacy of MBST in reducing suffering among patients with advanced cancer. The study included 73 patients with advanced cancer who exhibited a suffering score of ≥4/10 based on the Suffering Pictogram [74]. In the intervention group, patients received a 30-minute session of MBST from a palliative care doctor trained in MBST. In contrast, patients in the control group had a 30-minute supportive listening session conducted by a palliative care doctor who had no experience in MBST or mindfulness.

The results of the trial revealed a statistically significant improvement in overall suffering scores of The Suffering Pictogram, total scores of the Hospital Anxiety and Depression Scale (HADS), and the Functional Assessment of Chronic Illness Therapy–Spiritual Well-Being scale (FACIT-Sp) within the MBST group compared to the control group. These positive outcomes indicate that MBST not only reduced suffering but also had a positive impact on psychological well-being, including reduced anxiety and depression, and enhanced quality of life.

4.3 Application of MBST in the Clinical Setting

The application of MBST in the clinical setting involves three simple steps: directing attention, sustaining attention, and noticing distractions. The object of attention evolves from focusing on the breath to encompassing presence, listening, empathy, compassion, and boundaries.

Initially, attention is directed towards the breath, with individuals cultivating awareness of the in and out breath. The use of a mindfulness bell app can serve as a helpful reminder to periodically re-establish focus.

Subsequently, it involves expanding attention to include presence, wherein healthcare providers are aware of their breath and bodily sensations. This heightened awareness allows them to be fully present in the moment and engage with patients, family caregivers, and healthcare colleagues without a sense of haste or rush.

Then, attention is directed towards active listening. Healthcare providers employ open-ended questions and listen attentively, demonstrating awareness and refraining from interruptions. This mindful listening facilitates a deep understanding of patients', families', and healthcare colleagues' experiences without imposing one's own judgement or interpretations.

The next aspect involves cultivating empathy. Healthcare providers develop an empathetic stance by imagining themselves in the position of the patient, family caregiver, or healthcare colleague, seeking to comprehend the individual Fractal of quality of life, encompassing both suffering and well-being. This understanding guides healthcare providers to discern what patients, families, and healthcare colleagues 'want' in terms of verbal communication and actions. The concept of 'allowing' is recognised as a form of empathy, respecting and validating their needs and preferences.

Furthermore, healthcare providers cultivate compassion as they intentionally strive to alleviate suffering. This compassionate intention is complemented by aligning their words and actions with the desires and needs expressed by patients, families, and healthcare colleagues. The cultivation of awareness enables healthcare providers to navigate these interactions with a deep sense of compassion.

Finally, healthcare providers maintain awareness of boundaries throughout the therapeutic process. This includes acknowledging time constraints during presence, recognising countertransference in listening, being aware of vicarious traumatisation in empathy, and understanding the risk of compassion fatigue in compassion.

In summary, the application of MBST in the clinical setting involves directing and sustaining attention towards the breath, expanding awareness to encompass presence, listening, empathy, compassion, and being mindful of boundaries. Once the attention is distracted, healthcare providers can direct their attention back to their breath, then the five components of MBST.

5 Brief Guided Mindfulness Exercises (Second Phase)

Brief guided mindfulness exercises are derived from a series of mindfulness exercises specifically tailored for implementation within the palliative care setting [69–72]. The rationale behind their development stems from recognising that many patients and family caregivers lack the time or energy required to engage in a comprehensive eight-week mindfulness programme. These exercises are organised into four domains, namely body, feelings, mind, and reality, each serving a distinct purpose in cultivating mindfulness.

The core exercise revolves around mindful breathing, which comprises a 16-step process [72]. However, it can be simplified to a single step to accommodate the needs and limitations of patients or family caregivers, e.g. paying attention to the in-breath and the out-breath. The sixteen-step process can be divided into four tetrads, with each tetrad correlates with one of the four domains.

The initial tetrad within the mindful breathing exercise focuses on cultivating mindfulness of the body, primarily aiming to induce relaxation and ease within the physical being. The second tetrad centres on mindfulness of feelings, specifically referring to the affective qualities of pleasantness, unpleasantness, and neutrality. This exercise facilitates the recognition of habitual reactions to feelings, empowering individuals to interrupt automatic reactions.

The third tetrad emphasises mindfulness of the mind, enabling individuals to observe the arising and fading away of various mental states, rather than becoming entangled or absorbed in them. The fourth tetrad involves mindfulness of reality, wherein individuals learn to attentively observe the reality of their automatic negative thoughts without engaging in rumination or further elaboration.

In addition to mindful breathing, mindfulness exercises within the domain of the body encompass a range of other exercises, such as mindful postures, engaging in mindful activities, directing attention to body parts, contemplating body composition, and reflecting on the concept of death. Mindfulness of feelings involves directing awareness towards pleasant, unpleasant, and neutral feelings, as well as observing the arising of urges and recognising wholesome feelings, such as love, compassion, joy, gratitude, and peace, and unwholesome feelings. Mindfulness of the mind encompasses the observation of mental reactions, including those driven by greed and anger, as well as automatic reactions, and facilitating the cultivation of a mindful mind. Lastly, mindfulness of reality involves the exploration of hindrances that may impede mindfulness practice, as well as awakening factors that support and enhance mindfulness.

Therapists are required to complete an additional eight-week mindfulness training programme in addition to their initial MBST training, led by a trained palliative care specialist. Each session lasts approximately 2 hours. The training covers various topics such as focusing on the breath, integrating breath with body awareness, body scanning, mindful eating, walking mindfully, acknowledging body sensations, contemplating mortality, addressing emotions, recognising emotional impulses, cultivating love, practising self-compassion, fostering gratitude, contemplating inner peace, managing wandering thoughts, and becoming more attuned to sounds and thoughts, including the process of awakening from automatic thinking patterns.

5.1 *Evidence for Brief Guided Mindfulness Exercises*

The evidence supporting the use of brief guided mindfulness in palliative care is still emerging but shows promising results. Several studies have explored the efficacy of these exercises in improving various outcomes for patients in palliative care settings.

A pilot study demonstrated that a five-minute mindful breathing intervention resulted in a significantly larger reduction in distress scores compared to a 'listening' intervention among palliative care patients and family caregivers with distress, suggesting its potential as a useful tool for distress reduction in this context [75]. Another RCT demonstrated that five-minute mindful breathing effectively reduced distress among palliative cancer patients while also inducing significant physiological changes [76].

In several other RCTs, the efficacy of brief guided mindfulness was explored across various populations. One RCT showed that a three-month intervention of five-minute mindful breathing sessions three times daily reduced stress and enhanced mindfulness in stage I-III cancer patients [77]. In two RCTs, 20-minute mindful breathing demonstrated the ability to reduce suffering and bispectral index scores in palliative care patients and their families [78, 79]. A low bispectral index score in someone practising mindfulness generally indicates reduced brain activity and increased calmness and relaxation. Additionally, these 20-minute interventions were effective in reducing dyspnoea in patients with lung disease and heart failure, as observed in two other RCTs [80, 81]. Another RCT found that a 20-minute mindful breathing resulted in significant reductions in multiple symptoms measured by the Edmonton Symptom Assessment Scale (ESAS) [82]. Furthermore, a 30-minute mindful breathing intervention showed promise in reducing fatigue among haematological cancer patients in one RCT [83].

The benefits of mindfulness extended to other practices, with five-minute mindfulness of love and five-minute mindfulness of peace interventions in two RCTS reducing suffering and improving spiritual quality of life [84, 85]. Lastly, an RCT comparing mindful gratitude journaling for one week compared to routine journaling demonstrated reductions in suffering and improvements in quality of life with the mindful gratitude journaling approach [86].

5.2 *Application of Brief Guided Mindfulness Exercises in the Clinical Setting*

In contrast to MBST, where palliative care providers engage in mindfulness during patient care, brief guided mindfulness techniques are utilised by these providers to guide patients and family caregivers following MBST assessments. Applying brief guided mindfulness exercises in the context of palliative care to prevent suffering involves a structured approach encompassing briefing, exercise implementation, and debriefing, utilising the following key steps:

1. Briefing: Begin by providing a comprehensive explanation of mindfulness, emphasising its potential benefits in alleviating suffering. Engage in a discussion with the individual to understand their preferences and specific needs, informed by assessments from MBST. This collaborative process ensures the selection of an exercise tailored to their unique requirements.
2. Exercise: Initiate the exercise with an induction phase, guiding the individual to prepare for the practice by gently bringing their attention to the present moment, becoming aware of their breathing, posture, and gradually relaxing the body. Proceed to the main exercise phase, using a guided script to lead the individual through the practice. Pay careful attention to the rate, rhythm, tone, and silences within the script, creating a conducive environment for focused mindfulness. Conclude the exercise with a closing phase, transitioning to open awareness and allowing the individual to integrate the experience into daily life.
3. Debriefing: Provide an opportunity for the individual to share feedback and reflections on their mindfulness experience. Acknowledge their experiences with compassion and understanding, ensuring a safe and supportive environment. Offer an explanation of the potential mechanisms behind their experiences and the relevance to their well-being, addressing any questions or concerns they may have.

One notable aspect of brief guided mindfulness exercises is their inherent flexibility in terms of the number of sessions, ranging from a single session to a more extended programme of up to eight sessions. This flexibility allows for the adaptation of mindfulness interventions to accommodate varying needs, preferences, and constraints of individuals seeking mindfulness-based support in palliative care. The customisable nature of these exercises enables practitioners to tailor the intervention to the specific context and goals of the participants, ensuring a more personalised approach to mindfulness practice. The following case study in Box 2 will illustrate the utilisation of mindfulness in a practical context.

Box 2 Case Study

Mr. M, a 35-year-old gentleman facing the challenges of colon cancer and abdominal lymph node metastases. He found himself in the hospital due to intense back pain caused by enlarged retroperitoneal lymph nodes. When his oncologist shared his prognosis, he felt overwhelmed. At this crucial moment, his wife suggested a visit from a pastor, but he declined, which strained their relationship. Turning to her for support, he expressed his stress. It was during this time that they were referred to me for pain management and mindfulness exercises.

We began by addressing his pain with patient-controlled analgesia (PCA) morphine, later transitioning to a fentanyl patch of 150 mcg/h every 72 hours. After assessing his condition with Mindfulness-Based Supportive Therapy (MBST), I led the couple through a brief guided mindfulness exercise focused on sounds and thoughts. Surprisingly, this exercise revealed that their conflict was unnecessary and driven by their own thoughts. They were made aware that their thoughts are just thoughts, not facts.

Expanding upon this progress, a series of subsequent sessions were undertaken, encompassing distinct exercises. Among these was a body scan. The couple were guided to attentively focus on each of the body parts, 'breathing into' them, and 'breathing out' from them to release any tension, followed by sweeping the body with the rhythm of the breath. They emerged from this exercise with a profound sense of relaxation.

Continuing the practices, we delved into mindfulness of gratitude. They were directed to express gratitude towards their senses, the individuals surrounding them, their material possessions, the immediate present, and the invaluable opportunity to engage in mindfulness. Notably, they found themselves most deeply moved by the recognition of the opportunity to learn and embrace mindfulness itself.

Subsequently, the focus shifted to mindfulness of pain. Mr. M embarked on an exploration where he observed his pain devoid of judgement, cultivating a curious and open attitude. This approach allowed him to discern the nature of pain, its fluctuations, and the noticing of pain-free regions within his body. A significant breakthrough was achieved as he expanded his awareness, acknowledging the broader world around him where countless others also grappled with pain. This exercise proved to be a realisation, fostering a deeper connection between his personal experience and the universal human condition.

Remarkably, their relationship began to mend. Mr. M no longer placed undue stress on his wife, and his pain was significantly reduced and managed with a fentanyl patch of 75 mcg/h every 72 hours. Through the power of guided mindfulness exercises, they not only found relief from pain but also discovered a renewed harmony in their relationship, demonstrating the profound impact mindfulness can have on both physical and emotional well-being.

6 Conclusion

Overall, integrating mindfulness into The Fractals of Quality of Life provides a comprehensive and individualised approach to address suffering and enhancing well-being. It acknowledges the interconnectedness of human experience and empowers individuals to actively participate in their own healing and transformation.

Shantideva once said, '*Where is there enough leather to cover the surface of the Earth? But just having leather on the soles of one's feet is the same as covering the whole Earth. In the same way, it is not possible to control all external events; but, if we simply control our mind, what need is there to control other things?*' [87]

Therefore, attempting to control all external events to prevent suffering is an impossible task. However, the power to transform our inner experiences in the face of these events lies within us. Mindfulness emerges as a potent tool in this process of transformation, enabling us to cultivate a state of awareness and acceptance that can alleviate and prevent suffering. By directing our attention inward and practising mindfulness, we gain the capacity to navigate the challenges of life with resilience and inner peace.

References

1. Cherny N. The problem of suffering. In: Doyle D, Hanks G, Cherny N, Calman K, editors. Oxford textbook of palliative medicine. 3rd ed. New York: Oxford University Press; 2005. p. 7–14.
2. Sherman SW. Reciprocal suffering: the need to improve family caregivers' quality of life through palliative care. J Palliat Med. 1998;1(4):357–66.
3. Rokach A. Caring for those who care for the dying: coping with the demands on palliative care workers. Palliat Support Care. 2005;3(4):325–32.
4. Cherny NI, Coyle N, Foley KM. Suffering in the advanced cancer patient: a definition and taxonomy. J Palliat Care. 1994;10(2):57–70.
5. Vachon ML. Staff stress in hospice/palliative care: a review. Palliat Med. 1995;9(2):91–122.
6. Beng TS, Guan NC, Seang LK, Pathmawathi S, Ming MF, Jane LE, Chin LE, Loong LC. The experiences of suffering of palliative care patients in Malaysia: a thematic analysis. Am J Hosp Palliat Care. 2014;31(1):45–56.
7. Wilson KG, Chochinov HM, McPherson CJ, LeMay K, Allard P, Chary S, Gagnon PR, Macmillan K, De Luca M, O'Shea F, Kuhl D, Fainsinger RL. Suffering with advanced cancer. J Clin Oncol. 2007;25(13):1691–7.
8. Lobb EA, Clayton JM, Price MA. Suffering, loss and grief in palliative care. Aust Fam Physician. 2006;35(10):772–5.
9. McPherson CJ, Wilson KG, Murray MA. Feeling like a burden to others: a systematic review focusing on the end of life. Palliat Med. 2007;21(2):115–28.
10. McPherson CJ, Wilson KG, Murray MA. Feeling like a burden to others: exploring the perspectives of patients at the end of life. Soc Sci Med. 2007;64(2):417–27.
11. Chochinov HM, Kristjanson LJ, Hack TF, Hassard T, McClement S, Harlos M. Burden to others and the terminally ill. J Pain Symptom Manag. 2007;34(5):463–71.

12. Lee V, Loiselle CG. The salience of existential concerns across the cancer control continuum. Palliat Support Care. 2012;10(2):123–33.
13. Krause K. Contracting cancer and coping with it. Patients' experiences. Cancer Nurs. 1991;14(5):240–5.
14. Arman M, Rehnsfeldt A, Lindholm L, Hamrin E, Eriksson K. Suffering related to healthcare: a study of breast cancer patients' experiences. Int J Nurs Pract. 2004;10(6):248–56.
15. Oi-Ling K, Man-Wah D, Kam-Hung D. Symptom distress as rated by advanced cancer patients, caregivers and physicians in the last week of life. Palliat Med. 2005;19(3):228–33.
16. Thiagarajan M, Chan CM, Fuang HG, Beng TS, Atiliyana MA, Yahaya NA. Symptom prevalence and related distress in cancer patients undergoing chemotherapy. Asian Pac J Cancer Prev. 2016;17(1):171–6.
17. Portenoy RK, Thaler HT, Kornblith AB, Lepore JM, Friedlander-Klar H, Coyle N, Smart-Curley T, Kemeny N, Norton L, Hoskins W. Symptom prevalence, characteristics and distress in a cancer population. Qual Life Res. 1994;3(3):183–9.
18. Gramling R, Straton J, Ingersoll LT, Clarfeld LA, Hirsch L, Gramling CJ, Durieux BN, Rizzo DM, Eppstein MJ, Alexander SC. Epidemiology of fear, sadness, and anger expression in palliative care conversations. J Pain Symptom Manag. 2021;61(2):246–53.
19. Tan SB, Loh EC, Lam CL, Ng CG, Lim EJ, Boey CCM. Psychological processes of suffering of palliative care patients in Malaysia: a thematic analysis. BMJ Support Palliat Care. 2019;9(1):e19.
20. Balducci L. Beyond quality of life: the meaning of death and suffering in palliative care. Asian Pac J Cancer Prev. 2010;11(Suppl 1):41–4.
21. Hills J, Paice JA, Cameron JR, Shott S. Spirituality and distress in palliative care consultation. J Palliat Med. 2005;8(4):782–8.
22. Beng TS, Guan NC, Seang LK, Pathmawathi S, Ming MF, Jane LE, Chin LE, Loong LC. The experiences of suffering of palliative care informal caregivers in Malaysia: a thematic analysis. Am J Hosp Palliat Care. 2013;30(5):473–89.
23. Ortega-Galán ÁM, Ruiz-Fernández MD, Carmona-Rega MI, Cabrera-Troya J, Ortíz-Amo R, Ibáñez-Masero O. The experiences of family caregivers at the end of life: suffering, compassion satisfaction and support of health care professionals. J Hosp Palliat Nurs. 2019;21(5):438–44.
24. Rogalla KB. Anticipatory grief, proactive coping, social support, and growth: exploring positive experiences of preparing for loss. Omega (Westport). 2020;81(1):107–29.
25. de Graaff FM, Francke AL, van den Muijsenbergh ME, van der Geest S. 'Palliative care': a contradiction in terms? A qualitative study of cancer patients with a Turkish or Moroccan background, their relatives and care providers. BMC Palliat Care. 2010;9:19.
26. Milberg A, Strang P, Jakobsson M. Next of kin's experience of powerlessness and helplessness in palliative home care. Support Care Cancer. 2004;12(2):120–8.
27. Stajduhar KI, Cohen SR. Family carers in the home. In: Hudson P, Payne S, editors. Family carers in palliative care. Oxford: Oxford University Press; 2009. p. 149–68.
28. Tang ST, Liu TW, Lai MS, McCorkle R. Discrepancy in the preferences of place of death between terminally ill cancer patients and their primary family caregivers in Taiwan. Soc Sci Med. 2005;61(7):1560–6.
29. Docherty A, Owens A, Asadi-Lari M, Petchey R, Williams J, Carter YH. Knowledge and information needs of informal caregivers in palliative care: a qualitative systematic review. Palliat Med. 2008;22(2):153–71.
30. Ullrich A, Ascherfeld L, Marx G, Bokemeyer C, Bergelt C, Oechsle K. Quality of life, psychological burden, needs, and satisfaction during specialized inpatient palliative care in family caregivers of advanced cancer patients. BMC Palliat Care. 2017;16(1):31.
31. Beng TS, Chin LE, Guan NC, Yee A, Wu C, Pathmawathi S, Yi KT, Kuan WS, Jane LE, Meng CB. The experiences of stress of palliative care providers in Malaysia: a thematic analysis. Am J Hosp Palliat Care. 2015;32(1):15–28.
32. Jünger S, Pestinge M, Elsner F, Krumm N, Radbruch L. Criteria for successful multiprofessional cooperation in palliative care teams. Palliat Med. 2007;21(4):347–54.
33. Gardiner C, Cobb M, Gott M, Ingleton C. Barriers to providing care for older people in acute hospitals. Age Ageing. 2011;40(2):233–8.

34. Michtalik HJ, Yeh HC, Pronovost PJ, Brotman DJ. Impact of attending physician workload on patient care: a survey of hospitalists. JAMA Intern Med. 2013;173(5):375–7.
35. Peters L, Lee S, O'Connor M. Workplace stressors: a survey of palliative care nurses in Australia. End Life J. 2013;3(1):1–10.
36. Marcus JD, Mott FE. Difficult conversations: from diagnosis to death. Ochsner J. 2014;14(4):712–7.
37. Mpinga EK, Chastonay P, Rapin CH. End of life conflicts in palliative care: a systematic review of the literature. Rech Soins Infirm. 2006;86:68–95.
38. Rhee JJ, Zwar N, Vagholkar S, Dennis S, Broadbent AM, Mitchell G. Attitudes and barriers to involvement in palliative care by Australian urban general practitioners. J Palliat Med. 2008;11(7):980–5.
39. Miyashita M, Sanjo M, Morita T, Hirai K, Kizawa Y, Shima Y, Shimoyama N, Tsuneto S, Hiraga K, Sato K, Uchitomi Y. Barriers to providing palliative care and priorities for future actions to advance palliative care in Japan: a nationwide expert opinion survey. J Palliat Med. 2007;10(2):390–9.
40. Koh MYH, Gallardo MD, Khoo HS, Hum A. Burnout in palliative care—difficult cases: qualitative study. BMJ Support Palliat Care. 2022;13(e3):e1383–9. https://doi.org/10.1136/bmjspcare-2021-003347.
41. Hubik DJ, O'Callaghan C, Dwyer J. Strong emotional reactions for doctors working in palliative care: causes, management and impact. A qualitative study. Psychooncology. 2021;30(9):1582–9.
42. Sinclair S. Impact of death and dying on the personal lives and practices of palliative and hospice care professionals. CMAJ. 2011;183(2):180–7.
43. Beng TS, Chin LE, Guan NC, Ann YH, Wu C, Kuan WS, Jane LE, Khee SS, Meng CB. The experiences of well-being of palliative care patients in Malaysia: a thematic analysis. Am J Hosp Palliat Med. 2015;32(5):490–503.
44. Lau J, Khoo AM, Ho AH, Tan KK. Psychological resilience among palliative patients with advanced cancer: a systematic review of definitions and associated factors. Psychooncology. 2021;30(7):1029–40.
45. Beng TS, Xin CA, Ying YK, Khuen LP, Yee A, Zainuddin SI, Chin LE, Loong LC. Hope in palliative care: a thematic analysis. J Palliat Care. 2022;37(2):177–82.
46. Beng TS, Ghee WK, Hui NY, Yin OC, Kelvin KWS, Yiling ST, Huey TA, Capelle DP, Zainuddin SI, Chin LE, Loong LC. Happiness at the end of life: a qualitative study. Palliat Support Care. 2022;20(1):69–75.
47. O'Callaghan A, Bickford B, Rea C, Fernando A, Malpas P. Happiness at the end of life: a qualitative study. Am J Hosp Palliat Care. 2021;38(3):223–9.
48. Tavemark S, Hermansson LN, Blomberg K. Enabling activity in palliative care: focus groups among occupational therapists. BMC Palliat Care. 2019;18(1):17.
49. Aghaei MH, Vanaki Z, Mohammadi E. Emotional bond: The nature of relationship in palliative care for cancer patients. Indian J Palliat Care. 2020;26(1):86–94.
50. Kittelson SM, Elie MC, Pennypacker L. Palliative care symptom management. Crit Care Nurs Clin North Am. 2015;27(3):315–39.
51. Beng TS, Ying YK, Xin CA, Jane LE, Lin DC, Khuen LP, Capelle DP, Zainuddin SI, Chin LE, Loong LC. The experiences of well-being of family caregivers in palliative care: a qualitative study using thematic analysis. Progress Palliat Care. 2021;29(4):209–16.
52. Zimmermann C. Acceptance of dying: a discourse analysis of palliative care literature. Soc Sci Med. 2012;75(1):217–24.
53. Davis EL, Deane FP, Lyons GCB. Acceptance and valued living as critical appraisal and coping strengths for caregivers dealing with terminal illness and bereavement. Palliat Support Care. 2015;13(2):359–68.
54. Borelli E, Bigi S, Potenza L, Gilioli F, Artioli F, Porzio G, Porro CA, Efficace F, Bruera E, Luppi M, Bandieri E. Gratitude among advanced cancer patients and their caregivers: the role of early palliative care. Front Oncol. 2022;12:991250.

55. Holtslander LF, Duggleby W, Williams AM, Wright KE. The experience of hope for informal caregivers of palliative patients. J Palliat Care. 2005;21(4):285–91.
56. Henriksson A, Carlander I, Årestedt K. Feelings of rewards among family caregivers during ongoing palliative care. Palliat Support Care. 2015;13(6):1509–17.
57. Areia NP, Góngora JN, Major S, Oliveira VD, Relvas AP. Support interventions for families of people with terminal cancer in palliative care. Palliat Support Care. 2020;18(5):580–8.
58. Tan SB, Lee YL, Tan SN, Ng TY, Teo YT, Lim PK, Loh EC, Lam CL. The experiences of well-being of palliative care providers in Malaysia: a thematic analysis. J Hosp Palliat Nurs. 2020;22(5):407–14.
59. Tan SB, Ng JH, Lau XR, Mah ZL, Lim EJ, Loh EC, Lam CL. The ABCDE of good care: a thematic analysis of the art of caring for terminally ill patients in Malaysia. Adv Mod Oncol Res. 2017;3(S1):65–72.
60. Gillman L, Adams J, Kovac R, Kilcullen A, House A, Doyle C. Strategies to promote coping and resilience in oncology and palliative care nurses caring for adult patients with malignancy: a comprehensive systematic review. JBI Database System Rev Implement Rep. 2015;13(5):131–204.
61. Lowe MA, Gakumo CA, Patrician PA. Coping strategies of nurses in a palliative care unit. J Natl Black Nurses Assoc. 2016;27(2):50–4.
62. Fernando G, Hughes S. Team approaches in palliative care: a review of the literature. Int J Palliat Nurs. 2019;25(9):444–51.
63. Seccareccia D, Brown JB. Impact of spirituality on palliative care physicians: personally and professionally. J Palliat Med. 2009;12(9):805–9.
64. Webster J, Kristjanson LJ. Long-term palliative care workers: more than a story of endurance. J Palliat Med. 2002;5(6):865–75.
65. Mota Vargas R, Mahtani-Chugani V, Solano Pallero M, Rivro Jiménez B, Cabo Domínguez R, Robles AV. The transformation process for palliative care professionals: the metamorphosis, a qualitative research study. Palliat Med. 2016;30(2):161–70.
66. Kabat-Zinn J. Wherever you go, there you are: mindfulness meditation in everyday life. New York: Hyperion; 1994. p. 4.
67. Beng TS, Chin LE, Guan NC, Yee A, Wu C, Jane LE, Meng CB. Mindfulness-based supportive therapy (MBST): proposing a palliative psychotherapy from a conceptual perspective to address suffering in palliative care. Am J Hosp Palliat Care. 2015;32(2):144–60.
68. Beng TS. Mindfulness and care of the dying. Singapore: Partridge; 2018.
69. Tan SB, Capelle DP, Zainal NZ, Lim EJ, Loh EC, Lam CL. Mindfulness: a new paradigm of psychosocial care in the palliative care setting in Southeast Asia. Ann Acad Med Singap. 2017;46(9):339–46.
70. Beng TS. Mindfulness in palliative care. In: Beng TS, editor. The little handbook of palliative care. Singapore: Partridge; 2016. p. 519–28.
71. Beng TS. The little handbook of mini-mindfulness meditation. Pittsburgh: Dorrance; 2012.
72. Tung YZ, Tan SB. Mindful breathing for suffering. BMJ Support Palliat Care. 2023;13(2):241–2.
73. Beng TS, Guan NC, Jane LE, Chin LE. Health care interactional suffering in palliative care. Am J Hosp Palliat Care. 2014;31(3):307–14.
74. Beng TS, Ann YH, Guan NC, Chin LE, Loong LC, Ying NT, Teck TY, Li HL, Meng CBC. The suffering pictogram: measuring suffering in palliative care. J Palliat Med. 2017;20(8):869–74.
75. Beng TS, Ahmad F, Loong LC, Chin LE, Zainal NZ, Guan NC, Ann YH, Li LM, Meng CB. Distress reduction for palliative care patients and families with 5-minute mindful breathing: a pilot study. Am J Hosp Palliat Care. 2016;33(6):555–60.
76. Ng CG, Lai KT, Tan SB, Sulaiman AH, Zainal NZ. The effect of 5 minutes of mindful breathing to the perception of distress and physiological responses in palliative care cancer patients: a randomized controlled study. J Palliat Med. 2016;19(9):917–24.
77. Lei Chui P, Wai S, Lai LL, See MH, Tan SB. Mindful breathing: effects of a five-minute practice on perceived stress and mindfulness among patients with cancer. Clin J Oncol Nurs. 2021;25(2):174–80.

78. Beng TS, Jie HW, Yan LH, Ni CX, Capelle DP, Yee A, Guan NC, Hasan MSB, Seang LK, Chin LE, Loong LC. The effect of 20-minute mindful breathing on the perception of suffering and changes in bispectral index score in palliative care patients: a randomized controlled study. Am J Hosp Palliat Care. 2019;36(6):478–84.
79. Tan SB, Ching HC, Chia YL, Yee A, Ng CG, Hasan MSB, Lim KS, Ahmad SB, Capelle DP, Loh EC, Lam CL. The effect of 20-minute mindful breathing on the perception of suffering and changes in bispectral index score in palliative care informal caregivers: a randomized controlled study. Am J Hosp Palliat Care. 2020;37(8):606–12.
80. Tan SB, Liam CK, Pang YK, Leh-Ching Ng D, Wong TS, Wei-Shen Khoo K, Ooi CY, Chai CS. The effect of 20-minute mindful breathing on the rapid reduction of dyspnoea at rest in patients with lung diseases: a randomized controlled trial. J Pain Symptom Manag. 2019;57(4):802–8.
81. Ng DL, Chai CS, Tan KL, Chee KH, Tung YZ, Wai SY, Teo WJ, Ang BT, Lim MA, Tan SB. The efficacy of a single session of 20-minute mindful breathing in reducing dyspnoea among patients with acute decompensated heart failure: a randomized controlled trial. Am J Hosp Palliat Care. 2021;38(3):246–52.
82. Look ML, Tan SB, Hong LL, Ng CG, Yee HA, Lim LY, Ng DLC, Chai CS, Loh EC, Lam CL. Symptom reduction in palliative care from a single session mindful breathing: a randomized controlled trial. BMJ Support Palliat Care. 2021;11(4):433–9.
83. Ng DL, Gan GG, Anuar NA, Tung YZ, Lai NZ, Tan YW, Said SNM, Madihie A, Chai CS, Tan SB. The effect of a single session of 30-minute mindful breathing in reducing fatigue among patients with hematological cancer—a randomized controlled trial. BMC Palliat Care. 2021;20(1):160.
84. Lim MA, Ang BT, Lam CL, Loh EC, Zainuddin SI, Capelle DP, Ng CG, Lim PK, Khor PY, Lim JY, Huang SY, Low GQJ, Gan XY, Tan SB. The effect of 5-min mindfulness of love on suffering and spiritual quality of life of palliative care patients: a randomized controlled study. Eur J Cancer Care (Engl). 2021;30(5):e13456.
85. Yik LL, Ling LM, Ai LM, Ting AB, Capelle DP, Zainuddin SI, Beng TS, Chin LE, Loong LC. The effect of 5-minute mindfulness of peace on suffering and spiritual well-being among palliative care patients: a randomized controlled study. Am J Hosp Palliat Care. 2021;38(9):1083–90.
86. Tan TT, Tan MP, Lam CL, Loh EC, Capelle DP, Zainuddin SI, Ang BT, Lim MA, Lai NZ, Tung YZ, Yee HA, Ng CG, Ho GF, See MH, The MS, Lai LL, Pritam Singh RK, Chai CS, Ng DLC, Tan SB. Mindful gratitude journaling: psychological distress, quality of life and suffering in advanced cancer: a randomized controlled trial. BMJ Support Palliat Care. 2021;13(e2):e389–96. https://doi.org/10.1136/bmjspcare-2021-003068.
87. Shantideva. Guide to Bodhisattva's way of life. Ulverston: Tharpa Publications; 2002. p. 49.

Part VI
Training

Interprofessional Spiritual Care Education and Training for Palliative Care Staff

Roderick MacLeod and Richard Egan

Abstract The teaching of spirituality and spiritual care has often been neglected, although progress is being made. By understanding the nature of education, it is hoped that more effective methods of teaching and learning about the provision of spiritual care can be developed. Interprofessional education is an effective way of learning as such collaboration is an opportune context for the team working to 'learn from, with and about' each other for optimal patient care. Interprofessional education involves integration and shared learning throughout the continuum of professional education, training, and practice and is, therefore, particularly relevant to the care of people approaching the end of their life. A number of developments in the way spiritual care is taught and learned are outlined in this chapter, and the experience of a novel programme from Hospice New Zealand in Aotearoa New Zealand is explored in depth. That programme highlights the importance of understanding oneself and one's spirituality to be able to relate human to human first, with compassionate presence, then assessing expressions of spiritual needs, which may include religious needs. Interprofessional education in spiritual care effectively addresses these needs and aligns with the realities of providing comprehensive patient/family-centred care.

Keywords Interprofessional · Spirituality · Education · Training · New Zealand Palliative care · Spiritual care

R. MacLeod (✉)
General Practice and Primary Healthcare, Faculty of Medical and Health Sciences, University of Auckland, Auckland, New Zealand

The Violet Initiative, Sydney, NSW, Australia
e-mail: rd.macleod@auckland.ac.nz

R. Egan
Department of Preventive and Social Medicine, University of Otago, Dunedin, New Zealand
e-mail: richard.egan@otago.ac.nz

M. C. Best (ed.), *Spiritual Care in Palliative Care*,
https://doi.org/10.1007/978-3-031-50864-6_27

1 Introduction

The mandate for palliative care provision is unequivocal; addressing the spiritual needs of patients is a core aspect of care, and yet, these needs, for some, seem to be difficult to define. Research shows that the teaching of spirituality and spiritual care has often been neglected, although progress is being made [1]. This is almost certainly a universal phenomenon. In New Zealand, for example, a study by Egan et al. [2] examined spiritual care in hospices and discovered various obstacles, including 'inconsistent provision, limited understanding, lack of organisational commitment, resources, and professional development opportunities'. One surprising finding of Egan's study [3] was that 60% of the staff surveyed did not undertake formal spiritual assessments of their patients. It is hard to imagine that things are much different in other countries. Yet, as Ira Byock says, 'the confrontation with death lays bare the spiritual core of the human condition' [4].

Experienced clinicians would suggest that, in people facing a life-limiting illness, spirituality is as important as, or even more important than, other health domains. Cicely Saunders pointed out that 'attention to the achievements that a patient could still make in the face of his physical deterioration and awareness of the spiritual dimension of his final search for meaning' will help to bring about a good death [5]. This chapter considers spiritual care education for interprofessional palliative care staff by examining what underpins education and provides practical examples of existing education.

2 What Is Education?

> *'Education, then, can have no ends beyond itself. Its value derives from principles and standards implicitly. To be educated is not to have arrived at a destination; it is to travel with a different view'.* [6]

R.S. Peters was one of many who have tried to analyse the concept of education itself—in attempting to define what constituted education, he analysed the components of education separately to try to identify what it was that happened as people taught and learned. As a result of this, he claimed 'for education—as distinct from other things like training or indoctrination—to be taking place, three criteria must be met [6]. These are:

1. That "education" implies the transmission of what is worthwhile to those who become committed to it;
2. That education must involve knowledge and understanding in some kind of cognitive perspective, which are not inert;
3. That education at least rules out some procedures of transmission on the grounds that they lack willingness and voluntariness'.

Education, therefore, is an activity in its own right—worth pursuing for its own sake.

Wenger, in outlining his view of a social theory of learning, argues that because learning transforms who we are and what we can do, it is an experience in the development of our identity [7]. In order that we can maximise the experience for both ourselves either as teachers or as learners, we need to pay attention to what he calls the community of practice. That is, the way of clarifying the social configurations in which what we do (in our practice of palliative care, say) is seen as worth pursuing and our participation in that activity is recognisable as a form of competent practice. The other components of that particular social theory of learning (that are particularly pertinent to our learning about spiritual care) are:

1. Meaning—a way of talking about our abilities and our experiences that can be shared.
2. Practice—a way of talking about our shared histories and social frameworks that means we can understand each other.
3. Identity—a way of talking about how learning changes who we are.

Many writers, in reviewing what constitutes professional knowledge, emphasise the importance of reflective practice and stress that individual reflection in, on and about professional knowledge can be a powerful way of enhancing our understanding of it. Shared reflection with others who understand and can empathise with our experience and life world is especially valuable. This is why colleagues, mentors, teachers, and critical friends of all sorts are particularly valuable. Finding ways of encouraging collaborative reflection is an important professional development task that all those who work in palliative care should take seriously.

Parsell and Bligh [8] suggested that interprofessional approaches to learning were essentially about the integration and synthesis of knowledge to solve problems or explore issues. Since the 1990s, others (Carpenter and Hewstone [9], Wee et al. [10], for example) have looked at interprofessional training programmes for undergraduates and postgraduates in palliative care.

Interprofessional education is potentially different from uniprofessional education because the values and learning objectives of the participating professions may not be aligned.

Overall, in providing interprofessional care one might expect and hope for:

- Shared values, particularly with respect to patient (and family) outcomes
- Combined or integrated practices
- Discernible scopes of practice.

The first two could be the subjects of interprofessional learning, whereas the latter is more likely to be uniprofessional.

3 Interprofessional Education

Many years ago, there was evidence to support impressions that interprofessional education would be effective in overcoming barriers to education if it:

- Explored similarities and differences in roles, skills, knowledge, and ideology
- Recognised the complementary skills and resources of different disciplines
- Brought together course members of equal status in equal numbers
- Allowed communication in whole groups which are not too large
- Had full institutional support to ensure participants' involvement [9].

England's Institute of Community Studies for the Advancement of Interprofessional Education (CAIPE) has produced a useful review of interprofessional education with the following definition for the healthcare professions: 'Occasions when two or more professionals learn from and about each other to improve collaboration and the quality of care' [11]. In palliative care, interprofessional collaboration is an opportune context for the team working to 'learn from, with and about' each other for optimal patient care. Interprofessional education involves integration and shared learning throughout the continuum of professional education, training and practice [12] and is, therefore, particularly relevant to the care of people approaching the end of their life.

4 Developing a Curriculum

There are only a few examples of national initiatives that have utilised interprofessional learning in the pursuit of improving spiritual care.

4.1 United States of America

Puchalski and colleagues at the George Washington University Institute for Spirituality & Health (GWish) over the last ten years have developed a curriculum for education of healthcare professionals in spiritual care [13]. It was based on a consensus-derived generalist–specialist model of spiritual care, with all clinicians providing generalist–spiritual care and trained chaplains providing specialist spiritual care. In 2009, that team led the National Initiative to Develop Competencies in Spirituality in Medical Education (NIDCSME) for medical students, including teaching methods and assessment tools required to demonstrate student attainment of the competency behaviours [14]. They then developed an interprofessional pilot spiritual care training programme for clinicians, creating an online needs assessment survey in 2011 and collecting input from 441 physicians, nurses, and chaplains. In 2014, another needs assessment was completed through an online survey in a national sample of 119 clinicians from National Cancer Institute (NCI)-affiliated cancer centres and chaplains. Following this, interprofessional spiritual care education curriculum learning objectives were developed and named the *Interprofessional Spiritual Care Education Curriculum* (ISPEC) [13]. These were to:

1. Recognise the role of spirituality as an essential component of patient-centred care.
2. Review spiritual care guidelines and identify the basics of implementation of these guidelines.
3. Define spiritual distress in adults and children and distinguish the difference between spiritual distress and other types of distress.
4. Recognise skills for practising compassionate presence.
5. Identify communication strategies for eliciting spiritual issues.
6. Develop a whole-person assessment and treatment or care plan.
7. Recognise the clinician's spirituality as an integral component of professional development.

It was envisaged that these learning objectives would be achieved by participation in six learning modules.

Module 1 emphasises the theoretical, ethical, and evidence base for the role of spirituality in clinical care of seriously and chronically ill patients. The module provides an overview of the current state of the evidence to support the need for improvement in the provision of spiritual care.

Module 2 describes the nature of spiritual distress in adults and children and demonstrates the critical need for addressing and treating it. This module discusses how spiritual distress is associated with worse physical, social, and emotional distress, how it can negatively impact physical pain, cause poor emotional well-being, lower satisfaction with life, and increase risk for suicidal ideation.

Module 3 defines the elements of compassionate presence, identifies clinical models, and describes contemplative listening. It explores the nature and causes of suffering and attending to patients' and families' spiritual suffering. This module helps students understand different ways of demonstrating care for people who are suffering.

Module 4 presents communication strategies for uncovering spiritual issues and diagnosing spiritual distress; exploring spiritual screening, spiritual history, and spiritual assessment and the tools to use.

Module 5 addresses whole person assessment and treatment plans based on the biopsychosocial and spiritual model. Through case-based presentation, clinicians formulate a spiritual care plan, discuss how to document spiritual issues in the medical chart, and apply spiritual care interventions, including a host of interventions and practices.

Module 6 focuses on ethical standards in providing spiritual care and reflective or spiritual practice in clinician self-care. Learners are then given an opportunity to reflect on their own spirituality in practising compassionate presence, their professional call to serve, and their spiritual beliefs and self-care practices.

To facilitate these modules, the team at GWish developed a Train-the-Trainer course. Healthcare practitioners from different clinical professions were paired with chaplains and attended a two-and-a-half-day course which included didactic presentations, discussions, and lab sessions for each module.

Evaluations have been undertaken immediately after the course and again one year later and to date the response has been overwhelmingly positive [15].

So far, this programme has been undertaken in at least sixteen countries. Although the international dissemination has been continually evaluated to assure that it is appropriate across various settings and cultures, the authors recognise that 'this training needs to be carefully tailored for each specific use'. One example of this work in Australia is reported by Best et al. [16] and reports on an evaluation of the ISPEC training course administered to an Australian healthcare cohort using an online format. Their preliminary findings suggest that the ISPEC programme is effective in improving the ability of healthcare professionals to provide spiritual care but that 'more work is needed to improve the cultural relevance of the program in Australia'.

4.2 Europe

Building on that work in the United States, the European Association for Palliative Care (EAPC) Spiritual Care reference group, a former taskforce, was formed in 2010 to improve spiritual care in Europe, recognising the many and varied approaches in the different countries that make up that grouping. The group produced a White Paper to provide guidance on spiritual care education for all healthcare workers who provide palliative care, regardless of discipline and care context [17]. The target groups for that paper included healthcare workers involved in teaching or training palliative care and spiritual care, stakeholders, leaders, and decision makers responsible for training and education provided to all healthcare workers involved in palliative care and national and local curricula development groups. The reference group identified four broad areas to be included in spiritual care education.

1. Demonstrate the reflective capacity to consider the importance of spirituality in one's own life.

The first recommendation for training is developing the reflective capacity of staff to consider the importance of spiritual dimensions in their own lives. 'The greater the proportion of staff members who are not in touch with their spiritual needs, the more complicated provision of spiritual care becomes, and the less likely that the spiritual care needs of the patients are met' (p. 4). By addressing this first, the group identified the central importance of this aspect of ourselves in the delivery of compassionate spiritual care. They also noted that high personal spirituality and competence in spiritual care is associated with reduced burnout in palliative care professionals.

They acknowledged practical challenges in facilitating an intimate process such as self-reflection in a group of healthcare professionals but proposed several opportunities that may encourage such reflection. Their first suggestion was the development of regular voluntary informal forums where staff can discuss personal spirituality over a cup of coffee as being supportive of self-reflection. They also suggested the institution of Schwartz Rounds (a type of structured group forum where clinical and non-clinical staff meet regularly to discuss the emotional and social aspects of working in healthcare) as a means for staff from all backgrounds to come together to discuss the emotional and social challenges of caring for patients. Balint groups (a supportive and collaborative medical organisation of clinicians and teachers to help doctors understand the importance of the use of emotion and personal understanding in their work) are a further way for clinicians in a stable group to present clinical scenarios in order to improve and to better understand the clinician-patient relationship and to provide mutual support. They encouraged continuing professional development opportunities to address personal spiritual development, such as spiritual retreats.

The group include self-assessment tools such as the Spiritual Attitude and Involvement List (SAIL), the Spiritual Care Competency Scale (SCCS), the Spirituality and Spiritual Care Rating Scale (SSCRS), and the Spiritual Care Competence Questionnaire (SCCQ) and finally the Ars Moriendi ('Art of Dying') or Diamond-model from the work of Carlo Leget, one of the task force members [18].

2. Recognise the importance of spirituality in the life of the patients, and understand the patients' and families' spiritual, existential and religious needs, respecting their choice not to focus on this aspect of care.

In developing this recommendation, the authors emphasise how spirituality impacts the lives of people near the end of life. They suggest that staff need to provide opportunities for patients and families to express the spiritual dimensions of their lives in a supportive manner and to respect the patient's beliefs, regardless of our own. Sudden ill-health or significant loss may threaten a person's understanding of their world, as they are forced to confront their own limitations and mortality. This may potentially precipitate an existential crisis, and spirituality may become more important as they approach their own death.

Not everyone who cares for people near the end of life feels comfortable or equipped to take a spiritual history (the very presence of education outlined in this chapter, emphasises that). There may be team members who may be better placed initially to provide spiritual support. Ways to improve awareness of the importance of spiritual care may be to ensure the presence of spiritual care workers or specially trained volunteers; discussion of spirituality during handovers or ward rounds or in individual consultations; family meetings; music and art therapy; and symbolic acts in the palliative care unit when a patient has died. Spiritual care should be offered to all patients and families, but individuals may have their own resources and people who can help them, and these must be honoured and accepted. Others may decline the offer, but at least an offer should be made.

For many palliative care staff, there may be a number of barriers to providing spiritual care, including a lack of knowledge, confidence, and uncertainty in opening such a conversation. The task force outlines a number of reasons why these barriers may exist, such as a lack of appreciation of the need for spiritual care or difficulty in its provision.

To provide appropriate spiritual care, the task force recommends that a spiritual history be taken at the time of admission and suggests that any staff member can do this. However, without specific education in this area, many will feel uncomfortable. It is essential to understand the spiritual framework and values in which the person who is being cared for lives. To achieve this, practitioners must feel at ease with their own spiritual framework and understanding. Following this, they suggest some form of screening or triage for spiritual problems.

They outline a number of ways in which that spiritual history may be obtained.

1. The Ars Moriendi [18] or Diamond-model as noted above, is inspired by a medieval tradition that creates a common framework for communication and reflection on spirituality in palliative care within a secular and/or multi-faith society.
2. The FICA [19] is a spiritual history-taking tool that was developed to help healthcare professionals address spiritual issues with patients in all settings. It may be most effective for people who follow an organised religion.
3. The SPIRITual History [20] is a guide to identifying important components of the spiritual history for a broad range of patients.
4. HOPE [21] is a tool developed in a primary care context.
5. FAITH [22] is a spiritual history-taking tool that was developed for physicians and medical students.
6. Q2-SAM [23] is a model developed to ensure person-centred care in nursing. It is based on two simple questions: What's most important to you now? How can we help?

These tools may not suit everyone, and some will feel uncomfortable going through a routine list of questions, but over time most practitioners will develop their own ways of addressing these issues with questions such as 'What gives your life meaning?' or 'What helps you when things are difficult?' Even a simple question such as 'Are you at peace?" [24] may elicit a response to open the conversation.

The authors identify that screening 'may include enquiry about the main spiritual needs of the patient, and which spiritual resources the patient already accesses, so that the healthcare chaplain can work with what already exists. In the absence of a healthcare chaplain, this role may be temporarily filled by another staff member'.

Not all palliative care teams routinely record spiritual care needs in the health record, but it seems self-evident that doing so will enhance the care provision and help to address all the current needs of the people being cared for.

The culture and traditions of every person need to be understood and respected, particularly with regard to the provision of care. Recording what cultural as well as spiritual needs are, should be a given. If in doubt about aspects such as care around and after death, advice should be taken from the spiritual care expert.

Best et al. [17] also emphasise that the progression of spiritual care standards in palliative care 'will only be achieved through widespread and ongoing training of palliative care staff'. Such training should be available in all palliative care units, including opportunities for personal spiritual reflection. EAPC plans to develop online training modules to assist in providing such care.

In providing an overview of spiritual care education in various sites in Europe, Donia Baldacchino [25] suggests that the personal religiosity and spirituality of all of us, our mentors and other healthcare professionals we work with may foster a healthy spiritual clinical environment. She goes on to suggest that the organisation of spiritual retreats and/or prayer meetings for students and healthcare professionals may benefit both the caregiver and the recipient of their care. In this way, she suggests that health professionals may become change agents with the possible ultimate ripple beneficial effects of spiritual care:

If you reform your spiritual self, you will reform your professional care;
If you reform your professional care, you will reform your holistic care;
If you reform your holistic care, you will reform the care spiritually.

Establishing lasting effects of spiritual care education is challenging. However, numerous studies emphasise the need for ongoing education in spiritual care for healthcare professionals. Current literature indicates that spiritual care training is required for healthcare staff who have contact with patients [26]. However, while efforts have been made to integrate spirituality into nursing and other clinicians' curricula, data show that training is limited for nurses, increasing among physicians but non-existent among support, administrative, and ancillary staff. Austin et al. also recommend the further development of evidence-based models of spiritual care education like that developed in Aotearoa New Zealand by Morgan et al. [27], who describe an educational programme aimed at improving the understanding of spirituality and spiritual care of palliative care staff. This is a multi-disciplinary and collaborative learning programme addressing the learning needs of the whole team and is described below.

4.3 Foundations of Spiritual Care/Ngā Mātāpono O Te Manaaki Wairua: Hospice New Zealand/Te Kahu Pairuri o Aotearoa

Hospice New Zealand initially developed the *Fundamentals of Palliative Care* programme (https://www.hospice.org.nz/education-training/training-modules/) for any healthcare worker (registered and non-registered staff) caring for people with a palliative care need. The programme was initially launched nationally in 2012; since then, regular reviews have occurred, and in 2016 the *Introduction to Spiritual Care* package was added to the programme. Each year approximately 10,000 people nationally have taken part in one or more of the packages from the *Fundamentals* programme.

With the most recent review, in 2020–2021, Hospice New Zealand started work to make the *Fundamentals* programme available to a wider audience. Hospice New Zealand, in collaboration with its member hospices, now offers a new blended online learning *Fundamentals of Palliative Care* programme. Interest in the spiritual care component stimulated the development of a separate programme, *Foundations of Spiritual Care* [28], which aimed to produce a package of professional development resources targeting the spirituality training needs of New Zealand hospice teams (all staff and volunteers). Ultimately, the aim was to improve the understanding and knowledge of spirituality with and for the wider hospice team, thereby improving the spiritual wellbeing of their organisations and spiritual care for patients, families, and whānau.[1]

The programme was developed because Egan et al. [2, 3] showed spiritual care was inconsistent across hospices, to demystify spiritual care and provide resources for education in spiritual care. In this way, it was hoped to develop a more spiritually literate workforce, promote a 'spiritual culture' across hospice organisations, and develop strong relationships between hospices and key community cultural and spiritual advisors across Aotearoa New Zealand. The programme aims to enhance the provision of holistic palliative care in accordance with national/international standards and develop 'coalface' confidence in delivering spiritual care. There are extensive facilitator notes, a slide deck to accompany each session, and a workbook for each participant. Facilitators are commonly educators in the hospice team accompanied by Māori (the indigenous people of New Zealand) liaison staff. Accompanying this is a list of references and links to video presentations outlining aspects of spirituality as they are dealt with in each session [28].

The guiding principles are that this is a foundation programme—'starting the conversation'—that has been developed for all hospice team members (clinical, non-clinical, volunteer, governance, etc.). It is a professional development resource with reflective components intended to align with the principles of the *Te Tiriti o Waitangi*[2] and acknowledge the unique partnership with Māori—the intention is that this unique partnership will also form a bridge to many other cultural connections to spirituality. Of note, the programme encourages the facilitators to work with local Māori in providing the course, often as facilitators, particularly the session related to Māori death and wairua (spirituality).

The programme is non-sectarian, and the personal spiritual practice/s of participants are respected. Further aims are to uncover what participants already know, experience, and do; to draw out what is within each participant; to provide an opportunity for participants to explore and to ask, 'What do I bring to my work?'; to provide hospices with an ability to shape the programme to meet the local needs of the organisation and community and to allow identification and growth of spiritual care with and by organisations while acknowledging the challenges of delivering such care consistently and well.

---

[1] Whānau means extended family, family group, a familiar term of address to a number of people—the primary economic unit of traditional Māori society. In the modern context, the term is sometimes used to include friends who may not have any kinship ties to other members.

[2] The Treaty of Waitangi/Te Tiriti o Waitangi was signed in 1840 and was an agreement between the British Crown and many Māori chiefs. Today, the Treaty is widely accepted to be a constitutional document that establishes and guides the relationship between the Crown in New Zealand (embodied by our government) and Māori.

In total, there are four separate sessions. Learning outcomes to be achieved in the first session are that participants will be able to:

- Describe what spirituality may mean for people
- Differentiate between spirituality and religion
- Explain the importance of spiritual care in palliative care and end-of-life care
- Develop a deeper awareness of their own spirituality
- Describe attributes required to respond appropriately to others' spiritual need
- Describe existential suffering/spiritual distress/spiritual wellness.

Preparation for the first session asks participants to consider areas related to their own spirituality. Suggested reflective questions are included, such as:

- How do you feel about your own spirituality? (Who am I? Why am I here? What is life about?)
- What does spirituality mean to you?
- Consider your life experience and values and, therefore what values and beliefs you bring to the bedside/ organisation/board
- What and/or who gives ultimate and central meaning, purpose, and connection in your life?
- When you have been faced with difficult and challenging circumstances, what personal resource have you called on to get you through this time? Was there a spiritual aspect to this?
- What value does your hospice place on spirituality?
- How will you introduce yourself to the group?

The second part of this first session explores definitions of spirituality and caring in a spiritual way. 'Caring in a spiritual way is demonstrated in the way that we care and how we attend to a person's spiritual perspective and need. It is central to our practice; complementing, enhancing, and facilitating the care we provide and the interactions we have with people'. The third aspect of the first session is an exploration of the patient voice using a recording of a person approaching the end of life who was very much aware of his impending death. This session's final section explores the spiritual attributes needed to respond appropriately to spiritual needs. This is again undertaken as a facilitated group discussion.

The second session is devoted to *Wairuatanga i te ao Māori*—Spirituality in the Māori world. Participants are asked to read several resources and recordings, including Māori digital stories about caring for kaumatua (elders) at the end of life prior to attending. At the end of this session, it is hoped that participants will know, or be reminded of, some of the fundamentals of Te Ao Māori.[3] These include:

- Karakia—(prayer, incantation, blessing) the practice and its importance.
- Whanaungatanga—(acknowledgement of our relationships and connections) holistic connectedness to everything around us.

[3] Te Ao Māori refers to three key areas: te Reo Māori (Māori language), Tikanga Māori (protocols and customs) te Tiriti o Waitangi (the Treaty of Waitangi).

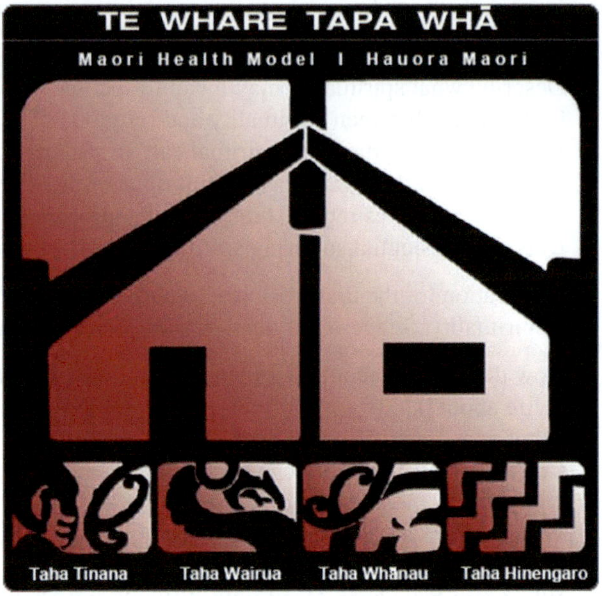

Fig. 1 Māori Health Model: Te Whare Tapa Wha, developed by Sir Mason Durie (image reproduced with permission of NZ Ministry of Health Māori Health Team, Manatū Hauora). https://www.health.govt.nz/our-work/populations/maori-health/maori-health-models/maori-health-models-te-whare-tapa-wha

- Tapu (sacred, protected, restricted) and noa—(unrestricted, ordinary, within one's powers, free from Tapu)—states of spiritual and physical protection and social order and daily living.
- Mauri—(life principle, source of emotions, protecting or radiating vitality and energy) the life force of everything—people, objects, and environment.
- Mana—(prestige, authority, control, power, influence, status, spiritual power, charisma) a supernatural force in a person, place, or object.

For many Māori, wairuatanga is considered core; they are connected to everything; it forms and directs their activities and ensures their safety. To examine wairuatanga is to examine every breath, every decision, every dream, every premonition, every meal, every ceremony, and every member of their whānau, hapū, and iwi[4]—before them, with them, and after them. Wairuatanga connects Māori to their natural environment and the universe. As this is a foundational course, the most it is thought that can be done is to provide participants with initial steps to begin to understand important wairuatanga concepts in te ao Māori. This is done by exploring personal attributes and understandings and group discussions. It is in this session that participants are reminded of the model of Te Whare Tapa Whā (Fig. 1) first introduced by Sir Mason Durie [29]. Briefly, this is the concept of the four sides of

[4]An iwi, or Māori tribe, is one of the largest kinship groupings and is generally made up of several hapū that are all descended from a common ancestor. Hapū are clusters of whānau where the whānau is usually an extended family grouping consisting of children, parents, often grandparents, and other closely related kin.

the house/whare, and attention must be given to the need of all sides for holistic health and wellbeing: Taha tinana—physical; Taha wairua—spiritual; Taha hinengaro—mental/intellectual; Taha whānau—connectedness/wider family connections. A recent addition was grounding the house on the land or whenua.

Session three explores *Te manaaki wairua hei te wā o te mate*—spiritual care at the end of life. At the end of the session, it is envisaged that participants will be able to:

- Reflect on communication skills
- Discuss the importance of a therapeutic relationship
- List potential spiritual needs/issues experienced at the end of life
- Appreciate the importance of a spiritual assessment
- Differentiate between spiritual screening/assessment/history
- Discuss the importance of documentation and care planning
- Describe the assessment methods and documentation used in the organisation
- Identify when a person needs a referral for specialist spiritual care.

This session is divided into four components: verbal and non-verbal communication; an overview; recognition of patient/family needs; developing a therapeutic relationship—use of self in spiritual care and screening, assessment, history, referral, and documentation. Participants are asked to discuss what questions people might ask when facing a life limiting condition. Have you seen a patient or family member troubled by spiritual issues? What did you notice? What drew you to this conclusion? What are some of the spiritual needs/issues patients face at the end of life? How comfortable are you exploring spiritual issues with patients, families, and whānau? What are the keys to developing a relationship with a patient within which spiritual issues/needs can be addressed safely? Facilitators are provided with guidance on how this group discussion session might develop.

The fourth session is focussed on *Te manaaki wairua o te tangata me te manaaki wairua whaiaro*—caring for others and caring for ourselves. At the end of the session, the participant will be able to:

- Discuss diversity and the needs of the groups and populations they work with
- Recognise burnout/compassion fatigue
- Describe strategies for self-care
- Describe ways to support colleagues and volunteers.

The session covers meeting the spiritual and cultural needs of diverse groups and populations; sharing of spiritually significant objects; sources of burnout/compassion fatigue; strategies for self-care and caring for others, including colleagues and volunteers. Once again, a host of resources are available for participants to refer to before the session. Much of this session is taken up once again by facilitated group discussion.

The programme's authors provide a post programme reflection that they recommend is completed 4–6 weeks after finishing the Foundations of Spiritual Care programme. Recommendations include:

- (Group) Develop a spiritual care plan for your service
- (Clinicians) Practice taking a spiritual history—either with a patient or with a colleague
- (Management) What policies need to be developed or reviewed?
- (Boards and Trustees) What is your responsibility around spiritual care for your organisation?

In summary, the programme suggests that addressing spiritual needs are not prescriptive and will vary according to individual patients. A 'one-size-fits-all' model for spiritual care is certainly not advocated, but there is a need for a clear framework to ensure that all patients have the opportunity to have their spiritual needs met. Participants are encouraged to reflect on their own feelings and beliefs. Reflection here is a deliberate process; it is not just thinking about something—it is purposeful consideration. It is a positive process allowing learning and change if necessary and can be used equally to highlight good practice. It makes the links between practice and theory.

An evaluation of the programme demonstrated that it positively influenced participants in both personal and professional areas. Personal influences included increased awareness and understanding of spirituality and spiritual care; it refreshed, affirmed, and validated prior spiritual knowledge and increased confidence. Regarding professional influence, the programme increased collegiality; increased health literacy and helped develop new skills. Some questions were raised by participants on the sustainability of experiences and outcomes, and mixed feelings were reported on the relevance of the entire programme for non-clinical participants [30].

5 Discussion: Best Practice

Hospice NZ's Foundations of Spiritual Care programme stands as an exemplary example of interprofessional spiritual care education. It embodies indigenous partnership, evidence-informed practices, inclusivity, skilled facilitators, patient engagement, and fosters participants' spiritual growth while emphasising evaluation. Indigenous spirituality offers a point of entry in many countries that counters (or compliments) biomedical and even biopsychosocial paradigms, with the latter dominating healthcare.

Interprofessional education needs to be evidence-informed to find purchase across the professionals, particularly in medicine, where evidence-based approaches are a priority. The Foundations programme came out of a national study that challenged hospice, suggesting it needed to attend to its stated objective of holistic care, particularly in relation to spiritual care. Then the Foundation programme's development included academics, clinicians, Māori experts and management, thus drawing on contemporary academic and pragmatic evidence.

Ethical spiritual care is also patient (and whānau) led, thus starting from a position acknowledging spirituality as a human universal but expressed, experienced, and cared for in a multitude of ways. By careful consideration of participants' own spirituality, the Foundations programme highlights understanding oneself and one's spirituality to be able to relate human to human first, with compassionate presence, then assessing particular expressions of spiritual needs, which may include religious needs.

Ideal spiritual care in the clinical context only happens when policy affirms its need and space is made available. One of the strengths of the Foundations programme is the facilitator training and resources, which are comprehensive in terms of written materials, links into multi-media (videos/recordings), and local expertise.

Regarding the inclusion of patient/whanau voices, today's healthcare context rightly emphasises participatory approaches such as co-design and co-production; thus, 'nothing to us without us' affirms the need to include end users in the development of healthcare. The Foundations programme did this reasonably well through the inclusion of patients' stories through audio and video. In many countries, such stories are likely to be available.

Naturally, there are challenges regarding interprofessional spiritual care education. Hospice NZ's programme is aspirational, expecting much from the teaching and learning experience. Teaching theory would suggest that a scaffolding approach with ongoing and increasing complexity would be useful to build on spiritual care competencies.

6 Final Words

At the core of comprehensive and compassionate care, spiritual care is significant in addressing the holistic needs of individuals and families, particularly in end-of-life settings [31]. Regardless of interpretation, failing to address the spiritual realm means neglecting holistic care. For over 50 years, the modern hospice and palliative care approaches have affirmed total care, including spiritual care [32], yet spiritual care is often implicit, thus missing explicit spiritual needs and distress. Spirituality underpins and is central to end-of-life care as it asks 'what matters most' of the institution, the staff, and the patient/family. Therefore, spiritual care is not just about the chaplain/spiritual care expert—it is everyone's business—it is expressed in all endeavours. Given the central role of spirituality, every member of the healthcare team possesses the capacity to influence the spiritual well-being of patients and their families, either in a positive or negative manner. Interprofessional training in spiritual care effectively addresses these needs and aligns with the realities of providing comprehensive patient/family-centred care.

References

1. Puchalski CM, Vitillo R, Hull SK, Reller N. Improving the spiritual dimension of whole person care: reaching national and international consensus. J Palliat Med. 2014;17:642–76.
2. Egan R, MacLeod R, Jaye R, et al. What is spirituality? Evidence from a New Zealand hospice study. Mortality. 2011;16:307–24.
3. Egan R, et al. Spiritual beliefs, practices, and needs at the end of life: results from a New Zealand national hospice study. Palliat Support Care. 2017;15(2):223–30.
4. Byock I. Contemplating mortality. www.onbeing.org/program/transcript/4655. Last Accessed 10 Mar 2023.
5. Foreword SC. In: Zimmerman JM, editor. Hospice: complete care for the terminally ill. Baltimore: Urban & Schwarzenberg; 1981. p. ix.
6. Peters RS. Education as initiation, inaugural lecture. London: University of London Institute of Education; 1967.
7. Wenger E. Communities of practice; learning meaning and identity. Cambridge: Cambridge University Press; 1998.
8. Parsell G, Bligh J. Interprofessional learning. Postgrad Med J. 1998;74:89–95.
9. Carpenter J, Hewstone M. Shared learning for doctors and social workers: evaluation of a programme. Brit J Soc Work. 1996;26:239–57.
10. Wee B, Hillier R, Coles C, et al. Palliative care: a suitable setting for undergraduate interprofessional learning. Palliat Med. 2001;15:487–92.
11. Barr H. Interprofessional education: today, yesterday and tomorrow. 2005. http://www.health.heacademy.ac.uk/publications/occasionalpaper/occp1revised.pdf. Accessed 13 Mar 2023.
12. Jones M, Thistlethwaite J. Interprofessional practice in palliative care. In: MacLeod RD, Van den Block L, editors. Textbook of Palliative Care. Cham: Springer Nature; 2019. https://doi.org/10.1007/978-3-319-77740-5_41.
13. Puchalski C, Jafari N, Buller H, Haythorn T, Jacobs C, Ferrell B. Interprofessional spiritual care education curriculum: a milestone toward the provision of spiritual care. J Palliat Med. https://doi-org.ezproxy.auckland.ac.nz/10.1089/jpm.2019.0375
14. Puchalski CM, Vitillo R, Hull SK, Reller N. Improving the spiritual dimension of whole person care: reaching national and international consensus. J Palliat Med. 2014;17(6):642–56. https://doi.org/10.1089/jpm.2014.9427.
15. Puchalski C, Ferrell BR, Borneman T, DiFrances RC, Haythorn T, Jacobs C. Implementing quality improvement efforts in spiritual care: outcomes from the interprofessional spiritual care education curriculum. J Healthcare Chaplaincy. 2021;28:431. https://doi.org/10.1080/08854726.2021.1917168.
16. Best MC, Jones K, Washington J, Sullivan J, Kearney M, Puchalski C. Evaluation of the interprofessional spiritual care education curriculum in Australia: online. Palliat Support Care. 2023;21(1):65–73. https://doi.org/10.1017/S1478951522000244.
17. Best M, Leget C, Goodhead A, et al. An EAPC white paper on multi-disciplinary education for spiritual care in palliative care. BMC Palliat Care. 2020;19:9. https://doi.org/10.1186/s12904-019-0508-4.
18. Leget C. Art of living, art of dying: spiritual care for a good death. Philadelphia: Jessica Kingsley Publishers; 2017.
19. Puchalski C. Spirituality and end-of-life care: a time for listening and caring. J Palliat Med. 2002;5(2):289–94.
20. Maugans T. The SPIRITual history. Arch Fam Med. 1996;5(1):11–6.
21. Anandarajah G, Hight E. Spirituality and medical practice: using the HOPE questions as a practical tool for spiritual assessment. Am Fam Physician. 2001;63(1):81–8.
22. Neely D, Minford E. FAITH: spiritual history-taking made easy. Clin Teach. 2009;6(3):181–5.
23. Ross L, McSherry W. The power of two simple questions. Nurs. 2018;19:439–47.
24. Steinhauser K, Voils C, Clipp E, Bosworth H, Christakis N, Tulsky J. "Are you at peace?": one item to probe spiritual concerns at the end of life. Arch Intern Med. 2006;166(1):101–5.

25. Baldacchino D. Spiritual care education of health care professionals. Religions. 2015;6:594–613. https://doi.org/10.3390/rel6020594.
26. Austin P, Macleod R, Siddall P, McSherry W, Egan R. Spiritual care training is needed for clinical and non-clinical staff to manage patients' spiritual needs. J Stud Spirit. 2017;7(1):50–63. https://doi.org/10.1080/20440243.2017.1290031.
27. Morgan A, Macleod R, Schumacher M, Egan R. Delivering spiritual care: a resource to train hospice staff in New Zealand. Europ J Palliat Care. 2015;22(3):130–2.
28. Foundations of Spiritual Care. Facilitator guide. Wellington: Hospice NZ; 2020.
29. Durie MH. A Māori perspective of health. SocSciMed. 1985;20:483–6.
30. MacLeod RD, Moeke-Maxwell T, Egan R. Foundations of spiritual care: report of an evaluation of an innovative programme. 2019. Unpublished manuscript.
31. Balboni TA, VanderWeele TJ, Doan-Soares SD, et al. Spirituality in serious illness and health. JAMA. 2022;328:184–97.
32. Saunders C. The evolution of palliative care. Patient Ed Couns. 2000;41(1):7–13.

Cultural Safety and Spiritual Care

Piret Paal

Abstract This chapter has an anthropological focus and looks at the evidence for culturally safe spiritual care in palliative care and suggests ways to advocate for non-discriminatory spiritual care education within palliative care. It introduces the concept of cultural safety and its link to the concept of power, which is not well understood by healthcare professionals seeking to provide culturally appropriate care. This also has implications for spiritual care education, which needs to consider the potential bias in the representation and understanding of spiritual care in current research and education. The case study adds an ethical dimension to the discussion of appropriate care versus culturally safe care that is helpful in opening up the discussion of cultural safety and culturally safe spiritual care.

Keywords Cultural safety · Appropriate care · Power · Spiritual care · Cultural competence · Cultural sensitivity · Cultural awareness · Palliative care · Self-assessment · Self-reflection

1 Introduction

Spiritual care and cultural safety are both terms that are heavily misunderstood, even if many regulations and guidelines state that it is the duty of healthcare staff to integrate religious, spiritual, and cultural competencies into their practice [1–5]. Simultaneously, the patient and their caregivers have the right to receive culturally

P. Paal (✉)
Institute for Palliative Care, Paracelsus Medical University, Salzburg, Austria

Department of Ethnology, Institute of Cultural Studies, University of Tartu, Tartu, Estonia
e-mail: piret.paal@ut.ee

M. C. Best (ed.), *Spiritual Care in Palliative Care*,
https://doi.org/10.1007/978-3-031-50864-6_28

safe care and spiritual care if they so wish. One of the four spiritual care competencies in palliative care encourages us to 'be conscious of the boundaries that may need to be respected in terms of culture, ritual and traditions' [6]. The European Association of Palliative Care (EAPC) white paper on spiritual care education [7] acknowledges that the evidence on culturally specific needs in palliative care is extremely limited; nevertheless, all healthcare staff need to be aware of the risk of prejudice, and training may be needed to promote inclusivity of all cultures within the palliative care service. As staff are aware of the cultural and religious diversity in the local population, all the measures listed below should be appropriate for both a secular and a religious culture as part of the cultural safety strategies:

- Patients tend to prefer healthcare structures and systems that make them feel safe and well-served.
- Respecting patients' culture-based aspirations may be encouraged and supported as long as they do not challenge the patient's well-being (and are not illegal).
- Staff should be trained to welcome family visitations, food-related rituals, or inviting (religious) leaders from the community into the hospital to support patients and their families.
- Ritual, if it helps patients to cope with illness, it is to be supported; however, if the patient agrees to this to please his/her family, it should be negotiated carefully, whatever culture is involved.
- Regular recording of cultural information that will impact on advance care planning, dietary requirements, or arrangements after death should be part of the care plan for the patient [7, 8].

The EAPC white paper expresses a concern that 'cultural taboos may not be observed if the staff is not aware of them—this is particularly an issue where new cultural populations, such as refugees, are present' [7].

Recent awakening in palliative care finally calls for recognising the structural disadvantages for racial and minority ethnic peoples which requires immediate action to make palliative care more accessible [9]. The implementation of cultural safety strategies requires institutional or organisational change. Because race, ethnicity, culture, and religion are constructs with significant overlap, all of which support structural othering, oppression, and discrimination at individual and systemic levels, they are considered in this chapter as phenomena that threaten patient safety and well-being. Ethically acknowledged strategies for appropriate spiritual care include listening, neutrality, and sensitivity to spiritual issues [10]. But are all patients approached with kindness and without judgement and stereotypes? There is sufficient evidence that health professionals who operate from assumptions and stereotypical attitudes place the health of the people they care for at risk and seriously impair service delivery [11].

As in palliative care [12], spiritual care research and training needs to look critically in the mirror and ask itself whether the spiritual care currently being promoted could be discriminatory and how the concept of cultural safety can help to overcome this. This chapter argues that it is crucial to promote practices that respect the rights and dignity of all people seeking spiritual care. Above all, it calls for comprehensive and culturally safe spiritual care education, research, and practice.

2 Cultural Safety—The Idea and Current Definition

The concept of cultural safety arose from the colonial context of New Zealand society. Formalisation of the concept of cultural safety began in 1988 at a *hui* (Māori term for gathering) in Christchurch, which was attended by nurse educators and Māori student nurses. A further hui was held during 1989 for Māori nurse teachers, and from this hui, a group of Māori nurses were nominated to prepare a set of cultural safety standards. The standards that were developed were known as *Kawa Whakaruruhau* which translates into 'cultural safety'. Cultural safety became a requirement for nursing and midwifery courses in 1992 [11].

The first definition of cultural safety provided by the Nursing Council of New Zealand was as follows:

> The effective nursing of a person/family from another culture by a nurse who has undertaken a process of reflection on own cultural identity and recognises the impact of the nurses' culture on own nursing practice. (*Nursing Council of New Zealand, Standards for registration of comprehensive muses from polytechnic courses. Glossary, Nursing Council of New Zealand, Wellington, 1992*)

This undertaking was heavily misinterpreted and ridiculed in New Zealand, as the quality of medical care that nurses trained in cultural safety would provide was questioned.

As with many new concepts introduced into healthcare practice, the best way to explain what it is, is to explain what it is not. Cultural safety is not about cultural sensitivity or awareness. It is not about learning the language and customs or worldviews of a particular ethnic, racial, or religious group. It is not transcultural care introduced and promoted by Madeleine Leininger, whose intercultural nursing experiences were largely based on her ethnographic studies conducted among the Gadsup people in New Guinea [13]. Widely used terms such as cultural sensitivity and cultural awareness both refer to knowledge of cultural and especially ethnic or racial or religious diversity. When the term culture is understood as ethnicity, race, or religion, it forms the basis for a misinterpretation of the concept of cultural safety [11]. Hence, many internationally relevant documents that stress the importance of culturally appropriate and acceptable healthcare within the increasing pluralism, diversity, and complexity of ethnic and cultural groups can be misleading, as healthcare providers establish interventions for their individual and professional definitions of 'appropriate' care. There is an ingrained assumption that healthcare professionals are solely responsible for the 'appropriateness of care' because of their expertise [14].

Power represents an essential distinction between cultural competence, sensitivity, transcultural, or culturally appropriate care and cultural safety [15, 16]. One of the first studies on cultural safety, conducted in a non-indigenous but pluralistic setting, among advanced nurse practitioners, found that nurses were unaware of their position of power in caring for their patients [17]. This indicates that nurses and other healthcare professionals should be taught to reflect on interpersonal power differences and acknowledge the power differences between nurses and patients. In 2019, the central role of power was highlighted in the consensus definition of cultural safety:

> Cultural safety deals with the balance of power between professional caregivers and people receiving care. Accordingly, professional caregivers must recognise that a person's dignity and right to self-determination have to be acknowledged and prioritised; address their own biases, attitudes, assumptions, stereotypes, prejudices, structures, and characteristics that may affect the quality of care; and engage in self-reflection. Healthcare organisations and authorities need to be held accountable for providing culturally safe care, as defined by patients and their communities, and as measured through progress towards achieving health equity. Cultural safety requires healthcare professionals and their associated organisations to influence healthcare to reduce bias and achieve equity within the workforce and working environment. [7, 15]

This definition demonstrates that cultural safety is a concept of general significance for all healthcare professionals [13].

3 Advancing Spiritual Care Education

Spiritual care training may help to challenge the spiritual vacuum in healthcare institutions [18]. Could it also enhance cultural safety in healthcare and reduce the discriminatory components of such training? Discriminatory spiritual care training refers to any form of education or training programme that promotes or exhibits bias, prejudice or discrimination based on a person's spiritual or religious beliefs, practices or affiliations. Examples of discriminatory spiritual care training are as follows: (1) Training in spiritual care can be discriminatory if only the major world religions are addressed; (2) Training in spiritual care can be discriminatory if the contribution of the major world religions is neglected in the curricula; (3) Spiritual care training can be discriminatory if it does not address the needs of agnostics or atheists; (4) Spiritual care training can be discriminatory if the multi-confessional content is unclear. It has been argued that spiritual care training programmes can have a negative impact on students by causing anxiety and pressuring them to change their views on spirituality, because of the tenuousness of students' spirituality. Therefore, any form of discriminatory spiritual care training is ethically or morally unacceptable as it undermines the principles of inclusivity, respect, and equality [19].

Box 1 Faculty Check—Making Spiritual Care Culturally Safe

1. Recognise and acknowledge the influences that may shape the spiritual or religious orientation of teachers.
2. Explain what spiritual care means. Point out that there are practices that discriminate against people based on their spiritual or religious beliefs, often resulting in unequal treatment, exclusion, or marginalisation.
3. Give specific examples of discriminatory practices such as favouring one religious tradition over another, stigmatising certain belief systems, imposing one's personal beliefs on others, or refusing to care for someone because of their spiritual or religious background.
4. Describe the negative consequences and effects of spiritual care. Explain that it perpetuates division, reinforces stereotypes, and hinders the development of trust and relationships between providers and those seeking spiritual support. It can lead to feelings of alienation, exclusion, and even harm for people who do not conform to prevailing spiritual or religious norms.
5. Emphasise the ethical concerns associated with discriminatory spiritual care. Discuss how this contradicts the fundamental principles of equality, human rights and the autonomy of individuals to freely practice and express their spiritual beliefs. Point out that this contradicts the principles of inclusive and person-centred care, which should respect people's different spiritual and religious backgrounds.
6. Explain that non-judgemental and non-discriminatory care promotes a sense of safety, trust, and open communication between caregivers and patients or clients, supporting overall well-being and holistic care.

4 Culturally Safe Approaches in Palliative Care

For rural Indigenous palliative care, culturally safe palliative care strategy includes involving patients and families in planning services, reflecting on individual and systemic racism, community ownership of services, and recognising the diverse worldviews that shape care [20]. In an urban, pluralistic context, healthcare professionals are faced with complex cross-cultural situations. Designing care pathways is much more complicated and has many pitfalls. Fox example, in Germany the introduction of 'migrant palliative care services', which are essentially seen as opening up services to 'others', but simultaneously create a barrier between 'us' and 'them' [8].

Box 2 A Case Study of Spiritual Needs and Best Care Leading to Clash of Cultures at the End of Life [21]

Mr. Saied is transferred from the oncology ward to the palliative care ward without prior consultation with his relatives. During the entire treatment period, his wife does not leave his side. Mr. Saied is 30 years old, was born in Tunisia and has been living in a large city in Germany with his wife of 27 years for 10 years. They have no children. Nothing is known about Mr. Saied's education or profession.

The staff know that the patient speaks Arabic, French, and fairly good German. His wife has little knowledge of German, and communication is difficult. Two older brothers live nearby and are very close to Mr. Saied. The whole family belongs to Islam and practices their faith.

Mr. Saied suffers from bronchial carcinoma. He is in a poor general condition and is bedridden (ECOG score 4). He is also cachectic and complains of dyspnoea (shortness of breath). His medication is reviewed and optimised on the palliative care ward. Nevertheless, Mr. Saied's general condition deteriorates rapidly. He is less and less responsive and hardly answers any questions.

Mrs. Saeid is informed that her husband will soon die. She reacts by crying profusely. Mrs. Saied stays with her husband and holds his hand. As the night progresses, the breathing noises increase and it seems as if Mr. Saied is having great difficulty breathing. For this reason, the nurse calls the doctor on duty, who orders more medication if necessary. Mr. Saied is also given oxygen and positioned with his upper body elevated. The shortness of breath seems to improve.

In the meantime, Mrs. Saied has called Mr. Saied's brothers, who enter Mr. Saied's room shortly afterwards. They are informed that the patient could soon die. They quickly flatten the bed, turn Mr. Saied on his side, fold his hands together and pray.

The nurse tries to straighten his upper body, but the brothers will not allow it. 'He belongs to us', 'he belongs to us now', they say—the staff have to leave the room. Mr. Saied himself is no longer conscious and therefore unable to express his wishes. The developing conflict between Mr. Saied's family and the staff is highly explosive.

Questions for self-reflection: Do you recognise this situation? What feelings does this case study trigger in you? What socio-economic or personal aspects are known about the patient? What medical and nursing aspects are known? What is the cause of the (intercultural) conflict? How could the conflict have been avoided? What is the power balance in this situation?

The EAPC White Paper calls for awareness of the boundaries that may need to be respected in terms of culture, rituals, and traditions. It argues that patients' cultural wishes should be respected and supported. On the other hand, it is equally important that the role of the healthcare provider is recognised to include the responsibility to protect patients from harmful culture-related activities. It can happen that cultural needs, as illustrated in the case study above, conflict with evidence-based medicine. This can be a source of stress for palliative care staff if it leads to increased suffering at the end of life, but it is equally stressful for family members who are forced to give up their autonomy [7].

5 Self-reflection

Healthcare professionals can apply Purnell's model [22] in practice to support the delivery of culturally safe care. In addition, this model can be used in self-assessment and is well suited for palliative care. The Purnell model for cultural competence provides a basis for understanding individual cultural needs in self-reflection and when in contact with patients and relatives, in order to provide holistic, culturally competent interventions in healthcare.

Purnell's model includes four circles of varying sizes as well as a 12-part inner circle that illustrates the various 'cultural domains'. The outer circles of the model are interconnected and are involved within the process of providing an individual with care. The circles represent global society, community, family, and the individual. The individual is described as a person with their own sense of self, cultural values and beliefs, which may or may not be affected by the outer domains.

The twelve inner pieces of the model are cultural domains that are composed of concepts that should be focused upon when evaluating self (or a patient). These domains focus on heritage, communication, family roles and organisation, workforce, biocultural ecology, high-risk behaviours, nutrition, pregnancy and childbearing, death rituals, spirituality, healthcare practices, and the healthcare practitioner.

Most importantly, the Purnell model includes a dimension for things that are unknown, as well as an indication of cultural competence associated with failures and successes, depending on the situation. This is consistent with the idea that cultural safety is not a skill that can be fully acquired in a training course, but that enabling cultural safety is a process that may or may not occur depending on personal openness and tolerance and is always affected by the particular situation.

6 Conclusions

Application of cultural safety requires that healthcare professionals care for people 'regardful' of those things which make them unique [3]. The problem is that even in countries where cultural safety is a well-established concept, the change in practice is complex, requiring leadership for a multi-system approach, critical pedagogy, and commitment [16]. Spiritual care is based on building relationships, which means that any perceived cultural or religious barriers hinder the care work. Working on one's own preconceptions [7] is therefore crucial and, perhaps, more important than acquiring knowledge about particular religious groups or ethnic minority traditions.

References

1. European Council. A New European Agenda for Culture – SWD (2018) 267 final. 2018.
2. International Council of Nurses. The ICN code of ethics for nurses. Geneva: ICN; 2021.
3. National Health Institutes. A practical guide to implementing the national CLAS standards: for racial, ethnic and linguistic minorities, people with disabilities and sexual and gender minorities. Washington, DC: National Committee for Quality Assurance; 2016.
4. World Health Organization. In: Office of the United Nations High Commissioner for Human Rights, editor. The Right to Health Fact Sheet No 31. Geneva: World Health Organization; 2002.
5. World Health Organization. In: Goals FA-AtuhcatSD, editor. Declaration of Astana. Astana: World Health Organization; 2018.
6. Gamondi C, Larkin P, Payne S. Core competencies in palliative care: an EAPC white paper on palliative care education: part 2. Eur J Palliat Care. 2013;20:140–5.
7. Best M, Leget C, Goodhead A, et al. An EAPC white paper on multi-disciplinary education for spiritual care in palliative care. BMC Palliat Care. 2020;19:9.
8. Paal P. Culturally sensitive palliative care research: what should we do with 'those people', or what should we do with ourselves? In: Kuehlmeyer K, Klingler C, Huxtable R, editors. Ethical, legal and social aspects of healthcare for migrants: perspectives from the UK and Germany. Routledge; 2018. p. 162–75.
9. Hussain JA, Koffman J, Bajwah S. Invited editorials. Palliat Med. 2021;35:810–3.
10. Polzer Casarez RL, Engebretson JC. Ethical issues of incorporating spiritual care into clinical practice. J Clin Nurs. 2012;21:2099–107.
11. Papps E, Ramsden I. Cultural safety in nursing: the New Zealand experience. Int J Qual Health Care. 1996;8:491–7.
12. Schrank B, Rumpold T, Amering M, et al. Pushing boundaries – culture-sensitive care in oncology and palliative care: a qualitative study. Psycho-Oncology. 2017;26:763–9.
13. Polaschek NR. Cultural safety: a new concept in nursing people of different ethnicities. J Adv Nurs. 1998;27:452–7.
14. Richardson S, Williams T. Why is cultural safety essential in health care? Med Law. 2007;26:699–707.
15. Curtis E, Jones R, Tipene-Leach D, et al. Why cultural safety rather than cultural competency is required to achieve health equity: a literature review and recommended definition. Int J Equity Health. 2019;18:174.
16. Wilson D. Indigenous and minority peoples and cultural safety: the role of nursing praxis. Nurs Prax N Z. 2014;30:2–4.
17. Pirhofer J, Bükki J, Vaismoradi M, et al. A qualitative exploration of cultural safety in nursing from the perspectives of advanced practice nurses: meaning, barriers, and prospects. BMC Nurs. 2022;21:178.
18. Paal P, Helo Y, Frick E. Spiritual care training provided to healthcare professionals: a systematic review. J Pastoral Care Counsel. 2015;69:19–30.
19. Brandstötter C, Grabenweger R, Frick E, et al. Die Kluft zwischen Training und Patientenversorgung: Maßnahmen und Möglichkeiten für eine nachhaltige Veränderung – ein Regenschirm Review. Spiritual Care. 2022;11:212–25.
20. Schill K, Caxaj S. Cultural safety strategies for rural indigenous palliative care: a scoping review. BMC Palliat Care. 2019;18:21.
21. Adam Y, Paal P, Pastrana T. Kultur- und migrationssensibler Umgang – kulturelle Sicherheit. In: Rolke S-NE, editor. Palliative Care multiprofessionell Fallbasiertes Lernen. Kohlhammer. Stuttgart. 2023.
22. Purnell L. A description of the Purnell model for cultural competence. J Transcult Nurs. 2000;11:40–6.

Self-Care for Palliative Care Staff

Jason Mills

Abstract Drawing from contemporary research, scholarship, and practice-based experience, this chapter provides an exploration of self-care for staff providing palliative care. Understanding self-care begins with appreciating what it is and why it is important. From that basis, due consideration can be given to the holistic nature of self-care in practice. Further, self-compassion, self-care planning, and compassionate leadership can enable self-care in both personal and professional settings. A key message of this chapter is that suffering and healing form part of the palliative care journey for both the living and the dying—those giving and receiving care—and that self-care for staff is a vital element of spiritual care in palliative care. Rather than relating to the care of self and others in dichotomy, self-awareness and insight to interdependence can serve as guides to 'total care' through ongoing reflection.

Keywords Death · Dying · Healing · Palliative care · Self-care · Self-compassion · Suffering · Wounded healer · Spiritual care

1 Introduction

Caring for others requires caring for oneself. [1]

In clinical settings, the concept of self-care is perhaps most familiar to practitioners in the context of patient self-management in chronic illness. Naturally, this form of self-care in clinical populations is necessary and widely promoted by those working across the healthcare disciplines. Patient self-care is both encouraged and

J. Mills (✉)
Research Centre for Palliative Care, Death, and Dying; College of Nursing and Health Sciences, Flinders University, Adelaide, SA, Australia
e-mail: jason.mills@flinders.edu.au

M. C. Best (ed.), *Spiritual Care in Palliative Care*,
https://doi.org/10.1007/978-3-031-50864-6_29

supported because it is understood and valued for its merits in promoting health and wellbeing. However, the same recognition and endorsement may not be so apparent in the case of self-care for practitioners providing palliative care. A lack of self-care in palliative care practice can be problematic because *caring for others requires caring for oneself* [1].

Drawing from contemporary research, scholarship, and practice-based experience, this chapter will provide an exploration of self-care for staff providing palliative care. In doing so, it will suggest that suffering and healing form part of the palliative care journey for both the living and the dying—those giving and receiving care—and that self-care for staff is a vital element of spiritual care in palliative care.

In exploring self-care for staff, it is helpful to consider the key questions pertinent to understanding its need and appreciating its place in contemporary palliative care. *What is self-care?* and *why is it important?* Further, *how can self-care be enabled?* and *what does self-care mean, and look like in practice?*

In this way, the chapter will first define and outline the importance of self-care. Next, it will discuss self-compassion, self-care planning, and compassionate leadership as enablers to self-care in both personal and professional settings. Then it will consider the holistic nature of self-care in practice. To conclude, a reflective narrative is shared from the perspective of a 'wounded healer', highlighting ways in which personal insight and self-awareness can guide ones' self-care through reflective practice.

2 Unpacking Self-Care

Providing care for others without caring for oneself is unsustainable. [2]

Effective and sustainable self-care requires that we first know what self-care is and understand, deeply, why it is important for practitioners providing palliative care.

2.1 What Is Self-Care?

The term 'self-care' came to great prominence with Dorothea Orem's Self-care Theory [3]. Self-care, in this context, relates to the identification of a patient's self-care deficit, and requires an appreciation of the agency, capacity, and responsibilities of patients in promoting their own health and wellbeing. Perhaps more importantly, Orem stressed that self-care was fundamentally a human endeavour.

It is in this broader context that self-care is situated within this chapter, given that practitioners providing palliative care are, themselves, human. In his seminal work *The Nature of Suffering and the Goals of Medicine*, Cassell [4] described the nature and causes of suffering in medical patients. In a corresponding text *The Nature of Suffering and the Goals of Nursing*, Ferrell [2] drew attention to the shared humanity and suffering of nurses, declaring that caring for others without caring for oneself was unsustainable. Thus, self-care is not only a matter of personal survival or optimal wellbeing; it also represents an important consideration for sustaining practitioners' capacity for patient care. This is reflected in Watson's [5] Theory of Human Caring and the Foucauldian concept 'care of the self' [6]. While noting that Foucault's philosophy of the self was not confined to the physical body, Perron [7] introduced the primacy of the self–self relationship as central to nursing and argued that care of the self was a fundamental condition for nurses to care for others.

Mills' [8] middle-range theory of self-care posits that: (i) Self-care is a relational aspect of healthcare practice; (ii) Self-compassion is a positive emotion that supports effective self-care practice in healthcare professionals; and (iii) The relationship between self-compassion and compassion for others varies according to individual compassion literacy. Taken together, self-care can be defined as the self-initiated behaviour consciously adopted to promote ones' own health and wellbeing.

While self-care is increasingly discussed in the general healthcare literature [9, 10], it is especially relevant to those providing spiritual care and palliative care. These practitioners represent a relatively small yet essential specialty area of clinical practice within healthcare systems, characterised by a holistic and team-based approach, as well as a central focus on therapeutic relationships with patients and their families to provide 'total care' [11, 12]. This total care requires an ongoing and, at times, intensive therapeutic use of self that demands constant attention to self-care to ensure a compassionate care for others that is sustainable [13, 14].

2.2 Why Self-Care?

> *The expectation that we can be immersed in suffering and loss daily and not be touched by it, is as unrealistic as expecting to be able to walk through water without getting wet.* [15]

While the extent to which one is 'touched' through daily immersion in suffering may vary, the need for self-care among staff providing palliative care remains constant. Ongoing exposure to death, dying, and loss while working in palliative care makes grieving and healing an important part of the journey for practitioners. It has been suggested that if one instead seeks to 'protect' oneself from loss and suffering, rather than engaging in self-caring grief and healing practices, over time these experiences may become a major cause of burnout [15].

Vachon [16] outlined a broad variety of occupational stressors that have featured over past decades. While suggesting that early recognition of the important role of self-care in the palliative care field may have gone some way towards alleviating the extent of stress experienced, Vachon cautioned that occupational stressors appear to be increasing, and thus, complacency must be avoided. This position is supported by research in international contexts of stress and burnout reported in studies of palliative care practitioners [17–19]. In a national study by Wang et al. [20], it was found that one third of palliative care physicians in Canada demonstrated a high degree of burnout. A systematic review and meta-analysis of burnout in palliative care nurses found the main variables associated with burnout were occupational and psychological [21].

The capacity of practitioners to provide high quality, compassionate care to patients is influenced, in part, by their own health status and level of wellbeing. The nature of human suffering is such that, based on a shared common humanity, the personal experience of health and illness among professional caregivers providing palliative care touches the collective health and wellbeing of those receiving that care. That is to say, professional roles do not protect against personal suffering, and care of self is relational to care for others. The importance of staff wellbeing to both care performance and patient experience of care has been established through large-scale studies of national health services staff, suggesting that staff wellbeing is an important antecedent of patient care performance [22, 23].

From their multi-site mixed-methods study using 498 patient experience surveys, 106 patient interviews, 427 staff wellbeing surveys, 86 staff interviews, and 206 hours of observation, Maben et al. [23] concluded that efforts to enhance the wellbeing of staff were not only important in their own right, but also for the quality of patients' experience of healthcare. The relationship between the quality of healthcare and the health and wellbeing of staff providing that care is therefore significant.

The benefits of staff self-care to their health and wellbeing are well supported by research. In a study of American chaplains, self-care practices were found to be a protective factor against risk of burnout; with low risk of burnout and higher professional quality of life observed in those practising a variety of self-care strategies on a regular basis [24]. These findings are consistent with other research focused solely on practitioners working in hospice care [25, 26]. Results from a study of Brazilian palliative care providers showed strong, statistically significant associations between self-care and resilience, self-reported professional life satisfaction, and lessened mental health impairment [27]. In studies of Spanish palliative care providers, self-care positively predicted competence in coping with death, self-compassion, and compassion satisfaction (pleasure derived from helping others), while negatively predicting compassion fatigue and burnout [28, 29].

It is therefore not surprising that the importance of, and need for, self-care is found reflected in professional palliative care practice standards used internationally [30–35]. Moreover, the maintaining of intentional self-care is mandated in national spiritual care frameworks such as the *Capabilities Framework for Spiritual Care Practitioners* developed by Spiritual Care Australia [36].

3 Enabling Self-Care

While knowing what self-care is and understanding its importance provides a solid foundation to support practitioners providing palliative care, appreciation of key enablers such as self-compassion, self-care planning, and compassionate leadership can optimise self-care practice.

3.1 *Self-Compassion*

> *Self-compassion is expressing the same kind of concern for our own pain and wellbeing as we would show for another in such a predicament.* [37]

In some ways, self-compassion can be understood as the oxygen that fuels the fire of self-care. It could thus be argued there is no self-care without self-compassion. At the same time, many might struggle with expressing or enacting it due to a fear of compassion for oneself [38]. For instance, it may be perceived and stigmatised as being selfish; or in highly self-critical individuals, one may be fearful that self-compassion will weaken performance and conflict with achievement. Others may believe that taking on suffering without self-compassionate care is their karma or spiritual 'cross to bear' in atoning for sinful actions. Citing words from the Bible, however, Wilhoit [37] argues that self-compassion can form a valuable element to spiritual practice. In this way, self-compassion may also contribute to spiritual wellbeing in practitioners providing palliative care [39]. Thus, acknowledging any reservations and embracing self-compassion may represent a powerful opportunity for transformation and authentic self-care.

Self-compassion involves directing compassion inwards to oneself with self-kindness, understanding, and positive regard [40]. As a pioneer in self-compassion research, Neff [41] conceptualised self-compassion as a six-factor construct comprising three positive sub-scales: (a) Self-kindness, (b) Common humanity, (c) Mindfulness; and three corresponding negative sub-scales: (d) Self-judgement, (e) Isolation, and (e) Over-identification. Thus, self-compassion encompasses (i) extending kindness and understanding to oneself—rather than harsh self-criticism and judgement; (ii) relating to one's negative experiences as part of the larger human experience—rather than as separating and isolating; and (iii) holding one's suffering in perspective through balanced awareness—rather than over-identifying with it [42].

Accordingly, self-compassion is associated with emotional intelligence [43], prosocial behaviour [44], and a broad range of benefits to health and wellbeing [45–49].

More importantly, quantitative and qualitative studies have found self-compassion to be a key enabler of self-care in palliative care providers [50, 51]. A study of Brazilian palliative care providers during the COVID-19 pandemic found positive and statistically significant correlations between self-compassion and self-care, and resilience [27]. In a national study of chaplains in the USA [24], self-compassion was found to be protective against risk of burnout and secondary traumatic stress. The results of a recent study of Spanish palliative care providers found that self-compassion was a strong predictor of self-care awareness and professional quality of life [28].

3.2 Self-Care Planning

If you fail to plan, you are planning to fail. [52]

Many have found the notion of planning for self-care to be useful in supporting their practice. Practitioners are proactive in formulating care plans for patients in a systematic way to ensure that all care needs are met, so it follows that self-care is best planned and guided in a similar way, rather than being reactive and ad-hoc.

This logic is also supported by studies among palliative care providers, with quantitative evidence linking self-care planning with self-care ability [53], and qualitative findings that self-care planning is an enabler to self-care practice [50]. Conversely, a lack of planning for self-care, or otherwise adopting an ad-hoc approach to self-care practice was found to be a barrier to effective self-care [50].

As highlighted by Adams and colleagues [52], self-care planning supports clinical care and contributes to 'total care'. Beginning with an evaluation of current self-care practice, a structured planning process can be used to support self-care planning (Fig. 1). While undertaking the planning process itself is considered more important than writing an actual plan [50], online resources are available to assist with documenting a self-care plan [54].

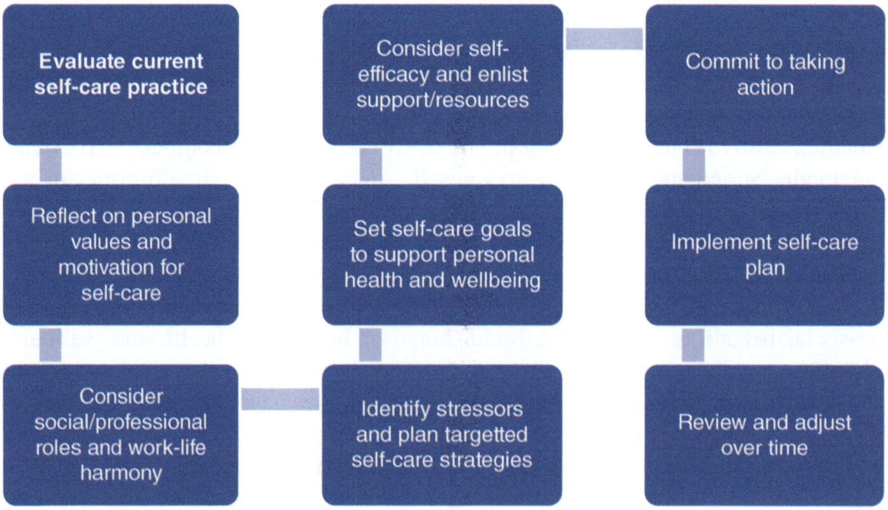

Fig. 1 Self-care planning process

3.3 Compassionate Leadership

Compassionate leadership is an important and often unrecognised enabler of self-care. As argued in the context of palliative care, 'compassionate leadership and organisational support are essential to supporting personal resources and sustaining capacity to meet professional outcomes that are achievable… in this way workforce wellbeing and resilience depend on self-care and staff support' [55].

An individual or team may struggle to implement self-care practices where a culture supportive of self-care is absent. Research suggests that positive workplace cultures supportive of self-care are vital to effective self-care practice. Normalisation of self-care is considered a key enabler that requires compassionate leadership from the top-down to effect positive change towards a culture more supportive of self-care [50].

4 Putting Self-Care into Practice

> *Practice doesn't make perfect; practice perfects a commitment to an ongoing work-in-progress.* [42]

With the requisite knowledge and understanding of self-care, together with appreciation of key enablers, one is able to consider the holistic nature of self-care in practice before exploring specific self-care strategies and closing with a final reflection.

4.1 The Holistic Nature of Self-Care in Practice

For palliative care practitioners, self-care is, by its very nature, relational. In this relational context, the holistic nature of self-care requires a recognition of interdependence and the enactment of a continuum of care between care providers and care recipients. In that way, authentic care for both self and others can be harmonised without the impediments to self-care that have arisen when they have been viewed as dichotomous [52].

From a qualitative study of Australian palliative care providers, the meaning of self-care was described as 'a proactive and holistic approach to promoting personal health and wellbeing to support professional care of others' [50]. The same study found the practice of self-care to encompass the management of barriers and enablers to self-care practice, as well as the maintenance of a range of personalised self-care strategies across both professional and non-professional contexts (Fig. 2).

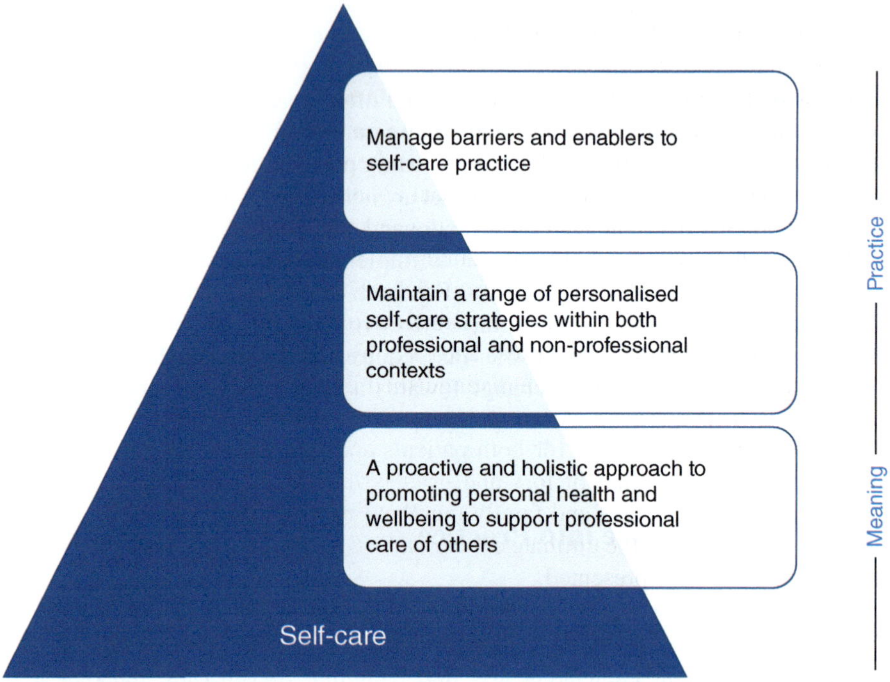

Fig. 2 The meaning and practice of self-care [50]. This article (Mills et al.) is published under the Creative Commons Attribution 4.0 License and is available at: https://bmcpalliatcare.biomedcentral.com/articles/10.1186/s12904-018-0318-0

4.2 *Self-Care Strategies*

Self-care strategies represent approaches and tangible actions for implementation as part of ones' self-care practice. They can be categorised into different groupings or domains for the purpose of evaluation and ongoing review. The number of self-care domains categorised in past studies have varied from six domains (physical, psychological, emotional, spiritual, professional workplace, and balance) [25] to ten domains (nutrition/hydration, exercise, soothing strategies, self-awareness/mindfulness, rest, relationships, physical and medical practices, environmental factors, self-compassion, spiritual practices) [56]. A mixed methods study of Australian palliative care providers [42] concluded that effective self-care practice involves the application of physical, social, and inner self-care strategies across both personal and professional contexts. These three domains of self-care (physical, social, and inner) align with the World Health Organisation's definition of health, as comprising physical, social, and mental wellbeing, while also encompassing spiritual health [42]. The application of specific self-care strategies across these domains in relation to the aforementioned meaning and practice of self-care is depicted in Fig. 3.

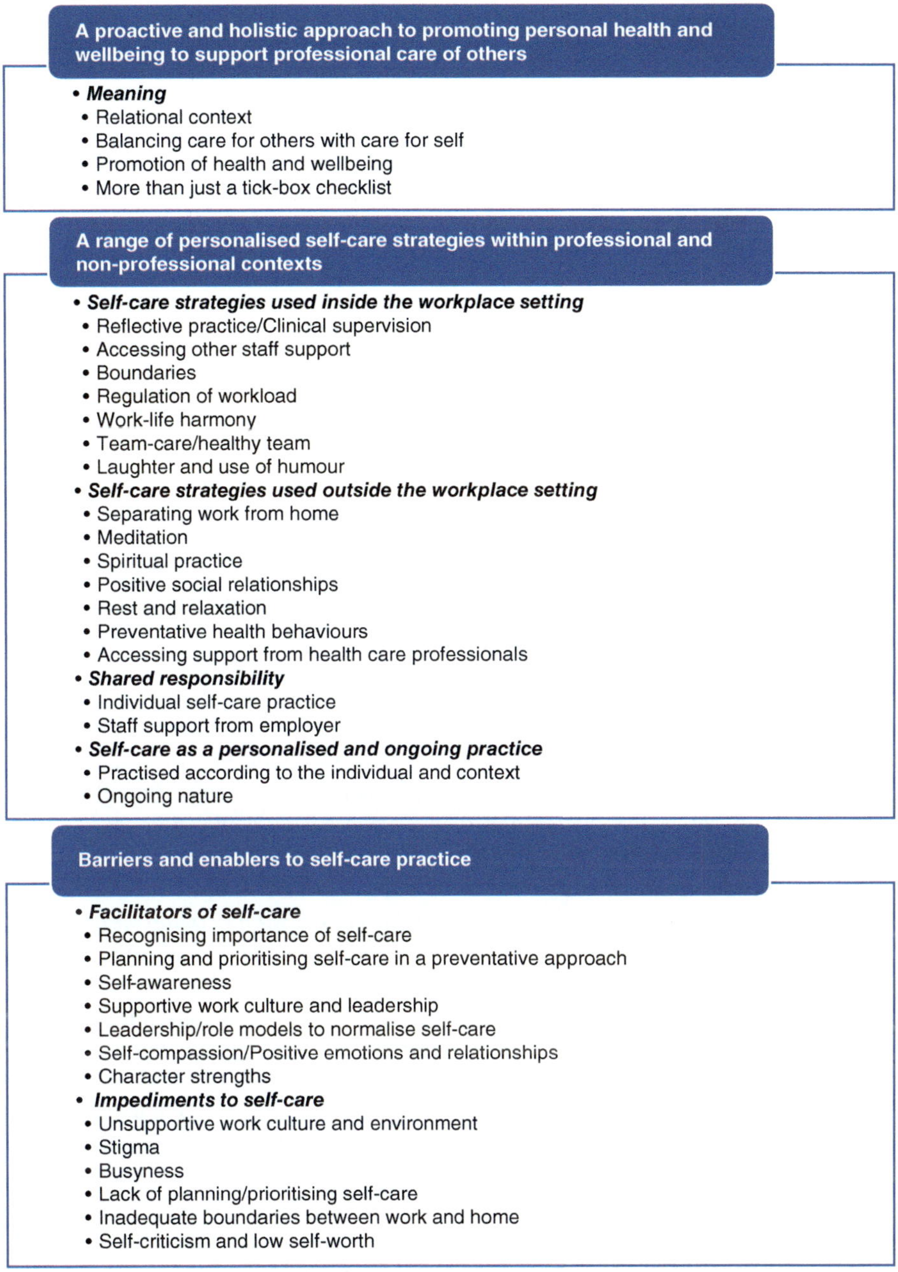

Fig. 3 Applying the meaning and practice of self-care [50]. This article (Mills et al.) is published under the Creative Commons Attribution 4.0 License and is available at: https://bmcpalliatcare.biomedcentral.com/articles/10.1186/s12904-018-0318-0

4.3 *Reflection*

Self-awareness and ongoing reflection are intertwined with effective self-care practice [50, 57, 58]. Therefore, to conclude, a reflective narrative is shared, drawing from perspectives of the 'wounded healer' [59], highlighting ways in which self-awareness and personal insight can support and guide ones' self-care through reflective practice (Box 1).

Box 1 Reflection: Self-Care and the Wounded Healer

It strikes me, just how deeply personal one's contemplation of self-care can be. Relating to oneself and discerning whether that reflection in the mirror paints a picture of compassionate care, or otherwise—self-judged, unforgiven. Truly confronting. And beyond the mere contemplative, how challenging it can be to put self-care into practice. Outside of any inward tensions, I've found the social stigma of attention to one's own needs being 'selfish' remains pervasive.

Beyond a basic survival instinct in times of potential threat, self-care is something that hasn't really come naturally to me. I don't recall learning about it in my formal nursing training, but then I guess that isn't too surprising, since becoming a nurse is very much about patient care rather than self-care.

It feels like a life-long project, constantly 'under construction'. Thankfully, I was encouraged (informally) by a mentor to think about self-care—and how it might be necessary to sustain myself while working as a nurse. I recall feeling both liberated and challenged at the same time, when being told 'you don't have to apologise when you're calling in sick—what is there to apologise for, being human'?

I guess I've always felt like I was letting the team down if I couldn't work my rostered shift. Being a 'team-player' is very important to me. I've always valued collaboration and collegiality. This is perhaps why self-care has felt challenging to me at times—reconciling the need to look after my own health and wellbeing with also not wanting to 'let the team down'. Of course, compassionate care for patients is also important to me. So, the relational aspect of care for self and others serves as a fulcrum in what seems for me an ongoing balancing act.

I'm heartened to recall the words of Carl Rogers: 'I have always been better at caring for and looking after others than I have in caring for myself. But in these later years I have made progress'.

While I have learned that neglecting self-care can have serious consequences to wellbeing, I have also learned of the need to not take oneself too seriously; at times, to instead be curious and playful as if a child in delight of encountering a new toy.

In my own experience, self-care can mean different things to different people and manifest in a variety of forms according to dynamic factors such as time, place, context, and personhood. It requires an ongoing commitment to self-awareness, self-acceptance, and self-compassion.

Much like self-care, self-compassion is something that did not come naturally to me. Raised in a Catholic family, it wasn't until exposure to Buddhist teachings in my early 20 s, that I became familiar with the notion of being compassionate with oneself; somehow this concept hadn't taken a strong hold on me. On reflection, perhaps a subtle yet strong resistance within me prevented this.

Somewhat poignantly, it was several years later—during a time of spiritual retreat and self-renewal in Assisi, the Umbrian town and birthplace of St Francis, that I fully embraced self-compassion as vital to my self-care and palliative care practice. The privilege and reward of companioning others in palliative care do not come without becoming touched by a shared suffering. With the rise and fall of the sun, each new day, I am grateful to be living, cognisant of my own mortality; with the reality of impermanence all around me.

In recognising and attending to my own woundedness (past and present), I have felt deeper and more authentic connections with those suffering alongside me. If it were not for my wounds, how could I begin to understand the suffering of others? A life tempered by chronic illness, at times not knowing how many more 'dark nights of the soul' could be endured, has enriched immeasurably my awareness and sensitivity to the suffering around me. More importantly, attending to my own wound has helped me realise the potential for healing and post-traumatic growth. Transformation and transcendence. Healing of self, healing in others.

Not that I consider myself, in any way, a 'healer' of anyone; more so that I am aware of our capacity to engage with ourselves and others in the spirit of acceptance, compassion, and loving kindness such that we can be companions on a journey of mutual healing. For me, this is the deeper meaning of total care. A continuum of care.

In practising self-care, may we share our lamp brightly while being aware of our shadow—such that it does not dim the eternal light in others?

5 Conclusion

Drawing from contemporary research, scholarship, and practice-based experience, this chapter has provided an exploration of self-care for staff providing palliative care. After defining and outlining the importance of self-care, it discussed self-compassion, self-care planning, and compassionate leadership as enablers to self-care in both personal and professional settings. It then considered the holistic nature of self-care practice, as manifest in a variety of self-care strategies used by practitioners providing palliative care.

In conclusion, a reflective narrative was explored, drawing from perspectives of the 'wounded healer', and highlighting ways in which personal insight and self-awareness can guide one's self-care through reflective practice. A key message of this chapter is that suffering and healing form part of the palliative care journey for both the living and the dying—those giving and receiving care—and that self-care for staff is a vital element of spiritual care in palliative care. Rather than relating to the care of self and others in dichotomy, self-awareness and insight to interdependence can serve as guides to 'total care' through ongoing reflection.

References

1. Lama D. Transforming the mind: teachings on generating compassion. London: Thorsons; 2003.
2. Ferrell BR. The suffering of nurses. In: Ferrell BR, Coyle N, editors. The nature of suffering and the goals of nursing. New York: Oxford University Press; 2008.
3. Renpenning KM, Taylor SG. Self-care theory in nursing: selected papers of Dorothea Orem. New York: Springer; 2003.
4. Cassell EJ. The nature of suffering and the goals of medicine. New York: Oxford University Press; 1991.
5. Watson J. Caring science and human caring theory: transforming personal and professional practices of nursing and health care. J Health Hum Serv Adm. 2009;31:466–82.
6. Foucault M. The ethics of the concern of the self as a practice of freedom. In: Rabinow P, Rose N, editors. The essential Foucault: selections from the essential works of Foucault. New York: New Press; 2003. p. 1954–84.
7. Perron A. Nursing as 'disobedient' practice: care of the nurse's self, parrhesia, and the dismantling of a baseless paradox. Nurs Philos. 2013;14:154–67. https://doi.org/10.1111/nup.12015.
8. Mills J. Theoretical foundations for self-care practice. Prog Palliat Care. 2021;29:183–5. https://doi.org/10.1080/09699260.2021.1952415.
9. Mills J, Chapman M. Compassion and self-compassion in medicine: self-care for the caregiver. Aust Med J. 2016;9:87–91. https://doi.org/10.4066/AMJ.2016.2583.
10. Mills J, Wand T, Fraser JA. On self-compassion and self-care in nursing: selfish or essential for compassionate care? Int J Nurs Stud. 2015;52:791–3.
11. Clark D. 'Total pain', disciplinary power and the body in the work of Cicely Saunders, 1958–1967. Soc Sci Med. 1999;49:727–36. https://doi.org/10.1016/S0277-9536(99)00098-2.
12. Canning D, Rosenberg JP, Yates P. Therapeutic relationships in specialist palliative care nursing practice. Int J Palliat Nurs. 2007;13:222–9.
13. Beng TS, Chin LE, Guan NC, et al. The experiences of stress of palliative care providers in Malaysia: a thematic analysis. Am J Hospice Palliat Med. 2013;32:15–28. https://doi.org/10.1177/1049909113503395.
14. Wakefield A. Nurses' responses to death and dying: a need for relentless self-care. Int J Palliat Nurs. 2000;6:245–51. https://doi.org/10.12968/ijpn.2000.6.5.8926.
15. Remen RN. Kitchen table wisdom: stories that heal. Sydney: Pan Macmillan; 2002.
16. Vachon MLS. Four decades of selected research in hospice/palliative care: have the stressors changed? In: Renzenbrink I, editor. Caregiver stress and staff support in illness. Oxford: OUP; 2011. p. 1–19.
17. Peters L, Cant R, Sellick K, et al. Is work stress in palliative care nurses a cause for concern? A literature review. Int J Palliat Nurs. 2012;18:561–7.
18. Peters L, Lee S, O'Connor M. Workplace stressors: a survey of palliative care nurses in Australia. End Life J. 2013;3:1–10.
19. Pereira SM, Fonseca AM, Carvalho AS. Burnout in palliative care: a systematic review. Nurs Ethics. 2011;18:317–26.
20. Wang C, Grassau P, Lawlor PG, et al. Burnout and resilience among Canadian palliative care physicians. BMC Palliat Care. 2020;19:169.

21. Gómez-Urquiza JL, Albendín-García L, Velando-Soriano A, et al. Burnout in palliative care nurses, prevalence and risk factors: a systematic review with meta-analysis. Int J Environ Res Public Health. 2020:17. https://doi.org/10.3390/ijerph17207672.
22. Boorman S. NHS health and well-being. Leeds: Department of Health; 2009.
23. Maben J, Adams M, Peccei R, et al. 'Poppets and parcels': the links between staff experience of work and acutely ill older peoples' experience of hospital care. Int J Older People Nursing. 2012;7:83–94. https://doi.org/10.1111/j.1748-3743.2012.00326.x.
24. Hotchkiss JT, Lesher R. Factors predicting burnout among chaplains: compassion satisfaction, organizational factors, and the mediators of mindful self-care and secondary traumatic stress. J Pastoral Care Counsel JPCC. 2018;72:86–98. https://doi.org/10.1177/1542305018780655.
25. Alkema K, Linton JM, Davies R. A study of the relationship between self-care, compassion satisfaction, compassion fatigue, and burnout among hospice professionals. J Soc Work End Life Palliat Care. 2008;4:101–19. Empirical/Quantitative. https://doi.org/10.1080/15524250802353934.
26. Hotchkiss JT. Mindful self-care and secondary traumatic stress mediate a relationship between compassion satisfaction and burnout risk among hospice care professionals. Am J Hospice Palliat Med. 2018; Online First; https://doi.org/10.1177/1049909118756657.
27. Garcia ACM, Ferreira ACG, Silva LSR, et al. Mindful self-care, self-compassion, and resilience among palliative care providers during the COVID-19 pandemic. J Pain Symptom Manag. 2022;64:49–57. https://doi.org/10.1016/j.jpainsymman.2022.03.003.
28. Galiana L, Sansó N, Muñoz-Martínez I, et al. Palliative care professionals' inner life: exploring the mediating role of self-compassion in the prediction of compassion satisfaction, compassion fatigue, burnout and wellbeing. J Pain Symptom Manag. 2022;63:112–23. https://doi.org/10.1016/j.jpainsymman.2021.07.004.
29. Sansó N, Galiana L, Oliver A, et al. Palliative care professionals' inner life: exploring the relationships among awareness, self-care, and compassion satisfaction and fatigue, burnout, and coping with death. J Pain Symptom Manage. 2015;50:200–7. Empirical/Quantitative. https://doi.org/10.1016/j.jpainsymman.2015.02.013.
30. Gamondi C, Larkin P, Payne S. Core competencies in palliative care: an EAPC white paper on palliative care education—part 2. Eur J Palliat Care. 2013;20:140–5.
31. Downing J, Ling J, Benini F, et al. A summary of the EAPC white paper on core competencies for education in paediatric palliative care. Eur J Palliat Care. 2014;21:245–9.
32. Hospice New Zealand. Hospice New Zealand standards for palliative care. http://www.hospice.org.nz/cms_show_download.php?id=647 (2012).
33. American Academy of Hospice and Palliative Medicine (HPM Competencies Project Work Group). Hospice and palliative medicine core competencies -version 2.3. (2009). American Academy of Hospice and Palliative Medicine.
34. Canning D, Yates P, Rosenberg JP. Competency standards for specialist palliative care nursing practice. http://www.pcna.org.au/images/documents/competystds.pdf (2005). Accessed 15 Sept 14.
35. Palliative Care Australia. Standards for providing quality palliative care for all Australians. http://palliativecare.org.au/wp-content/uploads/2015/07/Standards-for-providing-quality-palliative-care-for-all-Australians.pdf (2005). Accessed 24 June 2017.
36. Spiritual Care Australia. Capabilities framework for spiritual care practitioners. Spiritual Care Australia; 2023.
37. Wilhoit JC. Self-compassion as a christian spiritual practice. J Spiritual Formation Soul Care. 2018;12:71–88. https://doi.org/10.1177/1939790918795628.
38. Gilbert P, McEwan K, Matos M, et al. Fears of compassion: development of three self-report measures. Psychol Psychother Theory Res Pract. 2011;84:239–55. https://doi.org/10.1348/147608310X526511.
39. Best M, Vivat B, Gijsberts M-J. Spiritual care in palliative care. Religions. 2023:14(3):320. https://doi.org/10.3390/rel14030320.
40. Germer CK. The mindful path to self-compassion. New York: The Guilford Press; 2009.

41. Neff K. The development and validation of a scale to measure self-compassion. Self Identity. 2003;2:223.
42. Mills J. Self-care, self-compassion, and compassion for others. The University of Sydney; 2018.
43. Heffernan M, Griffin MTQ, McNulty SR, et al. Self-compassion and emotional intelligence in nurses. Int J Nurs Pract. 2010;16:366–73. https://doi.org/10.1111/j.1440-172X.2010.01853.x.
44. Lindsay EK, Creswell JD. Helping the self help others: self-affirmation increases self-compassion and pro-social behaviors. Front Psychol. 2014;5:5. https://doi.org/10.3389/fpsyg.2014.00421.
45. Arch JJ, Brown KW, Dean DJ, et al. Self-compassion training modulates alpha-amylase, heart rate variability, and subjective responses to social evaluative threat in women. Psychoneuroendocrinology. 2014;42:49–58. https://doi.org/10.1016/j.psyneuen.2013.12.018.
46. Hall CW, Row KA, Wuensch KL, et al. The role of self-compassion in physical and psychological well-being. J Psychol. 2013;147:311–23. https://doi.org/10.1080/00223980.2012.693138.
47. Neff KD, Dahm KA. Self-Compassion: what it is, what it does, and how it relates to mindfulness. In: Ostafin BD, Robinson MD, Meier BP, editors. Mindfulness and self-regulation. New York: Springer; 2015. p. 121–37.
48. Svendsen JL, Osnes B, Binder P-E, et al. Trait self-compassion reflects emotional flexibility through an association with high vagally mediated heart rate variability. Mindfulness. 2016;7:1103–13. https://doi.org/10.1007/s12671-016-0549-1.
49. Neff KD, Rude S, Kirkpatrick K. An examination of self-compassion in relation to positive psychological functioning and personality traits. J Res Personal. 2007;41:908–16.
50. Mills J, Wand T, Fraser JA. Exploring the meaning and practice of self-care among palliative care nurses and doctors: a qualitative study. BMC Palliat Care. 2018;17:63. https://doi.org/10.1186/s12904-018-0318-0.
51. Mills J, Wand T, Fraser JA. Examining self-care, self-compassion and compassion for others: a cross-sectional survey of palliative care nurses and doctors. Int J Palliat Nurs. 2018;24:4–11. https://doi.org/10.12968/ijpn.2018.24.1.4.
52. Adams M, Chase J, Doyle C, et al. Self-care planning supports clinical care: putting total care into practice. Prog Palliat Care. 2020;28:305–7. https://doi.org/10.1080/09699260.2020.1799815.
53. Mills J, Wand T, Fraser JA. Self-care in palliative care nursing and medical professionals: a cross-sectional survey. J Palliat Med. 2017;20:625–30. https://doi.org/10.1089/jpm.2016.0470.
54. Palliative Care Australia. Self-care matters: a self-care planning tool. https://palliativecare.org.au/download/15974/ (2020).
55. Mills J, Ramachenderan J, Chapman M, et al. Prioritising workforce wellbeing and resilience: what COVID-19 is reminding us about self-care and staff support. Palliat Med. 2020;34:1137–9. https://doi.org/10.1177/0269216320947966.
56. Cook-Cottone CP, Guyker WM. The development and validation of the mindful self-care scale (MSCS): an assessment of practices that support positive embodiment. Mindfulness. 2018;9:161–75. https://doi.org/10.1007/s12671-017-0759-1.
57. Germain A, Nolan K, Doyle R, et al. The use of reflective diaries in end of life training programmes: a study exploring the impact of self-reflection on the participants in a volunteer training programme. BMC Palliat Care. 2016;15:28. https://doi.org/10.1186/s12904-016-0096-5.
58. Salins N. Reflective practice in palliative care. Indian J Palliat Care. 2018;24:1–2.
59. Laskowski C, Pellicore K. The wounded healer archetype: applications to palliative care practice. Am J Hospice Palliat Care. 2002;19:403–7.

The Role of the Doctor in Spiritual Care

Megan C. Best

Abstract Doctors have a prominent role in patient care at the end of life, and patients express interest in having their doctor ask them about their spirituality as part of holistic patient care. However, this is done infrequently. The most significant barriers to including spirituality in the medical consultation are insufficient knowledge and training. Engagement with spirituality in the healthcare setting can have a positive impact on both the doctor and the patient. In this chapter, instruction on how to engage in spiritual care expands on the findings from a study of physicians from Australia and New Zealand who had experience in caring for advanced cancer patients. They described a delicate, skilful, and individualised procedure where the doctor can start to get to know the patient and encourage them to discuss their most important concerns. It was described as a way to provide a 'safe space' in which to discuss intimate topics.

Keywords Spirituality · Doctor · Physician · Primacy care provider · Spiritual care · Spiritual history · Palliative care · End of life

1 Introduction

Palliative care identifies four domains fundamental to patient care: physical, psychological, social, and spiritual. Regardless of the symptom being addressed, all four domains may need to be addressed to reduce suffering, and even non-religious patients express spiritual needs at the end of life [1, 2]. Spiritual wellbeing is as

M. C. Best (✉)
Institute for Ethics and Society, University of Notre Dame Australia, Sydney, NSW, Australia
e-mail: megan.best@nd.edu.au

M. C. Best (ed.), *Spiritual Care in Palliative Care*,
https://doi.org/10.1007/978-3-031-50864-6_30

important as physical wellbeing for quality of life according to both patients and their families [2, 3]. Acknowledgement of the spiritual dimension helps patients cope more effectively with terminal disease, and interventions to improve spiritual wellbeing can relieve patient suffering [4–6]. In this sense, healing can occur despite incurable disease.

Management of life-threatening disease almost invariably involves patient engagement with doctors [7]. While the World Health Organisation and the United Nations recommend that all individuals at the end of life have access to palliative care, it is recognised that this will not necessarily be provided by specialist palliative care or hospice services [8]. There are several reasons for this.

Generalist palliative care can be provided by adequately trained primary care providers (PCPs) who recognise it as an important aspect of their practice. Typically, PCPs have well-established relationships with their patients, providing insight into the patient's background and comorbidities, which contributes a good foundation for terminal care. Patients from many countries have expressed the desire for continued involvement of PCPs at the end of life, and their involvement is linked to several positive outcomes, including fewer emergency department visits and hospital admissions, and increased likelihood of a home death [9]. In many countries, PCPs also care for those who die in nursing homes, which in one international study was found to account for a fifth of all deaths of older people [7]. Furthermore, not all countries have yet fully developed palliative care services [10].

Even in countries where specialist palliative care is well established, with ageing populations and the increasing number of patients requiring end-of-life care, it is unlikely that there will be enough specialist palliative care doctors to see all patients. When available, consultation of specialist palliative care is preferred for patients with complex and severe problems. However, the association between spirituality and health outcomes [11] makes a compelling argument that doctors should have knowledge of this area, and it has been recommended that all doctors treating patients at the end of life should be able to provide a basic level of palliative care, which includes spiritual care [12].

2 Patient Desire for Spiritual Enquiry by Doctors

Although chaplains are the recognised specialist providers of spiritual care in healthcare, patients report a high level of interest in having their doctor ask them about spirituality, particularly in the context of terminal illness [13]. In one study of general hospital patients where over 90% patients were open to discussing spirituality (even though the term was initially unfamiliar to them) [14], the second most preferred staff member for this discussion was the doctor (22.4%) after the chaplain (32.9%) [15].

Research has shown that religious or spiritual direction is not what many patients have in mind when they verbalise interest in spiritual discussions with their doctor. Instead, they want the doctor to understand them holistically [2, 16], which necessarily requires the doctor to become familiar with their values, derived from the beliefs that inform their worldview. In such a way, the doctor is able to take these beliefs into account when recommending treatment, for example by modifying therapy to accommodate religious practices (such as adjusting diabetic care during the Ramadan fast) [17, 18].

These values also influence patient decision-making [19], and spiritual discussion gives the doctor insight into patient preferences in end-of-life care [20]. Acceptance even of patient decisions with which we do not agree is necessary within those healthcare systems which elevate patient autonomy to the highest ethical value. It is not essential to patients that their doctor share their views, but it is important that their values be respected [21].

Patients desire a close relationship with their doctors in which they feel known as individuals and which allow them to feel safe enough to discuss their fears and ask difficult questions, such as how long they have to live. Any patient is at risk of losing self-confidence in the medical system, where they can be made vulnerable by their dependent status, bedbound position, uncomfortable symptoms, and ignorance of medical jargon, and they often do not feel they have the close relationship they desire with their doctor [13].

Positive impacts on the doctor–patient relationship are found when the doctor addresses patient spirituality, independent of chaplaincy involvement. These include strengthening of the doctor–patient relationship, reinforcing the personhood of the patient, improved coping with physical symptoms, the ability to find meaning in terminal illness, satisfaction with medical care, improved quality of life, reduced suffering, less aggressive care at the end of life, and the opportunity for the patient to find peace at the end of life [5, 6, 19, 20, 22].

Once the link is formed between the doctor and patient, the subsequently improved communication allows further benefits such as shared decision-making [23], which is a factor that contributes to an increased feeling of control for the patient [24], and dying well [21]. Trust in the therapeutic relationship has many benefits, for example it has been shown to be a central factor in hospice enrolment for ethnic and racial minority patients in the USA [25]. Patients express a preference to be referred to a chaplain or community religious leader should spiritual problems exist [13]. This can be accommodated in countries where end-of-life care is supported by multidisciplinary services.

Similarly, patients want their doctor to understand the nature of their personal spiritual support system, for example family, religious community, or engagement with nature. We found that this knowledge allows the doctor to facilitate access to those supports during treatment and hospitalisation, for example, by increasing flexibility in visiting hours if the family's presence is important to patient wellbeing, or allowing a patient leave to spend time in the natural environment [14, 16]. The value of having access to spiritual supports and their role in helping patients cope with hospitalisation are well known [26]. It is therefore of concern that, in some studies, over half the sample of physicians tried to change the subject if patients started talking about spirituality and some would refuse to engage in the topic with the patient, even at the end of life [20]. In the hospital setting, doctors are often the gatekeepers regarding flexibility of visiting hours, gate leave or access to the ward by community spirituality leaders. By being unaware of patients' spiritual supports, doctors may inadvertently separate the patient from a crucial coping mechanism [27].

It should be noted that a small but significant proportion of patients do not want their spirituality addressed within healthcare. This does not correlate with patient spirituality or religious beliefs. These objections can be based on privacy concerns (particularly in the context of a shared ward), its perceived irrelevance to healthcare, or general discomfort regarding the topic [14, 22]. Some studies have found that the reason some patients did not want to discuss spirituality with hospital staff was because they already had a confidante outside the hospital, whether a family member, close friend or community faith leader [13, 15]. However, spiritual needs are known to fluctuate during the illness trajectory, and at the time of referral, patients may not anticipate spiritual needs that may arise in the future in association with health challenges [14]. This indicates that spiritual enquiry should not be limited to the first time a patient is seen, but be ongoing through the illness.

3 Frequency and Nature of Spiritual Enquiry by Doctors

Despite patients' desire for their doctors to ask them about their spirituality, literature suggests that the practice is infrequent and inadequate [13], although recent initiatives in spiritual care training may reverse this trend (see Chap. 27). Despite being recognised as a core competency of PCPs, discussion of existential issues is neglected in general practice [9, 28, 29] and when care is offered, it varies widely [30]. If discussion of religion and/or spirituality in the medical consultation is desired by patients and known to be beneficial, why is it uncommon?

It is not because doctors think spirituality is unimportant. A national survey of physicians in the United States found that 65% believed it was good practice for physicians to address patient's spiritual concerns at the end of life [31], and 89% thought that physicians should seek to relieve patients' spiritual suffering just as much as their physical pain [5]. A study of cancer physicians found that, although physicians held more negative perceptions of spiritual care than patients ($p < 0.001$), 71.6% thought regular provision of spiritual care by nurses or physicians would be at least slightly positive for patients [32]. However, this does not transfer to increased provision of spiritual care by doctors [33].

There may be a misunderstanding of what constitutes spiritual care. Despite extensive discussion of the meaning of spirituality in the healthcare literature, many clinicians appear to continue to confuse it with religion [32, 34]. Confusion between religiosity and spirituality can mean that rejection of the former leads to inadvertent rejection of the latter. Dominant paradigms in society change over time, and currently individualism and personal autonomy are highly valued in western societies. As a result, organised religions (as well as other authoritative institutions) are regarded with suspicion. Scandals on the international stage also contribute to the negative way religion is perceived [14]. This is unfortunate, as the condemnation of religion can obstruct spiritual care, which is really about helping patients find peace and meaning in their illness experience. However, separation of religion and spirituality does not mean that religious care is not important, merely that it can be different. Many patients, such as Muslim or Hindu patients, may equate spirituality with religion, and even very religious patients may still have low spiritual wellbeing.

Not many studies have examined what is actually discussed during spiritual discussions between doctors and patients. One review found that doctors reported encouraging the patient in their own spiritual beliefs and inquiring how faith influenced patient medical decisions. Other studies have found discussions focus on fear of death and dying and the search for peace [20, 35]. In a study of nursing home physicians, while 48.4% reported that they had provided spiritual end-of-life care to the last resident they cared for, 95.4% were found to have confused psychosocial and spiritual care [36]. The complexity of the relationship between spiritual care and other dimensions of care at the end of life has been previously explored [37]; however, this finding may partly explain why doctors can report a higher frequency of spiritual discussions than patients, even within the one study [20].

Many doctors report preferring chaplain referral to discussing spirituality with patients themselves, but the rates of doctors recommending chaplain referral versus actually making the referral differ [20]. The fact that chaplain referral is seen as preferable to personally discussing spirituality suggests that doctors do not see spiritual care as a relationship-building exercise in the same way as patients do. Most PCPs in a Dutch study were unaware of how to refer to a spiritual counsellor [28]. These findings could explain why prior training for doctors is the strongest predictor for discussions and provision of spiritual care—misconceptions are less likely as a result.

There is debate on whether the topic of spirituality should be raised by the doctor or the patient. Physicians may believe that it is always preferable for the patient to initiate the discussions, as it appears less intrusive [20], but our study examining transcripts of consultations with palliative care patients and their physicians found that discussions were 4.04 times more likely to occur if the doctor raised the topic [35]. Doctors with higher intrinsic religiosity are more likely to report that their patients mention spiritual issues, which suggests that an element of heightened awareness is required for doctors to recognise spiritual enquiry when it occurs. Doctors vary in how they respond to patient cues [20, 35].

4 The Role of Training

A survey of palliative care specialists found that, although just over half the sample thought it was their role to provide spiritual care, only 5% felt always able to do so [32]. Prior training is the strongest predictor of spiritual discussions and provision of spiritual care by doctors. Discussion of spirituality requires sensitivity, patience, tolerance for ambiguity and sensitivity to one's own spirituality, which does not always sit easily within a reductionist medical culture. These skills can be developed through training. A required spiritual care training programme run for hospital residents in the United States reduced barriers to addressing patients' spiritual needs and had lasting impact on the development of clinical skills. It reduced anxiety about provision of spiritual care and promoted personal formation. This impact did not appear to be related to personal beliefs [20, 38]. Doctors who have had training in palliative care have been found to experience fewer barriers to provision of spiritual care [20, 32, 36].

However, not all training is equal. Some studies of spiritual care training in medical school have not led to a significant increase of spiritual discussions with patients or retention of skills [39]. Some doctors blame their medical training for their marginalisation of the importance of spiritual care, resulting from exposure to supervisors who devalued its importance, stressing curing not caring as the role of the doctor [20, 40]. Concern has existed for some time regarding the impact of the 'hidden curriculum' in medicine, which may hinder or prevent the student's development of empathy for the subjective experience of others, openness to her own emotional experience, and ability to tolerate the uncertainty and limitations of medicine—all necessary components of the practice of spiritual care [41]. These findings suggest that learning the theory as a student may not be sufficient to transfer spiritual care skills, but that it needs to be modelled in real life, or perhaps that one needs to have engaged with patient suffering before appreciating its importance. Spiritual care skills certainly improve with experience [6].

Recommendations for spiritual discussions such as individualising care, listening well and becoming familiar with assessment tools are communication skills which can be taught. Training in communication skills is recognised as an important part of preparation. Doctors undergoing communication training reported that discussion of spirituality requires more advanced communication skills than other commonly taught skills, such as discussion of resuscitation orders [42]. Outcomes from spiritual care training in clinical practice include increased screening of patients and reporting of spiritual distress, increased multidisciplinary spiritual care and an improved working atmosphere, improved spiritual health, and reduced work-related stress and burnout of staff [43].

Some doctors have been found to respond to spiritual needs of patients intuitively, without a standardised approach. A study of Scottish PCPs found that their method of spiritual care was variable and related to personal attributes and previous experiences. While this tactic can have value, it is unclear to what extent such approaches are acceptable or effective for patients [28, 30].

5 Impact of Spiritual Care on the Doctor

The delivery of spiritual care is a dynamic relationship where the interaction with the patient can lead to spiritual growth for the doctor. Caring for the terminally ill impacts the carer. Palliative care physicians report that their work prompts them to think about their own mortality, facilitates self-reflection, and re-orientates their life by helping them prioritise the things that are important. Self-reflection prepares doctors to discuss spiritual matters with patients, reducing their death anxiety so they are not distracted by their own fears as they address patients' existential questions. At the same time, self-reflection encourages them to engage in self-care, for example through physical exercise, building supportive communities and pursuing spiritual self-education. Some doctors report that practising palliative care is itself spiritually fulfilling and that patient engagement is a source of wisdom [44, 45].

Through these avenues, the doctor becomes less vulnerable to compassion fatigue [46]. One possible moderator of this impact could be empathy—an association has been identified between the level of the doctor's empathy and spiritual care of patients ($p < 0.1$) [47] Integrating spirituality at work with self-actualisation can lead to increased job satisfaction. The self-awareness that develops with growing expertise in spiritual care allows doctors to establish shared meaning and relationships with their patients. Patients report that feeling cared for relies on displays of empathy, compassion, physicians recognising themselves and their patients as unique human beings, and being willing to develop an authentic human relationship [48]. A reciprocity of care is therefore demonstrated, with physicians reporting the need to address spirituality in order to provide holistic compassionate palliative care, the experience of which in turn positively shapes the growth and development of the doctor's own personal spirituality [44, 45]. Hospital patients identify characteristics such as empathy as more important than professional role when seeking spiritual discussion [15].

6 Engaging in Spiritual Care

While patients seek spiritual enquiry in order to build relationship, it is also important for the relief of suffering. Doctors need to see patients in their wholeness as human persons to understand the meaning of their suffering and determine appropriate treatment [49], and if doctors do not elicit information about a patient's most important beliefs, this will not occur.

The remainder of this chapter will focus on our study of a cohort of experienced physicians from Australia and New Zealand with experience in caring for advanced cancer patients. They described a delicate, skilful, and individualised procedure where the doctor can start to get to know the patient and encourage them to discuss their most important values. It was described as a way to provide a 'safe space'—a refuge where patients and doctors could be vulnerable with each other and discuss topics intimate for the patient [6]. Patients experiencing existential distress describe the need for such a space, describing a tension between the desire to discuss their sense of loss, and fear of the vulnerability they would experience in talking about it [50]. Difficulty in articulating distress is identified as a symptom of spiritual suffering. In the face of spiritual distress, sometimes what may be needed are not better communication techniques, but 'silence before the radical mystery of death' [51].

The study of 23 physicians identified six themes to describe their approach to spiritual care. They were (1) personal development; (2) developing one's attitude; (3) approaching the patient; (4) facilitators; (5) barriers; and (6) an important and effective intervention. These are discussed in relation to the literature below [49].

6.1 Personal Development

The physicians suggested that the most important component of developing the required skills for engaging in spiritual care was developing personal spirituality [6]. This correlates with the finding that doctors most likely to address spirituality in a medical consultation have strong intrinsic and extrinsic religion and spirituality [19, 20, 32]. In a separate cohort of palliative care physicians, we found that self-reported spirituality was significantly associated with: considering spiritual care to be important, having had training, having confidence in being able to provide spiritual care, and the likelihood of referring to another if unable to provide spiritual care themselves [32]. The doctor's level of ease with the content was considered to be a contributing factor in making patients feel comfortable enough to discuss personal subjects.

Understanding the self requires reflection and self-care, which many participants wished they had begun to work on earlier in their career, and now encouraged in younger doctors. It has been argued that doctors' spirituality cannot be enforced, but that opportunities for personal growth should be available for those in medical practice, and particularly in palliative care. Developing self-awareness, personal growth and wellbeing would also help medical students to learn how to become healers, treating patients holistically [52]. Perhaps opportunities to discuss personal responses to patient care should be routinely introduced into medical education to normalise the concept.

Experienced palliative care doctors recommend that self-reflection should be a lifelong practice for doctors caring for patients at the end of life as a way to promote personal spiritual growth. Indeed, spiritual care training is not successful without attending to one's own spiritual beliefs and needs, but spiritual care training can provide this opportunity [43].

The benefits of self-reflection for doctors have long been recognised [53]. These include providing the foundation for life-long learning in medical practice [54] as well as promoting wellbeing, improved coping with stress, maintaining empathy, developing personal maturity and providing a way to makes sense of emotional reactions to disturbing clinical scenarios [55]. Benefits are not dependent on personal existential orientation. Doctors have accessed self-reflection mechanisms through support mechanisms such as Balint groups, religious support groups, and institutional memorial services as well as formal supervision [56] [57, 58].

6.2 Developing One's Attitude

The doctors regarded spiritual care as a critical dimension of patient care, and this recognition was a prerequisite for providing it. The need to respect and value each patient and their beliefs was highlighted. Part of respecting the patient involved the doctor being honest and vulnerable during the patient interview. This was described as one of the most challenging aspects, because it involved opening oneself to intimacy with a patient. However, participants had found that by exposing themselves and making themselves vulnerable, patients were able to feel less vulnerable and open themselves to reveal what was distressing them most. Sharing oneself with patients to find common ground was seen not as manipulative but as a way of making the patient feel safe enough to discuss highly personal issues. However, it was acknowledged that there was a balancing act between connecting with a patient and over-connecting, which could lead to burnout. One way to find this balance was by letting the patient control the rhythm of the conversation rather than having a specific therapeutic goal: it meant you had to realise that spiritual care did not involve 'fixing things' or 'having all the answers', so much as being with patient and expressing committed attention.

One doctor reported: *'In a spiritual encounter…what I think has helped me is my belief in it, but also my willingness to be vulnerable and to sit in that space and not need to have to solve or fix and being able to live with the uncertainty and not having all the answers…it's more a healer model than a fixed medical model. So, for me, it's about me being truly myself in that space and allowing the patient to be truly themselves. It's a very deep thing really'.*

The doctors suggested that insight into human nature is needed to engage in spiritual discussions, and that this should be taught if personal hardship had not allowed the doctor to develop personal insight [6]. Familiarity with the humanities was the most commonly recommended route. The field of medical humanities originally emerged to counter the atomistic view of human nature on which modern medicine is predicated. Inclusion of the humanities in medical education has previously been recommended to help doctors learn to reflect on medical practice, develop empathy for those unlike themselves, awareness and understanding of their own emotional lives, and tolerance of ambiguity and uncertainty. Re-introduction of the medical humanities into the medical curriculum could also benefit the development of spiritual care [59].

6.3 Approaching the Patient

A trusting therapeutic relationship is a facilitator, and for some doctors a prerequisite, to spiritual discussion [22, 31, 36].

Experienced doctors demonstrated high-level communication skills related to experience over multiple patient encounters. They recognised patient cues, which were used to judge the appropriate timing and content of probing questions about spiritual concerns of patients. Cues for enquiring about spirituality could be visual or verbal: sacred texts at the bedside or religious figures on display can be commented on. Patient vocabulary may indicate a religious affiliation, such as mentioning prayer or blessings. However, a lack of cues did not mean that spirituality was not addressed, and experienced doctors develop their own approach.

Creating a safe space where a patient would be comfortable enough to reveal personal information can be challenging on a busy ward, but several techniques facilitate this process. A common process is to allow silence, allowing the patient to process their thoughts. Listening well is more important than 'doing it right'. Patient body language should be monitored to see how the patient is coping with the conversation. Doctors recognised that spiritual prompts could at times cause patient distress, but that this may be needed for them to deal with issues that, afterwards, can lead to peace. Conversations were individualised to patients' interests and timing.

Initiating a Spiritual Discussion

Taking a spiritual history fosters an environment open to sharing the existential, spiritual, and religious dimensions of illness. It is advised that doctor ask about the patient's spirituality as a part of the overall medical history. This could be done on first contact with the patient, although some patients express the desire to know the doctor well before discussing such intimate concerns. By asking about patient spirituality, the doctor is indicating her willingness to engage on spiritual topics in the future [34].

Many tools have been developed to assist doctors in asking about spirituality within the patient history [60, 61]. A recent analysis identified the 'HOPE' tool as the most comprehensively addressing important spirituality themes. 'HOPE' includes questions about (H) sources of hope, meaning, comfort, strength, peace, love, and connection, (O) organised religion, (P) personal spirituality/practices, and (E) effects of medical care and end-of-life issues [62]. Such tools have been criticised for limiting spontaneous discussions and the opportunity for patient to raise their own issues [63] although they can be helpful for the less experienced practitioner [20]. The experienced doctors in our cohort developed their own way of exploring a patient's spirituality, with questions such as 'what's important to you?' or 'what keeps you strong when times are tough?' Questionnaires enquiring about religion were particularly troubling for these doctors, as patients would often shut down when asked. This has been previously noted in other secular countries [64].

The physicians in this study also reported that, in discussing patient spirituality, it is important not to make assumptions:

KL was a church minister who was admitted with bowel cancer. His terminal diagnosis had precipitated a crisis of faith, which he had not discussed with anyone else, and he was assumed by his family to be spiritually strong. It was only when his doctor invited him to discuss his spiritual needs that he was able to reveal the source of his turmoil.

Screening for Spiritual Need

Spirituality was conceived as an ongoing conversation that evolved over time, thus supporting patients in their search for meaning. Doctors provide support by helping patients verbalise their existential questions and consider the answers. It is known that patients' spiritual needs fluctuate over time [15], so it is necessary to check with patients at regular intervals in case any new spiritual needs have arisen [32]. Short screening tools have been validated in palliative care populations [65, 66], although conversational prompts can also be effective within an established relationship [15].

Physicians in our study reported that sometimes a patient would indicate that they did not need spiritual assistance in preparing for death; however, doctors would still make a point of affirming the importance of this endeavour.

Interventions

If the physician identified any issue that required more intervention than she felt able to provide, a referral was made, which was a time-efficient option in busy units. Referrals could be made to a chaplain, faith leader, psychologist, psychiatrist, or other specialist caregiver, depending on patient need and staff availability. The high level of awareness in this cohort meant that doctors also realised that they were sometimes not the best person to speak to a particular patient. This could be the result of personality differences, time schedules, or a result of transference (going either way). Many participants talked about the benefit of multidisciplinary teams which meant that if one person was not appropriate, others were available.

AT was a young woman admitted to the palliative care unit who was scared of dying and had been sexually abused by her father. She didn't trust men, so the male doctor on the ward was not the one to explore her spiritual distress. Neither was the middle-aged male chaplain. The female social worker developed good rapport and was able to explore existential needs with this patient.

Empirical evidence for the most effective forms of spiritual interventions is still being gathered [67]. The suffering literature reports that when patients feel 'seen' by staff it can prompt their spiritual growth [68]. It is understood as an experience of connection and affirmation, which automatically increases the spiritual wellbeing of the patient. However, in the author's experience, patients do not need to be experiencing distress in order to benefit from being 'seen'. This suggests that interaction on a spiritual level is beneficial regardless of the level of spiritual wellbeing experienced by the patient at the time, and that doctors need to be educated in the benefits of addressing spiritual issues early in the trajectory of patients' illness.

6.4 Facilitators

Spiritual discussion was easier when doctor and patient shared spiritual and cultural backgrounds. Similar presuppositions and vocabulary make conversations easier, though lack of faith concordance was not necessarily a barrier, and research has shown that non-concordance of clinician beliefs may not influence the perception of quality of care [69]. However, participants noted that some patients benefited more from speaking to a community faith leader than a member of staff, which could be arranged.

Patients are more likely to be willing to talk about spiritual issues when they are comfortable. This depends on several factors, including the environment—level of privacy and who is present (spouses generally did not impede discussion but children often did). Conversations were more likely to be successful if they were one-on-one.

The physicians in our study never felt that discussing spirituality was a mistake, even when it was challenging. One doctor reported: *'Sometimes I say, 'I just don't know what to say, and I am so sorry, and I wish it was different for you'....I don't think, on the whole, that I'm making the patient feel worse, and I know that because when they leave, most of them look relieved or they hug me or say, 'thank you so much'.*

6.5 Barriers

The most commonly cited barrier for doctors contemplating spiritual care of patients is lack of time [20, 32]. However, lack of time is not a predictor of less spiritual care, and Ellis and colleagues found that a longer admission did not increase the provision of spiritual care by doctors to hospitalised patients [33, 70]. Clearly, lack of time is not the only factor operating.

Insufficient knowledge and/or training, including the fear that they would not know how to manage any spiritual issues raised, is also a common reason doctors give for avoiding spiritual discussion, once again reflecting misunderstanding of patient motives for desiring it. It is difficult to separate lack of training from other barriers (such as feelings of discomfort, concern that patients may be offended, etc.) [20, 22, 28] which suggest a lack of understanding regarding the role of spirituality in patient care.

We found that conversations were more likely to be successful if the doctor was not busy or distracted. However, time was not a significant barrier, in this cohort, as conversations about spirituality were viewed as a high priority, on a par with asking about pain levels. If the doctor felt rushed, she would reschedule the discussion, while emphasising the importance of addressing the matters raised, or refer to another staff member. It was perceived that patients could recognise when they had the doctor's attention and chose that time to raise questions of importance.

Both doctors and patients regularly confused spirituality with religion, but this was easily remedied once recognised. Some doctors were aware that their colleagues found references to faith and spirituality surprising, but not necessarily offensive. Religious doctors were conscious of a need to avoid proselytising, and this could lead to reduced spiritual care provision where the doctor feared overstepping the mark. However, strong faith was also recognised as beneficial in that it allowed the doctor to be more comfortable in discussing existential topics, to recognise the importance of spirituality, and to have a vocabulary available. The ethics of spiritual care are addressed in full in Chap. 42; however, it should be emphasised that spiritual care should always be voluntary and not prioritised over good medical care, nor should clinicians proselytise due to the power imbalance of the doctor–patient relationship.

Several of our participants discussed the problem of engaging with patients with whom they identified too closely:

HJ was a palliative care physician who had gone through a difficult divorce. She was aware that she did not have the ability to help patients whose spiritual distress was related to divorce, so she referred those patients to colleagues.

Finally, historical factors were considered a barrier to spiritual care. Even though our cohort was conscious of the importance of spirituality for patients at the end of life, they were aware that the medical focus on the biological and marginalisation of the spiritual that developed since the eighteenth-century Enlightenment meant that those things which could not be empirically proven, such as spiritual needs, were ignored by science. It is only with the re-introduction of the bio-psycho-social-spiritual model of the human being that the importance of spiritual care has been recognised [34]. However, even though spirituality has always been a domain of importance to palliative care, our participants were aware that it was not necessarily the case in mainstream medicine.

6.6 An Important and Effective Intervention

Finally, it was noted that exploration of patient spirituality improves care of the patient on all levels including symptom control and patient coping.

One doctor reflected: *The end of life is often a trigger …for hidden guilt and fears [to] surface…If you don't deal with this, you end up with terminal restlessness, where the patient is absolutely thrashing around, and it's too late then to tease out the hidden traumas. And the only option at that stage is heavy sedation, which is really sad.*

7 Conclusion: A Model for Spiritual Care with the Doctor as Provider

There is no doubt that spiritual care is of benefit to the patient. But in the end, does it matter who provides it? There is still lack of international consensus regarding whether this is a role for the doctor [71]. It makes sense for the doctor to be involved in a model of spiritual care for patients. Often the doctor sees a patient early in the disease trajectory, and in most healthcare models, the doctor sees all patients, which is not always the case for others in a treating team. Given the purpose of spiritual discussions for patients is largely to strengthen the therapeutic relationship, it seems reasonable to expect that all doctors should take at least a minimal interest in their patients' spirituality. Simple screening would suffice. Those with greater interest and skill can take it further as clinically appropriate. Many models of care would have a similar system in place for screening for patient needs which may require referral, for example to allied health staff.

This does not mean that spiritual screening is the role of the doctor alone. The generalist-specialist model of spiritual care [72] operates within a biopsychosocial-spiritual paradigm and works on the premise that the chaplain (or secular equivalent) is the specialist spiritual care provider, and all members of the multidisciplinary team have a role in providing holistic care to patient and identifying patients who would benefit from specialist referral. Chaplains cannot conduct all spiritual care themselves—inadequate staffing levels can necessitate screening by other staff to ensure they see the patients with the greatest spiritual need. And there is no doubt that there are benefits for patients receiving care from a doctor which cannot be replicated by other staff.

Attention to patient spirituality early in the disease trajectory has several potential advantages: there is evidence that spiritual needs may be higher soon after diagnosis, and improved patient spiritual wellbeing is associated with improved quality of life despite ongoing physical deterioration [3, 73]. While it is acknowledged that conversations about prognosis can be difficult, the doctor explaining to the patient that their illness is incurable could be considered the first step to providing spiritual care at the end of life. One important precipitant of the spiritual work of dying is the patient becoming aware of the proximity of death [74]. Delaying or denying the opportunity for patients to understand that their time is limited can rob them of the opportunity to enjoy the accelerated spiritual growth and transcendence which can be the outcome of spiritual care [49].

References

1. Alcorn SR, Balboni MJ, Prigerson HG, et al. "If God wanted me yesterday, I wouldn't be here today": religious and spiritual themes in patients' experiences of advanced cancer. J Palliat Med. 2010;13(5):581–8. https://doi.org/10.1089/jpm.2009.0343.

2. Steinhauser KE, Christakis NA, Clipp EC, McNeilly M, McIntyre L, Tulsky JA. Factors considered important at the end of life by patients, family, physicians, and other care providers. JAMA. 2000;284(19):2476–82. https://doi.org/10.1001/jama.284.19.2476.
3. Brady MJ, Peterman AH, Fitchett G, Mo M, Cella D. A case for including spirituality in quality of life measurement in oncology. Psychooncology. 1999;8(5):417–28. https://doi.org/10.1002/(SICI)1099-1611(199909/10)
4. Best M, Aldridge L, Butow P, Olver I, Price MA, Webster F. Treatment of holistic suffering in cancer: a systematic literature review. Palliat Med. 2015;29(10):885–98.
5. Smyre CL, Yoon JD, Rasinski KA, Curlin FA. Limits and responsibilities of physicians addressing spiritual suffering in terminally ill patients. Research support, N.I.H., extramural research support, Non-U.S. Gov't. J Pain Symptom Manag. 2015;49(3):562–9. https://doi.org/10.1016/j.jpainsymman.2014.06.016.
6. Best M, Butow P, Olver I. Creating a safe space: a qualitative inquiry into the way doctors discuss spirituality. Palliat Support Care. 2016;14(5):519–31. https://doi.org/10.1017/S1478951515001236.
7. Broad JB, Gott M, Kim H, Boyd M, Chen H, Connolly MJ. Where do people die? An international comparison of the percentage of deaths occurring in hospital and residential aged care settings in 45 populations, using published and available statistics. Int J Public Health. 2013;58(2):257–67. https://doi.org/10.1007/s00038-012-0394-5.
8. World Health Organization. Declaration of Astana: global conference on primary health care: Astana, Kazakhstan, 25 and 26 October 2018. 2019.
9. Liu JT, Kovar-Gough I, Farabi N, Animikwam F, Weers SB, Phillips J. The role of primary care physicians in providing end-of-life care. Systematic review. Am J Hosp Palliat Care. 2019;36(3):249–54. https://doi.org/10.1177/1049909118808232.
10. van de Geer J, Leget C. How spirituality is integrated system-wide in The Netherlands palliative care national programme. Prog Palliat Care. 2012;20(2):98–105. https://doi.org/10.1179/1743291X12Y.0000000008.
11. Balboni TA, VanderWeele TJ, Doan-Soares SD, et al. Spirituality in serious illness and health. JAMA. 2022;328(2):184–97. https://doi.org/10.1001/jama.2022.11086.
12. Periyakoil VS, van Gunten CF, Fischer S, Pantilat S, Quill T. Generalist versus specialist palliative medicine. J Palliat Med. 2022;25(2):193–9.
13. Best M, Butow P, Olver I. Do patients want doctors to talk about spirituality? A systematic literature review. Patient Educ Couns. 2015;98(11):1320–8. https://doi.org/10.1016/j.pec.2015.04.017.
14. Best MC, Jones K, Merritt F, et al. Australian patient preferences for the introduction of spirituality into their healthcare journey: a mixed methods study. J Relig Health. 2023;62(4):2323–40. https://doi.org/10.1007/s10943-022-01616-3.
15. Best MC, Jones K, Merritt F, et al. Australian patient preferences for discussing spiritual issues in the hospital setting: an exploratory mixed methods study. J Relig Health. 2023; https://doi.org/10.1007/s10943-023-01767-x.
16. Best M, Butow P, Olver I. Spiritual support of cancer patients and the role of the doctor. Support Care Cancer. 2014;22:1333–9.
17. Padela AI, Killawi A, Forman J, DeMonner S, Heisler M. American Muslim perceptions of healing: key agents in healing, and their roles. Qual Health Res. 2012;22(6):846–58.
18. Pathy R, Mills KE, Gazeley S, Ridgley A, Kiran T. Health is a spiritual thing: perspectives of health care professionals and female Somali and Bangladeshi women on the health impacts of fasting during Ramadan. Ethn Health. 2011;16(1):43–56. https://doi.org/10.1080/13557858.2010.523780.
19. Balboni MJ, Sullivan A, Enzinger AC, et al. Nurse and physician barriers to spiritual care provision at the end of life. Multicenter study research support, Non-U.S. Gov't. J Pain Symptom Manag. 2014;48(3):400–10. https://doi.org/10.1016/j.jpainsymman.2013.09.020.
20. Best M, Butow P, Olver I. Doctors discussing religion and spirituality: a systematic literature review. Palliat Med. 2016;30(4):327–37. https://doi.org/10.1177/0269216315600912.

21. Kehl KA. Moving toward peace: an analysis of the concept of a good death. Am J Hospice Palliat Med. 2006;23(4):277–86.
22. Phelps AC, Lauderdale KE, Alcorn S, et al. Addressing spirituality within the care of patients at the end of life: perspectives of patients with advanced cancer, oncologists, and oncology nurses. J Clin Oncol. 2012;30(20):2538–44. https://doi.org/10.1200/JCO.2011.40.3766.
23. Torke AM, Garas NS, Sexson W, Branch WT Jr. Medical care at the end of life: views of African American patients in an urban hospital. J Palliat Med. 2005;8(3):593–602.
24. Curtis JR, Patrick DL, Engelberg RA, Norris K, Asp C, Byock I. A measure of the quality of dying and death: initial validation using after-death interviews with family members. J Pain Symptom Manag. 2002;24(1):17–31.
25. Anandarajah G, Mennillo MR, Wang S, DeFries K, Gottlieb JL. Trust as a central factor in hospice enrollment disparities among ethnic and racial minority patients: a qualitative study of interrelated and compounding factors impacting trust. J Palliat Med. 2023;28:28. https://doi.org/10.1089/jpm.2023.0090.
26. Smith R. A good death: an important aim for health services and for us all. BMJ. 2000;320:129–30.
27. Pargament KI, Raiya HA. A decade of research on the psychology of religion and coping: things we assumed and lessons we learned. Psyke Logos. 2007;28(2):25.
28. Busser ST, Rens J, Thoonsen B, Engels Y, Wichmann AB. The GP's perceived role and use of language concerning the existential dimension of palliative patients: a Dutch interview study. BMC Prim Care. 2022;23(1):182. https://doi.org/10.1186/s12875-022-01789-6.
29. Evans N, Costantini M, Pasman HR, et al. End-of-life communication: a retrospective survey of representative general practitioner networks in four countries. Comparative study research support, Non-U.S. Gov't. J Pain Symptom Manag. 2014;47(3):604–619.e3. https://doi.org/10.1016/j.jpainsymman.2013.04.008.
30. Appleby A, Swinton J, Wilson P. What GPs mean by 'spirituality' and how they apply this concept with patients: a qualitative study. BJGP Open. 2018;2(2):bjgpopen18X101469.
31. Smyre CL, Tak HJ, Dang AP, Curlin FA, Yoon JD. Physicians' opinions on engaging patients' religious and spiritual concerns: a National Survey. Research support, Non-U.S. Gov't. J Pain Symptom Manag. 2018;55(3):897–905. https://doi.org/10.1016/j.jpainsymman.2017.10.015.
32. Best M, Butow P, Olver I. Palliative care specialists' beliefs about spiritual care. Support Care Cancer. 2016;24(8):3295–306. https://doi.org/10.1007/s00520-016-3135-0.
33. Ellis MR, Thomlinson P, Gemmill C, Harris W. The spiritual needs and resources of hospitalized primary care patients. J Relig Health. 2013;52:1306–18.
34. Best M, Butow P, Olver I. Why do we find it so hard to discuss spirituality? A qualitative exploration of attitudinal barriers. J Clin Med. 2016;5(9):77. https://doi.org/10.3390/jcm5090077.
35. Best M, McArdle MB, Huang YJ, Clayton J, Butow P. How and how much is spirituality discussed in palliative care consultations for advanced cancer patients with and without a question prompt list? Randomized controlled trial research support, Non-U.S. Gov't. Patient Educ Couns. 2019;102(12):2208–13. https://doi.org/10.1016/j.pec.2019.06.016.
36. Gijsberts M-JHE, van der Steen JT, Hertogh CMPM, Deliens L. Spiritual care provided by nursing home physicians: a nationwide survey. BMJ Support Palliat Care. 2020;10(4):e42. https://doi.org/10.1136/bmjspcare-2018-001756.
37. Rodin G, Lo C, Mikulincer M, Donner A, Gagliese L, Zimmermann C. Pathways to distress: the multiple determinants of depression, hopelessness, and the desire for hastened death in metastatic cancer patients. Soc Sci Med. 2009;68(3):562–9. https://doi.org/10.1016/j.socscimed.2008.10.037.
38. Anandarajah G, Roseman J, Lee D, Dhandhania N. A 10-year longitudinal study of effects of a multifaceted residency spiritual care curriculum: clinical ability, professional formation, end of life, and culture. Research support, Non-U.S. Gov't. J Pain Symptom Manag. 2016;52(6):859–872.e1. https://doi.org/10.1016/j.jpainsymman.2016.06.006.
39. Parikh PP, White MT, Buckingham L, Tchorz KM. Evaluation of palliative care training and skills retention by medical students. J Surg Res. 2017;211:172–7. https://doi.org/10.1016/j.jss.2016.11.006.

40. Tait GR, Hodges BD. Residents learning from a narrative experience with dying patients: a qualitative study. Research support, Non-U.S. Gov't. Adv Health Sci Educ Theory Pract. 2013;18(4):727–43. https://doi.org/10.1007/s10459-012-9411-y.
41. Barnard D, Quill T, Hafferty FW, et al. Preparing the ground: contributions of the preclinical years to medical education for care near the end of life. Working group on the pre-clinical years of the National Consensus Conference on medical education for care near the end of life. Consensus development conference research support, Non-U.S. Gov't review. Acad Med. 1999;74(5):499–505.
42. Ford DW, Downey L, Engelberg R, Back AL, Curtis JR. Discussing religion and spirituality is an advanced communication skill: an exploratory structural equation model of physician trainee self-ratings. J Palliat Med. 2012;15(1):63–70. https://doi.org/10.1089/jpm.2011.0168.
43. Paal P, Helo Y, Frick E. Spiritual care training provided to healthcare professionals: a systematic review. J Pastoral Care Counsel. 2015;69(1):19–30.
44. Penderell A, Brazil K. The spirit of palliative practice: a qualitative inquiry into the spiritual journey of palliative care physicians. Palliat Support Care. 2010;8(4):415–20. https://doi.org/10.1017/S1478951510000271.
45. Seccareccia D, Brown JB. Impact of spirituality on palliative care physicians: personally and professionally. J Palliat Med. 2009;12(9):805–9. https://doi.org/10.1089/jpm.2009.0038.
46. Holland JM, Neimeyer RA. Reducing the risk of burnout in end-of-life care settings: the role of daily spiritual experiences and training. Palliat Support Care. 2005;3(3):173–81. https://doi.org/10.1017/S1478951505050297.
47. Hamouda MA, Emanuel LL, Padela AI. Empathy and attending to patient religion/spirituality: findings from a National Survey of Muslim Physicians. Research support, Non-U.S. Gov't. J Health Care Chaplain. 2021;27(2):84–104. https://doi.org/10.1080/08854726.2019.1618063.
48. Janssen AL, MacLeod RD. What does care mean? Perceptions of people approaching the end of life. Palliat Support Care. 2010;8(4):433–40. https://doi.org/10.1017/S1478951510000301.
49. Best M, Aldridge L, Butow P, Olver I, Webster F. Conceptual analysis of suffering in cancer: a systematic review. Psychooncology. 2015;24(9):977–86. https://doi.org/10.1002/pon.3795.
50. Yang W, Staps T, Hijmans E. Existential crisis and the awareness of dying: the role of meaning and spirituality. OMEGA. 2010;61(1):53–69.
51. Okon TR. "Nobody understands": on a cardinal phenomenon of palliative care. J Med Philos. 2006;31(1):13–46. https://doi.org/10.1080/03605310500499161.
52. Novack DH, Epstein RM, Paulsen RH. Toward creating physician-healers: fostering medical students' self-awareness, personal growth, and well-being. Acad Med. 1999;74(5):516–20.
53. Zinn WM. Doctors have feelings too. JAMA. 1988;259(22):3296–8.
54. Driessen E, van Tartwijk J, Dornan T. The self critical doctor: helping students become more reflective. BMJ. 2008;336(7648):827–30. https://doi.org/10.1136/bmj.39503.608032.AD.
55. Puchalski CM, Guenther M. Restoration and re-creation: spirituality in the lives of healthcare professionals. Curr Opin Support Palliat Care. 2012;6(2):254–8. https://doi.org/10.1097/SPC.0b013e3283522223.
56. Benson J, Magraith K. Compassion fatigue and burnout: the role of Balint groups. J Article Aust Fam Physician. 2005;34(6):497.
57. McKee D, Worby M. Comparing a Christian physicians' support group with the Balint group. J Fam Pract. 1990;30(1):65–8.
58. Huggard P. Compassion fatigue: How much can I give? In: Communication, relationships and care. Routledge; 2004. p. 204–7.
59. Shapiro J. Whither (whether) medical humanities? The future of humanities and arts in medical education. J Learn Through Arts. 2012;8(1):n1.
60. Best M, Leget C, Goodhead A, Paal P. An EAPC white paper on multi-disciplinary education for spiritual care in palliative care. BMC Palliat Care. 2020;19(1):9. https://doi.org/10.1186/s12904-019-0508-4.

61. Lucchetti G, Bassi RM, Lucchetti AL. Taking spiritual history in clinical practice: a systematic review of instruments. Explore (NY). 2013;9(3):159–70. https://doi.org/10.1016/j.explore.2013.02.004.
62. Blaber M, Jone J, Willis D. Spiritual care: which is the best assessment tool for palliative settings? Int J Palliat Nurs. 2015;21(9):430–8. https://doi.org/10.12968/ijpn.2015.21.9.430.
63. Paal P, Frick E, Roser T, Jobin G. Expert discussion on taking a spiritual history. J Palliat Care. 2017;32(1):19–25. https://doi.org/10.1177/0825859717710888.
64. Vermandere M, Choi YN, De Brabandere H, et al. GPs' views concerning spirituality and the use of the FICA tool in palliative care in Flanders: a qualitative study. Research support, non--U.S. Gov't. Br J Gen Pract. 2012;62(603):e718–25. https://doi.org/10.3399/bjgp12X656865.
65. Steinhauser KE, Voils CI, Clipp EC, Bosworth HB, Christakis NA, Tulsky JA. "Are you at peace?": one item to probe spiritual concerns at the end of life. Comparative study multicenter study research support, Non-U.S. Gov't research support, U.S. Gov't, Non-P.H.S. Arch Intern Med. 2006;166(1):101–5.
66. King SDW, Fitchett G, Murphy PE, Pargament KI, Harrison DA, Loggers ET. Determining best methods to screen for religious/spiritual distress. Support Care Cancer. 2017;25(2):471–9. https://doi.org/10.1007/s00520-016-3425-6.
67. Best MC, Vivat B, Gijsberts M-J. Spiritual care in palliative care. Religions. 2023;14(3):320.
68. Langegård U. Consolation in conjunction with incurable cancer. Number. 2009;36(2):E99–E106.
69. Liefbroer AI, Nagel I. Does faith concordance matter? A comparison of clients' perceptions in same versus interfaith spiritual care encounters with chaplains in hospitals. Pastor Psychol. 2021;70(4):349–77. https://doi.org/10.1007/s11089-021-00947-4.
70. Balboni MJ, Sullivan A, Amobi A, et al. Why is spiritual care infrequent at the end of life? Spiritual care perceptions among patients, nurses, and physicians and the role of training. Research support, Non-U.S. Gov't. J Clin Oncol. 2013;31(4):461–7. https://doi.org/10.1200/JCO.2012.44.6443.
71. Harbinson MT, Bell D. How should teaching on whole person medicine, including spiritual issues, be delivered in the undergraduate medical curriculum in the United Kingdom? BMC Med Educ. 2015;15(1):96. https://doi.org/10.1186/s12909-015-0378-2.
72. Balboni MJ, Puchalski CM, Peteet JR. The relationship between medicine, spirituality and religion: three models for integration. J Relig Health. 2014;53:1586–98.
73. Moadel A, Morgan C, Fatone A, et al. Seeking meaning and hope: self-reported spiritual and existential needs among an ethnically-diverse cancer patient population. Psycho Oncol. 1999;8(5):378–85.
74. Coyle N. The existential slap–a crisis of disclosure. London: MA Healthcare; 2004. p. 520.

The Role of the Nurse in Spiritual Care

Wilfred McSherry and Christine Wright

Abstract Spiritual care has a long history in nursing and been a source of contention and debate over several decades. The chapter examines the development of spiritual care competence for nurses providing palliative care. The chapter provides a brief background to the historical development of spiritual care and some key definitions. It is argued that competence in the delivery of spiritual care requires nurses to be adequately prepared and educated to address this sometimes-overlooked dimension of palliative care. The chapter introduces the reader to the EPICC Spiritual Care Education Standard that comprises four competences. The integration of the EPICC Standard into programmes of nurse education will ensure a more standardised approach to teaching of this concept. Adoption of the EPICC Standard will make sure nurses have the requisite knowledge, skills, and attitudes to provide effective and safe spiritual care. The chapter provides some simple illustrations of how nurses can provide spiritual care within palliative care.

Keywords Nursing · Spirituality · Spiritual care · Competence · Palliative care
Assessment holistic care

W. McSherry (✉)
Department of Nursing and Midwifery, Staffordshire University, Stoke-on-Trent, Staffordshire, UK
e-mail: W.McSherry@staffs.ac.uk

C. Wright
Chaplaincy Department, University Hospitals of North Midlands NHS Trust, Stoke-on-Trent, Staffordshire, UK
e-mail: Christine.Wright@uhnm.nhs.uk

M. C. Best (ed.), *Spiritual Care in Palliative Care*,
https://doi.org/10.1007/978-3-031-50864-6_31

1 Introduction

The delivery of spiritual care has a long history in nursing, but it is only recently that any form of consensus has been reached regarding what preparation nurses require to be competent in this dimension of person-centred care [1]. Over the past three decades a considerable amount of time and 'ink' has been devoted towards achieving an authoritative definition of spirituality and what the implications of this might mean for the delivery of spiritual care. Attempts at defining spirituality have rumbled on with no real progress or conclusions being made. Analysis of these debates shows that there was a constant regurgitation and recycling of definitions which did not really advance the field but stifled growth and development. In fact, this endeavour probably led to a polarisation of opinions and differing schools of thought. One school that prevailed raised questions about the feasibility of teaching nurses about spiritual care. The question or argument was predicated on the following social learning theory: *is spiritual care something that can be taught to nurses or is it something best caught in practice* [2, 3]. This question raises important issues about the integration of theory and practice in the educational preparation of nurses and how these may inform the development of competence in spiritual care.

The preparation of nursing and indeed all healthcare professionals involved in the delivery of palliative care necessitates them developing competence both academically and practically. Often, the academic knowledge and practical skills are acquired through the completion of a validated programme of education. The academic component is normally provided through a Higher Education Institution while the practical elements are acquired through exposure to issues within the practice or clinical environment. An important concern that has challenged the development of spiritual care education is the fragmented and piece meal approach to how this is taught within programmes of nursing. There has not been a standardised approach to the integration of this within curricula. It has often been the case that if a member of the department had an interest in this aspect of care, then it often became their responsibility to include this at some point in the programme. The downside of this ad hoc approach was if there was no one with an interest then the subject was not taught, and the matter was neglected or deemed unimportant.

Reflecting on these historical and education developments reveals some significant omissions in the educational strategies employed and the methods used by educators, theorists, researchers, and practitioners. A major criticism of early attempts to define spirituality in nursing was that those involved in this task adopted a 'silo mentality' of working. This blinkered approach led to the exclusion or lack of dialogue with the classical disciplines, for example ethics, psychology, sociology, theology, philosophy, and religious studies. The effect was the construction of definitions not derived from the long traditions with an established track record of engaging with and researching this concept. This naivety meant that many definitions constructed and published during this period were not derived from empirical evidence but based on the conceptual and ideological understanding of an individual(s). One early definition that was embraced by nursing was the one developed by Murray and Zentner [4]:

> A quality that goes beyond religious affiliation, that strives for inspirations, reverence, awe, meaning and purpose, even in those who do not believe in any good. The spiritual dimension tries to be in harmony with the universe, and strives for answers about the infinite, and comes into focus when the person faces emotional stress, physical illness or death. (p. 259)

A criticism of early definitions was that they had been adopted by nursing uncritically meaning they lacked clarity and substance, making it difficult to apply them to the reality of nursing practice. [5, 6]

Another reason for drawing attention to these historical developments is that they have shaped and opened the path to a more inclusive and constructive discourse about the meaning and relevance of spiritual care both within nursing and its relationship with other disciplines. This is of fundamental importance when exploring how competency can be achieved in the delivery of spiritual care both generally in nursing and more specifically in palliative care. Competency in any field requires a clear foundation both conceptual and practical with strong evidence grounded in rigorous empirical research. This evidence informs and underpins the desired outcomes for effective, sensitive, and compassionate spiritual care. It also guarantees that the knowledge, skills, and attitudes acquired enable nurses to practice safely providing care based on the most up to date evidence and crucially within their scope of practice.

1.1 Aim of the Chapter

The primary aim of this chapter is to highlight the role of the nurse in the delivery of spiritual care. This will be achieved by highlighting those factors that can either enhance or inhibit the development of competence in this aspect of person-centred palliative care.

The chapter will draw upon the outputs from a European funded project titled *'Enhancing Nurses' and Midwives' Competence in Providing Spiritual Care through Innovative Education and Compassionate Care'* (EPICC), particularly the EPICC Spiritual Care Education Standard (See Boxes 1 and 2). This standard comprises four competences that underline what knowledge, skills, and attitudes are foundational and essential to provide effective, compassionate spiritual care. While these competences are generic, they are also relevant to nurses working in the field of palliative and end of life care. A full account of the EPICC project has been previously published [1, 7].

2 Nursing Mandate for Spiritual Care

It could be argued that, ever since its inception, nursing has possessed a clear mandate for the delivery of spiritual care. This is because care of the sick, dying, and destitute was primarily the responsibility of religious orders of men and women who saw this as a great work of charity and mercy [8]. Since the secularisation of nursing and healthcare, the responsibility for providing spiritual care has devolved particularly to the nursing profession.

This is reflected in the many professional codes of practice that outline the role and professional responsibility for nurses to address the holistic needs of the individual. This approach to care is considered of paramount importance in the delivery of palliative and end-of-life care in many countries. For example, the International Council of Nurses (ICN) in their recently revised '*Code of Ethics for Nurses*' [9] is explicit about the centrality of a spiritual dimension affirming:

> Inherent in nursing is a respect for human rights, including cultural rights, the right to life and choice, the right to dignity and to be treated with respect. Nursing care is respectful of and unrestricted by considerations of age, colour, culture, ethnicity, disability or illness, gender, sexual orientation, nationality, politics, language, race, religious or *spiritual beliefs*, legal, economic or social status. (p. 2)

'Nurses promote an environment in which the human rights, values, customs, religious and *spiritual beliefs* of the individual, families and communities are acknowledged and respected by everyone. Nurses' rights are included under human rights and should be upheld and protected' (p. 7).

However, this mandate is not always consistent or universally recognised across continents and countries. The Nursing and Midwifery Council in the United Kingdom in their present iteration of '*The Code*' makes no definite reference to the 'spiritual' dimension of the person. Instead, it promotes a bio-psycho-social model of care [10] which contradicts international thinking and practice. This omission certainly has implications for the delivery of high-quality palliative care. Failure to attend to the spiritual dimension of those in receipt of palliative care could result in a violation of the person's dignity and human rights as expressed by the ICN [9] and the World Health Organisation, which recognises this as a fundamental part of palliative care [11]. Furthermore, a recent systematic review published by eminent colleagues in the field of palliative care confirms the need for developing competences in this field of practice [12].

2.1 Defining Spirituality and Spiritual Care

The provision of spiritual care by nurses has long been a source of contention and debate both within and outside the profession. The contentious issues arise from several sources or challenges that have a direct impact on the provision of spiritual care. The first challenge is conceptual or theoretical: what do we understand or how do we define 'spirituality'.

As outlined above, for several decades, many attempts have been made to establish an authoritative definition of spirituality. The work of Pattison and Swinton in 2010 seemed to put an end to this ambition when they offered a solution and way forward to the perennial debate [13]. The solution they provide is based on a functional and contextual approach to understanding and applying spirituality within healthcare. They state:

> We suggest that instead of arguing about whether or not spirituality can exist in any realist, essential sense—a line of argument that has proven to be somewhat circular, controversial, and unhelpful—it is more useful to develop a thin, vague, and functional understanding of what this word and its cognates might connote and do in the world of health care. (p. 227)

Since the publication of this article there seems to have been less energy expanded on defining spirituality and more time and resource devoted to how this concept can be applied and addressed within practice. Table 1 presents a selection of definitions developed in the nursing and healthcare literature. Interestingly, the definition by Puchalski et al. is now the most cited and considered the most authoritative [14] having been adopted after some slight amendments [15] by the European Association for Palliative Care (EAPC) and The EPICC Project.

A review of the definitions in Table 1 affirms that spirituality is a broad umbrella concept comprising many different attributes that give life meaning, purpose, and

Table 1 Definitions of spirituality

European Association for Palliative Care (EAPC) [16] Available from https://eapcnet.eu/eapc-groups/reference/spiritual-care/	'Spirituality is the dynamic dimension of human life that relates to the way persons (individual and community) experience, express and/or seek meaning, purpose and transcendence, and the way they connect to the moment, to self, to others, to nature, to the significant and/or the sacred'. Spirituality and spiritual wellbeing are multidimensional, including: Existential challenges (questions and issues such as identity, meaning, suffering, despair, guilt, shame, reconciliation and forgiveness, freedom and responsibility, hope, love, and joy). Value based considerations and attitudes (what matters most to each person, such as relationships with oneself, and with family, friends, work, nature, art and culture, ethics and morals, and life itself). Religious considerations and foundations (faith, beliefs, and practices, relationship with God or the ultimate).
McSherry [29] (in McSherry and Smith [17, p. 118])	Spirituality is universal, deeply personal, and individual; it goes beyond formal notions of ritual or religious practice to encompass the unique capacity of everyone. It is at the core and essence of who we are, that spark which permeates the entire fabric of the person and demands that we are all worthy of dignity and respect. It transcends intellectual capability, elevating the status of all of humanity…
Puchalski et al. [14, p. 646]	'Spirituality is a dynamic and intrinsic aspect of humanity through which persons seek ultimate meaning, purpose, and transcendence, and experience relationship to self, family, others, community, society, nature, and the significant or sacred. Spirituality is expressed through beliefs, values, traditions, and practices'

fulfilment. They also underline how for many people spirituality involves connections and relationships with others, the sacred, and nature. They can be mapped on to Stoll's (1989) two-dimensional model of spiritual care [18] which suggests that spirituality is comprised of a vertical and horizontal dimension. The vertical axis signposts us to something transcendent that is a sense of something greater or outside our self. The horizontal axis concerns our relationship and connections with the physical and material world such as the environment, creation, and our personal relationships. It is an error to think that the two dimensions are distinct or separate from each other since there is intersection and synergy in this model.

While spirituality is acknowledged as being personal and unique to the individual, these definitions reveal that some elements are repeated or recurrent throughout the definitions. This means that they are universal and may have relevance to most people.

How nurses understand and define spirituality has a significant impact on how they recognise this within themselves and in other people. This self-awareness is of vital importance if this dimension of palliative care is going to be engaged with and supported in practice. There is a growing need for nurses and indeed all those involved in the delivery of palliative care to receive formal training and education in the spiritual aspect of care.

3 The Call for Educational Preparation

A recurrent theme in research findings addressing the delivery of spiritual care is that nurses do not feel sufficiently prepared to support patients with this dimension of care. The Royal College of Nursing (RCN) Spirituality (2010) [19] survey found that members felt inadequately prepared, and they called for more educational preparation. The RCN survey was replicated with a range of healthcare professionals, and it yielded very similar results [20]. These research findings are important because they affirm that many nurses working in palliative and end of life care may feel inadequately prepared to undertake this very important role confidently. Balboni et al. conducted a review of the evidence concerning spirituality in serious illness and the lack of training in spiritual care was a major theme in the research [21]. Furthermore, a recent survey conducted by members of the European Association of Palliative Care (EAPC) Spiritual Care Taskforce (SCTF) with those working in palliative care concluded 'Many respondents commented on the need for staff training and some for staff support, and several stated that more research is necessary, particularly in demonstrating the value of spiritual care' [22, p. 21].

Lack of training and education around spiritual care will continue to be a recurring theme in the nursing and palliative care literature until those responsible for commissioning and monitoring standards recognise the importance of this dimension for achieving high quality care. The recognition and call for more education and preparation must be addressed to ensure the safety of those receiving and those providing care. Failure to ensure nurses are adequately prepared to address this aspect of holistic and person-centred palliative care will perpetuate a cycle of neglect, misconception, and ignorance of the spiritual dimension of palliative care. This reinforces the need for all nurses to continually develop competence in the delivery of spiritual care. We do not want to provide a negative and distorted impression of nursing and spiritual care. There are many examples of excellent spiritual care being provided, education been delivered, and research conducted within this field (see EPICC Network under the section Research and Impact Epicc-network.org).

4 Competency Development in Spiritual Care

Several eminent scholars have devoted many years working in the field of spiritual care competence [23, 24]. Their contributions were the foundation or starting point for the construction of an EPICC Spiritual Care Education Standard (see Boxes 1 and 2). A detailed overview of how the EPICC Standard was constructed has been previously published [25].

Integration of the EPICC Standard in programmes of nurse education will ensure a more standardised approach to teaching these concepts and will ensure the acquisition of knowledge, skills, and attitudes to support the delivery of spiritual care. The EPICC Spiritual Care Education Standard was also developed into a 'Self-Assessment Tool' to enable nursing students and registered nurses to assess their own perceived level of competency against the four competences. A more detailed overview of this research has been previously published [26].

- **Before proceeding, read through the four spiritual care education competences presented in Boxes 1 and 2. Ask yourself, would you feel able to achieve these competences in your nursing practice?**

4.1 The EPICC Spiritual Care Education Standard

The first two competences in the EPICC Standard reinforce the centrality of 'self-awareness'. That is, being aware of your own 'Intrapersonal' spirituality and being open and sensitive to other peoples' 'Interpersonal' spirituality. Having this level of self-awareness is essential for supporting the spiritual needs of patients receiving palliative care. Self-awareness is necessary for nurses to be sympathetic to other people's worldviews and especially when supporting religious, personal, and spiritual beliefs. This is of particular importance when caring for people from diverse religious, ethnic, and cultural groups. In the delivery of spiritual care, great understanding and care must be provided when caring for indigenous populations who often feel marginalised, and their voices excluded from healthcare provision [27].

Box 1 EPICC Spiritual Care Education Standard

Competence 1: Intrapersonal spirituality		
Is aware of the importance of spirituality for health and wellbeing.		
Knowledge	**Skills**	**Attitudes**
Understands the concept of spirituality. Can explain the impact of spirituality on a person's health and wellbeing across the lifespan for oneself and others. Understands the impact of one's own values and beliefs in providing spiritual care.	Reflects meaningfully upon one's own values and beliefs and recognises that these may be different from other persons'. Takes care of oneself.	Is willing to explore one's own and individuals' personal, religious and spiritual beliefs. Is open and respectful to persons' diverse expressions of spirituality.
Competence 2: Interpersonal spirituality		
Engages with persons' spirituality, acknowledging their unique spiritual and cultural worldviews, beliefs, and practices.		
Knowledge	**Skills**	**Attitudes**
Understands the ways that persons express their spirituality. Is aware of the different world/religious views and how these may impact upon persons' responses to key life events.	Recognises the uniqueness of persons' spirituality. Interacts with and responds sensitively to the person's spirituality.	Is trustworthy, approachable, and respectful of persons' expressions of spirituality and different world/religious views.

Competences three and four concern the acquisition of knowledge, technical skills to provide nursing care through a systematic, problem-solving approach. This approach is commonly referred to as the 'nursing process' and means that the spiritual needs of those receiving palliative care are addressed in a comprehensive and holistic manner. The cyclic process means that the spiritual and palliative care needs of the patient are constantly assessed, planned, and evaluated and new priorities or goals set to meet identified needs. These competences also highlight the need to be aware of one's own strengths, resources, and limitations in addressing the spiritual needs of the patient. They also affirm the need to work collaboratively with other members of the multi-disciplinary team such as with referral to chaplaincy (who are the experts in spiritual care) or psycho-social services when necessary. There are some misconceptions surrounding chaplaincy and the services that they provide. Chaplains are not just present to care for people with a religious belief or who come from a particular faith tradition. They provide religious, pastoral, and spiritual care for people of all faiths and none. They are also a tremendous resource and asset for providing training and education on all aspects of spiritual care within the context of palliative care.

Box 2 EPICC Spiritual Care Education Standard

Competence 3: Spiritual care: Assessment and planning		
Assesses spiritual needs and resources using appropriate formal or informal approaches, and plans spiritual care, maintaining confidentiality and obtaining informed consent.		
Knowledge	**Skills**	**Attitudes**
Understands the concept of spiritual care. Is aware of different approaches to spiritual assessment. Understands other professionals' roles in providing spiritual care.	Conducts and documents a spiritual assessment to identify spiritual needs and resources. Collaborates with other professionals. Is able to appropriately contain and deal with emotions.	Is open, approachable, and non-judgemental. Has a willingness to deal with emotions.
Competence 4: Spiritual care: Intervention and evaluation		
Responds to spiritual needs and resources within a caring, compassionate relationship.		
Knowledge	**Skills**	**Attitudes**
Understands the concept of compassion and presence and its importance in spiritual care. Knows how to respond appropriately to identified spiritual needs and resources. Knows how to evaluate whether spiritual needs have been met.	Recognises personal limitations in spiritual care giving and refers to others as appropriate. Evaluates and documents personal, professional and organisational aspects of spiritual care giving, and reassesses appropriately.	Shows compassion and presence. Shows willingness to collaborate with and refer to others (professional/nonprofessional). Is welcoming and accepting and shows empathy, openness, professional humility and trustworthiness in seeking additional spiritual support.

Collectively, the four competences outline what is necessary for nurses to meet the spiritual needs of their patients and to provide effective spiritual care. In addition to self-awareness, there are some fundamental skills required to support patients, such as communication, professionalism, positive values, and attitudes, working according to one's level of competence and following national guidelines and codes of practice. Furthermore, nurses providing spiritual care need to work in an open and collaborative manner with colleagues across the multi-disciplinary team. An often-overlooked aspect of providing spiritual care is the need for 'Self-care'. This is of vital importance because we cannot give to others what we do not possess ourselves. Therefore, the development or roll-out of any spiritual care education programme or training must address this specific requirement to safeguard the emotional and spiritual wellbeing of those providing care (see Chap. 29). The successful acquisition of the four competences will ensure that spiritual care provided to those in receipt of palliative care is always holistic and person-centred. The next section highlights some examples that will help to support the delivery of spiritual care in practice.

5 Application to Palliative Care

The delivery of palliative care requires a combination of the 'artistic' aspects of care combined with the 'scientific', those technical and clinical skills required to practice safely and competently [28]. This means that those providing palliative care need to have those altruistic and humanistic skills (kindness, respect, approachable) that ensure care is provided sensitively and compassionately.

5.1 Treatment Versus Care

As part of his PhD studies, one of the authors (WMc) interviewed patients in a range of care settings, including those receiving palliative care [29]. The following reflection on a transcript from one of the patients provides some very important insights into the nurse's role around spiritual care.

The phrase—'Treatment versus care'—is an excerpt of transcript from an interview I held with an older gentleman who was dying from terminal lung cancer. The gentleman's words still echo in my ears—'Wilf'. He said: 'we get treatment in the hospital and care in the hospice'. These words are prophetic and have a relevance for nursing today.

The gentleman makes a clear distinction between 'treatment and care' pointing to some of the key issues associated with depersonalisation and over-medicalisation of care that some feel is present in palliative care. The gentleman's words imply 'treatment' is different to 'care' and 'care' or, more precisely, caring takes precedence or supersedes 'treatment'.

The gentleman described 'treatment' as the following: Someone who is technically proficient and good at their job, doing what they should, in a time and manner that is appropriate to the needs of the individual. In summary, a practitioner or carer worker who displays technical competence and proficiency with regards to the functional tasks and duties they perform. Yet, despite technical proficiency, the use of the word 'Treatment' presents the picture of someone almost robotic in their actions, someone detached and emotionally disconnected from the process of care. The word 'treatment' feels cold, scientific and, I would add, heartless, in that it appears to lack that human compassion and interaction.

Conversely, the word 'care', or the practical forms of knowledge, conjure up a picture of someone warm, someone who takes time and provides a presence. For the patient, 'care' is about being valued and accepted as a unique person with a unique set of needs. These needs may be expressed either physically, socially, psychologically or spiritually. This raises a question: can 'treatment' and 'care' be given synonymously when meeting the diverse needs of individuals?

5.2 Hard and Soft Nurse

The same gentleman elaborated and qualified his statement by adding: 'Wilf…, There is a hard and a soft nurse!' I asked, 'Can you explain this for me?' The response he gave was, 'The hard nurse approaches the patient with an opening such as, what's this pain in your chest?' The gentleman said '…instantly I know he or she is not concerned with me as a person but with the condition that has brought me into the hospital (the biological or the scientific)'. …While the soft nurse asks 'How you are this afternoon; how are your wife and family? They are concerned with me as person and my situation (the practical) not just the medical condition'.

This illustration tells us two fundamental things about patients: first, they want care, not just treatment, and second, importantly they can distinguish the type of nurse or practitioner who is likely to provide this. I think crucially the gentleman's phrase tells us that nursing and palliative care is a blend of the scientific and the artistic.

The challenge for the delivery of spiritual care is that nurses must become competent not just in the scientific and technical, but they must also be fluent at reading and responding to the emotional, psychological, and spiritual cues that are presented by patients. Health and palliative care services are often good at seeking prompt, real time patient satisfaction survey data from those attending their services. However, long before patients have been asked to complete, for example, a Friends and Family Test [30] (see Box 3), nurses are being audited by patients, carers, and visitors about the types of attitudes that they display. Are they welcoming, approachable, open, professional? The nurse's demeanour communicates something fundamental about the way they preserve and conserve the dignity of the patient. Dignity is a central thread that cannot be divorced or disassociated from the provision of spiritual care.

Box 3 The Friends and Family Test
The Friends and Family Test is an important feedback tool that supports the fundamental principle that people who use the National Health Service in the United Kingdom should have the opportunity to provide feedback on their experience. Listening to the views of patients and staff helps identify what is working well, what can be improved and how.

6 Dignity Conserving Care

Canadian psychiatrist Harvey Chochinov is a leading authority on dignity conserving care. In 2007, he published an article in the *British Medical Journal* presenting a very simple model for conserving dignity in care, entitled '*Dignity and the Essence of Medicine: The A, B, C, and D of Dignity Conserving Care*'. [31]

This simple model should be adopted by all those working in palliative care. The model is a very powerful reminder of what is important when caring for people and each other. A brief overview of the model can be found in Box 4.

Box 4 ABCD of Dignity Conserving Care

A = Attitudes	When nurses are addressing the spiritual needs of those receiving palliative care, they must be able to do this without any form or prejudice, assumption or discrimination. This can only be avoided or overcome by exploring and examining one's own attitudes towards death, dying, loss, and bereavement. This is why competences 1 and 2 deal with issues of self-awareness, encouraging personal reflection and introspection. Positive attitudes when we are caring for those receiving palliative care are of vital importance because they create caring environments that are open, respectful, and safe for the patient, family and all working in them. Chochinov [31, p. 185] captures this, stating: 'In other words, patients look at healthcare providers as they would a mirror, seeking a positive image of themselves and their continued sense of worth. In turn, healthcare providers need to be aware that their attitudes and assumptions will shape those all-important reflections'
B = Behaviours	Positive attitudes and values towards deeply personal aspects of human existence such as spirituality, death, and dying are of paramount importance. Holding positive attitudes are important because these in turn influence our behaviours and practices towards the delivery of spiritual care. Chochinov [31] tells us that our behaviour should always be centred on kindness and respect. The way that nurses display professionalism, which is reflected in one's demeanour, values, and attitudes, for example when meeting and welcoming patients, can have such a significant impact on those receiving palliative care. The smallest act of kindness, such as adjusting a patient's pillow, saying a 'good morning' or a 'how are you?', communicates something significant about our attitudes and the culture in a ward or department. The smallest act of kindness as outlined above can either validate a person's self-worth and self-esteem and dignity or it can destroy this in an instant for example with a frown or scowl or dismissal of need.

C = Compassion	Compassion is of overriding importance in the delivery of palliative care. Compassion enables the nurse to recognise the personal suffering and pain experienced by another person. This awareness and sensitivity moves the nurse to ease and relieve the problem for that person. This may involve utilising all the medical pharmacological and technical aspects of care at their disposal, but it also involves the nurse being present with the person. This means compassion is not something cerebral but something that draws on the humanity of each person, the patient, and the nurse. This synergy or symbiotic relationship between one human being and another is more than just something physical because it says something very deep about the nature of humanity connecting the persons at a spiritual level. This suggests that compassion is something intuitive and innate which develops through professional practice and life experience. Verbal and non-verbal communication are necessary channels for expressing and preserving compassion in all therapeutic relationships and interactions.
D = Dialogue	When teaching these concepts, WMc always reinforces that we cannot conserve dignity without attending to A, B, C, and D. Many assume D is for dignity and are a little taken aback when they learn D is for dialogue. Dialogue is so important in the delivery of palliative care because it communicates to the patient and their family that we are prepared to engage, listen, and create a safe space to gain a deeper understanding of their spiritual needs. Dialogue is about being prepared to listen so that we can be informed by the personal narrative and biography of the person. It is not about making assumptions about what the nurse feels the patient requires. Dialogue enables us to build a profile of the unique person capturing 'What is most important thing for you right now?' affording us the time and space to reply, 'How can we help?' This simple model developed by Ross and McSherry is known as the 2Q-SAM (2 Question Spiritual/Holistic Assessment Model) [32].

6.1 *Remember the Little Things*

One of the greatest obstacles to the provision of spiritual care is the overcomplication of the concept and how this can impact on care delivery. Separating out the spiritual dimension of palliative care as a discrete area for assessment, intervention, and support can make it appear as something very complex to accomplish. It also raises nurses' fears and anxieties regarding this area. Seeing the word 'spiritual' on an admission form or in a spiritual assessment can become a major obstacle and barrier to holistic person-centred care. Many nurses seeing the word 'spiritual' can become fearful and hesitant to engage with the dimension because it sounds complex and complicated when nothing can be further from the truth. Spiritual care is met in and through the everyday interactions and communications of the nurse. This is not to diminish or devalue the spiritual dimension, but to emphasise that spiritual care is all about the way we communicate, support, and come alongside the patient receiving spiritual care. This is reflected in the definition of spiritual care published by National Health Service Education for Scotland [33] in *'Spiritual Care Matters'* [32]:

> Spiritual care in its broad and inclusive sense can perhaps help give us a workable credo, as we acknowledge the importance of responding to spiritual need of all kinds in the health-care environment. Spiritual care is that care which recognises and responds to basic human needs and core beliefs when faced with trauma, ill health or sadness and can include the need for meaning-making, for self-worth, to express oneself honestly, for particular faith or belief group support, perhaps for rites or prayer or sacrament, or simply for a sensitive listener. Spiritual care begins with compassion in all of our human contacts, and especially in healthcare, and moves in whatever direction need requires.

This definition affirms that spiritual care must always be guided by the needs of the patient, and it stresses the relationship between dignity and personal beliefs that are fundamental to the individual. The final sentence underlines the centrality of having courage and compassion to come alongside the patient, responding and adapting spiritual care as needs change. The quotation confirms how it is that the small acts of care and the professionalism of the nurse that are crucial to the delivery of spiritual care.

Williams et al. [34] provide an excellent insight into the little things that become the big things for patients and the conservation of dignity [34]. These little things are central to communicating value, worth, presence and creating palliative care environments that feel safe and trustworthy for patients, families, and visitors. Some of the little things may be as follows:

- An introduction: hello my name is…
- A smile
- A warm word of welcome
- A 'how are you?'
- A 'please' and 'thank you'

When the above little things are absent or omitted from the delivery of palliative care, then the spiritual and humanistic aspect of care can be compromised leading to a loss of focus on the patient who is and should be the centre and priority of all care delivery.

7 Conclusion

Spiritual care is dependent upon the positive connections and relationship created between the nurse and patient that communicate care, concern, and compassion for the whole person. This type of relationship signifies to the patient that the nurse is prepared to listen, provide a presence, and offer support throughout the palliative care journey. Therefore, the nurse's role in the delivery of spiritual care is often not dependent on complex assessments, interventions, and procedures. It involves nurses developing their own self-awareness of this dimension both in themselves and others. This awareness is of vital importance for forming human relationships, attitudes, values, and behaviours that create environments that are caring, compassionate, and preserving the dignity of the person. This necessitates nurses to have the requisite competence in spiritual care by developing knowledge, skills, and behaviours that are founded on robust empirical evidence. The EPICC Spiritual Care Education Standard provides such a vehicle for the preparation of all nurses in the delivery of spiritual care. The four competences offer an in-depth account of the knowledge, skills, and attitudes necessary to engage in spiritual care safely, competently, and sensitively.

References

1. McSherry W, Boughey A, Attard J, editors. Enhancing nurses' and midwives' competence in providing spiritual care. Cham: Springer; 2021b.
2. Bradshaw A. Teaching spiritual care to nurses: an alternative approach. Int J Palliat Nurs. 1997;3(1):51–7.
3. Oman D. Spiritual modelling and the social learning of spirituality and religion. In: Pargament KI, Exline JJ, Jones JW, editors. APA handbook of psychology, religion, and spirituality (Vol. 1): context, theory, and research. Washington, DC: American Psychological Association; 2013. p. 187–204. https://doi.org/10.1037/14045-010.
4. Murray RB, Zentner JB. Nursing concepts for health promotion. London: Prentice Hall; 1989.
5. Paley J. Spirituality and nursing: a reductionist approach. Nurs Philos. 2008;9:3–18.
6. Clarke J. A critical view of how nursing has defined spirituality. J Clin Nurs. 2009;18:1666–73.
7. McSherry W, Ross L, Attard J, van Leeuwen R, Giske T, Kleiven T, Boughey A, the EPICC Network. Preparing undergraduate nurses and midwives for spiritual care: some developments in European education over the last decade. J Study Spiritual. 2020a;10(1):55–71. https://doi.org/10.1080/20440243.2020.1726053.
8. Bradshaw A. Lighting the lamp: the spiritual dimension of nursing care. London: Scutari Press; 1994.
9. International Council of Nurses. The ICN code of ethics for nurses. 2021. https://www.icn.ch/sites/default/files/2023-06/ICN_Code-of-Ethics_EN_Web.pdf. Accessed 6 Nov 2023.
10. Nursing and Midwifery Council. The Code. 2018. https://www.nmc.org.uk/standards/code/. Accessed 16 Nov 2023.
11. World Health Organization. Palliative care. 2020. https://www.who.int/news-room/fact-sheets/detail/palliative-care. Accessed 16 Nov 2023.
12. Gijsberts M-JHE, Liefbroer AI, Otten R, Olsman E. Spiritual Care in Palliative Care: a systematic review of the recent European literature. Med Sci. 2019;7:25. https://doi.org/10.3390/medsci7020025.
13. Swinton J, Pattison S. Moving beyond clarity: towards a thin, vague, and useful understanding of spirituality in nursing care. Nurs Philos. 2010;11:226–37. https://doi.org/10.1111/j.1466-769X.2010.00450.x.
14. Puchalski CM, Vitillo R, Hull SK, Reller N. Improving the spiritual dimension of whole person care: reaching national and international consensus. J Palliat Med. 2014;17(6):642–56.
15. Nolan S, Saltmarsh P, Leget CJW. Spiritual care in palliative care: working towards an EAPC task force. Eur J Palliat Care. 2011;18:86–9.

16. European Association of Palliative Care. Spiritual care. Spiritual care – EAPC. 2023. http://www.eapcnet.eu. Accessed 16 Jan 2023.
17. McSherry W, Smith J. Spiritual care. In: McSherry W, McSherry R, Watson R, editors. Care in Nursing Principles values and skills. Oxford: Oxford University Press; 2012.
18. Stoll RI. The essence of spirituality, Chapter 1. In: Carson VB, editor. Spiritual dimensions of nursing practice. Philadelphia: W B Saunders Company; 1989. p. 6–8.
19. Royal College of Nursing. RCN spirituality survey 2010: a report by the Royal College of Nursing on members' views on spirituality and spiritual care in nursing practice. London: Royal College Nursing; 2011.
20. Austin P, MacLeod R, Siddall P, McSherry W, Egan R. Spiritual care training is needed for clinical and non-clinical staff to manage patients' spiritual needs. J Study Spiritual. 2017;7(1):50–3.
21. Balboni TA, VanderWeele TJ, Doan-Soares SD, et al. Spirituality in serious illness and health. JAMA. 2022;328(2):184–97. https://doi.org/10.1001/jama.2022.11086.
22. Vivat B, Lodwick R, Merino MTG-B, Young T. What do palliative care professionals understand as spiritual care? Findings from an EAPC survey. Religions. 2023;14:298. https://doi.org/10.3390/rel14030298.
23. van Leeuwen R, Cusveller B. Nursing competencies for spiritual care. J Adv Nurs. 2004;48(3):234–46. https://doi.org/10.1111/j.1365-2648.2004.03192.xvan.
24. Attard J, Ross L, Weeks KW. Design and development of a spiritual care competency framework for pre-registration nurses and midwives: a modified Delphi study. Nurse Educ Pract. 2019;39:96–104. https://doi.org/10.1016/j.nepr.2019.08.003.
25. van Leeuwen R, Attard J, Ross L, et al. The development of a consensus-based spiritual care education standard for undergraduate nursing and midwifery students: an educational mixed methods study. J Adv Nurs. 2021;77:973–86. https://doi.org/10.1111/jan.14613.
26. Giske T, Schep-Akkerman A, Bø B, Cone PH, Moene Kuven B, Mcsherry W, Owusu B, Ueland V, Lassche-Scheffer J, van Leeuwen R, Ross L. Developing and testing the EPICC spiritual care competency self-assessment tool for student nurses and midwives. J Clin Nurs. 2022;00:1–15. https://doi.org/10.1111/jocn.16261.
27. Sivertsen N, Harrington A, Hamiduzzaman M. Two eyed seeing': the integration of spiritual care in aboriginal residential aged care in South Australia. J Relig Spiritual Aging. 2020;32(2):149–71. https://doi.org/10.1080/15528030.2019.1669515.
28. McSherry W, Ross L, editors. Spiritual assessment in health care practice. Keswick: M&K Publishing; 2010.
29. McSherry W. Treatment versus care!' Reintegrating spirituality and dignity' title of inaugural professorial lecture by Wilfred McSherry on Monday 27th April 2009, Staffordshire University, Shropshire Education and Conference Centre, Royal Shrewsbury Hospital, Shropshire. 2009.
30. National Health Service England. Friends and Family Test. 2023. https://www.nhs.uk/using-the-nhs/about-the-nhs/friends-and-family-test-fft/. Accessed 20 Nov 2023.
31. Chochinov HM. Dignity and the essence of medicine: the A, B, C, and D of dignity conserving care. Br Med J. 2007;335:184–7.
32. Ross L, McSherry W. The power of two simple questions. Nurs Stand. 2018;33(9):78–80.
33. National Health Service Education for Scotland (2021) Spiritual care matters. Available from https://www.nes.scot.nhs.uk/media/xzadagnc/spiritual-care-matters-an-introductory-resource-for-all-nhsscotland-staff.pdf [Accessed 16-07-20224]
34. Williams V, Kinnear D, Victor C. 'It's the little things that count': healthcare professionals' views on delivering dignified care: a qualitative study. J Adv Nurs. 2016;72(4):782–90. https://doi.org/10.1111/jan.12878.

The Role of the Palliative Care Chaplain in the United States

Edward Peñate, Allison Kestenbaum, and Sarah Byrne-Martelli

Abstract The authors are established palliative care chaplains in adult hospital-based palliative care programmes in the United States of America. In this chapter, we discuss the role of the chaplain from our own perspective, being aware that our social and geographical locations influence our perspective. As members of the interdisciplinary palliative care team, palliative care chaplains in the United States are in a unique position to provide team-based contributions. In this chapter, we describe emerging evidence-based models and current best practices in three realms (clinical, education/training, and leadership) in order to provide guidance to palliative care professionals on how the integration and strengthening of the role of the palliative care chaplain can be achieved.

Keywords Chaplain · Spiritual care · Communication · Assessment · Training Education · Clinical pastoral education (CPE) · Leadership · Advocacy Palliative care

E. Peñate (✉)
Section of Palliative Medicine and Spiritual Care & Education, Northwestern Memorial Hospital, Chicago, IL, USA
e-mail: epenate@nm.org

A. Kestenbaum
Spiritual Care & Clinical Pastoral Education, UC San Diego Health, CA, USA
e-mail: akestenbaum@health.ucsd.edu

S. Byrne-Martelli
Division of Palliative Care and Geriatric Medicine, Massachusetts General Hospital, Boston, MA, USA
e-mail: sbyrne-martelli@mgh.harvard.edu

M. C. Best (ed.), *Spiritual Care in Palliative Care*,
https://doi.org/10.1007/978-3-031-50864-6_32

1 Introduction

Since its origins, attending to the spiritual values and needs of patients has been a core component in the provision of quality palliative care [1]. Today, interprofessional consensus conferences have called for the integration of spiritual care as part of an interdisciplinary approach to comprehensive care for palliative care patients [2]. Additionally, National Consensus Guidelines in the United States and an expanding literature recognise the centrality of attending to spiritual aspects of care as part of palliative care [3–5]. This has prompted research on various fronts such as studying palliative care interdisciplinary collaborative care models [6].

As valued members of the interdisciplinary palliative care team in the United States, palliative care chaplains are in a unique position to provide team-based contributions in various realms [7]. For example, in the clinical setting, palliative care chaplains use their skills to support the delivery of value-based, person-centred, culturally sensitive care for patients and their families during complex medical decision-making discussions and supporting complex religious/spiritual needs [8–10]. As frontline healthcare professionals, palliative care chaplains are situated to contribute to policy change and advocacy due to their unique knowledge and insight into the lives of seriously ill patients.

As a specialty practice in the United States, palliative care chaplains, some of whom have advanced board certification in palliative care and hospice, offer skills in a variety of settings [7, 9–11]. In this chapter, we describe emerging evidence-based models and current best practices of chaplaincy care in three realms (clinical, education/training, and leadership) with the ultimate goal of guiding palliative care professionals through the integration and strengthening of the palliative care chaplain role. We approach this task by highlighting the published literature and drawing on anecdotal evidence from the three authors.

We have structured this chapter into three sections. The first section explores the clinical aspects of care, particularly responding to two questions—when should a palliative care clinician consult the chaplain, and if the clinician refers a patient to the chaplain, what can they offer? The second section explains how one becomes a palliative care chaplain in the United States, mainly highlighting the training trajectory. The third section briefly explores leadership opportunities for palliative care chaplains. We end this chapter with observations of barriers to chaplaincy care and suggested ways to address them.

2 Clinical

2.1 Screening, History-Taking, and Assessment

In the United States, palliative care chaplains are clinicians who function as an integral part of an interprofessional team, caring for seriously ill patients and their families and working alongside medical providers and social workers. In the

United States, interprofessional palliative care teams may include pharmacists, psychologists, psychiatrists, and bereavement care specialists. The interprofessional team provides care not only for the patient, but also for the family and caregivers. The interprofessional team views the seriously ill patient through the lens of 'Total Pain', a key palliative care concept which envisions the multidimensional nature of the patient's pain experience to include the physical, psychological, social, and spiritual dimensions [12]. The holistic and integrated nature of the palliative care philosophy recognises the dynamic nature of pain and suffering. At times, a patient's physical symptoms may be at the forefront of their concern, and at other times, a patient's existential questions or family concerns may be the priority. The chaplain takes the lead to address the patient and family's spiritual and existential pain, while communicating with the team to establish shared goals and a plan of care.

The palliative care team addresses spiritual needs through a combination of spiritual history, screening, and assessment. A spiritual history is generally taken as part of a thorough social history, wherein the medical team elicits demographic information about a patient's life, including religious/spiritual preference, family background, social supports, coping, language, cultural aspects of care, and other relevant information.

A spiritual screen is a more dynamic tool which is used to address the presence of spiritual concerns, distress, and resources. A screen is a 'quick determination of whether a person is experiencing a serious spiritual/religious crisis and therefore needs a referral to a professional chaplain' [13]. Just as with a spiritual history, a spiritual screen may be conducted by any member of a clinical team. However, a spiritual screen takes less time and is ideally conducted multiple times over the course of care and integrated into routine assessment. Just as a clinical team reassesses nausea, sleep, shortness of breath, and other symptoms that vary day to day, the clinical team should also readdress spiritual needs, which can change based on coping skills, new clinical information, improvement or worsening of symptoms, interpersonal dynamics, or personal reflection about one's illness trajectory, among other factors. New spiritual needs might arise and are more likely to do so in cases of serious illness [14].

Fitchett indicates that good models of spiritual/religious screening 'employ a few simple questions, which can be asked by any health care professional in the course of an overall screening' [13]. Examples of spiritual screening questions include: *Many people find comfort in their religious or spiritual practices. Is this true for you? If so, how can we support you while you are here? Where do you find strength? What's keeping you going through all of this?* and *What's the hardest part of this for you?*

Screening tools vary, necessarily, according to one's clinical setting, protocols, and interprofessional team structure and staffing. Examples designed to screen for religious/spiritual (R/S) struggles include the *Edmonton Symptom Assessment Scale* (ESAS-FS) and the *Rush Protocol* [15–17]. The ESAS-FS is a validated symptom screening tool developed for palliative care patients that lists, among physical symptoms such as drowsiness or fatigue, psychosocial and spiritual pain symptoms. It characterises spiritual pain as 'pain deep in your soul/being that is not physical' and is an example of a specialised scale that reflects a Total Pain model described above [15]. The Rush Protocol is a widely utilised spiritual screening protocol in the United States [17]. It screens for religious/spiritual struggle following an algorithm which asks about the importance of religion/spirituality in the person's life and, depending upon the response, two follow-up questions. The two possible pathways are illustrated in Fig. 1 [17]. The protocol was developed with medical rehabilitation patients but has also been used in oncology settings [18, 19].

It is important to note that any seriously ill patient, regardless of spiritual or religious background, may experience distress related to meaning-making, loss, existential concerns, fear of death or dying, legacy, family, and other concerns. Chaplains

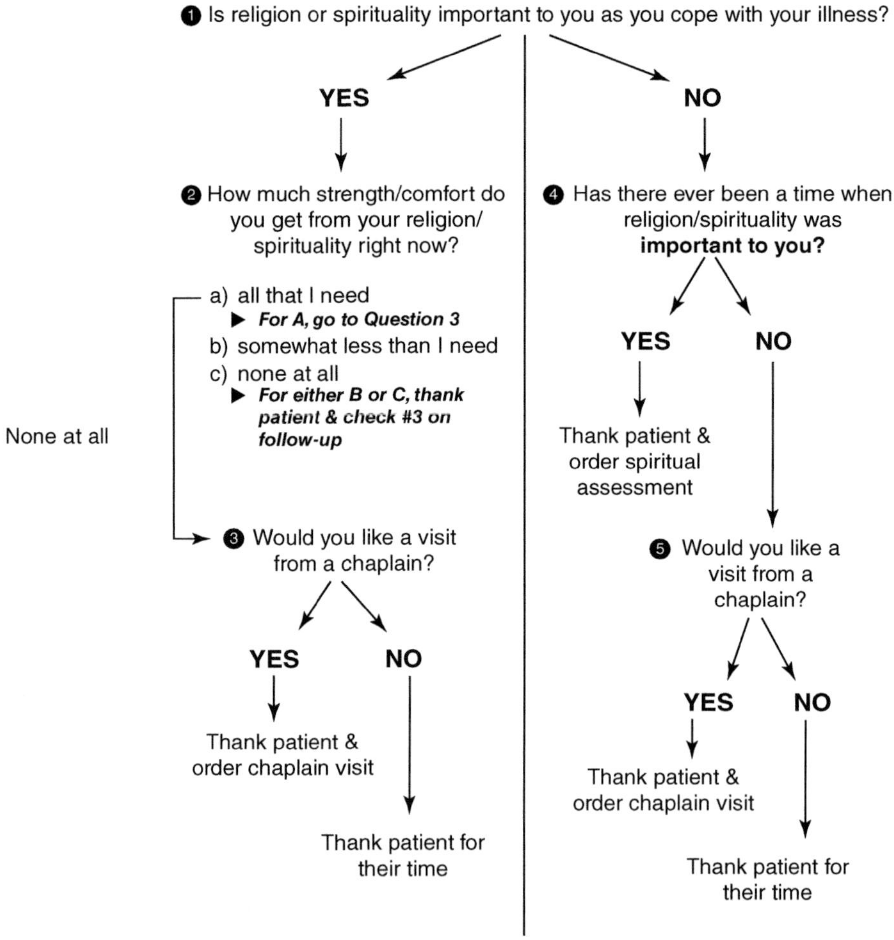

Fig. 1 Religious struggle screening protocol place around here

Table 1 PC-7 model

#	Theme	Indicator[a]
1	Need for meaning in the face of suffering	The patient is having difficulty coming to terms with changes in things that gave meaning to life.
2	Need for integrity, a legacy, generativity	The patient questions the meaning of life—whether the life he or she has lived has meaning.
3	Concerns about relationships: family and/or significant others	The patient has unfinished business with significant others.
4	Concern or fear about dying or death	The patient has concerns about dying or being unready for death. This may include explicit hesitation, reluctance, or avoidance to consider or discuss mortality, or associated issues.
5	Issues related to making decisions about treatment	The patient needs assistance with value-based advance care planning.
6	Religious/Spiritual struggle	The patient wonders whether he or she is being abandoned or punished by God.
7	Other dimensions	The patient identifies a need for assistance to perform important rituals, religious, or otherwise.

[a] Only one example of an indicator is listed per theme. For a full description of the indicators, please refer to Fitchett et al. (2020) [23]

provide care for patients struggling with these and other sources of distress. Spiritual care from a chaplain is not limited to patients who are 'religious'. Chaplains focus their assessment and interventions on areas of unmet spiritual needs.

In the United States, spiritual assessment is conducted by a professional chaplain. A spiritual assessment is an 'extensive (in-depth, on-going) process of actively listening to a patient's story as it unfolds in a relationship with a professional chaplain and summarising the needs and resources that emerge in that process' [13]. The chaplain's summary includes a 'spiritual care plan with expected outcomes which should be communicated to the rest of the treatment team' [13]. There are several well-established models of spiritual assessment including *Spiritual AIM* [20], the *Discipline for Pastoral Caregiving* [21], and the *Spiritual Distress Assessment Tool* (SDAT) [22]. For the specific setting of palliative care, the *PC-7* [23] is a quantifiable spiritual assessment tool that seeks to identify and describe areas of spiritual concerns related to seven key domains with suggestive indicators (see Table 1).

2.2 When to Consult a Chaplain?

A palliative care clinician should consult a chaplain when a patient or their family is facing spiritual or existential distress or concerns related to their illness or end-of-life care. Palliative care chaplains are trained to provide spiritual support to patients and their families, regardless of their religious or spiritual beliefs. They can help address existential concerns, offer guidance, facilitate communication, and assist with advance care planning.

From the experience of the three authors, the particular circumstances listed below are ones where a clinician could consider involving a chaplain.

1. When a patient or their family needs spiritual support or guidance.
2. When a patient struggles with questions of meaning, purpose, or faith in the face of illness.
3. When a patient or their family is experiencing grief, loss, or anticipatory grief.
4. When patients or their families deal with ethical or moral dilemmas related to their care.
5. When a patient or their family is experiencing conflicts or tensions related to their beliefs, values, or cultural practices.
6. When patients or their families seek rituals, prayers, or religious sacraments to provide comfort or solace.
7. When a patient or their family struggles with forgiveness, reconciliation, or unresolved issues.
8. When a patient or their family is experiencing distress related to end-of-life decision-making or advance care planning.
9. When a patient and family is facing a change in diagnosis, prognosis, or treatment.

2.3 *How Do Chaplains Contribute?*

Once a chaplain has assessed areas of spiritual distress or concern, the chaplain may employ interventions that include: identifying sources of spiritual strength or distress, identifying comforting prayers, music, readings, or poems; praying with the patient, facilitating end-of-life rituals; addressing existential fears; facilitating life review; celebrating positive news or lamenting difficult news; clarifying spiritual questions; deepening theological reflection; reconnecting with spiritual practices; providing guided meditation; normalising grief; affirming family relationships; and providing end-of-life education.

A Case Example: Addressing Existential Fears

John is a 60-year-old man who has been diagnosed with stage IV pancreatic cancer and was recently admitted for uncontrolled abdominal pain. He was recently referred to palliative care and has been receiving palliative care as part of a hospital-based programme for two months. During the palliative care inpatient encounter, John is experiencing intense existential fears and struggles with questions about the meaning of life and the afterlife. The palliative care chaplain, Fernando, is consulted by the attending physician to provide spiritual support.

Fernando meets with John in his room, and after an initial phase of introduction, rapport building, and Fernando listening attentively to John, John begins to share his existential fears, including his fear of dying and what comes after death.

Fernando acknowledges John's fears and validates his emotions. He reassures him that it is common to have these concerns and that many people facing serious illness grapple with similar questions. Fernando explains that exploring existential concerns is essential to the spiritual journey because it may help with meaning-making, connection, and resilience.

Fernando asks open-ended questions to encourage him to reflect on his life's meaning and purpose. He explores his spiritual and religious background and any spiritual practices or beliefs that have been meaningful to him in the past.

As John shares his thoughts and experiences, Fernando asks permission to share guidance and support. Fernando suggests engaging in practices that can help John find peace and meaning in the present moment. He introduces him to mindfulness meditation and guided imagery exercises, which can help calm the mind and cultivate a sense of inner peace.

Throughout their conversations, Fernando emphasises the importance of self-compassion and self-acceptance. He encourages John to be gentle with himself as he navigates these existential fears and reminds him that it is okay to have doubts and uncertainties.

Fernando regularly meets with John, providing ongoing spiritual support and reassurance. He helps him continue to explore his fears and concerns in a supportive environment. Fernando also collaborates with the interdisciplinary palliative care team, sharing his insights and observations to ensure that John's spiritual values and needs are integrated into his care plan.

A Case Example: Lamenting Difficult News

Ben is a chaplain who has been providing spiritual support to Emily, a patient in a skilled nursing facility with community-based palliative care services who has had cancer for several years. Emily had been stable for months. Recently, her medical team discovered that the cancer has spread, and the prognosis is now very poor, news which they shared with Emily and her family.

Ben schedules a visit with Emily. During the visit with Emily, Ben greets her and begins the conversation with a routine follow up; he then communicates his awareness of the recent family meeting between her and the medical team. He asks her to share her experience and understanding of the outcomes of that meeting. Emily shares the news about the prognosis, expressing her anger and sadness. As Emily talks about how she is feeling, Ben actively listens, acknowledging her sadness and anger and agreeing that receiving such news can be overwhelming and distressing. He acknowledges the pain and loss that she is experiencing and assures her that her emotions are valid and understandable.

Throughout the conversation, Ben reassures her that he or someone else from the spiritual care team will continue to accompany her, providing spiritual support and companionship during this difficult time. Ben also discusses the importance of self-care with Emily and encourages her to reach out to her loved ones for support. He also offers resources and suggestions for coping strategies, such as support groups or counselling services offered through the community-based palliative care organisation that may be helpful for her and her family.

After the conversation, Ben continues to check in with Emily regularly, providing ongoing support and reassurance. Ben remains present and available, offering a compassionate presence as Emily navigates the challenges of her prognosis and plans for the future.

In this case, Ben, the palliative care chaplain, laments difficult news with Emily, his patient. He acknowledges the weight of the news, providing space for her to express her emotions and offering ongoing spiritual support throughout her journey. These interventions are part of a spiritual care plan, one facet of the larger palliative care plan for the patient and family.

A Case Example: Hoping for a Miracle

One particular area where a chaplain's professional assessment and skillset can significantly impact medical care and decision-making is related to the topics of hope, healing, and miracles. When a patient and/or family employ spiritual, existential, and/or religious frameworks for decision-making, chaplains can engage them in discussions about spiritual distress, interpersonal dynamics, discernment, hope, and healing [24, 25].

More specifically, when patients and families express hope for a miracle, chaplains may facilitate deeper, more nuanced conversations about how the family envisions a miracle, whether they have experienced such miracles in the past, and how medical treatments might facilitate, change, or otherwise impact the process of hoping for a miracle [9, 24, 26–28]. Additionally, integrated chaplains participate in goals of care conversations with other members of the palliative care team and other service lines [8, 9, 26]. A case example is provided here.

Marie is a 50-year-old patient with lung disease and multiple co-morbidities, including complications from recent infections. The palliative care team has been consulted to provide symptom management as her condition worsens and she grows increasingly symptomatic. Marie has a supportive family, and they share a faith practice that includes daily prayer, community support, and a belief that 'God can work miracles'.

The palliative care chaplain meets with Marie and her brother as part of the interprofessional team. They state that 'this is all in God's hands', while they appreciate the medical interventions and care, they ultimately feel that 'God will have the last word'.

The chaplain understands that Marie's faith is her primary means of coping (through prayer and Christian Scripture), understanding suffering (that suffering is part of this life and God is omnipresent), and maintaining emotional stability amidst the many ups and downs of her disease process. The chaplain visits regularly to provide spiritual discussion and prayer and to develop trust with the family. In some conversations, Marie's brother states that they want to 'do everything' to allow God to heal Marie. The chaplain explores their understanding of God and what a miracle will look like. In addition to healing, they hope that Marie's sister can travel from abroad to see her.

During their visits, the team aligns with Marie, sharing their hope for a positive outcome and acknowledging the centrality of Marie's faith and supportive family. At the same time, the team is concerned that her condition will rapidly decline. They do not believe that aggressive measures such as intubation will help Marie and instead are of the opinion that they may cause her more suffering and harm. In light of these concerns, the team holds a family meeting. The chaplain, utilising her role as a trusted palliative care team member, facilitates a discussion about the family's understanding of Marie's illness along with their goals and values. The chaplain affirms their deep faith, trust in God, and daily prayers for healing.

Marie's family expresses that they feel heard and understood. The medical providers recommend that Marie be protected from aggressive interventions that would likely not be helpful. Though her family is deeply saddened at this prospect, they emphasise that they want Marie to feel comfortable, supported, and protected from harm.

Marie's condition declined, and she was provided with maximum comfort measures. As she begins dying, the chaplain keeps a prayerful vigil with her brother and Marie's sister, who has arrived after many hours of travel to be reunited with Marie. The chaplain notes, 'I know you have been hoping for a miraculous recovery. What is it like for you right now to see that she is approaching the end of her life?' The brother responds, 'We trust God. We did our best and always kept our hearts open for God's will. We prayed and hoped. We know that God is present. Our sister made it here in time, and we are all together. We appreciate how the team understood how important our faith is'. Marie dies peacefully with her family at her side, surrounded by music and prayer.

3 Training and Education of Palliative Care Chaplains

Due to the fact that there is not one central chaplaincy organisation that sets credentialing in the United States (as with medicine, nursing, and social work), chaplaincy education continues to be driven in part by job descriptions set by institutions that employ chaplains. Yet, hundreds of chaplains are affiliated with organisations that articulate preferred training and education pathways, including those required for board certification. Palliative care chaplains begin with a general educational pathway and focus on specialisation later in training. This route includes undergraduate education in any academic major subject, plus master's (post-graduate) level study in an academic discipline such as theology or spirituality. Supervised clinical education, known widely as *clinical pastoral education* (CPE), is common and required by various chaplaincy credentialing entities. CPE may occur during the period when a person is pursuing a master's degree or after completing it. Although many chaplains are ordained, commissioned, endorsed and/or supported by their denomination or spiritual community to train and work as a chaplain, the extent to which this is tied to required education depends on the denomination and spiritual tradition.

As mentioned above, the professional training and education pathway for professional chaplains seeking a board certification (professional recognition through an organisation such as the Association of Professional Chaplains in the United States) includes 1600 hours of CPE, accomplished in four single units or a year-long residency. CPE brings prospective chaplains, as well as other interested healthcare professionals, into supervised clinical encounters with people experiencing crisis such as a serious illness [29]. CPE takes place in a variety of settings, though the majority are in health systems in the United States. The degree to which a chaplain trainee encounters palliative care depends on whether their training site happens to have this medical specialty in affiliated inpatient, outpatient, or community-based settings. Furthermore, each healthcare institution's palliative care mechanism (e.g. division, service, agency) varies widely as does the extent to which a formal relationship exists with the spiritual care providers and chaplain trainees at the institution [10].

For example, some CPE programmes offer a brief clinical rotation in palliative care, where chaplain students shadow the interprofessional team, attend rounds, visit patients, and receive didactic training about palliative care [30]. There are approximately ten CPE programmes around the world that offer extensive curriculum about palliative care over a unit or residency [31, 32]. These programmes may assign CPE interns to palliative care as their primary placement for up to 300 hours per unit, as opposed to a brief rotation. This may occur at any point in CPE training or in the form of what is known as a second-year residency or fellowship, which some chaplains complete to specialise in palliative care. Due in part to the lack of centralised credentialing, there is no universal standardised palliative care curriculum in clinical pastoral education. Some CPE programmes in the United States have established CPE palliative care curricula informed by Domain 5 of the National Consensus for Quality Hospice and Palliative Care [3]. Internationally, the International Association of Hospice and Palliative Care provides resources in this area [33]. Programmes with palliative care CPE may also shape curricula related to the competencies that need to be demonstrated for Advanced Hospice and Palliative Certification [11].

The distinction between academic and clinical education for chaplains is important to note [34]. Many non-chaplain medical providers are surprised to learn that master's degree programmes (e.g. at a seminary, Master of Divinity) contain widely varying degrees of direct education in healthcare spiritual and pastoral counselling and care. It is rare for such an academic programme to include curricula about palliative care specifically. However, there are now emerging masters level programmes in the United States geared to spiritual leaders who intend to work as a chaplain; some of these have an interfaith orientation and an emphasis on spiritual care for seriously ill people and their loved ones.

The educational pathway for palliative care chaplains depends on whether the goal is advanced certification in hospice and palliative care or simply continuing education. For the former, in the United States, there are at least three courses that are approved for chaplains to complete to achieve advanced certification. These courses provide instruction in the fundamentals of palliative care along with specific skills and competencies for chaplains. Most of the existing courses are asynchronous and online, and they include a cohort of chaplains who comment on each other's work through a learning management system.

As for continuing education, regardless of whether a chaplain is board certified, what they deem appropriate for continuing education is left to their discretion. Board certified chaplains are typically required to submit continuing education activities to their certifying body, and those with advanced Hospice/Palliative Care certification must demonstrate a certain number of hours of ongoing learning that in this particular field. This may include interprofessional training, attending palliative care conferences hosted by any discipline (for example the American Academy of Hospice and Palliative Medicine), reading palliative care related research, or attending seminars focusing on discrete palliative care skills such as advance care planning [35].

4 Leadership

Leadership opportunities for chaplains in palliative care are infinite. Each individual chaplain can forge a path to develop their own leadership skills and foster their unique creativity and talents to help shape and advance the field [36].

The bullet points below provide examples of how chaplains can develop and demonstrate leadership in palliative care:

1. Chaplains may participate in leadership development programmes that provide mentorship to chaplains as part of the palliative care programme, for example, as Cambia Health Foundation Sojourns Scholar [35], or through the Interdisciplinary Curriculum in Oncology Palliative Education (iCOPE) [36] or the Interprofessional Spiritual Care Education Curriculum (ISPEC) [37]. These programmes will often be time limited, require application/acceptance, and entail a project that chaplains must complete, while receiving guidance from interprofessional palliative care leaders.
2. Some chaplains are employed as administrative and educational leaders in palliative care teams and departments, serving as director or associate director of clinical teams or educational fellowships.
3. The past two decades have seen a surge in palliative care chaplaincy quality improvement projects and research [38]. As a result, the practice paradigm within palliative care chaplains for the seriously ill has begun to shift to incorporate quality improvement and research practices. For example, in the United States, the Palliative Care and Hospice Advanced Certification (PCHAC) chaplain certification requires chaplains to conduct a quality improvement project [11].
4. Anyone can become a policy advocate; that is, any concerned person can express their opinions and advocate for change. Many dedicated and passionate palliative care chaplains have the opportunity to take it upon themselves to be involved with policy reform. Due to the direct clinical knowledge and insights from

patient narratives, palliative care chaplains are uniquely postured to collaborate with others to identify opportunities and priorities that can improve the delivery of palliative care, particularly in global regions where access to palliative care is underdeveloped. Philosophically, as part of the interdisciplinary approach and collaborative work in palliative care, like our palliative care colleagues in nursing, social work, and medicine who contribute to this realm (Policy and Advocacy), chaplains are encouraged to contribute to this work.
5. Chaplains can serve in leadership positions with interprofessional palliative care organisations as well as chaplain-specific organisations through board and steering committee service.
6. Through advocacy and public policy work, chaplains can foster and exhibit leadership in advancing palliative care. The Palliative Care and Hospice Education and Training Act (PCHETA) [39], developed by the American Academy of Hospice and Palliative Medicine (AAHPM) [40] aims to increase access to interdisciplinary palliative care education and training, educate patients and healthcare providers about the advantages of palliative care and the resources available to support patients facing severe or terminal illnesses, and allocate funds for palliative care research to enhance clinical practice and healthcare delivery.
7. Chaplains are leaders in their denominational /religious organisations; in this role they may facilitate clergy/community education, serve as advocates related to healthcare decision-making, and provide guidance in healthcare ethics.

5 Barriers

Spiritual care in palliative care faces several challenges due to barriers across healthcare settings. For our purposes, we define barriers as events or conditions within a palliative care chaplain's environment that prohibit the advancement and progress of the professional discipline of chaplaincy. We list a selection of common barriers that international colleagues have highlighted in the literature. There are several challenges, but we anticipate three to be especially pressing for the years ahead.

1. In areas where well-developed palliative care programmes are accessible, many patients are well provided for [41]. However, in places such as rural areas or where healthcare programmes are less developed, patients are less well served and have lower access to specialist-level palliative care, including spiritual care [41].
2. The American Hospital Association estimates that the healthcare system in the United States will have significant shortages in various discipline roles, such as physicians, nurses, and allied health professionals by 2033 [42]. These shortages impact everyone, but particularly patients already in areas where healthcare is underserved.

3. Integrating palliative care chaplaincy may be challenging to identify when many healthcare professionals need help understanding the role and scope of spiritual care and/or where professional chaplaincy is not a recognised discipline [43, 44].

6 Overcoming Barriers

The barriers identified above describe the notion of barriers as a complex system. Identifying specific types of barriers is necessary to devise specific intervention strategies. Below, we offer two modest solutions.

1. Build palliative care chaplaincy's knowledge and evidence base [45]. The palliative care chaplaincy we have described above is a relatively new subspecialty within a broader profession (institutional chaplaincy) that is also changing and becoming more professional. One important next step is researching to understand better what is working or not working in palliative care chaplaincy and then using the findings to improve the quality and results in various realms.
2. Empower specialised clinical palliative chaplaincy training [31]. There are several stages of learning, including specialised training. We must consider how such training is best achieved and how existing standards of practices and competencies are integrated into training programmes. Kestenbaum and others have made an initial effort to critically assess the effectiveness of a standardised training programme for those pursuing palliative care chaplain specialisation [31]. However, this assessment is made complex by the relative lack of studies in the published literature. There is a need to determine how much-specialised training is needed for palliative care chaplains to maintain competence and promote professional practice at the highest level.

7 Conclusion

This chapter examined the role of palliative care chaplaincy in the United States, with an awareness that the global community has more to share. In describing the role, the focus has been on delivering the best palliative care chaplaincy in three realms (clinical, training and education, and leadership). As palliative care chaplaincy matures, additional research is needed to help inform these and other realms relevant to the field. Key issues facing palliative care chaplaincy must be studied with a focus on outcomes that matter most to seriously ill patients and families. We must continue to assess and define critical factors such as professionalisation, staffing, programme funding, team structure, and advocacy while keeping in mind that our patients' spiritual values and needs are a core component of quality palliative care.

References

1. Connor SR. Hospice and palliative care: the essential guide. 3rd ed. New York: Routledge; 2017.
2. Puchalski CM, et al. Improving the quality of spiritual care as a dimension of palliative care: the report of a consensus conference. J Palliat Med. 2009;12:805–903.
3. Ferrell, et al. National consensus project clinical practice guidelines for quality palliative care, 4. J Palliat Med. 2018;21(12):1684–9.
4. Balboni TA, et al. State of the science of spirituality and palliative care research part II: screening, assessment, and interventions. J Pain Symptom Manage. 2017;54(3):441–53.
5. Steinhauser KE, et al. State of the science of spirituality and palliative care research part I: definitions, measurement, and outcomes. J Pain Symptom Manag. 2017;54(3):428–40.
6. Kang K. Models for spiritual care in Hospice and palliative care. J Hosp Palliat Care. 2018;21:41–50.
7. Dahlin C, Coyne P, Goldberg J, Vaughan L, et al. Palliative care leadership. J Palliat Care. 2019;1:21–8.
8. Wirpsa J, Pugliese K, Fitchett G, Walton M. Chaplains as partners in medical decision making: case studies in healthcare chaplaincy. Wirpsa J, Pugliese K, editors. Jessica Kingsley Publishers; 2020.
9. Jeuland J, et al. Chaplains working in palliative care: who they are and what they do. J Palliat Med. 2017;20(5):502–8.
10. McCann Klug L. The Specialty Chaplain on the Palliative Care Team: A Narrative Review. Am J Hosp Pallia Med. 2023;40(9):1021–8
11. Board of Chaplaincy Certification Inc (BCCi)–Palliative Care & Hospice Advanced Certification (PCHAC). http://www.apchaplains.org/bcci-site/advanced-certification/palliative-care-hospice-advanced-certification. Accessed 14 Aug 2023.
12. Saunders C. Into the valley of the shadow of death. A personal therapeutic journey. BMJ. 1996;313:1599–601.
13. Fitchett G, Canada AL. The role of religion/spirituality in coping with cancer: evidence, assessment, and intervention. In: Holland JC, editor. Psycho-oncology. New York: Oxford University Press; 2010.
14. Best MC, et al. Australian patient preferences for the introduction of spirituality into their healthcare journey: a mixed methods study. J Relig Health. 2023;62(4):2323–40.
15. Delgado-Guay M, et al. Frequency, intensity, and correlates of spiritual pain in advanced cancer patients assessed in a supportive/palliative care clinic. Palliat Support Care. 2016;14(4):341–8.
16. Hui D, et al. The Edmonton symptom assessment system 25 years later: past, present, and future developments. J Pain Symptom Manag. 2017;53(3):630–43.
17. Fitchett G, et al. Screening for spiritual struggle. J Pastoral Care and Counsel. 2009;63(1–2):1–12.
18. Blanchard JH, et al. Screening for spiritual distress in the oncology inpatient: a quality improvement pilot project between nurses and chaplains. J Nurs Manage. 2012;20(8):1076–84.
19. King SD, et al. Screening for religious/spiritual struggle in blood and marrow transplant patients. Support Care Cancer. 2013;21(4):993–1001.
20. Shields M, et al. Spiritual AIM and the work of the chaplain: a model for assessing spiritual needs and outcomes in relationship. Palliat Support Care. 2015;13(1):75–89.
21. Lucas AM. Introduction to the discipline for pastoral care giving. J Health Care Chaplain. 2001;10(2):1–33.
22. Monod SM, et al. The spiritual distress assessment tool: an instrument to assess spiritual distress in hospitalised elderly persons. BMC Geriatr. 2010;10:88.
23. Fitchett G, et al. Development of the PC-7, a quantifiable assessment of spiritual concerns of patients receiving palliative care near the end of life. J Palliat Med. 2020;23(2):248–53.
24. Cooper RS, et al. AMEN in challenging conversations: bridging the gaps between faith, hope, and medicine. J Oncol Pract. 2014;10(4):e191–5.

25. Shinall MC, et al. Addressing a patient's hope for a miracle. J Pain Symptom Manag. 2018;55(2):535–9.
26. Lyndes KA, et al. A survey of chaplains' roles in pediatric PC: integral members of the team. J Health Care Chaplain. 2012;18:74–93.
27. Cooper RS. The palliative care chaplain as story catcher. J Pain Symptom Manag. 2018;55(1):155–8.
28. Byrne-Martelli S, et al. Communication strategies when patients utilize spiritual language to hope for a miracle #433. J Palliat Med. 2022;25(3):506–7.
29. Hover M. The role of CPE in medical education. J Pastoral Care. 1984;38(3):226–32.
30. Ronald AH, et al. Insights and experiences of chaplain interns and social work interns on palliative care teams. Death Stud. 2020;44(3):141–51.
31. Kestenbaum A, et al. Improving access to palliative care clinical pastoral education. J Health Care Chaplain. 2023;15:1–16.
32. Jackson-Jordan E, et al. Evaluation of a chaplain residency program and its partnership with an in-patient palliative care team. J Health Care Chaplain. 2018;24(1):20–9.
33. International Association for Hospice & Palliative Care (IAHPC). https://hospicecare.com/home/. Accessed 14 Aug 2023.
34. Cadge W, et al. Chaplaincy and spiritual care in the twenty-first century: an introduction. Edited Chapel Hill: The University of North Carolina Press; 2022.
35. Cambia Health Foundation Sojourns Scholar Leadership. https://www.cambiahealthfoundation.org/focus-areas/sojourns-scholar-leadership-program.html. Accessed 3 Dec 2023.
36. Head BA, et al. The interdisciplinary curriculum for oncology palliative care education (iCOPE): meeting the challenge of interprofessional education. J Palliat Med. 2014;17(10):1107–14.
37. Interprofessional Spiritual Care Education Curriculum (ISPEC). https://gwish.smhs.gwu.edu/programs/transforming-practice-health-settings/interprofessional-spiritual-care-education-curriculum-ispecc. Accessed 3 Dec 2023. Fitchett G. Recent progress in chaplaincy-related research. J Pastoral Care Counsel. 2017;71(3):163–175.
38. Spiritual Care Association (SCA) Hospice Spiritual Care Leadership: Developing A Chaplaincy and Spiritual Care Education Department. www.spiritualcareassociation.org/docs/resources/hccn_sca_hospice_spiritual_care_leadership_2021.pdf. Accessed 14 Aug 2023.
39. Palliative Care and Hospice Education and Training Act (PCHETA). https://www.nationalcoalitionhpc.org/workforce/. Accessed 2 Dec 2023.
40. American Academy of Hospice and Palliative Medicine (AAHPM). https://aahpm.org. Accessed 2 Dec 2023.
41. Clark D, et al. Mapping levels of palliative care development in 198 countries: the situation in 2017. J Pain Symptom Manag. 2020;59(4):794–807.
42. American Hospital Association (AHA) Strengthening the Health Care Workforce [Fact Sheet]. https://www.aha.org/system/files/media/file/2021/11/strengthening-the-health-care-workforce-II.pdf. Accessed 14 Aug 2023.
43. Damen A, et al. What do chaplains do: the views of palliative care physicians, nurses, and social workers. Am J Hosp Palliat Care. 2019;36(5):396–401.
44. Puchalski CM, et al. Improving the spiritual dimension of whole person care: reaching national and international consensus. J Palliat Med. 2014;17(6):642–56.
45. Nolan S, et al. Spiritual care in palliative care: working towards an EAPC task force. Eur J Palliat Care. 2011;18:86–9.

Palliative *Caring*: The Essential Role of Social Work in Spiritual Care

Shirley Otis-Green, Debra Mattison, Kerry Irish, and Lisa Capparella

Abstract Social workers are an essential part of interprofessional teams providing palliative *caring* to diverse individuals facing serious illness, mortality, and end of life. Using biopsychosocial-spiritual assessments, advocacy, and clinical counselling skills to address a range of concerns including access and barriers to care as well as commonly occurring issues related to coping, life review and meaning making, social workers provide whole person care with a focus on the person in their environment.

Keywords Social work and spirituality · Biopsychosocial-spiritual care Palliative social work · Legacy work · Dignity therapy · Meaning-centred psychotherapy · Forgiveness · Gratitude · Existential care · Life review Palliative care · Spiritual care

S. Otis-Green (✉)
Collaborative Caring, Toluca Lake, CA, USA
e-mail: Shirley@CollaborativeCaring.Net

D. Mattison
School of Social Work, University of Michigan, Ann Arbor, MI, USA
e-mail: debmatt@umich.edu

K. Irish
Dempsey Centers for Quality Cancer Care, Lewiston, ME, USA
e-mail: kirish@dempseycenter.org

L. Capparella
Cancer Support and Welcome Center, Sidney Kimmel Cancer Center, Thomas Jefferson University, Philadelphia, PA, USA
e-mail: lisa.capparella@jefferson.edu

M. C. Best (ed.), *Spiritual Care in Palliative Care*,
https://doi.org/10.1007/978-3-031-50864-6_33

1 The Essential Role of Social Work: History and Values

Historically, care of the ill has been motivated primarily by religious and spiritual values for both providers and institutions [1]. Depending upon the culture and time period, 'wise women', shamans, and priests were typically the tenders of the sick, offering companionship, comfort, and ritualised support to their neighbours who either recovered, or quickly succumbed to their illness or injury. With the advances in science and medicine in the nineteenth century coupled with Descartes' arguments for the separation of body and spirit, the pendulum swung towards the medicalisation of healthcare. Illnesses were no longer ascribed to punishments from God, and prayers gave way to medical interventions performed by trained physicians. Further, as the 'business' of healthcare morphed from the earlier charity models of care into more formal profit-driven enterprises, healthcare became increasingly fragmented, hierarchical, and ever more specialised.

The modern hospice movement was an attempt to move the pendulum back towards a more individualised, 'whole person' perspective. Dame Cicely Saunders, a deeply religious woman, was dismayed by the suffering she witnessed patients experiencing at end of life. Integrating her background as a nurse, social worker, and physician, Dame Saunders founded St. Christopher's Hospice in Great Britain to transform the care of the dying [2]. She conceptualised the need to address a patient's 'total pain' using a collaborative team approach to better address the multidimensional aspects of suffering commonly experienced at end of life [3]. The United States of America's *National Consensus Project Guidelines for Quality Palliative Care* [4] identifies the core team for palliative care as physicians, nurses, social workers, and chaplains (supplemented with pharmacists, rehabilitation professionals, and others as appropriate) with the expertise needed to attend to the physical, psychological, social, and spiritual concerns impacting patient and family quality of life.

The field of social work followed a similar historical trajectory, with early social workers, (often religious women of means), motivated by a desire to serve the poor and marginalised. As social work became more 'academic', it too, moved away from its 'friendly visitor' roots to become more bureaucratic and less religiously focused. Concerns regarding proselytisation and a lack of formal spiritual training in social work's curriculum left many social workers uncomfortable addressing spirituality, turning instead to chaplains to provide spiritual care [5]. Unfortunately, this lack of confidence by many social workers left spiritual concerns often siloed and 'optional' rather than integrated into care as an essential aspect of a person's quality of life.

More recently, health social workers have returned to focusing more attention to, and a better integration of, people's spiritual concerns into their practice. Core social work values, including respect for each individual and a commitment to social justice, provide a solid foundation for spiritually sensitive social work practice [6]. Concern about the social drivers of health inequities and the need to provide contextualised care are motivated from the core belief in the inherent value of each person. Another shared perspective between social work and spiritual care is a focus on relationships [7]. Being fully 'present' as a 'companion' to those facing a serious illness is both a spiritual and social work principle. Social work, by definition, seeks social change—holding forth the belief that transformation in the person, organisation, community or world is possible [8]. This perspective is also an essential element in spiritual care [9] and sustains hope [10]. From this vantage point, social work can be seen as a discipline well poised to provide compassionate spiritual care [11].

Recognising the importance of spirituality in people's quality of life, [9, 12, 13] as well as the challenges that providers faced regarding this, leaders in palliative care came together to develop a consensus definition of spiritual care that could be understood by clinicians of diverse disciplines and faith traditions [14]. Although this definition has been adopted by many, and modified over time, the key elements remain:

> Spirituality is the dynamic dimension of human life that relates to the way persons (individual and community) experience, express and/or seek meaning, purpose, and transcendence, and the way they connect to the moment, to self, to others, to nature, to the significant and/or the sacred. [15, p. 88]

This individualised focus on a person's sense of meaning and purpose is consistent with the comprehensive biopsychosocial-spiritual assessment that palliative social workers perform in their development of contextualised care plans. This chapter offers context and guidance regarding the important role of social work as partners in the proactive provision of existential and spiritual care [16] with examples of evidence-informed interventions social workers may provide to enhance well-being and improve outcomes [17].

2 Integration of Spirituality in Social Work Practice

Comprehensive biopsychosocial-spiritual assessments are a bedrock of social work practice, providing a foundation for deeply seeing and attending to the whole person: body, mind, and spirit. Spirituality is an area of critical value in knowing who our patients and their families are, how they see the world, what it means to them to be sick or well and in exploring options for coping with life experiences. Spirituality is an integral part of palliative care [18, 19] and has been associated with increased quality of life for both patients and their families [20, 21]. Best and colleagues [22] reviewed empirical studies demonstrating benefits from addressing spiritual needs which included enhancement of therapeutic relationships with patients, and with patients feeling valued and affirmed by providers, all of which enhanced the ability to cope, improved meaning-making, increased satisfaction with care, and a reduction of healthcare costs.

Many people express a preference for care providers to initiate asking about their spirituality rather than expecting them to bring it up [23–25]. At the same time, some people voice fears that their providers will be uninterested, unreceptive to, or will pathologise their spiritual beliefs and experiences, which often leads them to avoid initiating these conversations themselves [26, 27].

Barriers remain to the consistent assessment of spirituality in social work practice [28]. A review of the most frequently cited barriers to engaging in spiritual discussions were *practitioner-related* barriers (e.g. lack of training or provider, discomfort, and perception that spirituality is not relevant) rather than *client-* or *agency-related* barriers [29]. Social work core values affirm that critical self-reflection and cultural humility are an expectation of social work practice. Introspection about one's own religious and spiritual beliefs, attitudes, and experiences is essential to ethical, competent practice when interacting with and responding to people while attending to their spiritual needs [30]. Acknowledging and avoiding both the potential *to impose one's spiritual and/or religious beliefs* on clients, as well as the corollary potential of *imposing one's avoidance*, neglect, or discounting of religion and spirituality, is essential to effective practice.

3 Social Workers as Providers of Spiritual Care

Effectively assessing and addressing spiritual needs of patients receiving palliative care cannot be simply relegated to one profession. Interprofessional practice affirms that people are best served by healthcare teams collaborating across the care-delivery spectrum [31, 32] to address core palliative care concerns in which multiple interprofessional team members are required to effectively meet clients' needs holistically. Quality interprofessional practice involves team members collaborating and contributing together based on their unique professional skills and training. These interventions may range from attentive listening for a patient's spiritual strengths, to referring to another team member for further assessment or intervention. Collaborative teamwork has also been shown to be beneficial to team members by fostering a feeling of work-related empowerment and that their work is meaningful [33]. It can also create opportunities for palliative care team staff to both increase their skills in responding to patient spiritual needs while also exploring their own personal spirituality, which may reduce professional burnout and moral distress [22].

4 Spiritual Distress and Existential Questions

Social workers working in hospitals, hospices, cancer centres, mental health settings, senior centres and in other diverse settings serve people who have the lived-experience of serious and/or chronic illness and will ultimately be confronted with the awareness of what Coyle [34, p. 520] calls the 'existential slap', in which one is faced with the reality of dying, often accompanied by multiple fears, questions, memories, and meaning making opportunities [35–38]. It is in these meaningful moments that social workers can use their extensive training in human relationships, transitions, and loss, to offer counselling. Skilled social workers enhance coping, and provide comfort, care, and compassionate, evidence-informed interventions.

The following sections provide practical application and clinical examples in four areas which often arise in the context of palliative care and end of life: forgiveness, gratitude, meaning making, and legacy. These examples demonstrate the vital role social work can have in addressing spiritual concerns with patients and their families.

5 Practical Applications

5.1 Forgiveness

At 73, five years after being diagnosed with stage IV ovarian cancer, Caroline's life was nearing its end. In many ways, Caroline was meeting the goals she had set early on in her counselling: to find meaning in, and gratitude for, each day; to freely express love towards the people in her life; and to continue to grow and deepen as a human being. During a counselling session with her social worker, Caroline shared, "The thing that disrupts my peace the most is that I haven't been able to forgive my mother." Caroline's mother had been severely abusive throughout her childhood and into her early adult years. Caroline had been through years of therapy to help heal the wounds of childhood trauma and had worked diligently to "live a life focused on love," an affirmation that she used daily. However, memories of her mother (who had died when Caroline was in her 30 s, and who had never apologised) elicited intense aversion. During counselling, Caroline's goals focused on forgiving her mother, exploring what forgiveness was and wasn't, and how she might proceed with "forgiveness work" over the coming weeks.

Supporting clients who are working on forgiveness can be a delicate, challenging, rich, and meaningful process, and there is abundant evidence for the positive impact of forgiveness on various health measures [39], and particularly on quality of life [40]. A meta-analysis of 103 independent samples consisting of 606 correlations with a total sample of 26,043 participants, including diverse samples and papers from 17 countries demonstrated a reliable overall association between forgiveness and both physical and psychological health outcomes. Measurements for physical health included blood pressure, cortisol levels, and bodily pain, and psychological health outcomes included depression, anxiety, and post-traumatic stress disorder. The association was stronger for psychological health than for physical health, though associations with cardiovascular health indicators (i.e. heart rate and blood pressure) were also robust [39].

When undertaking forgiveness work with clients, it is helpful to first clarify what forgiveness is and is not. Concepts drawn from Casarjian (2010) [41] are summarised here:

- *Forgiveness is not condoning negative, hurtful, abusive or inappropriate behaviour—one's own or anyone else's.*
- *Forgiveness is not pretending everything is just fine when it isn't.*
- *Forgiveness does not mandate communication directly with the person one has forgiven.*
- *Forgiveness is a decision to set oneself free*—to release holding on to resentment. It's a decision to open oneself to see the other person with deeper insight, beyond the limits of another person's personality, fears, and mistakes.
- *Forgiveness is a process.* It is rarely a 'one and done' type of event, especially when the hurt is deep.
- *Forgiveness is a way of life.* Casarjian [41, p. 25] elaborates: '*As a way of life, forgiveness involves a commitment to experiencing each moment uncluttered by past perceptions—seeing each moment freshly, clearly, and without fear. It is the fading away of the perceptions that cloud our ability to love*'.

While it is beyond the scope of this chapter to delve deeply into the methodology of addressing and facilitating forgiveness work with patients, both palliative social workers and chaplains are frequently called to do so. Serious illness, much like other major life experiences, often serves as a catalyst for healing in relationships, including with oneself, and healing relationships usually calls for forgiveness. Palliative care clinicians are well advised to read the literature and seek additional training to support those seeking to forgive themselves or others.

For Caroline, she was ready and able to release some of the long-held resentment she had carried for years towards her abusive mother. As a 'homework' exercise, she was invited to find two images, one that represented how she felt before she approached this work, and another that represented how she felt after. For the 'before' image, she presented a picture of a caged bird. For the 'after', she presented an image of a child who was smiling widely, riding a bicycle with no hands, as she uttered the word: 'Freedom'.

5.2 Gratitude

Over the past two decades, there has been increasing research regarding the effects of gratitude on well-being in both people facing health challenges as well as in the general population. This research demonstrates that gratitude is beneficial in improving physical, psychological, and relational well-being [42]. Specifically, gratitude interventions help reduce death anxiety, fear of cancer recurrence, and distress, [43, 44] while also enhancing resilience, higher psychological functioning, greater social support, life satisfaction, and post-traumatic growth, as well as overall well-being. [43–47] There is also an emerging body of research on the benefits of gratitude for the well-being of healthcare workers, and specifically those who work in palliative care, in mitigating the effects of stress and empathic distress [48].

While there are several well-researched gratitude interventions, the 'gratitude letter' is one that has demonstrated substantial impact [49]. While the impact of this intervention may be profound, the activity is a relatively simple one, and can be summarised by the following three steps [47, 50].

1. *Select an important person who has made a positive impact on your life, whether in the short- or long-term, towards whom you have never fully expressed your thanks.*
2. *Write that person a letter describing how you feel about what they have done for you and why you are grateful to them. The letter should be specific, concrete, and should mention how often you remember what they did.*
3. *While this may not always be an option, or at times may not be the right thing to do (for example, if safety is a concern), plan a visit with the recipient (either virtually or in person). Let them know you'd like to see them and that you have something special to share, but don't reveal the exact purpose of the meeting. The reason for this is that they may feel compelled to do the same for you, and then that changes the nature of the experience for both of you! When you meet, let the person know that you are grateful to them and would like to read a letter expressing your gratitude; ask that they refrain from interrupting until you've finished. Take your time reading the letter. While you read, pay attention to their reaction as well as your own. After you have read the letter, be receptive to the recipient's reaction and discuss your feelings together. Remember to give (or mail) the letter to the person when you leave.*

Research has shown that this act is correlated with a significant boost in positive emotions, lasting up to two months after doing a gratitude visit. Evidence suggests that while there are benefits simply to writing the letter, one reaps significantly greater benefits from delivering and reading it in person. A study involving 577 adult participants (42% male and 58% female) measured the impact of five different positive psychology interventions. Participants who completed the gratitude visit demonstrated the largest positive changes in the entire study, with a boost in happiness and decrease in depressive symptoms maintained at follow up assessments at one week and one month post-intervention. However, by three months, the participants who had completed the gratitude visit had returned to their baseline levels of happiness and depression [49]. In part, this is why it is suggested that the gratitude letter exercise be completed every six weeks, choosing a different person each time.

5.3 Legacy Work: Exploring Meaning and Purpose

In palliative care, the significance of legacy and meaning-centred work extends beyond medical treatments. Serious illness often acts as a catalyst for introspection, propelling individuals to seek solace, connection, and purpose amid uncertainty

[51]. Therapies like life review, dignity work, and meaning-centred psychotherapy aim to alleviate existential distress in patients facing serious illness [52].

Viktor Frankl's [53] ground-breaking work in *Man's Search for Meaning* laid the foundation for later therapeutic approaches such as life review therapy, dignity therapy, and meaning-centred psychotherapy. Life review therapy, a concise psychotherapeutic method, shares a common goal with dignity therapy in terms of enhancing feelings of meaning, purpose, and embracing one's life journey through a systematic review of significant life events and narratives [54]. Dignity therapy has emerged as a psychotherapeutic intervention backed by growing evidence of its effectiveness and acceptance, aiming to bolster the sense of meaning, purpose, and dignity among individuals as they approach the end of their lives, often achieved through the creation of a lasting legacy document. The short-term life review interview has demonstrated its effectiveness in enhancing spiritual well-being, reducing anxiety and depression, and promoting a sense of meaning in terminally ill patients. Further, it exhibits a similar level of feasibility as dignity therapy with lower withdrawal rates, and it may have higher efficacy in alleviating psycho-existential suffering [55]. In the early 2000s, building on Frankl's work, psychiatrist William Breitbart and his research team pioneered a care strategy known as meaning-centred psychotherapy which focuses on pain, symptom control and palliative care of cancer patients [56]. This approach combines psychological and spiritual elements with the goal of diminishing despair, demoralisation, hopelessness, and the desire for a hastened death. In a study of 253 individuals diagnosed with advanced cancer, meaning-centred group psychotherapy (MCGP) outperformed supportive group psychotherapy over eight sessions. MCGP led to better spiritual well-being, quality of life, and reduced depression, hopelessness, and physical symptoms, indicating a more positive overall impact [57].

By incorporating these therapeutic approaches into their practice, social workers can play a pivotal role in helping patients facing advanced illness rediscover a sense of purpose and fulfilment. With a strong foundation in empathy, active listening, and fostering open communication, social workers are uniquely positioned to engage sensitively with individuals facing a serious illness. Additionally, they often have expertise in addressing emotional and psychological needs, as well as the ability to navigate sensitive or charged topics.

Monique, a 53-year-old black woman, diagnosed with stage IV pancreatic cancer and triple-negative breast cancer, expressed a strong desire to produce a legacy video for her family. This took on greater urgency upon hearing from her doctor that her cancer had progressed and learning that her time was limited. When asked about what she wanted people to remember most about her, she conveyed:

> I hope they remember my constant presence and the legacy I leave—that my friends and family recognise my compassionate nature, my consistent pursuit of fairness, and my commitment to following God's path. I feel a sense of contentment, knowing that even after I'm gone, people will think positively about me. They'll recall me with warmth, knowing I prayed for them and offered assistance whenever possible.

Monique further reflected on the impact of cancer on her life and priorities, stating:

> In one aspect, cancer amplified my appreciation for life's value. It broadened my perspective, revealing the vast possibilities life holds. I've moved beyond self-pity and questioning 'why me.' I simply wish for a natural passing, to return home in a peaceful manner. I no longer desire further medical procedures; my ultimate wish is to find tranquillity.

Many patients facing an uncertain future and/or end of life express relief and gratitude for the opportunity to delve into topics for which other disciplines in healthcare have not been able to make space for exploring and expressing [58]. Legacy-related discussions may result in increased tranquillity and comfort and many report a decrease in feelings of depression and existential distress as a result [59]. Table 1 provides sample questions related to dignity therapy and meaning-centred approaches to incorporate into clinical practice. Dignity therapy and meaning-centred psychotherapy are manualised therapies with specific methodologies and questioning techniques. The sample questions in the chart below are adapted from these approaches.

Table 1 Sample Questions Adapted From Dignity Therapy and Meaning-Centered Therapy Approaches

Adapted Dignity Therapy Questions [60, p. 62] • *Tell me a little about your life history, particularly the parts that you either remember most or think are the most important. When did you feel most alive?* • *Are there specific things that you would want your family to know about you, and are there particular things you would want them to remember?* • *What are the most important roles you have played in life (family roles, vocational roles, community service roles,* etc.*)? Why were they so important to you, and what do you think you accomplished in those roles?* • *What are your most important accomplishments, and what do you feel most proud of?* • *Are there particular things that you feel still need to be said to your loved ones, or things that you would want to take the time to say once again?* • *What are your hopes and dreams for your loved ones?* • *What have you learned about life that you would want to pass along to others?* • *What advice or words of guidance would you wish to pass along to your (son, daughter, husband, wife, parents, others)?*
Adapted Meaning Centred Psychotherapy Questions [61, pp. 65–75] • *List one or two experiences or moments when life has felt particularly meaningful to you, whether it sounds powerful or mundane.* • *When you look back on your life, upbringing, and family history, what are the most significant memories, relationships, traditions, values,* etc.*, which have made the greatest impact on who you are today?* • *As you reflect upon who you are today, what are the meaningful activities, roles, or accomplishments that you are most proud of?* • *As you look toward the future, what are some of the life lessons you have learned along the way and values that you would want to pass on to others?* • *What is the legacy you hope to live and give?* • *What would you consider a 'good' or 'meaningful' death? How can you imagine being remembered by your loved ones?*

Empowering social workers to utilise sample prompts such as these to initiate these crucial conversations that engage the whole person including their spirituality can facilitate immense solace while creating profound meaning for the patients and families who are facing serious illness as well as for the social workers who are providing this comprehensive care [62].

6 Conclusion

Corpuz [18, p. 1] eloquently affirms that '*The integration of spirituality in palliative care is not only an essential component of comprehensive healthcare but is a reflection of our shared humanity and compassion towards those in need*'. Spiritual care is whole person care. Many say it is the 'heart of care' as it transcends what is happening to the body. Creating 'space' for the spirit (by whatever name one may call it) to seek meaning, comfort, connection, and peace is the essence of palliative *caring*.

In collaborative team practice with other skilled team members, social workers contribute their specialised skills of biopsychosocial-spiritual assessment with a unique multi-dimensional value-based framework that is focused on the inherent dignity of each individual, celebrating cultural diversity, cultivating social justice and recognising the 'person-in-environment'. Social workers bring clinical and mental health competencies to assess, advocate, counsel, and intervene to remove barriers in how care is both accessed and delivered and to assist with adapting to changing goals, options, and final end-of-life transitions. The compassionate provision of team-based spiritual care impacts not only how people die, but how they *live* until they die.

References

1. Puchalski C, Ferrell B. Making health care whole: integrating spirituality into patient care. West Conshohocken: Templeton Press; 2010.
2. Clark D. Cicely Saunders: a life and legacy. New York: Oxford University Press; 2018.
3. Otis-Green S. Cicely Saunders. In: Mizrahi T, Davis L, editors. Encyclopedia of social work, vol. 4. 20th ed. New York: Oxford University Press; 2008. p. 374–5.
4. National Consensus Project for Quality Palliative Care. Clinical practice guidelines for quality palliative care. 4th ed. Richmond: National Coalition for Hospice and Palliative Care; 2018. https://www.nationalcoalitionhpc.org/ncp. Accessed 27 Aug 2023.
5. Koenig HG. Spirituality in patient care: why, how, when, and what. 2nd ed. West Conshohocken: Templeton Foundation Press; 2007.
6. Holloway M. Social work. In: Cobb M, Puchalski CM, Rumbold B, editors. Oxford textbook of spirituality in healthcare. New York: Oxford University Press; 2012. p. 235–41.
7. Callahan AM. Spirituality and hospice social work. New York: Columbia University Press; 2017.
8. Altilio T, Otis-Green S, Cagle JG, editors. Oxford textbook of palliative social work. 2nd ed. New York: Oxford University Press; 2022. https://doi.org/10.1093/

med/9780197537855.001.0001, ISBN: 9780197537855 The Oxford Textbook of Palliative Social Work (Second Edition)
9. Singh KD. The grace in dying: a message of hope, comfort and spiritual transformation. San Francisco: Harper Collins Publishers; 1998.
10. Atlas M, Hart TL. Appraisals of cancer, religious/spiritual coping, and hope in patients with colorectal cancer. J Psychosoc Oncol. 2023;41(3):337–54.
11. Kellehear A. Spirituality and palliative care: a model of needs. Palliat Med. 2000;14:149–55.
12. Puchalski C. Spirituality in the cancer trajectory. Ann Oncol. 2012;23(3):iii49–55.
13. Balboni TA, VanderWeele TJ, Doan-Soares SD, Long KNG, Ferrell BR, Fitchett G, Koenig HG, Bain PA, Puchalski C, Steinhauser KE, Sulmasy DP, Koh HK. Spirituality in serious illness and health. JAMA J Am Med Assoc. 2022;328(2):184–97.
14. Puchalski C, Ferrell B, Virani R, Otis-Green S, Baird P, Bull J, Chochinov H, Handzo G, Nelson-Becker H, Prince-Paul M, Pugliese K, Sulmasy D. Improving the quality of spiritual care as a dimension of palliative care: the report of the consensus conference. J Palliat Med. 2009;12(10):885–905. https://doi.org/10.1089/jpm.2009.0142. PMID: 19807235.
15. Nolan S, Saltmarsh P, Leget C. Spiritual care in palliative care: working towards an EAPC task force. Eur J Palliat Care. 2011;18:86–9.
16. Otis-Green S. The transitions program: existential care in action. J Cancer Educ. 2006;21(1):23–5.
17. Schultz M, Baziliansky S, Mitnik I, Ulitzur N, Illouz S, Katra D, Givoli S, Campisi-Pinto S, Bar-Sela G, Zalman D. Associations between psycho-social-spiritual interventions, fewer aggressive end-of-life measures, and increased time after final oncologic treatment. Oncologist. 2023;28:e287–94.
18. Corpuz JCG. Integrating spirituality in the context of palliative and supportive care: the care for the whole person. Palliat Support Care. 2023;22:1–2.
19. Mesquita AC, Chaves ÉDCL, Barros GA. Spiritual needs of patients with cancer in palliative care: an integrative review. Curr Opin Support Palliat Care. 2017;11(4):334–40.
20. World Health Organization. Palliative care. 2020. Available online: https://www.who.int/news-room/fact-sheets/detail/palliative-care. Accessed on 10 July 2023.
21. O'Callaghan C, Seah D, Clayton JM, Welz M, Kissane D, Georgousopoulou EN, Michael N. Palliative caregivers' spirituality, views about spiritual care, and associations with spiritual well-being: a mixed methods study. Am J Hosp Palliat Med. 2020;37(4):305–13.
22. Best M, Vivat B, Gijsberts MJ. Spiritual care in palliative care. Religions. 2023;14(3):320.
23. Gomi S, Starnino V, Canda E. Spiritual assessment in mental health recovery. Community Ment Health J. 2014;50:447–53.
24. Harris KA, Randolph B, Gordon T. What do clients want? Assessing spiritual needs in counseling: a literature review. Spiritual Clin Pract. 2016;3(4):250–75.
25. Best M, McArdle M, Yi J, Josephine Clayton J, Butow P. How and how much is spirituality discussed in palliative care consultations for advanced cancer patients with and without a question prompt list? Patient Educ Couns. 2019;102:2208–13.
26. Gotterer R. The spiritual dimension in clinical social work practice: a client perspective. Fam Soc. 2001;82(20):187–93.
27. Furman LD, Perry D, Goldale T. Interaction of evangelical Christians and social workers in the rural environment. Hum Serv Rural Environ. 1996;19:5–8.
28. Oxhandler HK, Parrish DE, Torres LR, Achenbaum WA. The integration of clients' religion and spirituality in social work practice: a national survey. Soc Work. 2015;60(3):228–37. https://doi.org/10.1093/sw/swv018.
29. Oxhandler HK, Giardina TD. Social worker's perceived barriers to and sources of support for integrating clients' religion and spirituality in practice. Soc Work. 2017;62(4):323–32. https://doi.org/10.1093/sw/swx036.
30. Canda E, Furman L, Canda H. Spiritual diversity in social work practice: the heart of helping. New York: Oxford University Press; 2019.

31. Morgan S, Pullon S, McKinlay E. Observation of interprofessional collaborative practice in primary care teams: an integrative literature review. Int J Nurs Stud. 2015;52(7):1217–30. https://doi.org/10.1016/j.ijnurstu.2015.03.008.
32. Schot E, Tummers L, Noordegraaf M. Working on working together: a systematic review on how healthcare professionals contribute to interprofessional collaboration. J Interprof Care. 2020;34(3):332–42. https://doi.org/10.1080/13561820.2019.1636007.
33. Siekkinen M, Kuokkanen L, Kuusisto H, Leino-Kilpi H, Rautava P, Rekunen M, Seppänen L, Stolt M, Walta L, Sulosaari V. Work empowerment among cancer care professionals: a cross-sectional study. BMC Health Serv Res. 2021;21(1):1–11. https://doi.org/10.1186/s12913-021-06528-8.
34. Coyle N. The existential slap—a crisis of disclosure. Int J Palliat Nurs. 2004;10:520.
35. Egan R, MacLeod R, Jaye C, McGee R, Baxter J, Herbison P, Wood S. Spiritual beliefs, practices, and needs at the end of life: results from a New Zealand national hospice study. Palliat Support Care. 2017;15:223–30.
36. Kellehear A. Spiritual care in palliative care: whose job is it? In: Rumbold B, editor. Spirituality and palliative care: social and pastoral perspectives. New York: Oxford University Press; 2002. p. 166–77.
37. Puchalski C. Spirituality and end-of-life care: a time for listening and caring. J Palliat Med. 2002;5(2):289–94.
38. Breitbart W, Gibson C, Poppito SR, Berg A. Psychotherapeutic interventions at the end of life: a focus on meaning and spirituality. Can J Psychiatry. 2004;49(6):366–72.
39. Rasmussen KR, Stackhouse M, Boon SD, Comstock K, Ross R. Meta-analytic connections between forgiveness and health: the moderating effects of forgiveness-related distinctions. Psychol Health. 2019;34(5):515–34.
40. Kim J, Hulett J, Heiney S. Forgiveness and health outcomes in cancer survivorship: a scoping review. Cancer Nurs. 2021;44(4):E181–E192, 7/8. https://doi.org/10.1097/NCC.0000000000000809.
41. Casarjian R. Forgiveness: a bold choice for a peaceful heart. London: Bantam; 2010.
42. Emmons RA, Froh J, Rose R. Gratitude. In: Gallagher MW, Lopez SJ, editors. Positive psychological assessment: a handbook of models and measures. American Psychological Association; 2019. p. 317–32. https://doi.org/10.1037/0000138-020.
43. Otto AK, Szczesny EC, Soriano EC, Laurenceau J-P, Siegel SD. Effects of a randomized gratitude intervention on death-related fear of recurrence in breast cancer survivors. Health Psychol. 2016;35(12):1320–8. https://doi.org/10.1037/hea0000400.
44. Ruini C, Vescovelli F. The role of gratitude in breast cancer: its relationship with post-traumatic growth, psychological well-being and distress. J Happiness Stud. 2013;14:263–74. https://doi.org/10.1007/s10902-012-9330-x.
45. Cerezo MV, Ortiz-Tallo M, Cardenal V, de la Toree-Luque A. Positive psychology group intervention for breast cancer patients: a randomized trial. Psychol Rep. 2014;115(1):44–64. https://doi.org/10.2466/15.20.PR0.115c17z7.
46. Sztachańska J, Krejtz I, Nezlek J. Using a gratitude intervention to improve the lives of women with breast cancer: a daily diary study. Front Psychol. 2019;10:1365. https://doi.org/10.3389/fpsyg.2019.01365.
47. Niemiec RM. Character strengths interventions: a field guide for practitioners. Boston: Hogrefe; 2018.
48. Cheng S, Tsui PK, Lam JM. Improving mental health in health care practitioners: randomized controlled trial of a gratitude intervention. J Consult Clin Psychol. 2015;83:177–86. https://doi.org/10.1037/a0037895.
49. Seligman MEP, Steen TA, Park N, Peterson C. Positive psychology progress: empirical validation of interventions. Am Psychol. 2005;60:410–21.
50. Seligman M. Flourish: a new understanding of happiness and well-being and how to achieve them. London: Nicholas Brealey Publishing; 2011.

51. Connolly M, Timmins F. Spiritual care for individuals with cancer: the importance of life review as a tool for promoting spiritual well-being. Semin Oncol Nurs. 2021;37(5):151209. https://doi.org/10.1016/j.soncn.2021.151209.
52. Keall RM, Clayton JM, Butow PN. Therapeutic life review in palliative care: a systematic review of quantitative evaluations. J Pain Symptom Manag. 2015;49(4):747–61. https://doi.org/10.1016/j.jpainsymman.2014.08.015.
53. Frankl V. Man's search for meaning: an introduction to logotherapy. Boston: Beacon Press; 1992.
54. Vuksanovic D, Green H, Morrissey S, Smith S. Dignity therapy and life review for palliative care patients: a qualitative study. J Pain Symptom Manag. 2017;54(4):530–537.e1. https://doi.org/10.1016/j.jpainsymman.2017.07.016.
55. Ando M, Morita T, Akechi T, Okamoto T, et al. Japanese task force for spiritual care: efficacy of short-term life-review interviews on the spiritual well-being of terminally ill cancer patients. J Pain Symptom Manag. 2010;39:993–1002.
56. Breitbart W, Rosenfeld B, Gibson C, Pessin H, Poppito S, Nelson C, Tomarken A, Timm AK, Berg A, Jacobson C, Sorger B, Abbey J, Olden M. Meaning-centered group psychotherapy for patients with advanced cancer: a pilot randomized controlled trial. Psycho-Oncology. 2010;19(1):21–8. https://doi.org/10.1002/pon.1556. PMID: 19274623; PMCID: PMC3648880.
57. Breitbart W, Rosenfeld B, Pessin H, Applebaum A, Kulikowski J, Lichtenthal WG. Meaning-centered group psychotherapy: an effective intervention for improving psychological well-being in patients with advanced cancer. J Clin Oncol. 2015;33(7):749–54. https://doi.org/10.1200/JCO.2014.57.2198. PMID: 25646186; PMCID: PMC4334778.
58. Collins A. "It's very humbling": the effect experienced by those who facilitate a legacy project session within palliative care. Am J Hosp Palliat Med. 2019;36(1):65–71. https://doi.org/10.1177/1049909118787772.
59. Allen RS, Hilgeman MM, Ege MA, Shuster JL Jr, Burgio LD. Legacy activities as interventions approaching the end of life. J Palliat Med. 2008;7:1029–38.
60. Chochinov HM. Dignity therapy: final words for final days. New York: Oxford University Press; 2012.
61. Breitbart W, Poppito SR. Meaning centered psychotherapy for patients with advanced cancer. New York: Oxford University Press; 2014.
62. Buonaccorso L, Tanzi S, De Panfilis L, et al. Meanings emerging from dignity therapy among cancer patients. J Pain Symptom Manag. 2021;62(4):730–7. https://doi.org/10.1016/j.jpainsymman.2021.02.028.

Part VII
Special Groups

Spiritual Care in Neonatal Palliative Care

Victoria J. Kain and Christina Prinds

Abstract Neonatal palliative care is an essential component of healthcare services aimed at supporting infants with life-limiting conditions and their families. While physical and emotional aspects of care receive significant attention, the spiritual well-being of neonates and their families is often overlooked. The chapter is based on research highlighting how the end of life is strongly connected to parenthood transition and the beginning of life in neonatal palliative care. We discuss the role of spiritual care in neonatal palliative care, highlighting its significance, challenges, and potential approaches. By exploring the interplay between spirituality, neonatal palliative care, and ethical considerations, this chapter emphasises the importance of a holistic approach to care, acknowledging the spiritual needs of infants and their families during this vulnerable and sensitive period.

Keywords Palliative care · Neonatal · Spirituality · Infant newborn · Bereavement
Spiritual care

V. J. Kain (✉)
School of Nursing and Midwifery, Griffith University, Brisbane, QLD, Australia
e-mail: v.kain@griffith.edu.au

C. Prinds
Faculty of Health Sciences, University of Southern Denmark, Odense, Denmark

Department of Women's Health, University Hospital of Southern Denmark,
Aabenraa, Denmark
e-mail: cprinds@health.sdu.dk

M. C. Best (ed.), *Spiritual Care in Palliative Care*,
https://doi.org/10.1007/978-3-031-50864-6_34

1 Introduction

The complexities of defining and implementing spiritual care in neonatal palliative care cannot be underestimated. Unlike adult patients, neonates are unable to express their spiritual needs verbally, placing a greater responsibility on parents to discern and address these needs [1]. Moreover, their parents are also within the scope of care in a Neonatal Intensive Care Unit, and thus, the 'traditional' border between patient and relative is more unclear, compared to other areas of healthcare where the patient and relative are more clearly defined. Additionally, parents and healthcare providers may have differing interpretations and expectations of spiritual care, which can lead to misunderstandings and potential gaps in care provision [2]. Overcoming these challenges requires a clear understanding of the unique spiritual dimensions present in neonatal palliative care and how to foster effective communication between healthcare providers and parents [1].

Existing literature highlights the importance of addressing the physical, personal, and social needs of palliative care patients in adult contexts, with spiritual reflection becoming increasingly significant as individuals approach the end-of-life stage. However, understanding and delivering spiritual care in neonatal palliative care proves to be more complex due to differing interpretations and expectations of spiritual care among parents and healthcare professionals. This could be due to the fact that spiritual care encompasses the attentive consideration of patients' values and beliefs, necessitating proficient skills, and is fostered within a relationship between healthcare professionals and patients built upon trust and confidence [3]. The complexity of providing spiritual care in neonatal palliative care is heightened because neonates cannot speak for themselves. For neonates, who are unable to express their needs or beliefs, healthcare professionals must rely on their skills and intuition to interpret non-verbal cues and work closely with the families to understand the newborn's needs. The inability of neonates to communicate directly adds a layer of complexity, making the provision of spiritual care in this context both challenging and uniquely delicate. Therefore, this chapter emphasises the need to elucidate the concept of spirituality within neonatal palliative care to enhance effective communication, practice, education, and future research.

This chapter will explain spiritual care in the context of neonatal palliative care, aiming to foster effective communication, improve practice, advance education, and facilitate research efforts in this particularly vulnerable patient population.

2 The Transition to Parenthood in Neonatal Palliative Care

2.1 Spiritual Aspects of Parenthood Transition

Childbirth, a universally significant life event for parents, is characterised by a complex mix of emotions and experiences. While it is often associated with joy and relief, it can also bring about fear, loss of control, and feelings of vulnerability. Cultural, historical, and biological factors influence how childbirth and the transition to parenthood are understood and facilitated. From a spiritual perspective, individuals are tasked with exploring the meaning of their lives within their unique historical, cultural, and biological contexts. The transition to parenthood can elicit a range of paradoxical and complex emotions and experiences [4], which can be better understood by acknowledging existential and spiritual concerns related to life's vulnerability and the creation of meaning.

The experience of childbirth is sometimes described as a profoundly transcendent moment, where individuals feel a sense of connection to something greater than themselves [5]. It can be a transformative event that can evoke a sense of awe, wonder, and spiritual significance. The act of bringing new life into the world is, for some parents, seen as a sacred and even mysterious process that surpasses the boundaries of ordinary existence. In this context, the concept of birth transcending time or self suggests that during childbirth, individuals may enter a state where they feel a deep connection to the universal human experience of creation and renewal [6]. The experience of birth can feel timeless [7], as if one is participating in an infinite cycle of life and growth that has been repeated throughout history. It can also lead individuals to momentarily transcend their individual identity and merge with the collective experience of motherhood, fatherhood, and the human journey [8]. This idea of birth transcending time or self has been recognised in several studies [9, 10, 11], indicating that it is not an isolated perception but a common thread in the childbirth experience. These findings highlight the profound impact that childbirth can have on individuals' spiritual and existential perspectives.

Furthermore, it is noteworthy that personal interpretations of transcendent experiences during childbirth can vary significantly. While some individuals may attribute this transcendent experience to a personal God, others may find it difficult to associate it with a specific deity or religious framework [12, 13, 14]. Instead, they may view it as a more abstract and personal connection to their own inner self, the natural world, or a deeper understanding of their own destiny and purpose.

2.2 Transition to Parenthood Prior to the Need for Neonatal Palliative Care

Transition into parenthood is a significant life event and motherhood especially has been a focus of research, particularly within the field of psychology. Since the 1970s, a new paradigm of infant psychology emerged, taking a step away from the psychoanalytical tradition which had dominated the area since World War II [15]. A new more empirically founded tradition arose, dominated by scholars such as the infant psychologist Daniel N. Stern. He highlighted how a new way of navigating in life develops through the motherhood transition [16]. Motherhood is not merely a transitional period, but a continuous change in navigation, due to the 'motherhood constellation', a special mental approach where the mother gives preferential treatment to all issues related to motherhood (Stern [16], p. 33). Brudal [17] articulated, based on existential philosophy, motherhood transition as a 'borderland' (authors' translation), in which insecurity and new borders and rules arise [17].

Motherhood *transition* has been explored more sparsely in traditional health research, which is often trying to distinguish between health and disease, for example in relation to postnatal depression, post-traumatic stress disorder (PTSD) or post-traumatic growth (PTG) [18, 19, 20]. Motherhood transition per se has, furthermore, been explored in relation to experiences expected to be traumatising, for example giving birth preterm [21, 22].

Callister's research has revealed that mothers often experience shifts in perception such as a profound sense of change, feeling a connection to women across different generations, or a heightened alignment with their own bodies [23, 24, 21]. A scoping review focusing on existential meaning found that the motherhood transition is a paradoxical live event reorganising values and what makes life worth living, which for some women is interpreted as a spiritual experience [25].

In a more recent study that included both mothers and fathers, significant changes were identified which encompassed aspects such as shifts in the perception of life's meaning, transformations within relationships, and, for certain individuals, the emergence of transcendent beliefs. Additionally, a heightened awareness of mortality surfaced. Throughout the study, existential dimensions were meticulously explored and deliberated upon in intricate manners, revealing expressions of existential vulnerability [26]. These studies underline how transition to parenthood per se transforms life existentially and spiritually for some parents, and this awareness is important when caring for parents with a neonate in palliative care. They are already amid one of life's greatest transitions which is now embedded with paradoxical experiences and feelings. The mother especially may experience this, as she is also biologically transitioning from pregnancy to post-birth and sometimes nourishing the child as well [27].

2.3 The Intertwinement of Beginning of Life and End of Life

Birth and death are intrinsic aspects of the human experience. These pivotal life transitions are not only laden with profound significance but also give rise to complex and mixed emotions. Individuals navigate these transitions through a range of embodied, cultural, spiritual, and ritual practices, as highlighted in studies by Hallam et al. [28], Kaufman and Morgan [29], Mathijssen [30], and Wojtkowiak [31]. The liminal nature of birth and death, characterised by transitional and ambiguous states, engenders a profound need for rituals.

Rituals, observed across diverse cultures, accompany the processes of birth and death, acknowledging their transformative nature. These rituals serve important functions, such as welcoming the arrival of a child, honouring the expectant mother/parent through ceremonies that bestow names, or symbolically transitioning the departed into the realm of the deceased. They provide a structured framework for individuals and communities to mark and navigate these significant life passages, providing comfort, meaning, and a sense of continuity amidst the uncertainties and complexities inherent in birth and death [32].

When birth and death occur in close proximity, the spiritual effects on parents can be profound due to several interrelated factors [33]. Primarily, the loss of a baby is a deeply traumatic experience for parents, transcending cultural, religious, and personal beliefs. It shatters the parent's expectations of welcoming a new life and disrupts the natural order of their life events. This profound loss can cause parents to question the meaning and purpose of their own lives, as well as their beliefs about the divine or spiritual dimensions of existence. It challenges their understanding of the world and their place within it. If the baby dies in utero, death becomes part of women's living bodies in very concrete ways, difficult to comprehend in a rational sense [34].

The death of a baby also confronts parents with existential questions about the fragility and vulnerability of life in an unexpected way. They may grapple with the unfairness of the situation, questioning why their baby's life was cut short and searching for answers that may not be readily available. This search for meaning and understanding sometimes leads parents to explore their spirituality more deeply, seeking solace, comfort, and a sense of connection to something greater than themselves [35].

Additionally, the loss of a baby can profoundly affect parents' sense of identity and purpose. They may experience a sense of emptiness, guilt, or self-blame, questioning their abilities as parents or feeling a loss of direction in life. In these moments of profound grief, parents may turn to spirituality to find healing, strength, and a renewed sense of purpose. Spiritual beliefs and practices can offer a framework for processing and making sense of the overwhelming emotions and existential dilemmas that arise from such a devastating loss.

Furthermore, spirituality can provide a source of hope, comfort, and support during the grieving process. It offers a space for parents to connect with their baby on a spiritual level, even in the absence of a physical presence. Rituals, prayers, and other spiritual practices can provide a means of honouring and remembering the child, fostering a sense of continued connection and love.

3 Spiritual Care in Neonatal Palliative Care

3.1 Conceptualising Spirituality in Neonatal Care

A clear understanding of spirituality is crucial in neonatal palliative care, as it affects communication and care quality [36, 37]. Healthcare professionals need to align their perceptions with those of parents for effective spiritual care [38]. This understanding enhances interdisciplinary collaboration, education, and research, benefiting healthcare providers and families [39, 40].

In the realm of education, teaching healthcare professionals about spirituality in neonatal contexts helps them provide empathetic, personalised care and engage in sensitive spiritual discussions [41]. Research in this area informs strategies that address families' spiritual needs, improving their experience during challenging times [42].

For healthcare providers, engaging with families' spirituality enhances job satisfaction and reduces burnout, fostering a supportive work environment [43, 44]. Families benefit from this approach, as it provides comfort and a patient-centred care experience [45].

Overall, understanding spirituality in neonatal care leads to better collaboration, education, and research, creating a more compassionate and efficient healthcare environment for families during critical periods.

3.2 The Significance of Spiritual Care in Neonatal Palliative Care

The concept of spirituality in neonatal palliative care necessitates a comprehensive understanding that encompasses the unique circumstances and challenges faced by parents and infants who are unlikely to survive. Unlike in the adult population, where spiritual care predominantly involves personal beliefs, religious practices, and existential questions [46, 47], spirituality in neonatal palliative care incorporates broader elements of parental bonding, meaning-making, and navigating the grief and bereavement process. Parents' interpretations of spirituality may differ significantly from traditional definitions, emphasising the significance of exploring and acknowledging these perspectives to ensure a patient-centred approach.

3.3 Challenges and Barriers to Providing Spiritual Care

The diverse range of beliefs and interpretations of spirituality among parents and healthcare providers can create challenges in understanding and providing adequate spiritual care. Parents may have varying religious affiliations, spiritual beliefs, or philosophical views that influence their expectations and needs regarding spiritual support. Healthcare providers must navigate these differences sensitively and avoid imposing their own beliefs on families. Healthcare providers may be hesitant to address spiritual topics due to concerns about overstepping boundaries or offending families who hold different beliefs [48]. This fear can lead to a reluctance to initiate discussions about spirituality, leaving families without the support they may need.

Healthcare professionals often receive limited training in addressing spiritual needs and providing spiritual care, especially in neonatal care settings [49]. A Danish study investigated how health professionals in maternity care perceive the existential dimensions of transitioning to parenthood [50]. It revealed that while these professionals share some commonalities in their interpretations, they also have distinct perspectives in their professional versus personal lives. Typically, such existential elements come to the fore in traumatic instances or are associated with childbirth, where they manifest as a tangible yet silent connection between the mother, midwife, or partner. Recognition of these existential elements is rarer during the prenatal and postnatal stages. The language to describe these existential facets is notably absent from the professional dialogue in Danish maternity services. Health professionals involved in the study expressed appreciation for re-engaging with the significance of these existential elements in their work, likening it to uncovering a well-concealed treasure. From the viewpoint of existential philosophy, the journey through childbirth and into parenthood is fraught with a spectrum of contradictory and intricate emotions and experiences. These insights are echoed in the sentiments of maternity care workers [50].

The demanding nature of neonatal care, which involves medical interventions and monitoring, can create time constraints that hinder healthcare providers from engaging in meaningful conversations about spirituality. Focusing solely on medical aspects may lead to the overlooking of the spiritual needs of parents and families [51].

Neonatal care is primarily focused on medical interventions and ensuring the physical well-being of newborns. This emphasis on the medical aspect of care can sometimes overshadow the importance of addressing spiritual and emotional needs [52]. Spiritual care, on the other hand, involves families from diverse cultural and religious backgrounds, each with its own set of traditions, rituals, and beliefs. Healthcare providers need to be culturally sensitive and avoid making assumptions about the spiritual needs of families based on stereotypes or generalisations [53]. Spiritual care may be perceived as secondary to medical treatment by the healthcare team.

Engaging in conversations about spirituality within the neonatal context is a complex task that demands effective communication skills. Healthcare providers often find themselves grappling with the challenge of initiating and navigating these discussions in a manner that is not only respectful but also open and conducive to sharing spiritual concerns. This requires a delicate balance, as addressing the spiritual dimensions of care calls for a level of sensitivity and understanding that extends beyond medical interventions. Compounding this challenge are the structural limitations within some healthcare settings. These limitations manifest in the form of inadequate resources, guidelines, or protocols specifically tailored to address spiritual care in neonatal contexts [54]. The absence of a standardised framework for integrating spiritual care into neonatal practices can hinder healthcare providers' ability to provide consistent and comprehensive support to families. In such cases, the provision of spiritual care may become sporadic or overlooked altogether, despite its potential significance for parents facing the complexities of neonatal care.

Parents facing the challenges of neonatal care, especially in cases of palliative care, may be overwhelmed by distress and grief. This emotional burden can affect their ability to engage in spiritual discussions and hinder their capacity to find solace through spiritual practices [55]. This may be exacerbated by some healthcare providers perceiving spiritual care as irrelevant or unnecessary in a medical context, especially when dealing with critically ill infants [49]. This mindset can lead to the neglect of spiritual aspects and the potential benefits they offer to families.

Addressing these barriers requires a concerted effort to raise awareness, provide education, and foster a culture that values spiritual care as an integral component of neonatal care. By recognising the importance of spiritual well-being and equipping healthcare providers with the skills and sensitivity to address spiritual needs, neonatal care can become more holistic and supportive for both families and professionals involved.

4 Approaches to Spiritual Care in Neonatal Palliative Care

4.1 Assessing Spiritual Needs

Assessing spiritual needs in neonatal palliative care necessitates a considerate and sensitive approach that acknowledges the intricate and distinct nature of the neonatal context. Building a foundation of trust and empathy with parents or caregivers creates an atmosphere of openness, enabling them to share their spiritual beliefs, concerns, and requirements.

Initiating conversations about spirituality should be approached subtly, beginning with open-ended questions that allow parents to articulate their beliefs, values, and hopes [56]. Active listening is key to fully understanding the parents' perspectives, encompassing both verbal and nonverbal cues, while encouraging the sharing of personal stories and experiences [57]. Reflective and open-minded communications are teachable skills that can enhance professional work satisfaction [58, 59].

It's essential to be attuned to cultural and religious diversity, as spirituality often intertwines deeply with cultural practices and beliefs. Some healthcare settings employ specialised screening tools to systematically identify and address spiritual concerns. Examples of such tools include the FICA Spiritual History Tool [60] and HOPE Questions [61].

Gaining insight into parents' coping mechanisms, sources of strength, and how they find meaning and hope amid their child's condition can shed light on their spiritual resources [62]. Understanding any rituals, religious practices, or spiritual traditions that hold significance for the family can guide the provision of suitable support.

Engaging in discussions about the parents' beliefs concerning life, death, and the afterlife allows for comprehension of their spiritual framework. If parents are open to the idea, involving their spiritual leaders or clergy members can offer faith-specific guidance and support [41]. Given the dynamic and emotionally charged context of neonatal palliative care, acknowledging that spiritual needs may change over time is crucial. Continuously reassessing and revisiting these needs as circumstances evolve ensures ongoing support.

Spiritual assessment should be integrated seamlessly into the broader evaluation of the parents' and family's well-being, recognising the interconnectedness of spiritual, emotional, psychological, and physical aspects [41]. Documenting conversations and spiritual needs in medical records ensures the entire care team is informed and can provide consistent assistance.

Collaborating with other healthcare professionals like social workers, chaplains, and psychologists ensures a comprehensive approach to addressing the family's spiritual needs [63]. Respect for the parents' preferences in engaging in spiritual discussions and practices is paramount.

Assessing spiritual needs demands a gentle and non-judgemental demeanour. Acknowledge that each family's journey is distinct, and understanding their spiritual needs significantly contributes to delivering holistic and patient-centred care during this challenging period.

4.2 Communication and Collaboration

Communication and collaboration regarding spiritual care in neonatal palliative care play pivotal roles in ensuring comprehensive and compassionate support for families facing challenging circumstances. The dynamic and emotionally charged nature of neonatal care underscores the significance of effective communication and collaborative efforts among healthcare providers, families, and spiritual care professionals.

Collaboration among healthcare professionals is vital for addressing spiritual needs comprehensively. In a study about patients with lung cancer, it was emphasised that social workers, psychologists, chaplains, and medical staff should work collaboratively to ensure that all aspects of the family's well-being are considered [64], and this is no different in the neonatal context. Sharing insights from spiritual assessments and discussions can help the care team tailor interventions and support strategies. Furthermore, collaborating with families themselves is essential [65]. Parents possess unique insights into their spiritual beliefs and needs. By involving them in care planning and decision-making processes, healthcare providers can create care plans that align with the families' values and wishes.

Interdisciplinary collaboration extends to the development of protocols, guidelines, and resources for providing spiritual care [64]. Healthcare settings should establish frameworks that outline the roles and responsibilities of various professionals involved in spiritual care, ensuring that families receive consistent and well-coordinated support.

Effective communication and collaboration are integral to providing holistic spiritual care in neonatal palliative care. By fostering open dialogues, involving spiritual leaders, and promoting interdisciplinary teamwork, healthcare providers can create an environment that acknowledges and addresses the spiritual needs of families, enhancing their overall well-being during this challenging period.

4.3 Rituals, Symbols, and Practices

Rituals, symbols, and practices play a significant role in providing spiritual care within the context of neonatal palliative care. These elements offer avenues for families to find solace, meaning, and a sense of connection during the challenging journey of caring for a critically ill newborn.

Rituals are structured and symbolic actions that hold profound spiritual significance [66]. In neonatal palliative care, rituals can provide a framework for parents and families to commemorate their child's life, create lasting memories, and navigate the grieving process [67]. Rituals can range from personal and intimate moments, such as bathing or holding the baby, to formal ceremonies that involve family, friends, and religious leaders. These rituals offer a way for families to honour their child, acknowledge their emotional pain, and seek comfort in shared traditions. Rituals also provide a sense of continuity, allowing families to establish a connection between the life of their child and their broader spiritual beliefs [68, 69, 70].

Symbols hold deep meaning and can serve as visual representations of spiritual concepts. In children's palliative care, symbols can provide a way for parents to express their emotions, hopes, and connection to their child [71]. Common symbols include butterflies, doves, or stars, which can represent transformation, peace, and eternal life. Keepsakes such as handprints, footprints, or locks of hair are tangible symbols that hold sentimental value and enable parents to hold onto a physical connection with their child [72, 73]. These symbols offer a means of channelling grief, finding meaning, and expressing spiritual beliefs in a tangible way.

Spiritual practices encompass a range of activities that foster a sense of connection, reflection, and inner peace. Parents in neonatal palliative care may engage in practices like prayer, meditation, or mindfulness to find solace and connect with their child's spirit [1]. These practices can also be tied to religious traditions, offering families a familiar framework to navigate their grief and seek spiritual support. Additionally, engaging with a supportive community, whether through religious congregations, support groups, or online forums, can provide a sense of belonging and shared experiences. Spiritual practices in neonatal palliative care offer parents tools to cope with their emotions, find strength, and integrate their child's presence into their spiritual journey [1].

Incorporating rituals, symbols, and spiritual practices into neonatal palliative care requires sensitivity to each family's unique beliefs and cultural background. By offering opportunities for families to honour and connect with their child's spirit through these elements, spiritual care in neonatal palliative care becomes a way to provide comfort, understanding, and a sense of meaning during a profoundly challenging time.

4.4 Support for Religious and Cultural Diversity

Healthcare professionals need to develop cultural competence, which involves understanding the beliefs, practices, and values of different cultures and religions [74]. This enables them to provide care that is respectful and aligned with the families' preferences and traditions.

Considering the religious and cultural preferences of families when developing care plans is essential. This includes accommodating religious practices, rituals, dietary restrictions, and preferences for spiritual support, such as involving clergy members or spiritual leaders from their respective faith communities [1].

Establishing open communication with families about their religious and cultural needs is crucial. This involves creating an environment where families feel comfortable discussing their beliefs and practices, as well as any concerns they may have regarding spiritual care [75]. This collaboration ensures that spiritual care is provided in a manner that is consistent with the families' faith traditions.

While it's important to offer support in alignment with families' religious and cultural beliefs, it's equally crucial to respect their choices [1]. Some families may choose not to engage in certain religious practices or may have unique interpretations of their faith. Documenting families' religious and cultural preferences in their medical records ensures that all members of the care team are aware and can provide consistent support. This documentation also helps avoid inadvertently causing distress by going against families' religious or cultural wishes. Religious and cultural practices can vary widely even within the same faith tradition. Healthcare providers should approach each family with flexibility, recognising that there may be differences in interpretation and practice [1].

Given the diversity of the populations they serve, healthcare providers should engage in ongoing learning and self-awareness about various cultural and religious perspectives. This continual growth helps them adapt their approach to changing patient demographics and evolving healthcare environments. By embracing and supporting religious and cultural diversity in spiritual care, healthcare providers can ensure that families receive care that honours their beliefs, fosters a sense of cultural identity, and provides comfort during a challenging time.

5 Ethical Considerations in Spiritual Care

5.1 Cultural Sensitivity and Religious Beliefs

Cultural sensitivity and respect for religious beliefs are essential aspects of providing effective spiritual care in neonatal palliative care. Neonatal palliative care encompasses families from diverse cultural and religious backgrounds, each with their unique practices, values, and beliefs [76].

Cultural sensitivity involves understanding and appreciating the cultural norms, traditions, and values that shape families' lives [77]. Healthcare providers should approach spiritual care with an open mind, avoiding assumptions and stereotypes [78]. Taking the time to learn about the cultural background of each family allows healthcare professionals to tailor their approach to align with the family's preferences and beliefs.

Religious beliefs play a significant role in how individuals understand and cope with challenging circumstances [79], including neonatal palliative care. Healthcare providers must be aware of the diverse religious traditions and beliefs that families may hold. This knowledge enables them to engage in meaningful conversations about spirituality, respecting the family's faith-based practices and rituals.

Incorporating cultural and religious considerations into spiritual care requires sensitivity and flexibility. Some families may seek solace and meaning through prayers, rituals, or religious ceremonies. Others may draw strength from cultural practices that offer comfort during difficult times. Nevertheless, spiritual struggles can arise from ethical quandaries or doubts, such as wondering if suffering is a form of divine punishment. Research indicates that a number of bereaved parents harbour resentment towards God following the death of their child. Some perceive it as a punitive act, while others revaluate their faith in an all-knowing, all-powerful God, shifting instead to a belief in a fallible higher power [80, 81]. Meert et al. [82] reported that between 30% and 60% of grieving parents experience feelings of anger and self-blame, as well as directing blame towards God in the aftermath of their infant's or child's death.

Furthermore, respecting religious beliefs extends to end-of-life decisions and rituals. Families may have specific wishes regarding life-sustaining treatments, organ donation, and the handling of the baby's body after death [83]. Healthcare providers must collaborate with families and, when appropriate, religious leaders to ensure that these wishes are honoured to the best extent possible.

5.2 Addressing Existential and Ethical Dilemmas

Addressing existential and ethical dilemmas regarding spiritual care in neonatal palliative care involves navigating complex questions about the meaning of life, suffering, and the ethical considerations surrounding the provision of spiritual support to families facing the potential loss of their newborns.

Existential dilemmas arise as healthcare providers and families grapple with the profound questions about the purpose and significance of life, particularly when faced with the fragility of newborns. The challenge lies in understanding how to provide meaningful spiritual care that respects diverse beliefs and allows families to find comfort, hope, and a sense of purpose amidst the difficult circumstances [84].

Ethical dilemmas emerge when considering the boundaries of spiritual care and respecting families' autonomy and choices. Striking a balance between providing spiritual support and respecting families' decisions about their beliefs and preferences can be intricate [52]. Healthcare providers must navigate situations where their own beliefs may differ from those of the families they are caring for, requiring sensitivity and an unbiased approach [85].

Furthermore, ethical considerations extend to the potential influence of healthcare providers on families' beliefs. Providers must be cautious not to impose their own spiritual beliefs on families, ensuring that any spiritual support provided aligns with the families' values and wishes [45]. This requires a delicate understanding of the power dynamics in the healthcare relationship and a commitment to patient-centred care.

It is essential to foster an environment where families feel empowered to express their spiritual needs and preferences without fear of judgement or undue influence. Open and honest communication, as well as shared decision-making, plays a pivotal role in navigating these complex existential and ethical dilemmas.

Collaboration among healthcare providers, families, and spiritual care experts is crucial in addressing these challenges. Establishing clear policies and guidelines for providing spiritual care while respecting diverse beliefs can help healthcare providers navigate these dilemmas more effectively [41]. Regular ethical discussions and ongoing education for healthcare providers can promote a deeper understanding of the nuanced ethical considerations surrounding spiritual care in neonatal palliative care.

Incorporating the potential for spiritual distress, it becomes clear that tackling existential and ethical dilemmas within spiritual care demands a nuanced approach [86]. This includes fostering sensitive and open communication, embodying cultural competence, and steadfastly respecting the dignity and autonomy of families. Caregivers must recognise the spiritual turmoil that can be sparked by events such as the death of a child, where feelings of anger towards a deity or self-blame are manifestations of profound spiritual distress. It's imperative that spiritual care professionals provide empathetic support that navigates these complexities, aiding families through the arduous path of grief and potentially reshaped belief systems. This comprehensive support is essential in helping families confront and work through the spiritual dimensions of their experience during such pivotal moments of crisis.

6 Integration of Spiritual Care into Neonatal Palliative Care Guidelines

The integration of spiritual care into neonatal palliative care guidelines holds significant importance for fostering comprehensive and patient-centred support for families facing the challenges of neonatal palliative care. This integration enhances several critical aspects of neonatal palliative care.

Neonatal palliative care involves not only addressing the physical health of the infant but also supporting the emotional and spiritual well-being of both parents and families. By incorporating spiritual care into guidelines, healthcare providers ensure that families receive well-rounded and holistic support during this difficult journey. Recognising and addressing the spiritual needs of families aligns with the principles of patient-centred care [61]. It acknowledges that families bring their individual beliefs and values to their experiences, and tailors care to accommodate these unique perspectives. This approach fosters trust, empathy, and a sense of validation for families.

The challenges of neonatal palliative care can be overwhelming for families. Spiritual beliefs and practices often provide a source of comfort, hope, and strength during difficult times. Integrating spiritual care equips families with coping mechanisms and fosters resilience, supporting them in navigating their emotional journey [37]. Neonatal palliative care involves families from diverse cultural and religious backgrounds. Integrating spiritual care guidelines helps healthcare providers navigate cultural sensitivities and deliver care that respects and acknowledges the diverse spiritual beliefs and practices of families [52].

Guidelines for integrating spiritual care provide healthcare providers with a framework for initiating and conducting discussions about spirituality. This can lead to improved communication between healthcare providers and families, creating an environment where families feel heard and understood.

Healthcare providers often experience moral distress when they feel unable to address the holistic needs of their patients due to constraints or lack of guidance. Integrating spiritual care into guidelines can reduce moral distress by providing a structured approach to addressing families' spiritual concerns [87].

Spiritual care is not the responsibility of one discipline alone. Integrating it into guidelines encourages interdisciplinary collaboration, ensuring that chaplains, social workers, nurses, and physicians work together to provide comprehensive support. Formal integration of spiritual care into guidelines encourages research and evidence-based practices in this domain. It promotes the development of tools, assessment methods, and interventions that are backed by research, leading to more effective and impactful spiritual care.

7 Conclusion

Recognising the unique challenges and complexities of delivering spiritual care in neonatal palliative care is important. By addressing the conceptual ambiguities surrounding spirituality, healthcare professionals can better align their care practices with the needs and expectations of parents facing the loss of their infant. This chapter emphasises the importance of enhancing communication, practice, education, and research through clarifying the meaning of spirituality within neonatal palliative care. Such efforts will contribute to the development of patient-centred approaches that holistically support neonatal patients and their families during this profoundly difficult and sensitive period of their lives.

References

1. Kain VJ. Perinatal palliative care: cultural, spiritual, and religious considerations for parents-what clinicians need to know. Front Pediatr. 2021;9:597519.
2. Kain VJ, Chin SD. Conceptually redefining neonatal palliative care. Adv Neonatal Care. 2020;20(3):187–95.
3. Niels C, Hvidt K, Nielsen A, Kørup K, Prinds C, et al. What is spiritual care? Professional perspectives on the concept of spiritual care identified through group concept mapping. BMJ Open. 2020;10(12):e042142.
4. Cronin-Fisher V, Parcell ES. Making sense of dissatisfaction during the transition to motherhood through relational dialectics theory. J Fam Commun. 2019;19(2):157–70.
5. Olza I, Leahy-Warren P, Benyamini Y, Kazmierczak M, Karlsdottir SI, Spyridou A, et al. Women's psychological experiences of physiological childbirth: a meta-synthesis. BMJ Open. 2018;8(10):e020347.
6. Budin W. Birth and death: opportunities for self-transcendence. J Perinat Educ. 2001;1(2):38–42.
7. Crowther SA, Hall J, Balabanoff D, Baranowska B, Kay L, Menage D, et al. Spirituality and childbirth: an international virtual co-operative inquiry. Women Birth. 2021;34(2):e135–e45.
8. Hansen LB, Hvidt NC, Mortensen KE, Wu C, Prinds C. How giving birth makes sense: a questionnaire study on existential meaning-making among mothers giving birth preterm or at term. J Relig Health. 2021;60(1):335–53.
9. Babetin K. The birth of a mother: a psychological transformation. J Prenat Perinat Psychol Health. 2020;34(5):410–28.
10. Bartell SS. On becoming a mother: the psychological journey. Int J Childbirth Educ. 2005;20(1):28–30.
11. Crowther S, Smythe E, Spence D. Kairos time at the moment of birth. Midwifery. 2015;31(4):451–7.

12. Feeley C, Cooper M, Burns E. A systematic meta-thematic synthesis to examine the views and experiences of women following water immersion during labour and waterbirth. J Adv Nurs. 2021;77(7):2942–56.
13. Olza I, Uvnas-Moberg K, Ekström-Bergström A, Leahy-Warren P, Karlsdottir SI, Nieuwenhuijze M, et al. Birth as a neuro-psycho-social event: an integrative model of maternal experiences and their relation to neurohormonal events during childbirth. PLoS One. 2020;15(7):e0230992.
14. Taghizdeh Z, Ebadi A, Dehghani M, Gharacheh M, Yadollahi P. A time for psycho-spiritual transcendence: the experiences of Iranian women of pain during childbirth. Women Birth. 2017;30(6):491–6.
15. Mosbæk C. Det nyfødte barn – de nye forældre: om fødslens psykologi. København: Hans Reitzel; 1996. 209 sider p.
16. Stern DN, Bruschweiler-Stern N. The birth of a mother: how the motherhood experience changes you forever. New York: Basic Books; 1998.
17. Brudal LH. Psykiske reaksjoner ved svangerskap, fødsel og barseltid. Bergen: Fagbokforlaget; 2000.
18. Andersen LB, Melvaer LB, Videbech P, Lamont RF, Joergensen JS. Risk factors for developing post-traumatic stress disorder following childbirth: a systematic review. Acta Obstet Gynecol Scand. 2012;91(11):1261–72.
19. Hübner-Liebermann B, Hausner H, Wittmann M. Recognizing and treating peripartum depression. Dtsch Arztebl Int. 2012;109(24):419.
20. Sawyer A, Ayers S, Young D, Bradley R, Smith H. Posttraumatic growth after childbirth: a prospective study. Psychol Health. 2012;27(3):362–77.
21. Carvalho AEV, Linhares MBM, Padovani FHP, Martinez FE. Anxiety and depression in mothers of preterm infants and psychological intervention during hospitalization in neonatal ICU. Span J Psychol. 2009;12(1):161–70.
22. Shaw RJ, Sweester CJ, St. John N, Lilo E, Corcoran JB, Jo B, et al. Prevention of postpartum traumatic stress in mothers with preterm infants: manual development and evaluation. Issues Ment Health Nurs. 2013;34(8):578–86.
23. Callister LC. Making meaning: women's birth narratives. J Obstet Gynecol Neonatal Nurs. 2004;33(4):508–18.
24. Callister LC, Vehvilainen-Julkunen K, Lauri S. Giving birth: perceptions of Finnish childbearing women. MCN Am J Matern Child Nurs. 2001;26(1):28–32.
25. Prinds C, Hvidt NC, Mogensen O, Buus N. Making existential meaning in transition to motherhood – a scoping review. Midwifery. 2014;30(6):733–41.
26. Prinds C, Timmerman C, Hvidtjørn D, Ammentorp J, Hvidt NC, Larsen H, et al. Existential aspects in the transition to parenthood based on interviews and a theatre workshop. Sex Reprod Healthc. 2021;28:100612.
27. Palmér L, Carlsson G, Brunt D, Nyström M. Existential security is a necessary condition for continued breastfeeding despite severe initial difficulties: a lifeworld hermeneutical study. Int Breastfeed J. 2015;10:1–11.
28. Hallam E, Hockey J, Howarth G. Beyond the body: death and social identity. Routledge; 2005.
29. Kaufman SR, Morgan LM. The anthropology of the beginnings and ends of life. Annu Rev Anthropol. 2005;34:317–41.
30. Mathijssen B. Transforming bonds: ritualising post-mortem relationships in The Netherlands. Mortality. 2018;23(3):215–30.
31. Wojtkowiak J. Ritualizing pregnancy and childbirth in secular societies: exploring embodied spirituality at the start of life. Religions. 2020;11(9):458.
32. Wojtkowiak J, Mathijssen B. Birth and death: studying ritual, embodied practices and spirituality at the start and end of life. Religions [Internet]. 2022;13(9):820.
33. Jørgensen ML, Prinds C, Mørk S, Hvidtjørn D. Stillbirth–transitions and rituals when birth brings death: data from a danish national cohort seen through an anthropological lens. Scand J Caring Sci. 2022;36(1):100–8.

34. Damm MF, Jørgensen ML, Eklund MV, Hvidtjørn D, Prinds C. Carrying death: a qualitative study of women's bodily perceptions after their baby died in utero. OMEGA J Death Dying. 2023. https://doi.org/10.1177/00302228231190544.
35. Harris S. Motherhood and the traumatic death of one's child. In: Arnold-Baker C, editor. The existential crisis of motherhood. Cham: Springer International Publishing; 2020. p. 199–219.
36. Ettema EJ, Derksen LD, van Leeuwen E. Existential loneliness and end-of-life care: a systematic review. Theor Med Bioeth. 2010;31:141–69.
37. Reinert KG, Koenig HG. Re-examining definitions of spirituality in nursing research. J Adv Nurs. 2013;69(12):2622–34.
38. Ernecoff NC, Curlin FA, Buddadhumaruk P, White DB. Health care professionals' responses to religious or spiritual statements by surrogate decision makers during goals-of-care discussions. JAMA Intern Med. 2015;175(10):1662–9.
39. Nolan S, Saltmarsh P, Leget C. Spiritual care in palliative care: working towards and EAPC task force. Eur J Palliat Care. 2011;18:86–9.
40. van Randwijk CB, Opsahl T, Hvidt EA, Kørup AK, Bjerrum L, Thomsen KF, et al. Characteristics of religious and spiritual beliefs of Danish physicians: and likelihood of addressing religious and spiritual issues with patients. J Relig Health. 2019;58:333–42.
41. Swihart DL, Yarrarapu SNS, Martin RL. Cultural religious competence in clinical practice. Treasure Island (FL): StatPearls Publishing; 2023. http://europepmc.org/abstract/MED/29630268.
42. Rego F, Gonçalves F, Moutinho S, Castro L, Nunes R. The influence of spirituality on decision-making in palliative care outpatients: a cross-sectional study. BMC Palliat Care. 2020;19(1):22.
43. Morley L, Cashell A. Collaboration in health care. J Med Imaging Radiat Sci. 2017;48(2):207–16.
44. Wu X, Hayter M, Lee AJ, Yuan Y, Li S, Bi Y, et al. Positive spiritual climate supports transformational leadership as means to reduce nursing burnout and intent to leave. J Nurs Manag. 2020;28(4):804–13.
45. Fitch MI, Bartlett R. Patient perspectives about spirituality and spiritual care. Asia Pac J Oncol Nurs. 2019;6(2):111–21.
46. Benites AC, Rodin G, de Oliveira-Cardoso ÉA, Dos Santos MA. "You begin to give more value in life, in minutes, in seconds": spiritual and existential experiences of family caregivers of patients with advanced cancer receiving end-of-life care in Brazil. Support Care Cancer. 2021;30:2631–8.
47. Kukla H, Herrler A, Strupp J, Voltz R. "My life became more meaningful": confronting one's own end of life and its effects on well-being – a qualitative study. BMC Palliat Care. 2022;21(1):58.
48. Vigna PM, de Castro I, Fumis RRL. Spirituality alleviates the burden on family members caring for patients receiving palliative care exclusively. BMC Palliat Care. 2020;19(1):77.
49. Farahani AS, Rassouli M, Salmani N, Mojen LK, Sajjadi M, Heidarzadeh M, et al. Evaluation of health-care providers' perception of spiritual care and the obstacles to its implementation. Asia Pac J Oncol Nurs. 2019;6(2):122–9.
50. Prinds C, Timmerman C, Hvidtjørn D, Ammentorp J, Christian Hvidt N, Larsen H, et al. Existential aspects of parenthood transition seen from the health professionals' perspective – an interview and theatre workshop study. Sex Reprod Healthc. 2023;37:100884.
51. Scott HM, Coombes L, Braybrook D, Roach A, Harðardóttir D, Bristowe K, et al. Spiritual, religious, and existential concerns of children and young people with life-limiting and life-threatening conditions: a qualitative interview study. Palliat Med. 2023;37(6):856–65.
52. Isaac KS, Hay JL, Lubetkin EI. Incorporating spirituality in primary care. J Relig Health. 2016;55(3):1065–77.
53. Kaihlanen A-M, Hietapakka L, Heponiemi T. Increasing cultural awareness: qualitative study of nurses' perceptions about cultural competence training. BMC Nurs. 2019;18(1):38.

54. Schnall J, Hayden D, Wilkinson D. Newborns in crisis: an outline of neonatal ethical dilemmas in humanitarian medicine. Dev World Bioeth. 2019;19(4):196–205.
55. Eden LM, Callister LC. Parent involvement in end-of-life care and decision making in the newborn intensive care unit: an integrative review. J Perinat Educ. 2010;19(1):29–39.
56. Foster TL, Lafond DA, Reggio C, Hinds PS, editors. Pediatric palliative care in childhood cancer nursing: from diagnosis to cure or end of life. Seminars in oncology nursing. Elsevier; 2010.
57. Reis HT. Intimacy as an interpersonal process. In: Relationships, well-being and behaviour. New York: Routledge; 2018. p. 113–43.
58. Prinds C, der Wal JG-V, Crombag N, Martin L. Counselling for prenatal anomaly screening – a plea for integration of existential life questions. Patient Educ Couns. 2020;103(8):1657–61.
59. Timmermann C, Prinds C, Hvidt EA, Hvidt NC, Lau ME, Ammentorp J. Stimulating existential communication – first steps towards enhancing health professionals' reflective skills through blended learning. PEC Innov. 2023;2:100121.
60. Puchalski C. Spiritual care in health care: guideline, models, spiritual assessment and the use of the© FICA spiritual history tool. In: Spiritual needs in research and practice: the spiritual needs questionnaire as a global resource for health and social care. Cham: Springer; 2021. p. 27–45.
61. Kuckel DP, Jones AL, Smith DK. The spiritual assessment. Am Fam Physician. 2022;106(4):415–9.
62. Karaca A, Konuk ŞD. Spirituality as a coping method for mothers of children with developmental disabilities. Int J Dev Disabil. 2019;67(2):112–20.
63. Kruizinga R, Schuhmann C, Glasner T, Jacobs G. Enhancing the integration of chaplains within the healthcare team A qualitative analysis of a survey study among healthcare chaplains. Integr Healthc J. 2022;4(1):e000138.
64. Siler S, Mamier I, Winslow BW, Ferrell BR. Interprofessional perspectives on providing spiritual care for patients with lung cancer in outpatient settings. Oncol Nurs Forum. 2019;46(1):49–58.
65. Kokorelias KM, Gignac MAM, Naglie G, Cameron JI. Towards a universal model of family centered care: a scoping review. BMC Health Serv Res. 2019;19(1):564.
66. Sas C, Coman A. Designing personal grief rituals: an analysis of symbolic objects and actions. Death Stud. 2016;40(9):558–69.
67. Wyatt J, Hain R. Redirecting care: compassionate management of the sick or preterm neonate at the end of life. Children (Basel). 2022;9(3):344.
68. Carter BS. More than medication: perinatal palliative care, vol. 105; 2016. p. 1255.
69. Kolmar A, Hueckel RM, Kamal A, Dickerman M. Top ten tips palliative care clinicians should know about caring for children in neonatal and pediatric intensive care units. J Palliat Med. 2019;22(9):1149–53.
70. Wool C. Clinician confidence and comfort in providing perinatal palliative care. J Obstet Gynecol Neonatal Nurs. 2013;42(1):48–58.
71. Superdock AK, Barfield RC, Brandon DH, Docherty SL. Exploring the vagueness of Religion & Spirituality in complex pediatric decision-making: a qualitative study. BMC Palliat Care. 2018;17(1):1–14.
72. Denney-Koelsch E, Black BP, Côté-Arsenault D, Wool C, Kim S, Kavanaugh K. A survey of perinatal palliative care programs in the United States: structure, processes, and outcomes. J Palliat Med. 2016;19(10):1080–6.
73. Neville TH, Clarke F, Takaoka A, Sadik M, Vanstone M, Phung P, et al. Keepsakes at the end of life. J Pain Symptom Manag. 2020;60(5):941–7.
74. Shepherd SM, Willis-Esqueda C, Newton D, Sivasubramaniam D, Paradies Y. The challenge of cultural competence in the workplace: perspectives of healthcare providers. BMC Health Serv Res. 2019;19(1):1–11.

75. Harrad R, Cosentino C, Keasley R, Sulla F. Spiritual care in nursing: an overview of the measures used to assess spiritual care provision and related factors amongst nurses. Acta Biomed. 2019;90(4-s):44–55.
76. Bétrémieux P, Mannoni C. Neonatal palliative care and culture. Arch Pediatr. 2013;20(9):1000–5.
77. Schuster-Wallace C, Nouvet E, Rigby I, Krishnaraj G, de Laat S, Schwartz L, et al. Culturally sensitive palliative care in humanitarian action: lessons from a critical interpretive synthesis of culture in palliative care literature. Palliat Support Care. 2021;20:1–11.
78. Singh H, Haghayegh AT, Shah R, Cheung L, Wijekoon S, Reel K, et al. A qualitative exploration of allied health providers' perspectives on cultural humility in palliative and end-of-life care. BMC Palliat Care. 2023;22(1):92.
79. Krok D. The role of meaning in life within the relations of religious coping and psychological well-being. J Relig Health. 2015;54(6):2292–308.
80. Armentrout D. Living with grief following removal of infant life support: parents' perspectives. Crit Care Nurs Clin North Am. 2009;21(2):253–65.
81. Paris J, Kragt J. Bereavement and religion online: stillbirth, neonatal loss, and parental religiosity. Sociol Educ Scholarsh. 2013;11:657–74.
82. Meert KL, Thurston CS, Briller SH. The spiritual needs of parents at the time of their child's death in the pediatric intensive care unit and during bereavement: a qualitative study. Pediatr Crit Care Med. 2005;6(4):420–7.
83. Sarti AJ, Sutherland S, Meade M, Shemie S, Landriault A, Vanderspank-Wright B, et al. The experiences of family members of deceased organ donors and suggestions to improve the donation process: a qualitative study. CMAJ. 2022;194(30):E1054–e61.
84. Zumstein-Shaha M, Ferrell B, Economou D. Nurses' response to spiritual needs of cancer patients. Eur J Oncol Nurs. 2020;48:101792.
85. Rushton CH. Moral resilience: a capacity for navigating moral distress in critical care. AACN Adv Crit Care. 2016;27(1):111–9.
86. Velosa T, Caldeira S, Capelas ML. Depression and spiritual distress in adult palliative patients: a cross-sectional study. Religions. 2017;8(8):156.
87. Celano T, Harris S, Sawyer AT, Hamilton T. Promoting spiritual well-being among nurses. Nurse Lead. 2022;20(2):188–92.

Spiritual Care for Children in the End-of-Life Setting

Sara Stage Voetmann and Dorte Toudal Viftrup

Abstract Both healthy and life-threatened ill children and youth exhibit thoughts and feelings of a spiritual, existential, and/or religious nature. These thoughts and feelings increase when a child is confronted with serious illness and/or impending death. This chapter presents literature on how to care spiritually for children in an end-of-life setting, whether they are relatives of a dying family member or terminally ill themselves. We introduce cases from an ongoing empirical study. The study is based on 17 qualitative research interviews with children and youth from 6 to 23 years of age and numerous visits in hospices across Denmark from the fall 2021 until spring 2023. The children and youth are relatives of either a mother, a father, a grandparent, a great grandparent, or a spouse who is dying. Four aspects seemed particularly important in terms of providing spiritual care for children. These are: (1) The caring conflict, (2) The conversation, (3) The confrontation with death, and (4) Alone in my world. This chapter provides perspectives and concrete guidance on how to care for and communicate with children at different age stages about their existential concerns in an end-of-life setting.

Keywords Spiritual care · Spiritual communication · Existential communication Children · Youth · End-of-life care · Palliative care

S. S. Voetmann (✉) · D. T. Viftrup
Research Unit for General Practice, Department of Public Health, University of Southern Denmark, Odense, Denmark
e-mail: svoetmann@health.sdu.dk; dviftrup@health.sdu.dk

M. C. Best (ed.), *Spiritual Care in Palliative Care*,
https://doi.org/10.1007/978-3-031-50864-6_35

1 Introduction

When adults experience serious illness up close and death becomes imminent, thoughts and needs of an existential and spiritual nature increase [1, 2]. This is also the case for terminally ill children or children who are relatives of dying family members [3–5]. Both healthy and life-threatened ill children and youth exhibit thoughts and feelings of a spiritual, existential, and/or religious nature, for example about prayer, God, and the afterlife [6–8], and children's personal spirituality is important for their experience of hope and their ability to cope with severe illness [9]. There is evidence to suggest that spirituality contributes to positive functioning in childhood and adolescence [10, 11]. Spiritually engaged children may exhibit more prosocial behaviour and healthier coping mechanisms in dealing with life's challenges [12, 13]. It may lead to a sense of meaning and purpose in life, which contributes to children's motivation and overall life satisfaction, when adults nuture their spirituality [14].

Several studies emphasise the importance of caring for children's spirituality when they are confronted with severe illness or death [15]. Spiritual care is crucial to the well-being of children and adolescents in times of illness and hospitalisation when the goal is to provide holistic care [3, 16–18]. Older studies have found that children use spirituality to give meaning to their grieving process [19], and children's perception of an ongoing and personal relationship with God may be a primary component to effective coping [20]. Furthermore, studies indicate that children of seriously ill parents are more likely to develop emotional and behavioural problems than their peers with healthy parents, and their ability to perform and socialise in school and education are affected [21–23]. Parental death increases the risk of depression, post-traumatic stress, affective disorders, need for antidepressant medications, physical health problems, and increased mortality later in life [24–26]. It may be expected that these risks can be reduced if children are spiritually supported and cared for when they experience severe illness or risk of death themselves or among close family members. However, there seem to be several barriers for caring spiritually for children in healthcare settings.

2 Barriers for Spiritual Care

Several barriers for spiritual care and spiritual conversations with children have been reported by healthcare professionals (HCPs). A study found that even experienced nurses who are confident in discussing both death and end-of-life care goals with patients have reported great anxiety in discussing spiritual, religious, or existential concerns [29]. Several Danish qualitative studies show that spiritual care provided during parents' cancer illness is insufficient due to HCPs' fear of being emotionally overwhelmed and lacking practical training in communicating with children about spiritual concerns [30–32]. Although spiritual care is essential in paediatric palliative care, few providers receive training in communicating with ill children about spirituality [15]. A literature review highlighted a lack of knowledge and time as the main challenges in integrating spiritual care into the clinical practice of paediatric care [16]. A New Zealand qualitative study examining how HCPs working in paediatrics understand and practice spiritual care, found that there was a lack of training available in the spiritual care for children. The study suggested that more education and opportunities for peer- and self-reflection would support HCPs to develop an awareness of their own views on spiritual care and enhance their practice [33].

Evidence about how HCPs should talk to children and youth about their existential and spiritual thoughts and needs is limited [32, 34]. Furthermore, religiosity and spirituality are considered private and not a commonly shared topic of conversation in Denmark [35, 36], and studies have found limited resources among Danes for coping with spiritual, existential, and religious concerns when faced with crises [37–39]. This is thought to be linked to society's increased secularisation, detraditionalisation, and individualisation [40, 41], where even religious Danes exhibit a high degree of private and individualised spirituality [36, 42]. The limited spiritual and existential verbalization among Danish adults may affect children and youth. Although Danish children and youth wish to talk about existential and spiritual issues, only a few of them talk with their parents or other adults about death, the soul, the afterlife, the meaning of life, justice/injustice, identity, loneliness, belonging, or similar major life questions [4, 43]. Several Danish studies in spiritual care training point to the importance of increasing spiritual reflections and language among the HCPs to alleviate their experience of anxiety and feelings of helplessness, while providing highly needed spiritual conversations and care to patients and relatives [44–48]. These results suggest that children living in societies influenced by secularisation, detraditionalisation, and individualisation might have a great need, as well as limited possibilities, for spiritual care and conversation with HCPs when they experience serious illness or death up close.

The purpose of this chapter is to provide research-based knowledge for HCPs in low-religious contexts on how to best care spiritually and have spiritual conversations with children who are severely ill, dying, or relatives of terminally ill patients.

The chapter will present a 'how-to' approach to spiritual care and conversations with children. A Danish study on spiritual care for children who are relatives of patients in hospice is integrated to shed light on the barriers to caring spiritually for children and for anchoring the approach in the 'voices of the children'. This study is combined with definitions on spiritual care for children and recent published Danish guidelines on spiritual care in palliative care [49]. These guidelines are a Danish adaption of the Dutch guidelines [50]. Both guidelines are based on the international literature on spiritual care as well as input from patients in all phases of illness from HCPs and other relevant organisations.

3 Defining Spiritual Care for Children

Despite several definitions of spiritual care for children, research to date suggests that U.S., Canadian, Australian, Scandinavian, and several other European health care systems do not adequately meet the needs of seriously ill children or those with an affected relative [51–56]. Even though definitions do not facilitate spiritual care for children, they provide understanding of the purpose of spiritual care for children. For this chapter, we define spiritual care for children based on the World Health Organisation's (WHO) holistic concept of pain. The WHO defines *spiritual pain* as one of the four central focus areas in palliative care alongside physical, psychological, and social pain in their definition of *total pain* [57]. This understanding of total pain is evident in the Danish Health Authority's development of '*Recommendations for palliative care for children, youth, and their families*' where spiritual care is defined as: '*... attention to the existential suffering of the child and relatives, that means, attention to the degree to which the disease causes consideration of justice/injustice, meaning of life and death, or the existence or absence of a higher power. In addition, the focus is on how the family lives with the impotence caused by a life-threatening illness, whether the family manages to preserve or restore courage, hope, and meaning, and whether there are religious considerations'* [58]. This is in line with the definitions in both the Danish and the Dutch guidelines where *spiritual care* includes general psychosocial (secular), spiritual, religious, and existential aspects of patient support and care [57, 59–62].

4 The Empirical Study

The focus of the empirical study was to obtain specific knowledge about the existential and spiritual needs and resources which children and youth experience when they are relatives of a seriously ill or dying patient in hospice [63]. The study comprises 17 semi-structured, qualitative research interviews with children and youth from 6 to 23 years of age. All participants were relatives of either a mother, a father, a spouse, or a close grandparent who was seriously ill. The children were recruited via four Danish hospices. The initial contact with the children was facilitated by a contact person at the hospice, often a nurse, a psychologist, or the hospice chaplain, who knew the family well. We only include extracts from the data for illustrative purposes in this chapter. The study has been published in full elsewhere [64].

5 'How-to' Spiritually Care for Children

When reviewing the study data and existing literature, four aspects seemed particularly important to better understand and address the barriers experienced by the HCPs, and to provide spiritual care and conversations with children and youth when they are seriously ill, dying, or relatives of terminally ill patients. These are: (1) The caring-conflict, (2) The conversation, (3) The confrontation with death, and (4) Alone in my world.

5.1 The Caring Conflict: Intuitively Care, Intuitively Restrain

The most significant barrier for caring spiritually for children seems to be a reluctance among HCPs to discuss spiritual, religious, and/or existential concerns with children [29], and a Danish study points to HCPs' fear of being emotionally overwhelmed and lacking practical training in communicating with children about spiritual concerns [32]. However, as religious and spiritual matters are rarely talked about in public or in institutionalised contexts in the Nordic countries [65], adult Danes have a sparse vocabulary for spiritual concerns and may therefore find it difficult figuring out what to say or which words to use. Danes, and perhaps also people from other low-religious contexts, lack experience in communicating about spiritual concerns, and this may be one reason for the intuitive reluctance of HCPs to initiate spiritual conversations with children. It can be problematic if adults around children inadvertently leave them with unanswered questions, frustrations, and notions of a spiritual nature. When conducting the study among children who are relatives of patients in hospice, we also came across reluctance among the HCPs for involving children in the study.

We observed how the children's life circumstances seemed to trigger an intuitive caring response in the HCPs with a strong desire to support and help, but at the same time the HCPs might be concerned about increasing the child's pain by asking about thoughts and feelings of a spiritual nature and their life circumstances. The spiritual care and conversations with these children seemed to unfold in a field of tension between intuitive care on one hand and restraint on the other. The HCPs felt a professional or human responsibility to support and care spiritually for the child, and at the same time this intuitive caring response seemed to entail an insecurity about how to address the child, how to say the right things, and a general concern about upsetting the child and reinforcing their pain. It seems that HCPs experience a caring-conflict where they find it difficult to know how to best care spiritually for young children [32]. However, it is an important conflict, as children should not be left alone with their questions, worries, nor needs of a spiritual nature. These children are vulnerable because of their situation and age-related development [66], and therefore, to be concerned about not 'doing harm' seems highly relevant.

In order to address this caring conflict as well as the HCPs' lack of familiarity with spiritual conversations, the guidelines [49] suggest that HCPs explore and become aware of their personal spirituality, feelings, and values. For HCPs to be able to listen to the spirituality of the child, they need to be able to 'hear' their own spirituality, and it requires an openness towards spiritual issues to be able to care and converse spiritually with a child [49]. Courses involving spiritual self-reflection exercises are recommended, as well as shared spiritual reflections with peers and co-workers to develop a shared language for spiritual care and conversations [45]. Furthermore, it seems highly relevant to improve the HCPs' communication skills for attending to both sides of the caring conflict.

5.2 The Conversation

During the empirical study, we found that young relatives experienced relief when they participated in a research interview. They found their existential or spiritual concerns, ideas, and reflections neither foreign nor difficult to talk about. This might indicate that HCPs should be less reluctant to initiate spiritual conversations with children. A qualitative research interview resembles an ordinary conversation, but with the essential difference that the conversation is structured and somewhat controlled by the researcher. Qualitative research interviews allow the interviewees to express their experiences in their own words and thereby give the researcher the opportunity to be informed by what they feel, think, and experience [67]. When we, as qualitative researchers with health science and psychology backgrounds, talk to children and youth who are relatives of a dying family member at a hospice, we let ourselves be emotionally touched by their stories, both as researchers and as humans. We allow ourselves to be touched in order to be able to listen carefully, and to connect with the child and the story being told [68]. This curious, wondering approach that qualitative methods require entails that all good intentions to act and 'fix' must be set aside. We are present and listen without having any other agenda than to connect with the child, and to be touched by their stories. HCPs may be inspired by this approach to listening, when caring spiritually for children who are dying or are relatives of a dying family member.

The guidelines emphasise the importance of showing genuine interest in the story of the patient and what matters most to the specific human being when facilitating a spiritual conversation [49]. It is also important to use open questions, notice the non-verbal signals, and not answer one's own questions. The Danish psychologist Per Schultz Jørgensen [69] describes how meeting a child with nothing but oneself as a human being might impact how the child experiences and help them master their world [69]. He explains how adults can make a significant difference for the child through presence, authenticity, and by listening while the child share his or her stories and life circumstances [69]. It is not primarily through professional skills, experience, and competences, but as a fellow human being that the adult should relate to the child. Through the trusting relationship, the adult can contribute to creating a space where the child can reflect on and get to better understand her or his spiritual concerns, needs, and language. This 'relational space', which the adult creates, where the child feels valuable and understood, seems to be the foundation for spiritual care [70].

During an interview, Simon (aged 18, who is the son of a dying parent) confirmed how essential the sentient element and body language are in the relationship, and how much influence authentic presence has on his experience of care. Furthermore, Simon seemed to be able to differentiate between authentic interest and forced pity. Simon explained:

Interviewer	*It sounds like you're not too keen on that pity?*
Simon	*No. [...]*
Interviewer	*How do you know if they want to talk to you? Do you have a feeling about it?*
Simon	*That's like. You can kind of feel that when they start talking about it. [...] It's just like that, then they come 'oh it's such a shame and I feel so sorry for you, and I think about you so much'.*
Interviewer	*Yes. And those are the ones you feel you shouldn't talk to?*
Simon	*Yes.*
Interviewer	*What do those you want to talk to say? [...].*
Simon	*They don't really say anything.*

This extract illustrates how attention and presence are not to be equated with pity. Simon seemed to sense who he can talk to about his life circumstances in an authentic way. Likewise, the quote illustrates that spiritual care also has a sentient and non-verbal dimension [63]. With their body language and by being present, HCPs can contribute to building a relation in which the child experiences themself as valuable and significant.

5.3 The Confrontation with Death

Being confronted with death at an early age elicits thoughts and feelings in children which they should not be left alone with. Many of the children in the study had talked to their families about what they imagine will happen to the deceased after death—or what will not happen. Some of the children expressed the conviction that they 'don't believe in *that* way', but still they imagined that there is 'something' after death. Their stories and ideas about this afterlife may be rooted in Christian terminology about, for example, the resurrection, in ideas about reincarnation, or a transcendent connection to their deceased family member. Perhaps, growing up in a secularised, detraditionalised, and individualised society provides a broader and looser perspective on the afterlife; however, death and the afterlife are important topics of conversations for children [71]. The guidelines [49] present the model of *Ars Moriendi* [*The art of Dying*] [72] a as spiritual care model for discussing death and dying. It involves five themes where different relevant questions are suggested.

The themes are: (1) self—other (autonomy), (2) doing—allowing (suffering), (3) holding on—letting go (saying goodbye), (4) remembering—forgetting (unfinished business), and (5) believing—knowing (hope). We believe these themes are also relevant for children; however, they should be adapted to the child's age and general development. Based on a guide for spiritual care and conversations with children at three different age levels [64], it is recommended that adults support the preschool child by helping them show, express, and understand their feelings concerning death. The school-age child needs adults who listen to and acknowledge the child's understandings, experiences, and feelings as well as challenge their rigid thinking about death and other spiritual concerns. The teenager needs adults who are willing to be there for them physically, mentally, socially, and spiritually in a genuine relationship [64].

Being confronted with either one's own or a close family member's impending death may affect the way time is perceived [63]. This awareness about time is also evident in our empirical study, which suggested that the children became more aware of time and the quality of time they spend with their dying family member, as well as how this time was limited. For Simon, this realisation led to a desire to make the most of the time left, for example, through creating valuable memories for when his parent died.

> We have been good at creating memories. [...] We have been out traveling a few times. [...] And then we've also been eating out a lot, and just making memories, and just being more homely and such. [...] So really, we have been good at this, and that it doesn't have to be solely a miserable situation, but you can still turn it into something good. Create those extra memories instead of thinking the whole world is against you.

Many of the children aimed for the time spent with a dying family member to ideally be as good as possible. Twenty-one-year-old Agnethe explained:

> And a day wasted, that is, if you waste it on being mad or upset or something like that, you could just really feel that here [at the hospice], that if my mother or father have had a day like that, when they have been a little sad about it, then you will also be sad, if you have to leave it behind. If we have to go in the evening. [...] Then it's like that—it's the kind of day you don't want to end life on. Or you know. End on.

The presence of death seemed to stimulate spiritual conversations in some families, although the confrontation with death is frightening. In this way, the confrontation with death becomes an entrance to deeper relationships and conversations. These conversations can be about what happens to us when we die, what it means to love and to be loved, what makes us happy, and about what matters in life. Per Schultz Jørgensen [66] describes how the child and adult together can create a relational space of trust where the child can share her or his concerns and where these will be met and understood. Through the conversation about death, adults can help and support children to discover the resources of being able to better understand and handle the challenge and crisis of being confronted with imminent death [66].

The children in the empirical study expressed much uncertainty associated with having a dying family member. Particularly in relation to the HCPs, the child would sense things that were unsaid, and concerns and notions about whether there was something that the adults were not telling were often elicited. Thirteen-year-old Vilhelm explained:

Vilhelm	*And there haven't really been any of the doctors who wanted to say anything to us. So, we have had the thing about whether it [death] would happen soon, all the time. That uncertainty.*
Interviewer	*So, the uncertainty. What does uncertainty mean?*
Vilhelm	*That you don't always know when it [death] will happen.*
Interviewer	*Yes.*
Vilhelm	*And that you really want to know, but you don't get to know anything.*

The children were sensitive to the adults around them. They expressed wanting to be involved and informed in a way that suited them, so that they did not have to sense or guess how their mother or father was feeling at the current stage of their illness. Involving and informing children is highly important when caring for children, and it should be done at a level that is adapted to the child's age and current situation [64].

5.4 *Alone in My World*

We have learned from the interviews with children and youth who were relatives of dying parents and other close family members, that they often experience being the only one in the world living with a dying relative. Many of the children describe how they must navigate new, unknown feelings and thoughts, often without having others with whom to reflect or discuss their situation. They often experience being in the world in a different way than their peers. Agnethe, aged 21, who was the daughter of a dying parent, described it this way:

Agnethe	*It has been a very strange presence [existence]. It is also, you could say, right here and now life is developing the fastest.*
Interviewer	*Yes*
Agnethe	*This age group I am in.*
Interviewer	*Exactly.*
Agnethe	*There is a lot of identity and a lot of expression that I haven't had the same opportunity to be a part of. Or whatever you say.*
Interviewer	*Could you try to tell a little more about this, Agnethe? How have you thought about this?*
Agnethe	*Well, everyone, now I say with goosebumps, but all 'normal' young people are out and have lots of friends. Has lots of contact. Um. They go to parties. They go to school. And they have things to attend to. Um. And. Uh. You [long pause] you need that now.*

Agnethe's quote illustrates how she and other children with a dying family member are required to exist on a continuum between ordinary everyday life with school and friends, at the same time as they are confronted with major existential concerns and the impending death of a close family member. This will also be the case for children who are terminally ill themselves in end-of-life care. To live and be in a world that keeps on going, while dying yourself or losing a parent or close family member is a hard task, in which no child should be left alone. The themes (3) holding on—letting go (saying goodbye) or (5) believing—knowing (hope) of the Ars Moriendi model [72] seem highly relevant for facilitating spiritual conversation when a child feels alone in their world. However, it is important that the age of the child is considered. The insights into existential and spiritual concepts in life naturally depend on the age and maturity of the child. A spiritual conversation will vary both in terms of the level of abstraction and duration depending on whether the child is 6 years old, like Dagmar below, or 21 years old like Agnethe. What they have in common is that they want to talk about their experiences and thoughts about death and other spiritual topics. Younger children may alternate between, for example, talking about death and something more daily and concrete. Dagmar says:

Dagmar	*And they have numbers [on the doors] and grandpa's number that's number four.*
Interviewer	*Yes. That's true. He lives in room number four. And then you get the help you need. But the thing with these patients who are here, like your grandfather, is that they have an illness from which they cannot recover.*
Dagmar	*Really! […] And if my grandfather dies somewhere, where should we bury him? Do they have a bury place here?*
Interviewer	*No, they actually they don't have a cemetery, but they have a priest who will help with things like that.*
Dagmar	*But how do you get a person like out [of the house] if they are dead? […]*
Interviewer	*For example, now that your grandfather is here at the hospice, um, what would you say, what is important to you, for example, if someone here, any of these nurses or adults, they have to be really nice to you? Can you name some things? Maybe three or four things you'd like them to do for you?*
Dagmar	*Lollipop. Or not lollipop. Popsicle stick. And do you have lollipops?*

Preschool children do not yet understand that death is permanent, and they think adults talk about death literally and concretely. Therefore, they will not understand metaphorical phrases like: 'He finally had peace' or 'she passed away'. When it comes to grief reactions, the little child has not yet developed a wide repertoire of emotional expression nor a clear perception of their own emotions. Therefore, preschool children need adults who can help them show, express, and understand their feelings related to death and loss, as well as meeting them with positive emotions, understanding their logic, and concrete care [64].

Older and more mature children may express themselves philosophically and reflect on symbolism in relation to what was significant for their dying relative. Agnethe talked about how she saw a connection between her mother's room at the hospice, which faced the garden, and the symbolism the garden represented for her mother's life:

Agnethe	*My mother got [room] number nine with a view over the garden and she has always been such a real garden person. [...] Really green fingers and knows the names of all flowers and very garden loving.*
Interviewer	*Is this significant or can you say something more about it?*
Agnethe	*Mmm. Um. Yes. So, I just think it's a bit of, what do you say, existential reflection.*
Interviewer	*Yes?*
Agnethe	*Of what happens in one's life. So that my [mother] gets the view and the ending she wants. Um. Which can also represent her life. Um. And like that her whole existence, she just kind of 'of course she has to have a garden view', when that's what she likes.*

Teenagers and young adults understand and think more abstractly and personally about life and death than the younger child. They begin to grasp the complexity of life, the world, death, and spirituality. Therefore, they need spiritual care to be personal and connected to their concrete reality and understanding of self [64]. The teenagers' and young adults' increased existential and abstract thoughts are highly centred on themselves. This also influences their grief reactions and how they deal with death. They may become more preoccupied with how others see them, and their external self-perception becomes overactivated, and it can lead to social isolation and a sense of loneliness, where they often feel that nobody understands who they are and how they feel. The teenagers or young adults need adults who are willing to be there for them physically, mentally, socially, and spiritually, who will provide care, challenge, and support them by engaging in conversations about their existential and spiritual thoughts. The teenager or young adult needs HCPs who bring themselves and their own existential and spiritual thoughts, doubts, experiences, and reflections into the conversation and into a genuine relation [64].

6 'Are You Coming Back Tomorrow'?

In this chapter, we have integrated existing knowledge on spiritual care and communication with children and youth with proposals on 'how to' provide spiritual care for children at different age stages combined with empirical examples from a current research study [63]. By the time you read this chapter, the children whose voices you have heard will all have lost someone they loved dearly. Prior to the death, they might have been confronted with shorter, longer, or several episodes of illness which have influenced their daily life and who they are. Not all life-threatening illness ultimately results in death. This points to the importance of integrating and being aware of existential and spiritual dimensions of life not only in palliative care, under the auspices of hospice or another end-of-life setting, but also in serious illness which involves children.

The caring conflict is real and the HCPs are required to navigate it. Existing knowledge points to benefits for HCPs investigating their own spirituality (spiritual self-reflection) both individually and with colleagues. Through this, HCPs may increase and refine their language for spiritual matters which may entail facilitating and initiating conversations about spiritual concerns more easily. Likewise, creating the relational spaces where the child or youth experiences a trusting atmosphere and feels valued and understood seems to be the foundation for spiritual conversations. Without being able solve the complexity of the caring conflict, this chapter argues that children and youth needs relationships and relational spaces for conversations about their spiritual concerns. Perhaps that is why we have sometimes been asked: 'Are you coming back tomorrow?' after an interview with a child who was relative of a patient in a hospice. The first contact and initiative for conversation may seem like the biggest challenge. Do it! Vilhelm, aged 13 years, talked about how it had become a little easier for him to talk about his parent's cancer because he was given opportunities to talk about it with adults and peers.

Vilhelm	*Well, It was very difficult for me in the beginning. [...] But now after I have opened up more to people. Having been in Shadow Children [grief group for children and young people] and talking to different people and such, it has become much easier.*
Interviewer	*Yes. And what does it do? How does it feel?*
Vilhelm	*So, there is not the same lump in the throat as there was the first time we had to talk about it.*

Death and the afterlife are important conversation topics for children, even though children in low-religiosity societies have a more broad and loose perspective on the afterlife. The Ars Moriendi model [72] can be adapted to children's ages and function as a spiritual care approach. Confrontation with death can affect the way children perceive time, and it can become an entrance to deeper relationships and conversations where adults can support the child. Involving and informing the children about their parents' or another close family member's illness is highly important when caring for them.

Children confronted with death often experience being alone in their world, while having to navigate new, unknown feelings and thoughts. They live on a continuum between an ordinary everyday life with school and friends, at the same time as they are confronted with major existential concerns and impending death. It is important that no child should be left alone in that, but when facilitating spiritual care and conversation, the age of the child should be considered.

The most touching and motivating moments we have experienced in our interviews with children who are relatives of hospice patients were, how these children find it meaningful to be able to contribute by telling their story and thereby help other children in a similar situation. One interpretation could be that this gesture might be an expression of finding something meaningful in what otherwise seems a meaningless situation. We will let the young relatives have the last word, because if you ask them what their best advice is for another child in a similar situation, they answer: '*Find someone to talk to*'.

Acknowledgements The authors wish to send a warm word of gratitude to the participating children and youth. Thank you for your courage, your willingness to share your experiences, and giving us your time when it was most precious.

References

1. Jones JM, Cohen SR, Zimmermann C, Rodin G. Quality of life and symptom burden in cancer patients admitted to an acute palliative care unit. J Palliat Care. 2010;26:94–102.
2. Thune-Boyle IC, Stygall JA, Keshtgar MR, Newman SP. Do religious/spiritual coping strategies affect illness adjustment in patients with cancer? A systematic review of the literature. Soc Sci Med. 2006;63:151–64.
3. Hart D, Schneider D. Spiritual care for children with cancer. Semin Oncol Nurs. 1997;13:263–70.
4. Larsen I, Sørensen PG. Gudsforestillinger I Folkeskolen (god-images in primary school children). In: Højsgaard MT, Iversen HR, editors. Gudstro I Danmark (faith in god in Denmark). København: Anis; 2005.
5. Pandya SP. Spirituality for wellbeing of bereaved children in residential care: insights for spiritually sensitive child-centred social work across country contexts. Child Adolesc Soc Work J. 2018;35:181–95.
6. Coles R. The spiritual life of children. Boston: Houghton Mifflin Company; 1990.
7. Pehler SR. Children's spiritual response: validation of the nursing diagnosis spiritual distress. Nurs Diagn. 1997;8:55–66.
8. Smith J, Mcsherry W. Spirituality and child development: a concept analysis. J Adv Nurs. 2004;45:307–15.
9. Lima NNR, Do Nascimento VB, De Carvalho SMF, Neto MLR, Moreira MM, Brasil AQ, Junior FTC, De Oliveira GF, Reis AOA. Spirituality in childhood cancer care. Neuropsychiatr Dis Treat. 2013;9:1539–44.
10. Bryant-Davis T, Ellis MU, Burke-Maynard E, Moon N, Counts PA, Anderson G. Religiosity, spirituality, and trauma recovery in the lives of children and adolescents. Prof Psychol Res Pract. 2012;43:306.
11. Cotton S, Larkin E, Hoopes A, Cromer BA, Rosenthal SL. The impact of adolescent spirituality on depressive symptoms and health risk behaviors. J Adolesc Health. 2005;36:529.
12. Koenig HG. Research on religion, spirituality, and mental health: a review. Can J Psychiatry. 2009;54:283–91.
13. Koenig HG. Religion, spirituality, and health: the research and clinical implications. ISRN Psychiatry. 2012;2012:278730.
14. Wong P. Positive psychology 2.0: towards a balanced interactive model of the good life. Can Psychol. 2011;52:69–81.
15. Ferrell B, Wittenberg E, Battista V, Walker G. Nurses' experiences of spiritual communication with seriously Iii children. J Palliat Med. 2016;19:1166–70.
16. Alvarenga WA, De Carvalho EC, Caldeira S, Vieira M, Nascimento LC. The possibilities and challenges in providing pediatric spiritual care. J Child Health Care. 2017;21:435–45.
17. Elkins M, Cavendish R. Developing a plan for pediatric spiritual care. Holist Nurs Pract. 2004;18:179–84; Quiz 185–6.

18. Feudtner C, Haney J, Dimmers MA. Spiritual care needs of hospitalized children and their families: a National Survey of Pastoral Care Providers' perceptions. Pediatrics. 2003;111:E67–72.
19. Andrews CR, Marotta SA. Spirituality and coping among grieving children: a preliminary study. Couns Values. 2005;50:38–50.
20. Hassan M, Mehta K. Grief experience of bereaved Malay/Muslim youths in Singapore: the spiritual dimension. Int J Child Spiritual. 2010;15:45–57.
21. Grabiak BR, Bender CM, Puskar KR. The impact of parental cancer on the adolescent: an analysis of the literature. Psycho-Oncology. 2007;16:127–37.
22. Huizinga GA, Visser A, Van Der Graaf WT, Hoekstra HJ, Stewart RE, Hoekstra-Weebers JE. Family-oriented multilevel study on the psychological functioning of adolescent children having a mother with cancer. Psychooncology. 2011;20:730–7.
23. Osborn T. The psychosocial impact of parental cancer on children and adolescents: a systematic review. Psychooncology. 2007;16:101–26.
24. Appel CW, Johansen C, Christensen J, Frederiksen K, Hjalgrim H, Dalton SO, Dencker A, Dige J, Boge P, Dyregrov A, Mikkelsen OA, Lund LW, Hoybye MT, Bidstrup PE. Risk of use of antidepressants among children and young adults exposed to the death of a parent. Epidemiology. 2016;27:578–85.
25. Appel CW, Johansen C, Deltour I, Frederiksen K, Hjalgrim H, Dalton SO, Dencker A, Dige J, Boge P, Rix BA, Dyregrov A, Engelbrekt P, Helweg E, Mikkelsen OA, Hoybye MT, Bidstrup PE. Early parental death and risk of hospitalization for affective disorder in adulthood. Epidemiology. 2013;24:608–15.
26. Berg L, Rostila M, Saarela J, Hjern A. Parental death during childhood and subsequent school performance. Pediatrics. 2014;133:682–9.
27. Melhem NM, Walker M, Moritz G, Brent DA. Antecedents and sequelae of sudden parental death in offspring and surviving caregivers. Arch Pediatr Adolesc Med. 2008;162:403–10.
28. Rod NH, Bengtsson J, Budtz-Jørgensen E, Clipet-Jensen C, Taylor-Robinson D, Andersen A-MN, Dich N, Rieckmann A. Trajectories of childhood adversity and mortality in early adulthood: a population-based cohort study. Lancet. 2020;396:489–97.
29. Malloy P, Virani R, Kelly K, Munévar C. Beyond bad news: communication skills of nurses in palliative care. J Hosp Palliat Nurs. 2010;12:166–74.
30. Dencker A, Kristiansen M, Rix BA, Bøge P, Tjørnhøj-Thomsen T. Contextualisation of patient-centred care: a comparative qualitative study of healthcare professionals' approaches to communicating with seriously ill patients about their dependent children. Eur J Cancer Care. 2018;27:E12792.
31. Dencker A, Murray SA, Mason B, Rix BA, Bøge P, Tjørnhøj-Thomsen T. Disrupted biographies and balancing identities: a qualitative study of cancer patients' communication with healthcare professionals about dependent children. Eur J Cancer Care. 2019;28:E12991.
32. Dencker A, Rix BA, Bøge P, Tjørnhøj-Thomsen T. A qualitative study of doctors' and nurses' barriers to communicating with seriously ill patients about their dependent children. Psycho-Oncology. 2017;26:2162–7.
33. Parkinson S, Bray Y, Kool B. How do health professionals provide spiritual care to seriously ill children? Int J Child Spiritual. 2020;25:64–77.
34. Buchwald D, Delmar C, Schantz-Laursen B. How children handle life when their mother or father is seriously ill and dying. Scand J Caring Sci. 2012;26:228–35.
35. Andersen PB, Lüchau P. Individualisering Og Aftraditionalisering Af Danskernes Religiøse Værdier. In: Gundelach P, editor. Små Og Store Forandringer. Danskernes Værdier Siden 1981. København: Hans Reizels Forlag; 2011.
36. Viftrup DT, Hvidt NC, Buus N. Religious coping in a Christian minority group: a qualitative study among Pentecostal Danes. Nordic J Relig Soc. 2017;30:115–35.
37. La Cour P. Danskernes Gud I Krise [the Danes' god in crisis]. In: Højsgaard MT, Iversen HR, editors. Gudstro I Danmark [Belief in god in Denmark]. København: Anis; 2005.
38. Pedersen HF, Pedersen CG, Pargament KI, Zachariae R. Religious coping and quality of life among severely ill lung patients in a secular society. Int J Psychol Relig. 2012;23:188–203.

39. Pedersen HF, Pedersen CG, Pargament KI, Zachariae R. Coping without religion? Religious coping, quality of life, and existential well-being among lung disease patients and matched controls in a secular society. Res Soc Sci Study Relig. 2013;24:163–92.
40. Stimpel BB, Raakjær O. Religiøsitet, Spiritualitet Og Død [Religiosity, spirituality and dead]. In: Steenfeldt VØ, Hansen FT, editors. Hospice – Æstetik, Eksistens, Omsorg. København: Munksgaard; 2017.
41. Zuckerman P. Society without god. What the least religious nations can tell us about contentment. New York: New York University Press; 2008.
42. Viftrup DT, La Cour P, Buus N, Hvidt NC. Religious transformation among Danish Pentecostals following personal crisis and group psychotherapy: a qualitative study. J Spiritual Ment Health. 2016;18:1–23.
43. Thomsen IH, Mejdal S. Hospice I Børnehøjde [Online]. Skive: Hospicelimfjord; 2020. Available: Https://Hospicelimfjord.Dk/Hospice-I-Boernehoejde/. Accessed: 08/07/24.
44. Roessler KK, Lindemann F-W. How to cope with anxiety in hospital settings: evaluation of a professional training. Expository Times. 2014;126:63–70.
45. Viftrup DT, Laursen K, Hvidt NC. Developing an educational course in spiritual care: an action research study at two Danish hospices. Religions. 2021a;12:827.
46. Viftrup DT, Nissen R, Søndergaard J, Hvidt NC. Four aspects of spiritual care: a phenomenological action research study on practicing and improving spiritual care at two Danish hospices. Palliat Care Soc Pract. 2021b;15:26323524211050646.
47. Viftrup DT, Rosenbæk F, Damgaard HH, Hemdrup M, Nielsen M, Nissen RD. Caring spiritually: a study on spiritual care training in a hospice setting. J Hosp Palliat Nurs. 2023;25:156–64.
48. Voetmann SS, Hvidt NC, Viftrup DT. Verbalizing spiritual needs in palliative care: a qualitative interview study on verbal and non-verbal communication in two Danish hospices. BMC Palliat Care. 2022;21:3.
49. Hvidt NC, Madsen LD, Ogstrup AJ, Sandborg-Olsen AM, Stimpel BB, Villadsen B, Pedersen CL, Kragh CF, Vibe CL, Mathiesen D, Viftrup DT, Hansen H, Kopp K, Bonde S, Hansen MB, Adsersen M, Lassen TH. Eksistentielle Og Åndelige Aspekter I Palliativ Indsats. In: Dmcg-Pal, editor. 1.0. Sekretariatet For Kliniske Retningslinjer På Kræftområdet; 2023.
50. Iknl 2018. Existential and spiritual aspects of palliative care. In: Iknl (Ed.) 2.0.. Netherlands Comprehensive Cancer Organisation.
51. Johnston DL, Nagel K, Friedman DL, Meza JL, Hurwitz CA, Friebert S. Availability and use of palliative care and end-of-life services for pediatric oncology patients. J Clin Oncol. 2008;26:4646–50.
52. Morrison RS, Maroney-Galin C, Kralovec PD, Meier DE. The growth of palliative care programs in United States hospitals. J Palliat Med. 2005;8:1127–34.
53. Van Aerde J, Gorodzinsky F, Society CP, Fetus & Committee, N. Guidelines for health care professionals supporting families experiencing a perinatal loss. Paediatr Child Health. 2001;6:469–77.
54. Weber M, Alvariza A, Kreicbergs U, Sveen J. Communication in families with minor children following the loss of a parent to cancer. Eur J Oncol Nurs. 2019;39:41–6.
55. Wickramasinghe LM, Yeo ZZ, Chong PH, Johnston B. Communicating with young children who have a parent dying of a life-limiting illness: a qualitative systematic review of the experiences and impact on healthcare, social and spiritual care professionals. BMC Palliat Care. 2022;21:125.
56. Widger K, Davies D, Drouin DJ, Beaune L, Daoust L, Farran RP, Humbert N, Nalewajek F, Rattray M, Rugg M. Pediatric patients receiving palliative care in Canada: results of a multicenter review. Arch Pediatr Adolesc Med. 2007;161:597–602.
57. World Health Organization. Definition of palliative care [Online]. Available: Http://Www.Who.Int/Cancer/Palliative/Definition/En/. Accessed: 08/07/24.
58. Sundhedsstyrelsen. Anbefalinger for Palliative Indsatser Til Børn, Unge Og Deres Familier. København: Sundhedsstyrelsen; 2018.

59. Greasley P, Chiu LF, Gartland M. The concept of spiritual care in mental health nursing. J Adv Nurs. 2001;33:629–37.
60. Puchalski C, Romer AL. Taking a spiritual history allows clinicians to understand patients more fully. J Palliat Med. 2000;3(1):129–37.
61. Puchalski CM, Lunsford B, Harris MH, Miller RT. Interdisciplinary spiritual care for seriously ill and dying patients: a collaborative model. Cancer J. 2006;12:398–416.
62. Paal P, Roser T, Frick E. Developments in spiritual care education in German – speaking countries. BMC Med Educ. 2014;14:1472–6920.
63. Voetmann SS. Ongoing PhD project: Children and youth' spiritual and existential needs and vocabulary - spiritual and existential care for children who are relatives of lifethreateningly ill family members. University of Southern Denmark. 2021.
64. Viftrup DT, Voetmann SS. Caring existentially and spiritually for young children and close grandchildren of life-threatened cancer patients in secularized Denmark. Semin Oncol Nurs. 2023;39:151484.
65. La Cour P, Hvidt NC. Research on meaning-making and health in secular society: secular, spiritual and religious existential orientations. Soc Sci Med. 2010;71:1292–9.
66. Jørgensen PS. Robuste Børn: Giv Dit Barn Ansvar, Livsmod Og Tiltro Til Sig Selv, Kbh., Kristeligt Dagblad; 2017.
67. Kvale S, Brinkmann S. Interview. København: Hans Reitzels Forlag; 2009.
68. Hansen FT, Thorsted AC. Den Fænomenologiske Attitude. In: Berørthed NOU, editor. At Tænke Med Hjertet – En Grundbog I Eksistentiel Praksisfænomenologi. 1st ed. Aarhus: Forlaget Klim; 2022.
69. Jørgensen PS. Broen – Til Det Andet Menneske: Fra Den Første Kontakt Til Den Dybe Samhørighed, Kbh., Kristeligt Dagblad; 2016.
70. Viftrup DT, Hvidt NC. Det Relationelle Som Fundament For Omsorg. In: Hvidt EA, Søndergaard J, Grønning A, editors. Relationer I Sundhedsvæsenet: Hvorfor Og Hvordan? 1st ed. Frederiksberg: Samfundslitteratur; 2021.
71. Viftrup DT, Andersen AH, Nissen RD. Det Var Sgu Meget Dejligt At Snakke Om Døden: Et Studie Om At Tale Med Børn Om Døden. Omsorg. 2022;2022:69–73.
72. Leget C. Art of living, art of dying: spiritual care for a good death. Jessica Kingsley Publishers; 2017.

Spiritual Care for Adolescents and Young Adults

Suvi-Maria Saarelainen and Jonna Ojalammi

Abstract Spiritual care needs are rarely met among adolescents and young adults (AYA) whose lives have been affected by serious illness. The chapter discusses the significance of spirituality for AYAs in palliative care in the context of cancer. By reviewing the literature and introducing notions about both young adult cancer studies and more general palliative care studies, the chapter reveals that the need for information and honest discussion lingers among AYAs in palliative care. Such need for dialogue includes a spiritual and existential component. Furthermore, reflections are required for the formation of mortality salience to allow a dying patient to let go of self-blame and to form the required new identity. Various religious and spiritual elements may provide consolation and comfort in proximity to death. In palliative care, close relationships foster hope, but the proximity of death also challenges important relationships. For those for whom spirituality matters, this creates an opportunity to support an individual in this turmoil and may improve quality of life. As spirituality is a culturally bound term and difficult for young adults themselves to use, it is suggested that future research utilise concepts such as meaning, purpose, and hope.

Keywords AYA · Spirituality · Religion · Meaning · Cancer · Palliative care Spiritual needs · Existential needs · Adolescents · Young adults · Spiritual care

---

S.-M. Saarelainen (✉) · J. Ojalammi
School of Theology, Philosophical Faculty, University of Eastern Finland, Joensuu, Finland
e-mail: suvi-maria.saarelainen@uef.fi; jonna.ojalammi@uef.fi

M. C. Best (ed.), *Spiritual Care in Palliative Care*,
https://doi.org/10.1007/978-3-031-50864-6_36

1 Current State of the Art

Although the overall cure rate for adolescent and young adult (AYA) cancer is 80%, cancer is the most common cause of disease-related death among young people. Annually, 70,000 young people in the United States of America (USA) and 20,000 in Europe are diagnosed with cancer [1–3]. Being diagnosed with cancer as an AYA is especially challenging because the occurrence of cancer at this stage of life disturbs hopes and dreams for the future [4]. From the care perspective, it is known that the age-specific needs of young patients are rarely met [5, 6]. Unmet needs for religious and spiritual counselling have been reported in both the European [7] and USA contexts [8–10]. In the age group of 30–39 years, 21.5% reported unmet needs [8]. Additionally, a qualitative study from Finland found that only a few young adults had any spiritual counselling during their cancer treatment even though most of the interviewees had religious or spiritual struggles during their cancer trajectory. Furthermore, some identified only after the treatment and meetings with the chaplain that they would have appreciated that kind of support much more [7]. In the end-of-life care setting, 38% of caregivers report unmet religious/spiritual needs in the process of letting go of their AYA relative [10]. Many of the young patients report that they do not have religious or spiritual needs during the treatment process: the younger the patient, the less these needs are reported [8]. Based on these notions, this chapter examines current research focusing on studies of AYAs whose lives have been seriously affected by cancer. These findings are likely to be relevant to the experiences of young patients with other diseases undergoing palliative care.

A review of the literature in the field of spiritual and religious coping among AYAs with cancer indicates that the majority of existing studies are quantitative, and the focus is on the USA context [11, 12]. Studies scrutinising the end of life among young patients from the perspective of spirituality are even more limited. For this chapter, we ran a keyword scan in the PubMed database to gain a general understanding of the existing literature. Seventy-four papers were returned with the keywords 'young adult' + 'cancer' + 'end of life' or 'palliative care' + spirituality. Based on the abstract reading, only 11 focused on spirituality in the palliative or end-of-life care of AYAs with cancer. We decided to add 'existential' to the keywords, resulting in an additional 24 papers. Another paper was identified after duplicates were excluded.

To grasp the range of significance of spirituality among AYAs with cancer in palliative care, this chapter ties the identified articles to a larger body of research focusing on young adults' cancer. Additionally, in our keyword scan and literature searches, we identified palliative care papers in which young adults belong to the research group. When relevant, we draw ideas from the scarce studies of spirituality in studies of young adults coping with cancer. This allows us to delve more deeply into the spirituality of AYAs with cancer receiving palliative care.

2 Spirituality, Religiosity, and Existential Aspects Matter

In the few studies focusing on young cancer patients' end-of-life care, the role of spirituality has been discussed especially in relation to the patient's concerns about their own death and dying [13]. In this context, it has been shown that existential themes of meaning and purpose in life and hope can be activated [10, 14–17]. Questions about the reasons for suffering—for example, guilt—may arise [18]. Although death and dying are central themes of spirituality in the end-of-life care of AYAs, there are also many other significant concerns. For example, the stage of life constitutes a unique situation for AYAs compared to significantly older cancer patients: cancer especially interrupts AYAs' lives at a time of significant psychosocial, including spiritual, change [19, 20]. In the AYA years, an individual is still in the process of developing and forming personally significant values. Values and spiritual views are still very fragile at this stage of personality development [21, 22]. Therefore, a cancer diagnosis in the AYA years is likely to impact the personal path of forming spiritual views.

Research has even suggested that younger patients have more religious and spiritual needs than older patients. They may have an increased need for experiencing connection with the transcendent, searching for meaning in life and/or using religious coping practices such as prayer [23]. For those for whom spirituality matters, spiritual well-being is positively correlated with some aspects of psychological adjustment. For instance, increased experience of meaning and peace contributed to better mental health and lowered cancer-related stress. In the long run, personal faith seemed to be the factor to support cancer-related growth among the survivors [24, 25]. A Finnish project has shown that even in secular northern Europe, religious beliefs and practices such as prayer or intercession may unexpectedly become a source of hope for young adults with cancer [16, 26].

AYAs who have been affected by cancer may undergo religious and spiritual struggles. Religious seeking becomes vivid in the narratives of young adults, who describe cancer as prompting a religious process that makes them consider their personal relationship with God. Some even believe God has chosen to give them cancer [11, 27]. AYAs are driven to think about how and what to believe. For example, a personal relationship with God or a higher power through prayer and intercession is found supportive and comforting. Prayer is reported to be especially helpful for young adults when they are afraid or suffering from insomnia or nausea, for example. Cancer prompts young adults to find consolation in turning to God or the supernatural, even if they are unsure as to whom it is that they are turning [11, 26]. At a general level, some young adults experience their religious belief as the power that helps them cope mentally with the disease, and that the significance of religion increases after their diagnosis [11, 12]. Yet, spiritual struggles are also associated with problems with adjustment [24] and the misuse of alcohol [28].

A growing body of research in cancer care and palliative medicine aims to understand the existential problems that may arise, including those of AYAs [29]. Being constantly confronted with disease and the experience of loss may trigger existential concerns about life's finality, isolation, and meaninglessness [30]. Existential suffering with cancer contributes to severe anxiety and depression, as well as the feeling that one is a burden for others, leading to a poor quality of life [31–35].

Support may be needed in facing such uncertainties, such as confirming the realities inherent in a changed life situation, giving emotional support, providing the possibility of being heard and space for reflective discussions of values and existential appraisals, and meaning in life. These all ground the existential care of young adults with cancer [36]. Ragsdale and others [27] found that AYAs who had experienced spiritual struggles addressed their problems through prayer or other religious rituals. Furthermore, Saarelainen has reported individually meaningful religious rituals to bring comfort with cancer. For example, some found that small angel figurines provided God's protection during treatment. One even had a blessed piece of linen that was given from a local charismatic church to provide tactile presence of God's comfort and care during the treatment [11]. An international literature review indicated that religiosity was found to provide a sense of coherence for patients at different ages. Elements such as bible reading, prayer, personal spirituality, and reconciliation reinforce an experience of tranquillity and peace of mind [37].

Nevertheless, AYAs with a life-threatening disease are not necessarily interested in spiritual issues or may find their discussion uncomfortable [38–40]. Moreover, AYAs with cancer seem rarely to turn to health care chaplaincy [7, 28]. Those rare individuals who turn to pastoral care find meetings very fruitful [7], but hospital chaplains are an underused resource for adolescents with cancer [18]. According to researchers, chaplains are too often connected only with 'spiritual emergency' situations such as approaching death. Studies suggest that even though death and dying are important discussion topics to cover, support for and reflection on existential concerns in general is highly beneficial, for cancer patients' ease with existential questions and existential well-being is a strong predictor of health-related quality of life [41–44]. Therefore, hospital chaplains can be a resource for young adults in many ways and in various phases of the illness [33]. Current models of spiritual care suggest that meeting spiritual needs and existential concerns should be addressed by multidisciplinary teamwork in which varieties of professionals offer the possibility of person-centred care, allowing compassion to become a source of spiritual care [45].

3 Call for Information and Honest Discussions

It has been suggested that the deep need to have more information about a cancer diagnosis has existential and spiritual elements for AYAs. Timely provided information could possibly provide existential support in different phases of the cancer trajectory [36]. Before diagnosis, AYAs report searching the internet for information about the possible diagnosis, but the internet seems to often reveal all the worst possible scenarios [16, 28]. From the care perspective, it seems the waiting time to confirm the diagnosis varies from a couple of weeks to several months. Before the official diagnosis, they are rarely given further information, support, or possible explanations for their health condition [36].

In palliative care, patients of different ages highlight the value of honest face-to-face dialogue where information and diagnoses are provided [46]. Patients value honest discussions, as they are eager to learn and understand their prognosis [47]. Previous studies among AYAs report that diagnoses are commonly delivered over the phone, and this is questioned by some, whereas others appreciate receiving the diagnosis in their chosen location. Wherever the diagnosis is given, the lack of empathy seems to be the issue that affects the experience of receiving information inappropriately. AYAs also describe challenges in receiving sufficient information about treatment outcomes [36]. The value of open dialogue is significant for end-of-life care planning and the recording of legal wishes. Legal planning promotes dying patients' autonomy [48]. Palliative care studies advocate that both end-of-life care and funeral planning can be found meaningful, so it is also likely to be important to young adults [40, 47–49].

It seems the more everyday information required can partly be supported by utilising a mobile app. With a portable support connection, palliative care patients can avoid extra hospital trips and are allowed more freedom and flexibility in their daily lives [50]. Among young cancer survivors there are early indications that eHealth solutions create opportunities to meet a variety of mental and physical needs [51]. Both social media [52] and the internet [53] are used as sources of information and networking among AYA patients. Although the possibility of eHealth supporting the spiritual needs of young adults in palliative care has been little studied, there are indications that a co-created mobile app may positively affect quality of life: AYAs in remission reported a significant improvement in general quality of life after their treatment ended [54, 55]. More specific studies are needed to determine whether app use offers benefits in young adult palliative care.

4 Facing Death

As news and social media have presented realistic narratives about what it means to die, the sociological taboo regarding discussions about death and dying has reduced. The psychological taboo of what it means that *I* am dying, however, lingers. It is difficult for an individual facing death to comprehend and reflect on the boundaries of human life [56]. This type of psychological taboo is at the core of existential concerns of humanity [57], and therefore, we could also call it an existential taboo around personal mortality. Based on secondary analysis of four different datasets gathered from cancer patients, it has been suggested that mortality salience is particularly difficult for young people, and young individuals require a time of reflection to comprehend that dying is an inevitable part of life [58].

AYAs' difficulty with communication and reflection affect many areas. First, the fear of death prompts anxiety about how loved ones will cope and a desire to protect family members from certain thoughts [4, 47]. Second, professionals and family members are often uncertain and anxious about discussing death with a young patient. Research suggests, however, that discussing death openly is important for young patients' spiritual well-being. This should be done at an earlier stage of the illness than is the current practice [32, 40, 59, 60]. For instance, in a literature review by Bell and colleagues, they noted that it was common for discussions on death to take place during the last 30 days of life. This was interpreted as leaving a dying individual without opportunities to deal with their personal emotions nor to take care of other preparations linked to end-of-life care [61]. Even when death is close, it is important for the young person to have an opportunity to take a break from constantly thinking about cancer and to and to have the opportunity to talk with people who are open to honest discussion and reflection about reality [4, 17, 26].

Challenges in facing the fear of death seem strong even for young adults undergoing treatment with the aim of a cure. For instance, AYAs highlighted the need to have time off from constant thoughts about cancer. The fear of death is particularly strong during treatment: There is still a high probability that cancer will lead to death for some. Studies report that some young adults feel ready to face the seriousness of their situation only after treatment [4, 11]. This is similar to older patients, who have also been reported to wish to avoid actively thinking about their own approaching of death: If one does not actively contemplate death's inevitability, an experience of living fully, even during hospice care, is possible [47].

Fear of death seems to linger also among AYAs in cancer remission, as many discover their future is unpredictable: Thoughts of an early death from a relapse of cancer often remain. Closeness of individual death was vivid when a remission patient in the very last months before her check-up depicted an idea of death. She is even reported to have some sort of end-of-life care planning as she requested death: 'boots on, no agony'. She was convinced that she would face early death no matter what: either she expected to have a cancer relapse or secondary cancer that would make her life short [4]. Such wishes about quick death are usually those of dying patients [58].

The understanding of time changes with a cancer diagnosis [62]. AYAs have reported experiencing cancer diagnoses as the end of a fairy-tale of childhood, or as a forced process of maturation in which they had to examine and evaluate their life differently [11]. A study in which AYAs with cancer portrayed their life experiences with an art assignment found that several participants did not finish the top of their drawing of a tree. These individuals said that cancer meant it was impossible or too painful to consider what the future might bring. Insecurity about the future was grasped in the life tree drawings composed by AYAs and interpreted as being linked to experiences of crises concerning the meaning in life [12, 62].

In palliative care, future perspectives become limited for AYAs. Long-term goals are replaced by shorter-term and more realistic ones [63]. A study in which some of the interviewed patients were young adults confirmed that holding on to everyday life was important as each day spent together with the loved ones was found to be worth cherishing. Even when personal capacities decreased, it was meaningful to cling to ordinary activities in which one could still participate [46]. The courage to live each day and to appreciate the present moment can be found in individual inner strength that supports an encounter with harsh emotions and accepts that death cannot be avoided [37].

There is little explicit research on hope and its significance for AYAs with terminal cancer. It seems that an awareness of the remaining time and the nature of hope are interconnected. A study that included AYAs' ideas reported that awareness of death was connected with eschatological hope—the hope of eternal life—comforting those of a religious or spiritual orientation [15]. Hope may become a spiritual resource for young adults [14, 63]. Religiosity may alleviate religious individuals' sense of emptiness caused by the approach of death [46]. Some have reported acceptance of the approaching death based on God's will and increased faith [23]. However, religion does not often provide solutions to difficult questions; instead, in the context of pastoral care, chaplains' ability to be present alleviates suffering [33].

5 Appearance of Guilt

Studies suggest that a judgemental attitude towards the self is harmful for cancer patients, as it can cause psychological stress and reduce quality of life [64–66]. Guilt and self-blame are also reported among young adults with cancer [14, 18]. When the first suspicions of cancer emerge, AYAs can be driven to blame themselves. After the diagnosis is confirmed, some try to find a reason for their cancer in their previous behaviour [67]. Furthermore, the phenomenon of blame is relational by its nature, as it has been discovered that criticism of the patient's lifestyle choices does not necessarily arise from the person themselves but from other people [35].

For religiously oriented individuals, the relational element of self-blame and guilt may have religious tones. Some AYAs who are confronted with the question 'why?' find an answer in God's punishment. Cancer is then viewed as the consequence of personal evil deeds. This indicates that religious and spiritual struggle can cause stress and agony for young people facing serious health problems. Some may channel their anger, bitterness, and disappointment towards God [11, 26]. Yet, AYAs also turn to God in a religious and spiritual struggle to solve these issues [11, 24]. Spirituality is therefore reported to have the potential to release patients from these harsh emotions and positively affect their quality of life [66].

There are indications that self-blame is particularly active in the early stages of cancer [68]. Self-forgiveness interventions are effective at reducing self-loathing and improving quality of life, even in its late stages. Although more studies are required to develop specific forgiveness practices and interventions in palliative care, all adult patient groups seem to benefit from forgiveness and conflict resolution, which allow peace of mind in the last stages of life [69].

6 Renewal of Self and View of Life

AYAs with serious health conditions are likely to face change related to identity, which creates distress and existential concerns. For example, cancer engenders a consideration of who *I* am, and what *my* core values and worldview are [34]. The religious, spiritual, and existential are often intertwined in this process [12, 26].

The mental level sees the formation of a new identity, from being a healthy to a dying person, which requires a reflective mindset and a readiness to face varieties of emotions [46]. As the number of AYA cancer patients is relatively small compared to other patient groups, the experience of being different among other patients is highlighted in hospital, where the other patients are usually old, or at least significantly older [36]. This minority position makes AYAs with cancer especially vulnerable [35] as being diagnosed with a serious illness at a young age means an individual belongs to a minority among both their own peer group and among those diagnosed with an illness [9, 11, 70]. At the same time as they are trying to comprehend everything that is changing in their life, they may undergo physical changes that make it difficult to identify with one's own body. Losing hair, undergoing weight change, and having physical scars make it difficult to identify 'this' as really 'me' [35, 62].

At the level of values, an intensified quest for individually important ways of living is reported. For example, a willingness and capacity to live in the moment is described. Living in the moment seems to be strongly connected with a greater appreciation of the small things in life. As already observed, those diagnosed in their adolescent years find themselves suddenly having to mature [34]. Religious seeking becomes vivid in the narratives of AYAs, who describe cancer as prompting a religious process that makes them consider their personal relationship with God. They are driven to think about how and what to believe. For example, a personal relationship with God or a higher power through prayer and intercession is found supportive and comforting. Prayer is reported to be especially helpful for young adults when they are afraid or suffering from insomnia or nausea, for example. Cancer prompts AYAs to find consolation in turning to God or the supernatural, even if they are unsure as to whom it is that they are turning [11, 26]. At a general level, some AYAs experience their religious belief as the power that helps them cope mentally with the disease, and that the significance of religion increases after their diagnosis [11, 12].

7 Relational Aspect of Living and Dying

Social networks have a special capacity to foster hope in multidimensional ways for AYAs in palliative care [16, 26]. Close relationships are described as one of the most meaningful sources of support, particularly the family [11, 46]. A new understanding of the fragility of life and an intensified relational network led AYAs to a new appreciation of family and friends. Furthermore, many formed new relationships when meeting peer patients and supporters during the treatment process [34].

Friendships are further intensified during the last stages of life [46]. The experience of coherence in close relationships provides a sense of security during palliative care: one's nearest and dearest provide the experience of being loved and encountered also in the last stages of life which is found comforting [37].

Yet, dilemmas in the relational network are manifold. AYAs with cancer find it distressing to consider their loved ones' experience of their illness. Some AYAs feel cancer is such a heavy burden on their family members that they should keep their most painful thoughts to themselves. It has even been reported that AYAs are unable to cry in front of their parents because of their desire to protect them [4, 67]. Still, studies have also found that young patients experience overprotectiveness by their parents. As many of AYAs moved back to their parents' house after some time of independent living, moving back to childhood home was not always easy. For instance, participants in a study by Kent and colleagues reported 'helicopter parenting' to explain how much the parents were trying to easy up daily living and reduce stress and difficulties of daily living [70]. Becoming dependent on others was found difficult among AYAs with cancer: Becoming newly dependent after living independently was found to be connected with despair [4, 12].

There is a fear of encountering social exclusion among AYAs with cancer [35]. Young cancer patients easily become socially isolated due to fear of infections and stigma of being different from others. Isolation is very harmful, as it can lead to behavioural problems like smoking, misuse of alcohol, and risky sexual behaviour [71]. Moreover, difficult questions are also faced in romantic relationships, as broken and strongly challenged relationships and difficulties in sexual relations are reported [12, 67]. For instance, in Saarelainen's study, a female participant shared a narrative of how cancer was such a huge crisis to her spouse as well as herself that he totally froze. In his fear of losing her to cancer, he withdrew from the relationship for a while. After two weeks of being out of contact, they were able to communicate again. When the couple were trying to get counselling to support their relationship that was going through difficulties, they were told to sort the argument out as any other argument [67]. It could be suggested that the stress that cancer brings to intimate relationships is not well recognised as the divorce rate is higher among young cancer survivors than in the general population [3, 70, 72].These notions underline the fact that cancer and even more drastically the move to palliative care is a crisis for both the patient and others important to them. To support the patient, it is crucial to support the family as well. To make the relational network supportive for the one facing death in their immediate future, the significant others also need to be supported.

8 Spirituality and Beyond

The impact of cultural context has been emphasised in previous studies of AYAs' spirituality in palliative care: spirituality means different things in different life and living contexts [73, 74]. Most existing studies in this field have been conducted within the framework of psychosocial needs. In these studies, spirituality is defined and measured in various ways, making the comparison of results difficult. In many studies, however, the distinctive nature of spirituality and religiosity in relation to psychological needs is recognised, and it has also been considered important to distinguish between religiosity and spirituality [14, 18, 33, 75].

The concept of spirituality remains blurry, entailing tautology and overlapping with other factors associated with well-being [76, 77]. The only agreement is that no easy definitions exist, and that these concepts are poorly transferable culturally [78]. The term *spirituality* has very different connotations in English compared to other languages in which the term may simply not exist or carries a purely religious connotation. However, when studying the experiences of AYAs with cancer, it has been considered important to separate between religiosity and spirituality [18, 79]. Young adults with cancer need time and space to reflect on their religious and/or spiritual needs without pressure from outside such as parents or hospital staff [79]. Furthermore, a large-scale and cross-sectional European Values Study points out that religious and spiritual attitudes are in flux. As one national example, in Finland, the quickest changes in values can be seen among people that would currently be AYAs (millennials, Y- and Z-generations). The largest changes seen are how connectedness to religiosity decreases among younger generations [80]. Yet, academics utilise the concepts such as religiosity and spirituality in their research contexts, even though it is unlikely to encapsulate the understandings of the research participants themselves [14]. We need to find terminology that captures research participants' self-understanding, [77] otherwise researchers are at risk of providing identifications to participants' ideas which they do not recognise themselves. More importantly, we need to utilise and discover terminology that meets the self-understanding of a suffering human being to facilitate and structure care that meets various spiritual, religious, and existential care needs.

More than 20 years ago, it was noted that existentiality was likely to be at the core of the debated definitions of religion and spirituality [81]. The current research indicates that cancer at a young age engenders a deeply existential process in which the spheres of religion, spirituality, and the secular intersect [7, 11, 14, 26]. During palliative and end-of-life care for young adults, religious and spiritual resources can be used to verbalise existential concerns [10]. Instead of explicitly using the concepts of religion and spirituality, it may be helpful to use concepts such as guilt, self-image, meaning, purpose, and hope [14].

9 Conclusion

In summary, we have showed that AYAs with cancer are driven to varieties of religious, spiritual, and existential quests after being diagnosed with cancer. Palliative care and end-of-life care particularly are a delicate time for both AYAs and their nearest and dearest. Aspects found in research discussed under the terminology of religion, spirituality, and existential aspects are likely to be included in the process.

To be able to meet the multifaceted care needs rising from these perspectives, open and honest discussions about realities of life, death, and values are needed.

When having a cup of coffee with AYAs with cancer, the first author of this article asked the group, how would they like their possible religious or spiritual or various of kinds of needs to be addressed. They instantly grasped what is needed:

> *Just ask what we need. Just ask how we see the world and what is meaningful. It does not hurt us to be asked.*

References

1. Vassal G, Fitzgerald E, Schrappe M, Arnold F, Kowalczyk J, Walker D, et al. Challenges for children and adolescents with cancer in Europe: the SIOP-Europe agenda. Pediatr Blood Cancer. 2014;61(9):1551–7.
2. Nass SJ, Beaupin LK, Demark-Wahnefried W, Fasciano K, Ganz PA, Hayes-Lattin B, et al. Identifying and addressing the needs of adolescents and young adults with cancer: summary of an Institute of Medicine Workshop. Oncologist. 2015;20(2):186–95.
3. Docherty SL, Kayle M, Maslow GR, Santacroce SJ. The adolescent and young adult with cancer: a developmental life course perspective. Semin Oncol Nurs. 2015;31(3):186–96.
4. Saarelainen SM. Landscapes of hope and despair: stories of the future of emerging adults in cancer remission. J Pastor Theol. 2019;29(2):67–84.
5. Wong AWK, Chang T t, Christopher K, SCL L, Beaupin LK, Love B, et al. Patterns of unmet needs in adolescent and young adult (AYA) cancer survivors: in their own words. J Cancer Surviv. 2017;11(6):751–64.
6. Cheung CK, Zebrack B. What do adolescents and young adults want from cancer resources? Insights from a Delphi panel of AYA patients. Support Care Cancer. 2017;25(1):119–26.
7. Saarelainen SM. Meeting the spiritual care needs of emerging adults with cancer. Religions. 2019;11(1):16.
8. Zebrack BJ, Block R, Hayes-Lattin B, Embry L, Aguilar C, Meeske KA, et al. Psychosocial service use and unmet need among recently diagnosed adolescent and young adult cancer patients: AYA cancer patients. Cancer. 2013;119(1):201–14.
9. Zebrack B, Kent EE, Keegan THM, Kato I, Smith AW, Aya Hope Study Collaborative Group. "Cancer sucks," and other ponderings by adolescent and young adult cancer survivors. J Psychosoc Oncol. 2014;32(1):1–15.
10. Currie ER, Johnston EE, Bakitas M, Roeland E, Lindley LC, Gilbertson-White S, et al. Caregiver reported quality of end-of-life care of adolescent and young adult decedents with cancer. J Palliat Care. 2022;37(2):87–92.
11. Saarelainen SM. Coping-related themes in cancer stories of young Finnish adults. Int J Pract Theol [Internet]. 2016;20(1):69–96. [cited 2023 May 25]. https://www.degruyter.com/document/doi/10.1515/ijpt-2014-0045/html
12. Saarelainen SM. Meaningful life with(out) cancer: coping narratives of emerging Finnish adults. Helsinki: University of Helsinki; 2017.
13. Abdelaal M, Avery J, Chow R, Saleem N, Fazelzad R, Mosher P, et al. Palliative care for adolescents and young adults with advanced illness: a scoping review. Palliat Med. 2023;37(1):88–107.
14. Barton KS, Tate T, Lau N, Taliesin KB, Waldman ED, Rosenberg AR. "I'm not a spiritual person." How hope might facilitate conversations about spirituality among teens and young adults with cancer. J Pain Symptom Manag. 2018;55(6):1599–608.

15. Baczewska B, Block B, Kropornicka B, Niedzielski A, Malm M, Zwolak A, et al. Hope in hospitalized patients with terminal cancer. Int J Environ Res Public Health. 2019;16(20):3867.
16. Juvakka T, Kylmä J. Hope in adolescents with cancer. Eur J Oncol Nurs. 2009;13(3):193–9.
17. Flavelle SC. Experience of an adolescent living with and dying of cancer. Arch Pediatr Adolesc Med [Internet]. 2011;165(1):28–32. [cited 2023 Jun 15]. http://archpedi.jamanetwork.com/article.aspx?doi=10.1001/archpediatrics.2010.249
18. Proserpio T, Ferrari A, Veneroni L, Giacon B, Massimino M, Clerici CA. Spiritual aspects of care for adolescents with cancer. Tumori J. 2014;100(4):e130–5.
19. Quinn G, Goncalves V, Sehovic I, Bowman M, Reed D. Quality of life in adolescent and young adult cancer patients: a systematic review of the literature. Patient Relat Outcome Meas. 2015;6:19.
20. Wein S, Pery S, Zer A. Role of palliative care in adolescent and young adult oncology. J Clin Oncol. 2010;28(32):4819–24.
21. Parks SD. Big questions, worthy dreams: mentoring emerging adults in their search for meaning, purpose, and faith. San Francisco: Jossey Bass; 2011.
22. Saarelainen SMK. Lack of belonging as disrupting the formation of meaning and faith. J Youth Theol. 2018;17(2):127–49.
23. Alcorn SR, Balboni MJ, Prigerson HG, Reynolds A, Phelps AC, Wright AA, et al. "If God wanted me yesterday, I wouldn't be here today": religious and spiritual themes in patients' experiences of advanced cancer. J Palliat Med. 2010;13(5):581–8.
24. Park CL, Cho D. Spiritual well-being and spiritual distress predict adjustment in adolescent and young adult cancer survivors: spirituality in adolescent/young adult survivors. Psychooncology. 2017;26(9):1293–300.
25. Yanez B, Edmondson D, Stanton AL, Park CL, Kwan L, Ganz PA, et al. Facets of spirituality as predictors of adjustment to cancer: relative contributions of having faith and finding meaning. J Consult Clin Psychol. 2009;77(4):730–41.
26. Saarelainen SM. Emerging Finnish adults coping with cancer: religious, spiritual, and secular meanings of the experience. Pastor Psychol. 2017;66(2):251–68.
27. Ragsdale JR, Hegner MA, Mueller M, Davies S. Identifying religious and/or spiritual perspectives of adolescents and young adults receiving blood and marrow transplants: a prospective qualitative study. Biol Blood Marrow Transplant. 2014;20(8):1242–7.
28. Park CL, Edmondson D, Hale-Smith A, Blank TO. Religiousness/spirituality and health behaviors in younger adult cancer survivors: does faith promote a healthier lifestyle? J Behav Med. 2009;32(6):582–91.
29. Lemay K, Wilson K. Treatment of existential distress in life threatening illness: a review of manualized interventions☆. Clin Psychol Rev. 2008;28(3):472–93.
30. Chan HY, Pang SM. Quality of life concerns and end-of-life care preferences of aged persons in long-term care facilities. J Clin Nurs. 2007;16(11):2158–66.
31. Tang ST, Chang WC, Chen JS, Chou WC, Hsieh CH, Chen CH. Associations of prognostic awareness/acceptance with psychological distress, existential suffering, and quality of life in terminally ill cancer patients' last year of life: impacts of prognostic awareness/acceptance for dying cancer patients. Psychooncology. 2016;25(4):455–62.
32. Lyon ME, Jacobs S, Briggs L, Cheng YI, Wang J. A longitudinal, randomized, controlled trial of advance care planning for teens with cancer: anxiety, depression, quality of life, advance directives, spirituality. J Adolesc Health. 2014;54(6):710–7.
33. Cooke L, Chung C, Grant M. Psychosocial care for adolescent and young adult hematopoietic cell transplant patients. J Psychosoc Oncol. 2011;29(4):394–414.
34. Shaha M, Bauer-Wu S. Early adulthood uprooted: transitoriness in young women with breast cancer. Cancer Nurs. 2009;32(3):246–55.
35. Williams BR. Dying young, dying poor: a sociological examination of existential suffering among low-socioeconomic status patients. J Palliat Med. 2004;7(1):27–37.
36. Saarelainen SM. Existential care in cancer – perspective of emerging adults. In: Ta vare En bok om diakoni, sjelesorg og eksistensiell helse [Internet]. Oslo: VID; 2022. p. 199–214. (VID Rapport). https://hdl.handle.net/11250/3001282.

37. Saukkonen M, Viitala A, Lehto JT, Åstedt-Kurki P. Syöpäpotilaan ja hänen läheisensä selviytymistä edistävät tekijät palliatiivisen hoidon aikana – systemaattinen kirjallisuuskatsaus. Hoitotiede. 2017;29(3):195–206.
38. Mack JW, Fisher L, Khalaj A, Altschuler A, Chao CR, Kushi LH, et al. Quality indicators for adolescents and young adults with advanced cancer: a modified Delphi process with patients, family members, and clinicians. J Pain Symptom Manag. 2023;66:54–61. S0885392423004220.
39. Sansom-Daly UM, Zhang M, Evans HE, McLoone J, Wiener L, Cohn RJ, et al. Adapting the voicing my CHOiCES advance care planning communication guide for Australian adolescents and young adults with cancer: appropriateness, acceptability, and considerations for clinical practice. Cancers. 2023;15(7):2129.
40. Wiener L, Ballard E, Brennan T, Battles H, Martinez P, Pao M. How I wish to be remembered: the use of an advance care planning document in adolescent and young adult populations. J Palliat Med. 2008;11(10):1309–13.
41. Shin HW, Noh DY, Lee ES, Nam SJ, Park BW, Ahn SH, et al. Correlates of existential well-being and their association with health-related quality of life in breast cancer survivors compared with the general population. Breast Cancer Res Treat. 2009;118(1):139–50.
42. Laubmeier KK, Zakowski SG, Bair JP. The role of spirituality in the psychological adjustment to cancer: a test of the transactional model of stress and coping. Int J Behav Med. 2004;11(1):48–55.
43. Cohen SR, Mount BM, Tomas JJN, Mount LF. Existential well-being is an important determinant of quality of life: evidence from the McGill quality of life questionnaire. Cancer. 1996;77(3):576–86.
44. Edmondson D, Park CL, Blank TO, Fenster JR, Mills MA. Deconstructing spiritual well-being: existential well-being and HRQOL in cancer survivors. Psychooncology. 2008;17(2):161–9.
45. Sharp J, Nash S. Spiritual teamwork within end of life care. In: Spiritually competent practice in health care. London: CRC Press, Taylor & Francis Group; 2017. p. 145–59.
46. Viitala A, Saukkonen M, Lehto JT, Palonen M, Åstedt-Kurki P. The coping and support needs of incurable cancer patients. J Hosp Palliat Nurs. 2018;20(2):187–94.
47. Viitala A, Åstedt-Kurki P, Lehto JT, Palonen M. 'I am still valuable' – a qualitative study of incurable cancer patients coping in hospice care. Scand J Caring Sci. 2023;37:720–31. https://doi.org/10.1111/scs.13160.
48. Mäki-Petäjä-Leinonen A, Saarelainen SM. Funeral wills and the autonomy of a dying person: experiences of older people in palliative care and their carers. Int J Law Policy Fam. 2021;35(1):ebab034.
49. Wiener L, Zadeh S, Battles H, Baird K, Ballard E, Osherow J, et al. Allowing adolescents and young adults to plan their end-of-life care. Pediatrics. 2012;130(5):897–905.
50. Viitala A, Åstedt-Kurki P, Lehto JT, Palonen M. Online follow-up with a mobile device improves incurable cancer patients' coping – a qualitative study. Eur J Oncol Nurs. 2021;55:102047.
51. Ramsey WA, Heidelberg RE, Gilbert AM, Heneghan MB, Badawy SM, Alberts NM. eHealth and mHealth interventions in pediatric cancer: a systematic review of interventions across the cancer continuum. Psychooncology. 2020;29(1):17–37.
52. Perales MA, Drake EK, Pemmaraju N, Wood WA. Social media and the adolescent and young adult (AYA) patient with cancer. Curr Hematol Malig Rep. 2016;11(6):449–55.
53. Schiffman JD, Csongradi E, Suzuki LK. Internet use among adolescent and young adults (AYA) with cancer. Pediatr Blood Cancer. 2008;51(3):410–5.
54. Elsbernd A, Hjerming M, Visler C, Hjalgrim LL, Niemann CU, Boisen KA, et al. Using cocreation in the process of designing a smartphone app for adolescents and young adults with cancer: prototype development study. JMIR Form Res. 2018;2(2):e23.
55. Elsbernd A, Hjerming M, Visler C, Hjalgrim LL, Niemann CU, Boisen K, et al. Cocreated smartphone app to improve the quality of life of adolescents and young adults with cancer (Kræftværket): protocol for a quantitative and qualitative evaluation. JMIR Res Protoc. 2018;7(5):e10098.

56. Walter T. What death means now: thinking critically about dying and grieving. Bristol: Policy Press; 2017.
57. Yalom I. Existential psychotherapy. New York: Basic Books; 1980.
58. Little M, Sayers EJ. While there's life …. Soc Sci Med. 2004;59(6):1329–37.
59. Keim-Malpass J, Erickson JM, Malpass HC. End-of-life care characteristics for young adults with cancer who die in the hospital. J Palliat Med. 2014;17(12):1359–64.
60. Pritchard S, Cuvelier G, Harlos M, Barr R. Palliative care in adolescents and young adults with cancer. Cancer. 2011;117(S10):2323–8.
61. Bell CJ, Skiles J, Pradhan K, Champion VL. End-of-life experiences in adolescents dying with cancer. Support Care Cancer. 2010;18(7):827–35.
62. Saarelainen SM. Life tree drawings as a methodological approach in young adults' life stories during cancer remission. Narrat Works. 2015;5(1):68–91.
63. Bennett CR, Coats H, Hendricks-Ferguson VL, Gauthier K, Sousa K. The lived experiences with hope from adolescents and young adults who have advanced cancer. J Pain Symptom Manag. 2022;63(4):581–9.
64. Toussaint L, Barry M, Angus D, Bornfriend L, Markman M. Self-forgiveness is associated with reduced psychological distress in cancer patients and unmatched caregivers: hope and self-blame as mediating mechanisms. J Psychosoc Oncol. 2017;35(5):544–60.
65. Toussaint L, Barry M, Bornfriend L, Markman M. Restore: the journey toward self-forgiveness: a randomized trial of patient education on self-forgiveness in cancer patients and caregivers. J Health Care Chaplain. 2014;20(2):54–74.
66. Friedman LC, Barber CR, Chang J, Tham YL, Kalidas M, Rimawi MF, et al. Self-blame, self-forgiveness, and spirituality in breast cancer survivors in a public sector setting. J Cancer Educ. 2010;25(3):343–8.
67. Saarelainen SM. Anteeksianto ja sovinto syopaa sairastaneiden nuorten aikuisten narratiiveissa. Teol Aikakauskirja. 2018;123(4):321–34.
68. Romero C, Friedman LC, Kalidas M, Elledge R, Chang J, Liscum KR. Self-forgiveness, spirituality, and psychological adjustment in women with breast cancer. J Behav Med. 2006;29(1):29–36.
69. Silva RS, Caldeira S, Coelho AN, Apóstolo JLA. Forgiveness facilitation in palliative care: a scoping review. JBI Evid Synth. 2020;18(11):2196–230.
70. Kent EE, Parry C, Montoya MJ, Sender LS, Morris RA, Anton-Culver H. "You're too young for this": adolescent and young adults' perspectives on cancer survivorship. J Psychosoc Oncol. 2012;30(2):260–79.
71. Patterson P, McDonald FEJ, Zebrack B, Medlow S. Emerging issues among adolescent and young adult cancer survivors. Semin Oncol Nurs. 2015;31(1):53–9.
72. Warner EL, Kent EE, Trevino KM, Parsons HM, Zebrack BJ, Kirchhoff AC. Social well-being among adolescents and young adults with cancer: a systematic review: social well-being of AYAs with cancer. Cancer. 2016;122(7):1029–37.
73. Sansom-Daly UM, Wakefield CE, Patterson P, Cohn RJ, Rosenberg AR, Wiener L, et al. End-of-life communication needs for adolescents and young adults with cancer: recommendations for research and practice. J Adolesc Young Adult Oncol. 2020;9(2):157–65.
74. Upshaw NC, Roche A, Gleditsch K, Connelly E, Wasilewski-Masker K, Brock KE. Palliative care considerations and practices for adolescents and young adults with cancer. Pediatr Blood Cancer [Internet]. 2021;68(1):e28781. [cited 2023 Jun 13]. https://onlinelibrary.wiley.com/doi/10.1002/pbc.28781
75. Beerbower E, Winters D, Kondrat D. Bio-psycho-social-spiritual needs of adolescents and young adults with life-threatening illnesses: implications for social work practice. Soc Work Health Care. 2018;57(4):250–66.
76. Visser A, Garssen B, Vingerhoets AJ. Existential well-being: spirituality or well-being? J Nerv Ment Dis. 2017;205(3):234–41.
77. la Cour P, Hvidt NC. Research on meaning-making and health in secular society: secular, spiritual and religious existential orientations. Soc Sci Med. 2010;71(7):1292–9.

78. Hermans CAM. From practical theology to practice-oriented theology. Int J Pract Theol [Internet]. 2014;18(1):113–26. [cited 2023 May 26]. https://www.degruyter.com/document/doi/10.1515/ijpt-2014-0009/html
79. McNeil SB. Spirituality in adolescents and young adults with cancer: a review of literature. J Pediatr Oncol Nurs. 2016;33(1):55–63.
80. Ketola K. Uskonto ja kulttuurin murros. In: Uskonto arjessa ja juhlassa: Suomen evankelis-luterilainen kirkko vuosina, Kirkon tutkimuskeskus, Tampere. 2020;2016–2019.
81. Stifoss-Hanssen H. Religion and spirituality: what a European ear hears. Int J Psychol Relig. 1999;9(1):25–33.

Spiritual Care of Family Carers in Palliative Care

Michael Connolly

Abstract Palliative care enhances not just the quality of life of the individual living with a life-limiting condition but their family carer as well. In palliative care practice, it is essential to understand the spiritual dimension of family carers in order to provide meaningful emotional support at a significant time of need. Key to this understanding is the ability to communicate well and listen attentively. It is also important to recognise the role of impeccable assessment of the spiritual needs of family carers and to ensure that this assessment services to plan for effective emotional support, meaning making, and preparation for bereavement. Presence, attentiveness, and support will all aid in providing for the spiritual needs of family carers.

Keywords Family carer · Spiritual dimension of family care · Emotional support
Making meaning · Spiritual care · Palliative care

1 Introduction

Palliative care aims to enhance the quality of life of individuals living with a life limiting condition, focusing on providing support and comfort, while managing pain and other complex symptoms. Palliative care by its very nature centres on holistic attention to physical, psychological, social, and spiritual needs. Importantly palliative care also focuses on the care of the individual's family. Family should be seen as whoever the individual says it is and is not only a relationship of sanguinity

M. Connolly (✉)
School of Nursing, Midwifery & Health Systems, University College Dublin, Dublin, Ireland

Education & Research, Our Lady's Hospice & Care Services, Dublin, Ireland
e-mail: michael.connolly@ucd.ie

M. C. Best (ed.), *Spiritual Care in Palliative Care*,
https://doi.org/10.1007/978-3-031-50864-6_37

or contract. In the context of palliative and particularly end-of-life care, a specific focus of family care is the provision of spiritual care during what can be a challenging time for family members, witnessing their loved one receiving palliative care. It is worth noting that in their study, Chua et al. [1] found that often family carers needed more support than the patient. Family carers can encounter a range of spiritual problems such as trying to find meaning in the current situation, coping with uncertainty about the future, and in some cases living with sense of hopelessness, while others are trying to come to terms with their sense of relief [2]. While, sadly, spiritual care is often an unmet need for family carers, it is important to recognise the place of spiritual care for the family carers of those receiving palliative care, as a space where the emotional and existential needs which arise as end-of-life approaches can be addressed.

2 Understanding the Spiritual Dimension for Family Carers

Spirituality encompasses a broad range of beliefs and/or practices that give to the individual a sense of meaning, purpose, and connection to what can often be described as something greater than themselves. Importantly, spirituality is not confined to religious affiliation but goes beyond to personal philosophy, values, and beliefs about living and dying. In the context of palliative and end-of-life care, spirituality is the place where hope is found and existential questions can be explored.

When someone loved is diagnosed with a life-limiting condition and is referred for palliative care, family carers may experience a range of emotions including fear, anxiety, grief, sadness, anxiety, and in some cases relief [3–5]. At this time, family carers are faced head on with having to come to terms with their own mortality while trying to cope with potential changes in the dynamics of the family and navigating a quite often complex healthcare system. Coping with such an emotional burden can easily become overwhelming and so spiritual care can be a vital source of support [6, 7].

The goal when providing spiritual care to family carers is to first of all recognise the spiritual needs of the family carers and demonstrate a genuine concern to address these needs [8]. In doing so, the healthcare professional can positively impact the family carers' experience and their spiritual well-being [8].

3 What Does Spiritual Care of Family Carers Entail?

Spiritual care of family carers needs to be tailored to individual needs due to its subjective and multifaceted nature [9]. That said, there are several key components that should be considered.

3.1 Communication and Active Listening

Providing effective spiritual care begins with communication that is both open and empathetic. Communicating with family caregivers of a palliative care patient about their own spiritual care needs is a delicate but important aspect of holistic care.

Establishing a trusting and empathetic relationship with the family carers is an important tool to demonstrate genuine concern for well-being and to emphasis support. This is best done in a quiet and comfortable place where a safe space for open communication can be created.

Using open-ended questions that allow carers to share their thoughts and feelings is key.

This type of open communication with families provides a space for family carers to feel at ease expressing their feelings, fears and hopes for what lies ahead. When combined with empathy, open communication enables the family carer to express their own spiritual beliefs, while trying to find meaning in what is happening to their loved one as they journey with them [3, 4].

Active listening is how healthcare professionals can demonstrate they understand the family carer's values, beliefs and hopes for them and their loved ones. Being fully present to the conversation and using the family carer's own words to reflect what they say show understanding of both their concerns and emotions. Sometimes healthcare professionals need to be present but do not need to use words all the time. Being with, while sitting in silence, can be an effective means to communicate understanding. It sometimes helps for healthcare professional to stop and "WAIT"—"Why Am I Talking?" If the healthcare professional is continually talking, then how are the family carer's spiritual needs known?

Understanding the unique spiritual values and needs allows for a more nuanced and personal approach to the support that can be provided to family carers.

3.2 Assessment and Identification of Spiritual Needs

Not only should the spiritual needs of the patient be assessed but so too the spiritual needs of family carers. Therefore, healthcare professionals need to be knowledgeable in the assessment and identification of the spiritual needs of family carers. Gently inquire about their spiritual beliefs and values. In doing so, sensitivity about the diverse spiritual and cultural backgrounds of the family carers can be acknowledged. At all times, respect for expressed beliefs and practices is demonstrated and, where necessary, care and support are tailored to meet individual needs. These needs may include assistance with end-of-life decisions, desire for prayer or engaging with other religious rituals, or simply a safe place to talk through fears and anxieties about what is to come as end of life is approaching. Given the nature of palliative care, including the care of the patient and their family, it is worth considering using such assessment tools when conducting family meetings where wishes and preferences for care, or changes in focus of care, may be discussed.

Impeccable assessment is a corner stone of palliative care for any individual, so that physical, psychological, social, emotional, and spiritual needs are identified, and a plan of care can be implemented and evaluated. The same impeccable assessment is also needed to ensure family carers' needs are identified. Several spiritual assessments have been developed which have tended to focus on spiritual needs of patients. These can be easily adapted to suit the assessment spiritual needs of family carers. A selection of spiritual assessment tools has been identified with some suggested issues and questions to focus on (Table 1).

Table 1 Spiritual assessment tools

Assessment tool	Key issues and questions to focus on with family carers
AMEN—Affirm, Meet, Educate, No matter what (Cooper et al. [10])	Affirm the family carers' beliefs and ensure that their role as a carer and a support to the patient is validated Meet the family carer member where they are. It is important to avoid giving a false sense of hope while also ensuring that hopelessness does not manifest and take over Educate the family carer about your role within the healthcare team and ensure they know that the team is available to address their questions and concerns about what the future holds for their loved one No matter what; assure the family carer of your commitment to be with them at this point in time
The FICA (Faith, Importance, Community, Address) Spiritual History Tool (Krakowiak and Fopka-Kowalczyk [11])	F—Faith and Belief—It is important to understand the existing faith and beliefs of the family carer. Open questions can be used to ascertain this information: "Do you consider yourself spiritual or religious?" or "Do you have spiritual beliefs that help you cope with stress?" If the family carer responds "No," the healthcare provider may ask: "What gives your life meaning?" I—Importance—"What importance does your faith or belief have in your life?" Have your beliefs influenced how you take care of yourself as you care for your loved one? What role do your beliefs play in understanding your loved one's illness currently? If the family carer indicates no faith or belief—the question can focus on how their meaning in life helps you to understand what is important for you at this time C—Community Are you part of a spiritual or religious community? Is this a support to you and how? If the family carer indicates there are not part of a spiritual or religious community, the healthcare provider can ask: Is there a group of people who are important to you, who can provide support to you at this time? A—Address in Care How would you like me, as your healthcare provider, to address these issues for you at this time?

Table 1 (continued)

Assessment tool	Key issues and questions to focus on with family carers
HOPE (H—sources of hope, strength, comfort, meaning, peace, love and connection; O—the role of organised religion for the patient; P—personal spirituality and practices; E—effects on medical care and end-of-life decisions). (Anandarajah and Hight [12])	Sources of hope, meaning, comfort, strength, peace, love and connection I was wondering, what is there in your life that gives you internal support? What are your sources of hope, strength, comfort and peace? What do you hold on to during difficult times? What sustains you and keeps you going? Organised religion Do you consider yourself part of an organised religion? How important is this to you? What aspects of your religion are helpful and not so helpful to you? Are you part of a religious or spiritual community? Does it help you? How? *If the family carer is not part of organised religion move to personal spirituality* Personal spirituality/practices Do you have personal spiritual beliefs that are independent of organised religion? What are they? What aspects of your spirituality or spiritual practices do you find most helpful to you personally? (e.g. for those part of organised religion—prayer, meditation, receipt of the sacraments of religion; reading sacred texts. For example, for those not part of organised religion—meditation, listening to music, hiking, communing with nature) Effects on medical care and end-of-life issues Has seeing your loved one being sick (or your current situation) affected your ability to do the things that usually help you spiritually? (For those who are part of organised religion—Or affected your relationship with God?) As part of the team caring for your loved one, is there anything that I can do to help you access the resources that usually help you? Are there specific care needs to be considered for your loved one, over the next few days/weeks/months?

3.3 *Providing Emotional Support*

At the heart of spiritual care for family carers is the need for healthcare professionals to recognise their role is offering emotional support, which includes the acknowledgement of the pain and suffering that both the patient and their family carers are going through. An often-overlooked way to provide this emotional support is through the simple act of being present to the individual. Quite often in the business that is healthcare, there is tendency to avoid sitting in silence and simply being present to the other person. Emotional support can also be provided through engaging in meaningful conversations and, where needed, directing to supportive counselling. For many family carers, there is a sense of helplessness due in part to the uncertainty of what to expect as their loved one grows more ill and weaker and begins to die. Taking time to provide information is a sensitive and emotionally supportive way to family carers can help to validate their spiritual needs and concerns and ensure that they feel heard and, importantly, understood.

Another key consideration is to encourage the family carer to attend to their own self-care needs, which may have been neglected because of their care responsibilities. Remind the individual that self-care is not being selfish but is something necessary that they need to do to continue to provide effective care and support to their loved one.

Providing emotional support to family carers of those receiving palliative care is another example of the holistic and compassionate approach that can contribute significantly to the well-being of both family carers and the loved ones receiving palliative care [3, 4].

3.4 Facilitating Rituals and Traditions

As alluded to earlier, for some individuals, their spiritual wellness is dependent and fed by the engagement in religious or cultural rituals and traditions. Healthcare professionals may need to assist in supporting the facilitation of these rituals. This may include arranging for a spiritual leader to visit the inpatient unit with the family carers, or simply creating a space in the hospital where the family can attend to their rituals and customs.

It may be helpful to work with family carers to develop a plan that incorporates their meaningful rituals into the caregiving routine. This could include daily rituals, special occasions, or cultural observances. A particular focus may be on significant rituals and traditions that have been sources of strength and endurance in the past and which may be of help now at this difficult time for family carers [3, 4].

3.5 Meaning Making

For family carers of a loved one receiving palliative or end-of-life care, trying to find meaning is an important aspect of their journey. Finding meaning is a key aspect of spiritual care. Often, help is needed by family carers to reflect on the life of their loved ones, while also reflecting on their own values and beliefs. At such times, it can be difficult to recognise what is being learnt during these difficulty journeys for patients and their family carers.

Meaning making can help to provide comfort and an indeed a sense of purpose for both the patient and their family carer. One way of meaning making may be to encourage family caregivers to engage in life review activities with their loved one. This can involve reminiscing about positive memories, sharing stories, and celebrating the life of the individual receiving palliative care. This life review can also provide a space to have neglected conversations and perhaps speak with family about things that have been difficult in the past in order to attain closure [13]. As part of this life review, the family carer can be encouraged to engage in activities that hold personal significance, and may include creating rituals, participating in favourite hobbies, or spending quality time together. It can also afford family carers a time to understand and fulfil any end-of-life goals or wishes their loved one may have. This can provide a sense of purpose and accomplishment for the family carer when their loved one has died.

3.6 Offering Bereavement Support

Spiritual care for family carers will extend beyond their loved one's death. After their loved one has died, family carers may continue to seek answers to spiritual and existential questions. Healthcare professionals should be open to providing support and work to connect family carers with counselling and bereavement support services. Even at this difficult time for family carers, it is important to offer information about grief and bereavement resources. Preparing caregivers for the grieving process and providing ongoing support can contribute to their ability to find meaning in their caregiving experience. Bereavement care following death can include some very simple things that can be mean a lot. For example, a card sent to family carers a month after the death of their loved providing some information about local bereavement support services that might be possible. Some hospice services host annual memorial events that can provide a space where family carers can come together to share their grief in solidarity with one another. Importantly this can only be achieved if there is early engagement in assessment of needs in the pre-bereavement period to best support the family carer in post-bereavement period [14].

Box 1: Case Study

Bernadette is 68 years old and has been admitted to the Intensive Care Unit due to complications related to end-stage heart failure. Her heart failure was a result of radiotherapy-related damage to heart valves caused when she was treated for Hodgkin's disease at the age of 25 years. Over the last three years, she has had multiple admissions for exacerbation of her heart failure symptoms. Her husband was her main family carer and is assisted by two adult children.

Bernadette was accompanied by her husband and children at admission. It is noticeable that the family are close and following an initial family meeting, the current treatment plan and potential prognosis are shared. They have also been advised to alert the wider family to the current situation.

Initial interventions were reviewed at another family meeting after 24 hours. At this meeting, Bernadette's deteriorating condition was discussed, and a change in focus of care was agreed on due to her worsening health. Although upset, her family accepted that Bernadette was beginning to die and would now be provided with palliative and supportive care.

Bernadette and her husband both expressed a religious faith while their children, although not religious, were anxious that their mother be seen by a minister of religion while she was still able to speak. For them, it was important that rituals associated with their mother's beliefs were attended to and seeing this happen did seem to ease their anxiety and provided an opportunity for much needed emotional support. It was obvious to all staff that there was a strong emotional bond within the family and it was important that this be maintained.

Bernadette's condition deteriorated over the remainder of the day, and she died with her extended family round her.

How Did Spiritual Care Help Family Carers?

- Family carers knowing that staff were attentive to their loved one's needs was important. Knowing that a loved one's spiritual needs were being met reduced the emotional burden on them and tended to reduce anxiety.
- Staff taking time to explain what to expect over the coming hours, while also giving time for family carers to talk about their concerns, was appreciated.
- Staff enabling family carers and wider family to be present throughout her final hours was important as it ensured that they all had an opportunity to have important conversations that aided final memory making.
- Ensuring time and space and availability of a minster of religion enabled rituals to be observed which began the bereavement and grief journey.

4 Conclusion

Spiritual care is a fundamental part of palliative care and focuses on emotional and existential needs of the patient, but also of family carers. As a loved one is receiving palliative care and nearing the end of life, the support provided to family carers can influence how they cope with their loved one's impending death and their subsequent grieving. All healthcare professionals play a role in ensuring family carers receive the spiritual care they need. Being present, listening, assessing need, and providing support can serve to address the spiritual needs of family carers.

References

1. Chua GPPG, Yee ACP, et al. Supporting the patients with advanced cancer and their family caregivers: what are their palliative care needs? BMC Cancer. 2020;20:768.
2. Pepin E, Herbert J. Needs of caregivers of patients receiving in-home palliative and end-of-life care. Can Oncol Nurs J. 2020;30(2):147–52.
3. Kurtgöz A, Edis EK. Spiritual care from the perspective of family caregivers and nurses in palliative care: a qualitative study. BMC Palliat Care. 2023;22:161.
4. Benites ACRG, de Oliveira-Cardoso ÉA, et al. "You begin to give more value in life, in minutes, in seconds": spiritual and existential experiences of family caregivers of patients with advanced cancer receiving end-of-life care in Brazil. Support Care Cancer. 2022;30(3):2631–8.
5. Vigna PM, de Castro I, Fumis RRL. Spirituality alleviates the burden on family members caring for patients receiving palliative care exclusively. BMC Palliat Care. 2020;19(1):77.
6. Rocha RCNP, Pereira E, Silva RMCRA, et al. Spiritual needs experienced by the patient's family caregiver under oncology palliative care. Rev Bras Enferm. 2018;71:2635–42.
7. Selman LE BL, Sinclair S, et al. Patients' and caregivers' needs, experiences, preferences and research priorities in spiritual care: a focus group study across nine countries. Palliat Med. 2018;32(1):216–30.
8. O'Callaghan C, Seah D, Clayton JM, et al. Palliative caregivers' spirituality, views about spiritual care, and associations with spiritual well-being: a mixed methods study. Am J Hosp Palliat Care. 2020;37(4):305–13.
9. Wikert JTM, Theochari M, et al. How does spirituality manifest in family caregivers of terminally ill cancer patients? A qualitative secondary analysis. Palliat Support Care. 2022;20(1):45–54.
10. Cooper RSFA, Bodurtha JN, et al. AMEN in challenging conversations: bridging the gaps between faith, hope, and medicine. J Oncol Pract. 2014;10(4):e191–5.
11. Krakowiak P, Fopka-Kowalczyk M. Faith and belief, importance, community, address in care spiritual history tool by C. M. Puchalski as an instrument for an inter-disciplinary team in patient care. J Perspect Econ Polit Soc Integr. 2015;21:117.
12. Anandarajah G, Hight E. Spirituality and medical practice: using the HOPE questions as a practical tool for spiritual assessment. Am Fam Physician. 2001;63(1):81–9.
13. Connolly M, Timmins F. Spiritual care for individuals with cancer: the importance of life review as a tool for promoting spiritual well-being. Semin Oncol Nurs. 2021;37(5):151209.
14. Aoun SM, Ewing G, Grande G, et al. The impact of supporting family caregivers before bereavement on outcomes after bereavement: adequacy of end-of-life support and achievement of preferred place of death. J Pain Symptom Manag. 2017;55(2):368–78.

Spiritual Care of the Elderly

Elizabeth B. MacKinlay

Abstract This chapter focuses on spiritual development that occurs in later life, and ways in which spiritual development can be supported at the end of life. Therefore, the chapter addresses the spiritual dimension and especially a model of Spiritual Tasks and Process of Ageing to describe the final life career or journey into death from a spiritual perspective. A broad basis is used for discussion of the spiritual dimension, taking account of both religious aspects and secular understandings of the spiritual in later life. The chapter explores factors such as narrative, self-transcendence, suffering, relationship, searching for final meanings, and hope. Examples of people experiencing the final life journey are provided with excerpts from research that have explored the importance of inner strength in this final stage of life. Examples are mostly drawn from older frail people, who were living and dying from mainly chronic and complex disease conditions, common to later life.

Keywords Ageing · Spirituality · Dying · Inner strength · Spiritual tasks Spiritual care · Palliative care

1 About Growing Older, Dying, and Death

The journey towards death is the last important journey that each of us takes in life. In ageing western societies in the twenty-first century, most people die in older age. Therefore, many people have not witnessed the dying or death of anyone close to them until they themselves are possibly into mid-life or even later. This journey

E. B. MacKinlay (✉)
Centre for Ageing and Pastoral Studies, Australian Centre for Christianity and Culture, Charles Sturt University, Barton, ACT, Australia
e-mail: emackinlay@csu.edu.au

M. C. Best (ed.), *Spiritual Care in Palliative Care*,
https://doi.org/10.1007/978-3-031-50864-6_38

towards death is a journey that we each want to get 'right', but without personal experience of dying, we may lack a clear pattern on how best to travel this final life journey. Too often dying is about the loved ones and *their* journey, rather than the journey of the person who is dying. While the journey of those who accompany the one who is dying is important, the central experience of dying can only be known by the person who is dying. Kastenbaum and Moreman [1], Barbato [2], Heinz [3], and others have emphasised the purpose of this journey as a time to reflect on life and to prepare for death. Still others, including Frankl [4], have focused on the importance of coming to terms with the final meanings of our life: Why have I been here? What has my life been about? Have I fulfilled my purpose? Each life journey is unique to that individual, and at the same time, each journey has similarities with the dying of many others.

Palliative care has wide application for older people who are dying from progression and complications of chronic health conditions and disabilities. Therefore, palliative care is offered far more widely to older people than those who have a cancer diagnosis [5]. I see the spiritual dimension, importantly, underlying the palliative approach to dying. The approach in this chapter will address the spiritual dimension of ageing, and ways in which spiritual growth and spiritual care may continue into later life and until death. My central and primary concern is the life experience of the person who is travelling the journey into death. An important guiding question is, 'what does it feel like to be facing my own death?' Some people will not wish to ask or explore that question, while others wish to engage with all of life, for as long as they are able.

1.1 Grief and Loss as Part of Life: Attitudes to Dying of Older People

People bring their whole life experience to the process of dying. Yet, as Heinz wrote in 1995, the perception that older people first die a social death and become removed from awareness of the wider society well before they finally die has become even more prevalent in our communities now, several decades later.

> If people have been losing their own dying, giving their death away, the last passage becomes a lost passage. A life heading nowhere loses its depth dimension. And the connection between the living and the dead, between the living and aging, between the aging and their important last career, is broken and lost. [3, p. 5]

Heinz has starkly placed the dying of older people in a sharply defined position—outside of the rest of the society. He called for a reemphasis of the last (final) life career into the trajectory of dying. Now, in the twenty-first century, we may ask, what may this last career look like? Hudson, writing in 2022 (p. 206), alluded to the important role that care staff in residential aged care have to affirm the residents in their care, that their social selves continue to be upheld even as they approach bodily death; their spiritual selves also need affirmation.

The 'final life career' is a time of indefinite length, preparing for this journey into death, and it is also a time of handing over to the coming generations. It can be a time of struggle, but also of joy and completion; a journey that, at best, is travelled together with loved ones and carers. This chapter explores spiritual aspects of the final life career of older people, and the term final life career is used deliberately to indicate that this last stage is still an important part of life.

1.2 The Final Life Career: The Journey into Death

This final life career is important, and its significance was captured in a quotation from Metzger:

> What I ask from my death, is that at the last minute I will be able to look back over my life and know, without any doubt, the entire story I have been living... Then I will know, despite pain, disappointment, and limitation, that this life of mine has been a good and meaningful work. [6, p. 137]

Metzger's goal of finding final meaning seems to have been left unfulfilled for numbers of older people dying in societies that see the whole of life bounded by medical interventions. Another way of considering the journey towards death is to acknowledge the individual's life story and their ability to connect with this story, because story underpins identity and is of vital concern in the final life career and in the process of dying. During this process, the individual's life story may become almost a sacred treasure of what has taken one's whole life to achieve. It is only at this time, as Metzger has written, that we can become assured that it was all worthwhile, or to the contrary, if we are unable to find meaning in our story, life may seem to end in despair. By understanding more about the spiritual process of ageing and dying, it may be possible to prepare more appropriately for dying and death, while engaging in life until the end.

2 How Spirituality Is Mediated

The way that older people access or mediate their spiritual dimension does not differ markedly from other points in the life span. Connecting to the spiritual is always mediated through one or more of these modes of: relationship; creativity/creation; the arts and through religious or secular modes of prayer, sacred texts, meditation, rituals, and symbols. These are human ways of expressing the spiritual, as described by MacKinlay [7, 8]. I outline each of these four ways of mediating the spiritual dimension below (see Fig. 1). In reality, the content of each of these components varies at different points across the lifespan and according to life experience of the individual. In this chapter, I will concentrate on how the spiritual dimension can be mediated in ageing, before going on to describe a model of Spiritual Tasks and Process of Ageing (STPA) [7].

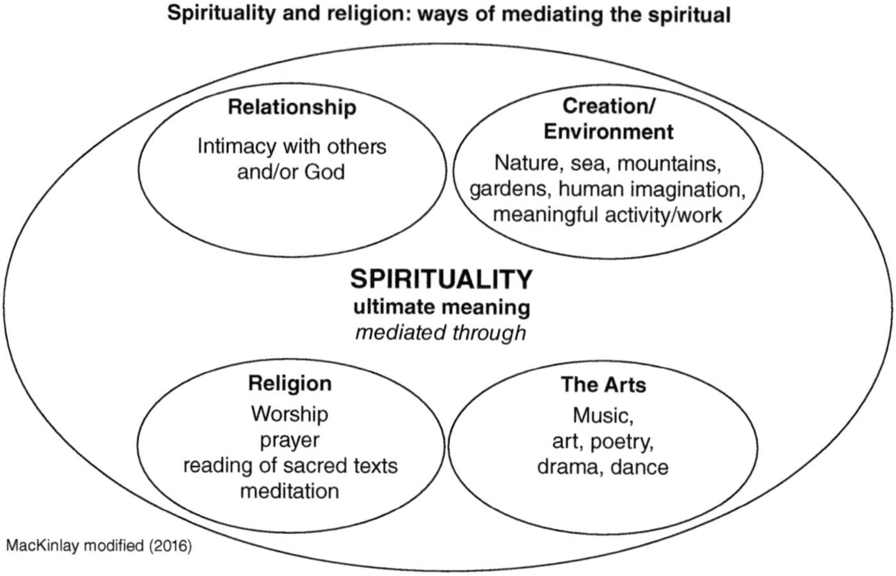

Fig. 1 How spirituality is mediated. (Reprinted with permission MacKinlay [7] revised)

2.1 *Relationship, Spirituality, Growing Older, and Preparing for Death*

Relationship (Fig. 1) is vital for human flourishing. Relationship or connectedness is important for all human beings, but in the process of dying there may be barriers to accessing these vital connections. Some years ago, when I first began to listen to stories of older frail people in high level residential care, I realised that numbers of these people had few living relations. But it was even more complex, as I often heard of the problems of connections with others due to geographical separation among family members, and stories of breakdown in relationships over time. When I asked these frail and elderly people, 'who or what is most important in your life now', a not uncommon response was 'God' or 'Jesus' (the sample of older people I was accessing at that time were mostly of Anglo Celtic background) [9].

Relationship remained important. However, what had changed for some was a move from connecting through human relationship to divine relationship, for those who held a religious faith. In writing of relationship and spirituality, I wish to differentiate between psychological and spiritual aspects of relationship. If we address the spiritual dimension through the lens of psychology, we use psychological means of addressing the spiritual. The spiritual dimension needs the use of spiritual lenses to appreciate this dimension. Understanding of relationship in the spiritual dimension takes on a different meaning. This is obviously evident in religious faiths, for example the Abrahamic faiths, where relationship is between the person and their God, and with other human beings. But it is not only people of faith who connect with the spiritual. It is generally recognised that the human being has a spiritual dimension, as well as body and mind.

In a Christian context, God's Spirit connects with the human spirit. This may be of such depth that Paul in the New Testament wrote of how, at times of our need or weakness, the Spirit prays within us, '*with sighs too deep for words*' (Rom 8: 26). Older people without a religious affiliation still need relationship with others, at deep and meaningful levels. Failure to thrive in later life may in part be due to loss of meaningful human relationships. Added to these losses are the physical ones of vision and hearing deficits, loss of energy and loss of mobility. In residential care, lack of time for staff to listen to older people, and a shortage of special palliative care skilled staff, result in lack of opportunity for deep relationships, and the resulting loneliness may become dire.

2.2 Creativity, Creation, and the Natural Environment

Creativity and the natural environment remain important to older people (see Fig. 1). Hospices pay a great deal of attention to the effects of the therapeutic built and natural environments and how these can provide a peaceful place of connection with nature. For older people who are dying, such environments can provide memories and feelings of peace and joy, and times of relief. Special places can provide a sacred space or atmosphere for the person. However, in pastoral practice, such places do not need to be outside, but may also be created through the relationship between a couple of people, or a small group with the person who is dying. The natural environment can bring joy and insight to people who are dying, for example, I remember an instance when my son's godmother, Mary, was dying, I had visited her in palliative care in a local hospital about two hours' drive away from my home. I had taken her some camellia blooms from my garden. A couple of days later one of the registered nurses phoned to tell me that Mary had died that day, and that a few hours before her death, while the nurse was with her, one of the flowers had fallen off the camellia, and Mary noticed and remarked, how sad, 'but look, another bud is coming out—new life'.

Creativity is regarded as having divine origins; however, it is also recognised that human beings have creative capacities and imagination, and these do not diminish in later life. In the next section, I will discuss the place of mediating spirituality, through the arts.

2.3 The Arts

The arts are ways that humans respond to meaning, and with imagination, engage in music, dance, art, poetry, drama, and much more. Often as older people lose physical abilities, engaging actively in the arts becomes more challenging. However, at any point in the journey towards death, the arts can be engaged to benefit those on this final life journey. This occurrence is especially so in regard to music, which can provide great comfort for the person who is dying, right to the point of death. Music may also provide rich connecting points for people who live with dementia.

2.4 Religion

Aspects of religion connect with deep needs within all human beings, regardless of whether the person has a religious affiliation. All people may respond to meaning through symbol, rituals and liturgies, religious and non-religious. There are secular rituals and liturgies, and we should be careful not to restrict these only to people of religious faith. There is a deep-seated need and corresponding response within humans to meaningful rituals and liturgies [10]. Symbols can become vehicles of meaning for the individual and/or family or community. Prayer is used by numbers of people who would not regard themselves as 'religious' or as 'pray-ers' as they negotiate critical life experiences and face death. The great religious faith traditions have used these modes of connecting humans with God or other deities in all sorts of situations; it is simply part of being human. Religions that are functioning effectively will use the arts, including music, art, dance, silence, and symbols, to bring their religious adherents into greater connection with the divine. Rituals and symbols are regularly used and developed in non-religious settings by individuals to connect to meaning as they grapple with life.

These four means of mediating the spiritual dimension are still relevant for older people who are dying. I want to turn now, to consider more specifically the final life career and the spiritual dimension.

3 The Spiritual Dimension in Ageing

There remains a final life career which takes in the spiritual dimension. In my research and care of older people, I have found that often the spirit becomes reawakened as the person moves towards death and an increased awareness of life meaning is triggered. But what shape does this later life spiritual awakening take? Story is often the vehicle of meaning, should the person have a story listener. That story listener may be a staff member, a family member, or a trained pastoral volunteer. In residential care, where there is often a shortage of people with time to sit and listen, trained volunteers can be of great value as story listeners, encouraging the story to emerge from the storyteller [11, 12].

3.1 *A Model of Spiritual Tasks and Process of Ageing Applied in a Palliative Approach to Dying in Later Life*

A pattern of spiritual development can be seen in many older people. One way of understanding changes and development that may occur in older people has been described in the Spiritual Tasks and Process of Ageing (STPA) [7]. While there are many differences between people, major themes can be seen and mapped. For each spiritual theme, there is a corresponding spiritual task or process.

The Spiritual Tasks and Process of Ageing

The process is based on research by MacKinlay [13–15]. The STPA describes six spiritual tasks, common to older people, whether or not they hold a religious affiliation (see Fig. 2). The first four tasks comprise:

- Self-transcendence or, according to Frankl [4], self-forgetting
- The process of searching for meaning
- Finding intimacy with God and/or others
- Finding hope

'The remaining two spiritual tasks both influence and are influenced by these four tasks. Thus, at the core of our being are found the outcomes of our searches for meaning.

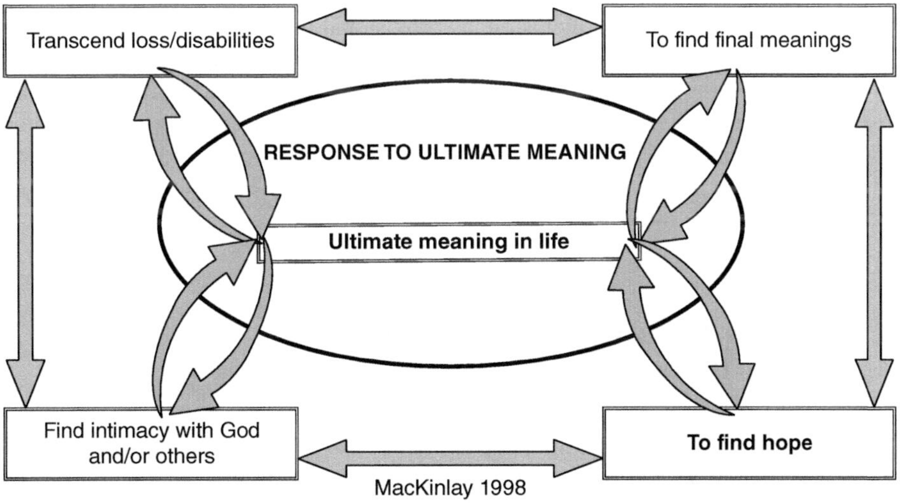

Fig. 2 Spiritual tasks and process of ageing (and dying)—a continuing process. (Reprinted with permission from MacKinlay, E. [7], Fig. 5.3, p. 116)

- The task (outcome) of finding ultimate or final meaning.
- Response to meaning and the outcome results in how we respond to all of life' [15, p. 152].

These six spiritual tasks will be further explained in relation to the continued development and movement into the final life career.

3.2 *The Spiritual Themes of Ageing and Associated Spiritual Tasks and Process of Ageing*

The STPA model was developed from the themes of ageing and spirituality identified in the narratives of independent living older people [13]; surveys were analysed and factor analysis applied to identify participant themes. The spiritual tasks and process of ageing potentially continue through life and include the process of dying (final life career), with death completing the life cycle. The final life career forms a continuum until death.

4 The Spiritual Tasks of Ageing and Dying

The first four tasks outlined above [7] link the physical and psychosocial processes of ageing and the spiritual dimension, and these tasks are naturally occurring in older people; indeed, some of these changes may also be seen in younger people who are dying. In this final journey towards death, the human narrative can take its final shape and draws to a conclusion, as provisional meanings, assigned to earlier life events, are finally re-examined and realisation of final meanings is reached. It is at this stage that the process of spiritual accompaniment in the model of the midwife may be of value in the dying process. Journeying with a dying person is a privileged journey. Of course, as Frankl wisely noted [4], not everyone comes to find the meaning of their lives before death; in fact, some people come to death without having discerned that there might be meaning to their life.

4.1 *Self-Sufficiency Versus Vulnerability and Self-Transcendence Linkages*

The process of spiritual development that may be stimulated by a loss of self-sufficiency and greater perceived vulnerability, leads to development of self-transcendence (see Fig. 3). It is at this point that the spiritual dimension has its greatest likelihood of producing a late 'Spring' in life. Erikson and Erikson have written wisely of this development, focusing on the psychosocial, but also on the

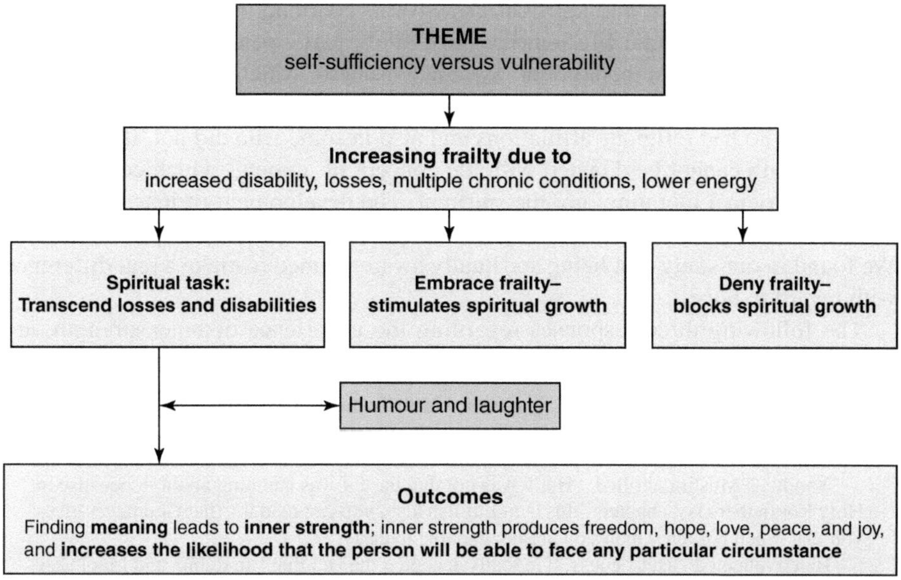

Fig. 3 Self-sufficiency versus vulnerability. (Figure based on MacKinlay model of spiritual themes, tasks, and process of ageing [7], described p. 116–120; MacKinlay et al. [19], Taylor & Francis Ltd, reprinted by permission of the publisher (Taylor & Francis Ltd, http://www.tandfonline.com))

spiritual dimension, culminating their important work while in their own ageing of late 80s to 90s [16, 17]. The Eriksons recognised a ninth stage of psychosocial development, that of self-transcendence, or gerotranscendence, linking to Tornstam's [18] theory.

One of the signs of transcendence is gratitude which is visible in inner peace and strength. Diana had numerous physical health issues, and yet she was able to say to the interviewer: 'So you know really, I've got a million things to be thankful for, so why would I complain? I'm truly blessed, honestly'. In the following section, I will address matters of self-transcendence and inner strength.

The Getting of Inner Strength

What is this 'inner strength' that is perceived in self-transcendence? What has happened when people are said to have moved towards self-transcendence or transformation, or sanctification? It becomes clear to others that the person who is experiencing self-transcendence is showing a sense of being relaxed and at peace and being other centred. There may be a deep sense of joy in their demeanour, joy that remains even when the person is facing difficult times and decisions, and/or loss. In the terms of the model of spiritual tasks and process of ageing [7], this change is the move towards self-transcendence—moving beyond oneself. In Frankl's [4] understanding, it is the ability of the person to 'self-forget'. It is at this stage that fear recedes, and spiritual growth can continue. In our work with frail older people in this final life journey [19], study participants often responded to questions of what 'kept them going' as 'inner strength' which allowed them to continue to keep going almost against all expectations. This inner strength was present in people who had religious affiliations and also in some who did not. It seems that inner strength cannot be equated with the concept of 'coping' which comes out of the psychological literature, not the spiritual. The development of inner strength is what could be termed a 'meta change' in the person, which is of a spiritual nature. We found in our study that being spiritually aware seemed to make a real difference with regard to hope.

The following three responses regarding the experience of inner strength, are from participants in a study of frailty, ageing, and the spiritual dimension:

> For Margaret, a Christian, it was: "I suppose basically just trusting God, I mean, he's there all the time and you know that God the Father, he loves us, he's not going to test us beyond our means. So, whatever happens, you just trust, and I think you can get through it."
>
> Xanthe, a Muslim, replied: "But it was not that hard. I was laughing about it, because in Holy Koran there is a chapter – this is in English also, you can read it – that God never gives you that much burden which you are not capable to carry."
>
> Helen reflected: "But I guess, I've really accepted the fact that I'm dying, and I feel very comfortable with that. So now I'm just enjoying the trip". [20, p. 245]

Helen expressed a readiness to face her dying, and it is with that in mind that I write now about the spiritual in those final times of moving towards death.

Walking with People in the Final Life Career

Two modes of enquiry and intervention in the spiritual domain are of value in working with and caring for older people who are entering their final life career. Ideally, the first meeting of the person will be early enough to be able to take a spiritual history or assessment. It may also be possible to engage in spiritual reminiscence, which is a special way of communicating with older people that focuses on supporting the person in their search for the meaning of their unique life events, rather than simply an historical account of their lives. It is in the process of spiritual assessment [9] and spiritual reminiscence [7, 14, 21] that people can have the opportunity to continue or renew their spiritual growth or can be assisted to address spiritual distress. It can be valuable to work on these processes early in the final life career; however, if the person is nearer to death, then spiritual assessment can certainly identify spiritual needs as they arise, so that these can be appropriately addressed.

For those of us who share the privileged ministry and care of older people who are dying, each death is different because the person who is dying is a unique human being, and their hopes and fears will be reflected in their final life journey. Sometimes, the dying person may not even speak a word, but there is a heightened sense of being in the room and being with them. I well remember when my mother, who had dementia, was dying. She had not spoken for something like two years prior to her death, and I was the geographically distant daughter who travelled overnight with my daughter to visit one last time. Although my mother said nothing in our presence, she was very present to us, and her eyes seemed fixed on us, seemingly drinking in all she could see, as my daughter and I each had our own time with her saying our own 'thank you' and 'goodbye', before we both came back to be together with her. Then, quietly Mum stopped breathing, and both her daughter (me) and granddaughter were there with her, in the moment, with Mum's favourite music playing in the background. This was a special and sacred moment to each of us, with eye contact being a vital connecting point for us. The senses are very important at these times, and it seems there can be a heightened awareness in the person dying of what is going on around them. At such times, words may be extraneous. Touch, eye contact, assurance, and hope mingle with the type of rituals and symbols that are relevant to the dying person, in the best of these deaths. So, it is important for the person providing spiritual care near death to be aware of the type of rituals and symbols that will speak to the dying person and their loved ones who may be present, so that these events will be meaningful and connect with them. I have experienced that deepness of connection as spiritual on many occasions as I have ministered to older people who were dying.

Situations around dying became so much more complex during the COVID-19 pandemic, when the process of dying meant the chaplain would be required to wear full protective clothing to restrict infection. This action led to diminished physical contact and difficulty for the person dying to hear what was being said through use of masks, or to see faces of those who were ministering to them, nor were family allowed to be present in residential care. Prevention of infection spread must always be held in balance with being able to connect person-to-person, in what is true person-centred care.

4.2 The Process of Searching for Meaning

This task is life-long, sometimes more consciously pursued while at other times the search may be almost subconscious [22]. Importantly, meaning is concerned with identity, and one's sense of identity evolves over a lifetime. Frankl [4] wrote of the way in which human beings process memories of the significant events of their lives. Whether and how deeply an event is processed at the time depends on the meaning and significance of that event to the individual. According to Frankl, these are provisional memories, and it is not until a person becomes aware of their own mortality, that they are moved to re-process their life story in relation to meaning as deep questions of life emerge: 'What has been the meaning of my life?' or perhaps simply, 'why was I here?' This process is a component of the spiritual dimension that seemed to occur naturally in many people. How deeply the spiritual dimension played out in the life of any individual depends on several factors, such as significant events in one's life, the individual's personality, and potentially social factors as well. In societies where instant gratification and technology are prized, opportunities for reflection on life and the search for meaning are likely to be compromised. Butler [23] first realised the importance of reminiscence among older people through his work as a psychiatrist in mental hospitals in the 1960s in the United States of America. In later life, he continued to highlight the importance of reminiscence. Butler subsequently wrote these words on the relevance of reminiscence for older people in his foreword in Haight and Webster [24]:

> As one's life nears an end, the opportunity to confront lifetime conflicts and acts of omission and commission which warrant guilt as well as opportunities for atonement, resolution and reconciliation is precious, because this is the last opportunity one had. (p. xxi)

There is a tendency for the search for meaning to become more focused as people grow older and is accentuated with rising awareness of mortality. Kimble reflected on Frankl's understanding of the spiritual dimension of 'being', noting that according to Frankl [4], it is 'the energy within the person that strives for meaning and purpose' [25, p. 35]. Further, Frankl described the spiritual dimension as 'the unifying and integrating dimension of being that includes the experience of transcendence and the mystery of the holy' [25, p. 35]. Kimble suggested that in light of this, understanding of the older person needs to be enlarged to be understood as the 'essence of one's very being'. The crucial question then arises, asked of this search for meaning: 'Is growing old worth one's whole life to achieve?' [25, p. 36].

In my model, I have separated out two tasks around meaning. First is the lifelong task and *process* of searching for and assigning meaning to events during one's life (provisional meanings), while the second is the *outcome* of finding ultimate or final meaning. The knowledge of the outcome is deposited at the very core of my being, at the heart. Even this final life meaning is subject to change until death.

4.3 Finding Intimacy with God and/or Others

Depth of relationship lies within the spiritual dimension in the sense of understanding intimacy, and being known at my depth, accepted as I am at the very core of my being [26]. This sense of intimacy can be of divine and/or human experience. In a sense, we human beings are made for relationship. It is well recognised that sometimes people remain alive, against all odds, to see someone or to be reconciled to someone before they die. Among older people facing their final life career, the relationship with God may become more central, given the loss of most of the closest human relationships an older person has. The time of approaching death can become, for some, one of the thin places of moving between the human, physical world and that of eternity.

Margaret, reflecting on her journey of faith remarked: 'My faith has been the, how would you say—without it I think I wouldn't be able to live my life this way. I always believe, I have strong faith whatever comes'. Margaret explained the nature of her faith and her relationship with God: 'I think my faith has given me strength and love of God'. He knows. I always say, 'Help me to be worthy of his love'.

4.4 *Finding Hope*

I placed hope as the fourth of the four main spiritual tasks of ageing. My reason was that, unlike the other tasks, hope is not so much a doing, but rather, it is a mode of being and an outcome of spiritual development in later life. Finding hope is a function of the spiritual dimension and occurs even in the face of dying; hope is found in the culmination self-transcendence, finding final meanings, and in the depth of spiritual connectedness in relationship. So, hope becomes evident in the person who has learned to transcend the self and reach out to others, hope is evident in the person who is working on their search for life meaning, hope is evident in the person who has effective relationships, with others and/or with God or the divine. These spiritual tasks are continuing, to the point of death, so they are always becoming, never finished.

The older person who 'has hope' loses a sense of fear. Often the person who has hope will show a deep-seated sense of joy, that transcends life crisis and hardships, joy that others may witness but not necessarily understand. Hope is seen among people of the Abrahamic faiths (Jews, Christians, and Muslims) in their scriptures, rituals and doctrines, beliefs, and the ways they live their lives. For most, there is some form of belief of an afterlife, and hope is based on this belief, not only on the current life. Buddhists and Hindus also see hope within their scriptures and beliefs in the continuity of life.

5 The Fifth and Sixth Spiritual Tasks and Outcomes

I now turn to the remaining two spiritual tasks that both influence and are influenced by these four tasks, already described. Thus, at the core of our being are found the outcomes of our searches for meaning.

- 'The task (outcome) of finding ultimate or final meaning
- Response to meaning and the outcome results in how we respond to all of life' [15, p. 152].

It seems that these two spiritual tasks are of a different character than the other four tasks already described. While the other four tasks are life-long, these two tasks are dependent on the first four tasks, and, yet, at the same time, they feedback to the other tasks. The spiritual process is highly interactive. For instance, it is difficult to see beyond oneself, without some development of self-transcendence and self-transcendence is necessary for the person to be able to reach out and respond to others. For example, the person who remains focused on their own physical illness and conditions is likely to remain self-focused and unable to self-forget, and therefore become compromised in their ability to take on a self-transcendent perspective of life. Erikson [16], wrote of developing the ability to transcend one's life problems that is evident in some older people, that is seen as letting go and moving beyond the anxieties and fears around dying. This is associated with these two spiritual tasks of ageing, finding ultimate life meaning and responding to these final meanings. I describe these two tasks further below.

5.1 The Outcome of Finding Ultimate or Final Life Meaning

During our years of developing maturity, we can lay down memories and understandings of life events as we have perceived the events at the time. It is as Frankl [4] has written, that when we become aware of our personal mortality we are moved to re-visit and re-evaluate significant life events as we experienced them earlier in life. This is the time of the connections, of 'Ah ha'—and the sudden awareness of—'so that is what it all means!' Ultimate or final meaning lies at our hearts. When I raised questions of where he found meaning, one of my study participants said: 'you're touching the deep things now'. This participant's simple statement was also profound. His statement went to the very core of his being, to ultimate meaning. We may even get to revise the provisional meanings we have carried for many years. For the first time, we may confront our needs for confession, forgiveness, and reconciliation, but also, may come to appreciate our life final meanings and experience satisfaction of having completed the tasks set before us in life, as we come to see in whole, not in part (1 Corinthians 13:12). Coming to this place brings with it the realisation that we are ready for facing our own deaths. Often this journey is accompanied by a sense of peace, joy, and hope [4]. This spiritual task of searching for meaning in life has come to its natural conclusion, as the process has come to an end. Of course, this experience of journey will not be so for some older people, who may fight dying until the very end of life, to die in distress, such as in '*Do not go gentle into that good night*', the poem by Dylan Thomas [27, p. 283], written of his father going blind near the end of his life. This is a poem of struggle, of sadness and grief. Grief no doubt, to some extent, expressed by the son who sees, from the outside, his father's increasing loss of sight, darkness and disability, and his response to this outcome. The responses of adult children to the death of parents may be similar, or different from the perception of the parent. Grief certainly forms an important component of this scenario. But certainly, there are situations where at the end of a long life, the person dying does not die at peace and where struggle continues until death.

5.2 Response to Meaning: The Outcome Drives How We Respond to All of Life

If the spiritual task of finding meaning is to come to awareness of one's final life meaning, then the spiritual task of response to meaning will entail how we respond to final life meaning. If we come to our dying with an assurance of fulfilment in life, having found, even to some extent, the answers to why we were here, then we are likely to respond to others in relationship with a new openness, characterised by love, joy, and a sense of freedom; our response to life and death will be other-centred. As humans, we respond to others out of what lies at our hearts, whether it is a sense of love, or joy or peace, or anger, fear and distrust. In many instances, liturgies relevant to the dying person will be supportive for them and their families in this final journey. Symbols will be vehicles of meaning. At times, symbols that connect with the dying person may even become therapeutic in helping shape meaningful outcomes and a change of heart for the person who is dying [10]. These will need to be tailored to the needs of the individual. Spiritual and pastoral care practitioners have opportunities for creative care at this time.

The six spiritual tasks and process of ageing are interactive and continue the work of spiritual growth to the point of death; thus, at no time is spiritual care irrelevant. In fact, during the time of dying, spiritual care becomes paramount to the well-being of the dying person.

6 Conclusion

In this chapter, I have outlined two ways of considering the spiritual dimension among older people. First, I have outlined a figure that presents the ways that humans may mediate spirituality in their lives, at any point across the lifespan, whether of religious or secular perspective. Secondly, I have described a model of spiritual tasks and process of ageing [7], that can be applied to developmental changes in the spiritual dimension in ageing. I have applied this model to the final life career that encompasses the life journey of older people, culminating in death. I note that this model is not a model of 'successful ageing', but rather that it attempts to outline processes involved in developmental growth of the spiritual dimension among older people. The model seeks to embrace all experiences of ageing and dying; fears, struggles, grief, hopes, laughter, the searching for and finding of final life meanings.

The model and the figure were based on western concepts of the Spiritual dimension, religious and secular, since the research on which they were based collected data from mainly Anglo-Celtic participants, and it might be seen to be culture-bound to western societies. However, during subsequent workshops I was invited to conduct in Japan and Singapore, the model was seen by participants to be applicable to people of their cultures and faiths. In a very real sense, the model of spiritual tasks and process of ageing lies at a deep level of the individual, at the spiritual depths, so that cultures become the overlay of the spiritual dimension.

It is a privilege to accompany an older person who is spiritually aware and dying on this final life journey, to see them grappling with the deep questions of life, to see them coming to acceptance and readiness for dying and death. Too often, it seems that the medical priorities around yet more investigations and treatment overtake and impinge upon the work of the spiritual in the dying process. The spiritual dimension is the essence of the palliative approach to dying that should be fought for as strongly as some fight for 'the right to die' through voluntary assisted dying.

References

1. Kastenbaum R, Moreman C. Death society and human experience. New York: Routledge; 2018.
2. Barbato M. Caring for the dying patient. Intern Med J. 2005;35(10):636–7. https://doi.org/10.1111/j.1445-5994.2005.00911.x.
3. Heinz D. Finishing the story: aging, spirituality and the work of culture. J Relig Gerontol. 1995;9(1):3–19. https://doi.org/10.1300/J078V09N0102.
4. Frankl VE. Man's search for meaning. New York: Washington Square Press; 1984.
5. Hudson R. Ageing in a nursing home: foundations for care. Cham: Springer; 2022.
6. Metzger D. Writing for your life. In: Morgan RI, editor. Remembering your story: creating your own spiritual autobiography. Nashville: Upper Room Books; 1993.
7. MacKinlay E. The spiritual dimension of ageing. 2nd ed. London: Jessica Kingsley Publishers; 2017.
8. MacKinlay E. A narrative of spirituality and ageing: reflections on the ageing journey and the spiritual dimension. Religions. 2022;13:463. https://doi.org/10.3390/rel1305046.
9. MacKinlay EB. Spiritual growth and care in the fourth age of life. London: Jessica Kingsley Publishers; 2006.
10. Niven A. What ritual teaches about life, humour and ageing. J Relig Spiritual Aging. 2021;33(2):223–35. https://doi.org/10.1080/15528030.2020.1850604.
11. Kenyon GM. Telling and listening to stories: creating a wisdom environment for older people. Generations. 2003;27(3):30–3.
12. Kenyon GM, Clark P, de Vries B, editors. Narrative gerontology: theory, research, and practice. New York: Springer; 2001.
13. MacKinlay EB. The spiritual dimension of ageing: meaning in life, response to meaning, and well-being in ageing [Dissertation]. La Trobe University; 1998.
14. MacKinlay E, editor. Palliative care, ageing and spirituality. London: Jessica Kingsley Publishers; 2012.
15. MacKinlay E. Spiritual reminiscence in later life. In: Gibson F, editor. International perspectives on reminiscence, life review and life story work. London: Jessica Kingsley Publishers; 2019. p. 143–59.
16. Erikson J. The life cycle completed: extended version. New York: W.W. Norton & Co; 1997.
17. Erikson E, Erikson J, Kivnick H. Vital involvement in old age. New York: W.W. Norton & Co; 1986.
18. Tornstam L. Gerotranscendence: a developmental theory of positive aging. New York: Springer Publishing Company; 2005.
19. MacKinlay E, Burns R, Mordike S. The lived experience of frailty: what does it mean to be frail? J Relig Spiritual Aging. 2023. https://doi.org/10.1080/15528030.2023.2223156.
20. MacKinlay E. Ageing and frailty: a spiritual perspective of the lived experience. J Relig Spiritual Aging. 2021;33(2):236–49. https://doi.org/10.1080/15528030.2020.1845279.
21. MacKinlay E, Trevitt C. Spiritual factors in the experience of Alzheimer's disease and other dementias. In: Dick-Muehlke C, Li R, Orleans M, editors. Psychosocial studies of the individual's changing perspectives in Alzheimer's disease. Hershey: IGI Global Publishing; 2015.
22. Damasio A. Self comes to mind: constructing the conscious brain. New York: Pantheon Books; 2010.

23. Butler RN. The life review: an interpretation of reminiscence in the aged. In: Neugarten BL, editor. Middle age and aging: a reader in social psychology. Chicago: The University of Chicago Press; 1963. p. 497–508.
24. Butler RN. Foreword. In: Haight B, Webster J, editors. The art and science of reminiscing. Washington, DC: Taylor & Francis; 1995. p. pxxi.
25. Kimble M. Beyond the biomedical paradigm: generating a spiritual vision of ageing. J Relig Spiritual Aging. 2002;12(3–4):31–4. https://doi-org.ezproxy.csu.edu.au/10.1300/J078v12n03_03
26. Carroll LP, Dyckman KM. Chaos or creation: spirituality in mid-life. New York: Paulist Press; 1986.
27. Ferris P. Dylan Thomas. New York: Paragon House Publishers; 1989. p. 283.

Spiritual Care for People Living with Dementia

Chris Swift

Abstract A diagnosis of dementia (in its different forms) represents the identification of a disease which (if no other illness or event supersedes it) will eventually result in death. Altered behaviour and capabilities vary considerably among people living with the illness. This chapter identifies and explores approaches to spiritual care which have the greatest constructive impact on people living with dementia, their carers, families, and friends. Drawing on the personal experience of the author, along with a range of relevant literature, it sets out ways in which the agency and engagement of people can be enabled and enhanced by skilfully delivered spiritual support.

Keywords Dementia · Palliative care · Spirituality · Pastoral care · Agency
Ritual · Spiritual care

1 Introduction

My mother lived for 4 years with a diagnosis of dementia before she died in 2017. To a limited extent, her illness was managed and shielded by my father before her diagnosis. Like many people in the Western world, his desire to cope independently meant that help was not sought until a late stage in the first phase of her illness. When she spent hours every day packing belongings and stacking them in the hallway, he spent every evening returning things to their original place. My mother

C. Swift (✉)
School of Health, Science and Wellbeing at Staffordshire University,
Stoke-on-Trent, Staffordshire, UK
e-mail: Christopher.Swift@staffs.ac.uk

M. C. Best (ed.), *Spiritual Care in Palliative Care*,
https://doi.org/10.1007/978-3-031-50864-6_39

recognised the furniture in their home because they had owned it for decades. Some items of furniture she had known her entire life. But the house where they lived was newer, and my mother came to believe that it was not their home. As her mind worked to reconcile these perceptions, she determined that they were on holiday, but was perplexed as to why their furniture had come with them. This period of daily packing was intended to presage a journey home. It was distressing for both of them.

Many readers will recognise this situation, and many variants of what I experienced. A new generation of neuroscientists, including Anil Seth, believe that our consciousness is 'a special kind of controlled hallucination that has been shaped by evolution to regulate and control the living body' [1]. There are other theories of consciousness, but Seth's work offers an interesting approach to understanding what happens during the progress of dementia. As changes take place in the brain, people lose varying degrees of ability to cohere the world around them—to sustain the kind of consciousness they experienced previously. For example, my mother knew the furniture was hers—but the growing gaps in knowledge meant that she did not believe the house to be their home. There was still an attempt to reconcile this disparity, to generate plausible meaning. When are we in a house which is not our home? When we are on holiday. It is unsurprising that anxiety is a feature often found in the stages of living with dementia, often exacerbated by the stigma attached to the condition [2]. As people attempt to interpret their reality, with notable gaps in their memories emerging, it can become harder and harder to perceive a world that 'makes sense'.

For my mother, gradually gaps became more abundant, and the ability to hold together a sense of what is generally understood as reality, dwindled. Very familiar figures were misperceived as long-dead relatives (such as her father). My mother entered a care home and conversation became increasingly limited. Breaking the news that my father had died brought a moment of lucidity. 'I wondered where he'd gone', she said, as a single tear rolled down her cheek. It was the only moment when she appeared to recognise and understand her loss.

Providing spiritual care in these circumstances requires considerable patience and insight. It can be advantageous if there is knowledge about the person living with dementia which comes from an earlier stage in life. Material supplied by friends and relatives can be a great help—covering issues such as early life and personal preferences. However, it should also be recognised and understood that people may change significantly through the process of living with dementia. What may have been helpful and supportive once, might no longer receive the same reception as the illness progresses. One indication of this may be the expression of frustration. For example, when someone has previously enjoyed reminiscing about their working life becomes disengaged from conversation. It may be necessary to explore whether the focus of memory has changed and other topics for reminiscence have become more meaningful.

2 Knowledge and Engagement

As referenced above, due to a fluidity of temporal awareness, people living with dementia can experience memories of past events, places, and people in a way that is vivid and expressed as contemporaneous. A visitor's family resemblance may be recognised by someone living with dementia, but the precise association may be misplaced. For example, a niece might be addressed and related to as her mother. There is considerable value, given these manifestations of dementia, to provide past and present links with people close to the person experiencing these effects. For example, the *Famileo Gazette* [3] is one example of a tool that organises photographs and information provided by friends and family into a personalised newspaper with current and historic material relevant to the older person. In a care setting, this serves not only to maintain connections with a wider community but allows staff members to understand more about the past life of the person in their care.

Material that has been prepared with the resident in advance, such as information about their preferences approaching the end of life, is essential in meeting the needs of someone no longer able to express these preferences with the clarity they once expressed. However, care needs to be taken to ensure that current preferences are also regarded. There may have been a significant development in the spiritual and emotional life of the person living with dementia and it may no longer be appropriate to meet the needs as previously described. For example, while someone may once have wished to be surrounded by photographs of family members, this may become a cause for distress if the person can no longer identify the people. Being surrounded by images of strangers could be unnerving or alarming. It may, tacitly, convey the impression that the person is in the room of someone else.

A systematic review and meta-synthesis of the experience of spirituality from the perspective of people living with dementia noted both the valuable part spirituality can play [4]. For someone brought up within a particular religion or spiritual tradition from a young age, elements of iconography and text may have an enduring resonance through the progress of dementia. It is not unusual for people who find it difficult to speak—and may be silent for extended periods—to participate with verbal clarity when someone recites the Christian 'Lord's Prayer'. Similarly, the material nature of spirituality, including images and the use of colour during different parts of the year, may orientate someone's sense of the season. Christmas, particularly in Western cultures, has a very wide range of sensory expressions that enable people to respond and participate. This can include food; music; decorations; costume and liturgy.

However, the authors also note the risk that, in societies that are increasingly secular, this significance may be overlooked or poorly understood:

> Overall, the studies included indicated that people with dementia experience a deep understanding of spirituality, often enhanced by their remembrance of early life experiences. Faith, belief and rituals over the life-course were shown to sustain the person through the challenges they encounter in living with dementia. [4]

Given the rapid nature of change in matters of religion in Westernised nations (in particular), there is often a gulf between the place of religion in the childhood of carers and in the early years of people living with dementia. For this reason, carers may often be unaware of the spiritual landscape in which older people are living, or what steps or actions might be welcomed as supportive and meaningful. A central approach to spiritual care must therefore include active listening and a willingness to follow up on themes or concepts that are unfamiliar. Family members, and older residents who are able to articulate their memories, may assist in this process. Given the established significance and benefit of reminiscence, this should be a purposeful activity on the part of care staff [4].

It is probable that, in many instances, palliative care is provided at the point when someone is in the more advanced stages of dementia. This will mean that there is less likelihood that needs and wishes can be obtained through contemporaneous discussions. Peter Kevern has written about the paucity of research and publication concerning spirituality in these later stages of the condition. There are, understandably, reasons why this is the case—especially when it may be difficult to obtain consent to participate in research and when it is hard to validate the perception of spiritual needs. However, this review of the literature [5], and critical analysis of the data, poses interesting questions about an understanding of spirituality which is largely individual; interior; and of the moment. In contrast, Kevern suggests that in late-stage dementia it is necessary to view spirituality as the ingrained convictions and practices that we have exercised over time, and which remain part of us even as we lose the ability to communicate in ways that others can understand easily. Secondly, Kevern argues for the relational significance of spirituality. At a point when we can no longer sustain the sharing of memories and stories, others who have accompanied us during parts of our life are able to ensure that we remain connected to our spiritual identity. This may give added importance to the visits of friends and family and also to the place of religious texts, images, sounds, and rituals. The latter are significant because they can connect us through multi-sensory means to a long tradition of practices conveying a sense of the sacred and our value and place within a broader scheme of existence.

3 Ritual

Ritual can be difficult to define. It is recognised that there is a long history of human religious ritual, which may be connected to mammalian ritual during the process of evolution. It is deeply rooted in many human cultures and there may continue to be forms of ritual which are intrinsically spiritual even when someone identifies as 'non-religious'. Generally speaking, religious rituals are traditional acts or patterns of structured practice, when physical posture, artefacts, and voice may be used to foster a particular form of connection or association with the transcendent. As rituals are multi-sensory (and may have been familiar in childhood), they can have a particular potency when it comes to engagement with people who are experiencing the effects of dementia.

> The recurrent components of ritual, including exaggerated formality, sequencing, invariability, and repetition, have been selected to facilitate communication by eliciting arousal, directing attention, enhancing memory, and improving associations. [6]

There is a risk in the identification of someone's beliefs and convictions of giving excessive weight to some kind of confessional assent. In other words, that a person is religious because they give cognitive assent to a particular creed or formal statement of faith. It is notable that in the seventeenth century, the governing body of one of the United Kingdom's (UK) largest hospitals for mental health patients debated whether a chaplain should be employed. The body concluded that if people were incapable of 'receiving instruction', they could not benefit from the presence of a chaplain [7]. Although this explicit discussion is in the distant past, there continue to be religious groups that lay considerable emphasis either on cognitive assent to a credal statement, or to the value of an articulated personal testimony.

One example of this comes from the Methodist Church in the UK. One of the primary hymn books of this Christian denomination is entitled *Singing the Faith.* This reflects the fact that Methodist spirituality in particular has a deep tradition in music and congregational singing. It is in the act of singing, with texts often drawn directly from the Bible, that many Methodists feel their spirituality most clearly [8].

For many people, religion is as much a part of their identify and daily practices as the language they speak. People who have a religious upbringing may choose a different path when they become an adult but, as with language, aspects of their formative spirituality will always be their mother tongue. Through the process of ageing and the development of dementia these early experiences may return to the foreground of their concerns and wishes. In research using a standardised instrument of assessment for spirituality [9], researchers found that both carers and people living with dementia scored equally for their levels of belief. They also noted the value stated by people living with dementia for routines of spiritual practice, concluding that spirituality should be included in the general assessment of people living with dementia [10].

There is an important caveat to the re-emergence of childhood memories and associations. Many childhoods were not happy or positive, and in some cases, religious experiences may have been damaging and destructive. The extensive evidence and literature concerning abuse in churches provides an important basis for being alert to responses to spiritual rituals and expressions that may indicate distress. This may be particularly difficult if it is no longer possible or advisable to discuss what may lie behind a certain reaction.

In providing spiritual care and support for people coming to the end of life through dementia, an iterative approach is often required. Even close family and friends may not be familiar with the early life of the person who is dying, and it may be these earliest memories which hold the greatest significance for someone at this point in their lives. It is therefore essential that a person's response to initiatives of spiritual care is evaluated carefully in order to focus on rituals that bring a sense of peace, uplift, connection or other positive animation.

Many practitioners and researchers argue for the importance of multi-sensory approaches to engage people who are living with dementia [11]. For this reason, early memories, or spiritual formation at any stage in life, may be meaningful and important assets in the life of someone experiencing cognitive changes, providing moments of coherence, participation, and connection. In turn, all this can enhance the dignity of someone participating in religious or spiritual activities. In many world faiths, physical or mental illnesses may give someone increased significance and value within the community. During collective worship, it is not uncommon that the only people to be mentioned in prayer by name (with consent) are the sick and those who are at the end of life.

The potency of participation in religious and spiritual practices should not be underestimated. As one paper found: 'Participants repeatedly attributed engaging in religious activities with moments of clarity, lucidity, or "coming back"' [12]. Working with longstanding and deeply embedded personal/communal practices can enable a level of participation which is rewarding and satisfying for both the person living with dementia, and their carers.

4 Relatives and Friends

One of the most contentious elements of the COVID-19 pandemic, in relation to hospitals and care homes, was the denial or limitation of access for relatives when someone was receiving palliative care or at the end of their life [13]. People normally expect that close relatives and friends will be present with someone during their final days and hours of life. Religious or spiritual leaders may also be asked to attend in order to say prayers, conduct rituals or offer a blessing. During the pandemic, some of this support was offered remotely, but this was generally felt to be less satisfactory than being physically present not least because, as with ritual, the multi-sensory nature of presence is seen as particularly helpful for someone coming to the end of life while living with dementia [14].

The pandemic accelerated and widened the use of digital forms of communication, and this at least facilitated some connection between relatives and staff. Care workers became intermediaries for family and friends, especially when it came to care at the end of life. However, there were inevitable limitations to this. During an outbreak of the virus, with staff who tested positive for COVID-19 away from work, and poorly patients requiring more care, it was often very difficult for staff on duty to answer calls or engage in conversations.

The experience of visiting an older relative in a formal care setting can be difficult for younger family members. In some cases, the older person, typically a grandparent, may have been involved in the care of the younger relative. As changes take place during the course of dementia, it may be that a young visitor is not recognised or identified as a different child from the person's past. This can be upsetting for a younger person. Spiritual care can be an important way to enable links across the generations and to provide moments of sharing. For example, someone living with dementia may recall and be able to sing religious songs which have been learned in childhood. In some cases, these songs may be known to the younger person as well. Prayers, such as in the Christian faith 'The Lord's Prayer', may also be recalled and participated in. A partnership between three charities in the UK has seen the production of a story book designed for younger people which helps contextualise and explain the people and circumstances that might be encountered in a care home. A central linking figure in this story is the chaplain in the residential facility [15].

5 Health and Social Care Service Integration for Holistic Dementia Care

As the foregoing makes clear, knowledge and understanding of the history, preferences, and wishes of people living with dementia is vital for the provision of excellent care. This can be challenging as spirituality may have significant links to the deep past of the person receiving care, and the number of contemporaries able to assist with information about that period of life is likely to be limited. Consequently, an early indication of preferences, including the identification of people who are needed for support and involvement, can make the progress of care smoother and more effective. While recognising the reality of personal change over the course of the illness, personal knowledge of the person enables the accurate interpretation of communication (verbal and non-verbal) in order to meet need and preferences most meaningfully. There is probably no equivalent substitute for a friend or family member to be present during the final phase of life in order to support the best possible care. However, this is not always possible. Written notes from previous interviews with the person before their dementia precluded that opportunity, and also notes from family and friends that may have been recorded in care plans, are an essential resource in order to ensure the continuity of care.

There is a mixed picture about the degree of fragmentation in health services for people living with dementia in the last year of their life. It is possible that this group has a smaller ecosystem of health services than a comparator group of older adults with serious health conditions, but without dementia [16]. However, it is also noted in the literature that hospital admissions in the last months of life are associated with poor quality care for people living with dementia:

> People with dementia are at high risk of multiple hospital admissions at the end of life and preventing these admissions is a policy priority. This study found that people with dementia who had better continuity of care with GPs were less likely to have multiple hospital admissions in the last 90 days of life, in particular if they lived at home and had multiple comorbidities. People living in care homes and with an identification of palliative care needs in their primary care records were less likely to experience these admissions. [17]

One of the conclusions of this research was that an earlier designation of palliative care may aid the continuity of support, while recognising that with dementia, finding the right moment for such a designation can be challenging.

In the UK, there is no systematic way to ensure that records of spiritual care can, with consent, be passed to a hospital chaplain or hospital ward during an admission. Usually, the person normally linked with the care of a patient—either a local religious leader or care home chaplain—will seek individual or family consent to call the hospital chaplain. Preferences for care would then be shared verbally with the expectation that the chaplain would follow-up on the patient and provide support. In the UK, it is rare to find funded chaplaincy roles in care, nursing, and residential homes. Similarly, in the community, there is a wide disparity in the training, staffing, and organisation of pastoral care provision. One exception to this has been the growth of 'Anna Chaplaincy', a community service that is based in the local church and focused on the needs of older people [18]. This form of chaplaincy ensures a common standard of recruitment, selection, and practice.

6 End-of-Life Lucidity

Over the course of 30 years of chaplaincy work I have met many relatives and friends of people who died with/of dementia who tell of a sign or words of lucidity just before death. For a long time, I wondered if this was a perception shaped by desire, and that some final gesture of recognition by the person who was dying met an understandable need. Researchers term this kind of process as 'memory distortions'. However, research which has sought to exclude the influence of distortions concludes that there is something here that requires further attention and study. When all the caveats have been applied, and recognising the limits of present understanding, researchers nevertheless concluded:

> an unknown number of dementia patients appear to experience full spontaneous remission of their cognitive function and verbal ability shortly before their death. [19]

In the United States, the National Institute on Aging has released tranches of research funds to explore this phenomenon further, with the hope that understanding the mechanism of temporary lucidity may open a path to novel forms of treatment for dementia [20].

Given the growing evidence about lucidity close to the time of death, it suggests that there may be a moment of opportunity for people to engage more cognitively in spiritual care at this defining moment in their life. For example, and with great care, it may be possible during a period of lucidity to ascertain someone's preferences for particular prayers to be said; religious texts to be read; or final wishes to be honoured. Greater understanding of this phenomenon should inform the discussion about how best to provide spiritual care in the final days and hours of life. This may include the need to prioritise visits by family members and religious leaders if and when a period of lucidity emerges.

7 Conclusion

Spiritual care is usually a bespoke form of support, shaped by the spirituality of the person for whom the care is provided. Typically, this means that a patient or care facility resident discusses their spiritual heritage and current commitments with a member of staff. In the case of people living with dementia, this may have been documented in the past or can be ascertained via relatives and friends. In some cases, it may be very difficult to gain a full picture of the person's spirituality or wishes. In all events, an iterative approach that builds on available knowledge is the best way to develop a pattern of spiritual support. The use of religious and spiritual texts, rituals and worship alongside others may provide care that animates the person in a positive way. This can increase their agency, sense of dignity and connection with practices that have been familiar across their life. At the end of life, this kind of knowledge on the part of carers can ensure that forms of spiritual care are used which bring comfort to the person who is dying, as well as support for family members and friends.

References

1. Seth A. Being you: a new science of consciousness. New York: Penguin; 2021.
2. Riley RJ, Burgener S, Buckwalter KC. Anxiety and stigma in dementia: a threat to aging in place. Nurs Clin. 2014;49(2):213–31.
3. Familio Gazette UK. https://www.famileo.com/famileo/en-GB/?utm_source=google_ads_search_marque&utm_medium=cpc&gad=1&gclid=EAIaIQobChMIyY6mts2pgQMVcWHmCh0MggjxEAAYASAAEgId5PD_BwE. Accessed 14 Sept 2023.
4. MacKinlay E, Trevitt C. Living in aged care: using spiritual reminiscence to enhance meaning in life for those with dementia. Int J Ment Health Nurs. 2010;19(6):394–401.
5. Kevern P. The spirituality of people with late-stage dementia: a review of the research literature, a critical analysis and some implications for person-centred spirituality and dementia care. Mental Health Relig Cult. 2015;18(9):765–76.
6. Sosis R, Alcorta C. Signaling, solidarity, and the sacred: the evolution of religious behavior. Evol Anthropol. 2003;12(6):264–74.
7. Swift C. Hospital chaplaincy in the twenty-first century: the crisis of spiritual care on the NHS. London: Routledge; 2015.
8. Kimbrough ST. Lyrical theology: theology in hymns. Theol Today. 2006;63(1):22–37.
9. King M, Speck P, Thomas A. The Royal Free interview for religious and spiritual beliefs: development and standardization. Psychol Med. 1995;25(6):1125–34.
10. Jolley D, Benbow SM, Grizzell M, Willmott S, Bawn S, Kingston P. Spirituality and faith in dementia. Dementia. 2010;9(3):311–25.
11. Smeaton E, Maher C. Supporting spiritual engagement for people living with dementia. Health Soc Care Chaplain. 2016;4(2):130–41.
12. Carr TJ, Hicks-Moore S, Montgomery P. What's so big about the 'little things': a phenomenological inquiry into the meaning of spiritual care in dementia. Dementia. 2011;10(3):399–414.
13. Siesage H, Sams L, Ellis NJ, Swift C. Exploring the changing experiences of chaplains employed in care and residential homes during the COVID-19 pandemic: a longitudinal qualitative study. Health Soc Care Chaplain. 2023;11(2):220.

14. Swift C. Being there, virtually being there, being absent: chaplaincy in social care during the COVID-19 pandemic. Health Soc Care Chaplain. 2020;8(2):154–64.
15. Bacon J, Parmenter S. Finding nana: an MHA special places book. London: Methodist Publishing; 2023.
16. Nothelle S, Kelley AS, Zhang T, Roth DL, Wolff JL, Boyd C. Fragmentation of care in the last year of life: does dementia status matter? J Am Geriatr Soc. 2022;70(8):2320–9.
17. Leniz J, Gulliford M, Higginson IJ, Bajwah S, Yi D, Gao W, Sleeman KE. Primary care contacts, continuity, identification of palliative care needs, and hospital use: a population-based cohort study in people dying with dementia. Br J Gen Pract. 2022;72(722):e684–92.
18. Thrower D. Anna chaplains. Rural Theol. 2017;15(2):124–7.
19. Batthyány A, Greyson B. Spontaneous remission of dementia before death: results from a study on paradoxical lucidity. Psychol Conscious Theory Res Pract. 2021;8(1):1.
20. Eldadah BA, Fazio EM, McLinden KA. Lucidity in dementia: a perspective from the NIA. Alzheimers Dement. 2019;15(8):1104–6.

Deathbed Visions and the Moment of Death

Michael Barbato

Abstract Once considered a sacred and hallowed time, the moment of death has become destabilised within our secularised, medicalised world with the focus moving from the profound to the practical. Death may represent the end of life as we know it, but unbeknown to many, this time may be punctuated by transcendent phenomena, leading one scholar to suggest these events spiritualise death by bringing comfort and a sense of wonder to the person dying and their family. This chapter will review recent animal and human research that focuses on the end of life. It will probe the empirical and neuroscientific literature in an attempt to uncover meaningful information about the lived experience of dying and two of the now well-described, but poorly understood, accompaniments of dying, namely deathbed visions and terminal lucidity. Although at times speculative, the inquiry will show that deathbed visions and terminal lucidity occur at and around the time of death. These end-of-life phenomena are predominantly covert, yet they are considered by many to be instruments of healing for the person dying and a potential source of comfort for grieving family and friends. Based on what we know, and despite our limited understanding of unconsciousness, this chapter will conclude with broad recommendations concerning the holistic care of unresponsive dying patients.

Keywords Deathbed visions · Terminal lucidity · The moment of death · End-of-life dreams and visions · Unresponsiveness · Lived experience of dying · Palliative care · Spiritual care

M. Barbato (✉)
Honorary Research Fellow, Palliative Care Services, Illawarra Shoalhaven Local Health District, Wollongong, NSW, Australia

M. C. Best (ed.), *Spiritual Care in Palliative Care*,
https://doi.org/10.1007/978-3-031-50864-6_40

1 Deathbed Visions

In her dying memoir, Cory Taylor declares that death has been demoted to that of a medical event, a failure of treatment or an unmentionable thing [1]. Believing this unforeseen shift is a conversation the palliative care profession should engage in, Robert Kastenbaum laments that the mere mention of research around the moment of death leads to resistance and a closing of minds and doors [2]. Death may represent the end of life as we know it, but unbeknown to many, this time is punctuated by transcendent phenomena, leading Stafford Betty, Professor of Religious Studies at California State University, to suggest that visions at or near the end of life spiritualise death by bringing comfort and a sense of wonder to the person dying and their family [3].

My interest in Deathbed Visions (DBVs) was aroused early in my career by one single event. Stella was in her late 70s and had been admitted to our palliative care unit for end-of-life care. She was gaunt from the ravages of cancer and on the occasion of my final visit she had been unresponsive for more than 36 hours. Her hands were cold, her breathing shallow and her pulse barely palpable. Knowing death was imminent, I stayed hoping her family who had been notified would arrive before she died. Without any provocation, Stella suddenly opened her eyes and literally sprung to life. Unassisted, she sat bolt upright and gazed straight ahead. Her arms were outstretched as if reaching for someone or something she alone could see. She did not acknowledge her family when they arrived and remained engrossed in what I could only assume was a vision that had captured her attention as well as her imagination. She remained mute, motionless, and mesmerised for several minutes before lying back on the bed. Her breathing ceased the moment her head hit the pillow [4, p. 136].

Although rarely seen now [5], experiences such as Stella's were once a common occurrence and were well described at the turn of the last century by Sir William Barrett in his classic text, *Deathbed Visions* [6]. Apart from some notable exceptions [7, 8], descriptions of visions at the moment of death have all but disappeared from the contemporary palliative care discourse while reports of end-of-life dreams and visions (ELDVs) in conscious patients nearing death have increased dramatically [9–15].

There is every reason to believe that visions occurring moments before death have a phenomenology, cause, and effect similar to that of ELDVs. What makes them so unusual and mysterious, however, is that they occur when the person's body is about to give up the ghost. Rather than introduce a new descriptor I will refer to these near-death dreams or visions as a deathbed vision (DBV) on the understanding it's the classical form of an ELDV that occurs immediately before death that I'm describing.

If indeed DBVs occur in patients at the edge of death, one can only wonder about the clarity and potency of dreams that jolt them from what Shakespeare called the 'sleep of death'. Why they occur when they do has bewildered clinicians, artists, poets, neuroscientists, and theologians alike. The door into this hitherto mysterious field of DBVs has opened somewhat following recent research demonstrating unexpected neurophysiological changes immediately before death. These changes posit a possible explanation for DBVs as well as other experiences such as ELDVs, near-death experiences (NDEs), out-of-body experiences (OBEs), and terminal lucidity (TL) [16, 17]. This observation has renewed neuroscientists' interest in changes that occur in the dying brain and raises questions about the lived experience of patients at the edge of death.

For ethical, philosophical, and practical reasons, research into the lived experience of unresponsive palliative care patients has always been considered taboo. The first of a small number of such studies took place at the start of this century when processed electroencephalography (EEG) was used to track the level of awareness in 12 consenting palliative care patients from the moment they became unresponsive until their death [18]. The EEG instrument, known as the Bispectral Index (BIS) monitor, had until then been used almost exclusively with anaesthetised patients to measure their level of sedation [19]. The monitor's size, ease of operation and an algorithm that generates a continuous numerical measure of awareness (the BIS score) from a single frontal sensor makes it the ideal instrument for use in the palliative care situation.

One of the many serendipitous findings from that original study was a sudden increase in BIS scores in four of the 12 patients immediately before death (Fig. 1). In the anaesthetic situation, this change would be attributed to an increase in a patient's level of awareness, but the absence of a noticeable change in demeanour in any of the four dying patients calls for an alternative explanation (we will explore this later). This observation generated little interest at the time, but similar BIS findings in subsequent studies [20–23] led to further speculation about the cause and significance of the surge. Nurses and doctors who witnessed DBVs first-hand wondered if the sudden unexplained increase in BIS scores was somehow related.

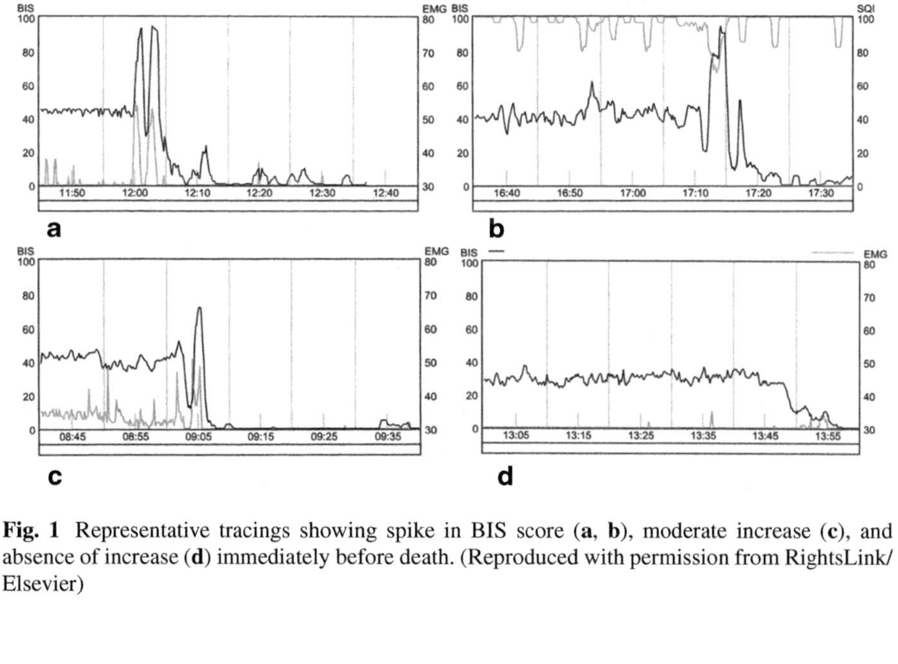

Fig. 1 Representative tracings showing spike in BIS score (**a**, **b**), moderate increase (**c**), and absence of increase (**d**) immediately before death. (Reproduced with permission from RightsLink/Elsevier)

Neuroscientists, however, remained convinced the surge represented little more than the agonal throes of a dying brain.

The very same neuroscientists were obliged to review their stance following research that scrutinised raw EEG data in rats undergoing experimental cardiac arrest [16]. The finding of neural correlates of heightened consciousness immediately before death came as a surprise and for the first time afforded a scientific explanation for NDEs reported by some near-death survivors. This shift in thinking reached seismic proportions when later research described raw EEG changes in patients who died in an intensive care unit (ICU) after withdrawal of ventilator support [24, 25]. These changes were observed in three of five patients in the last minutes of life and were characterised by high frequency gamma wave oscillations and functional connectivity, similar to that seen in the animal study. Not only do the changes occur at the same time as the BIS spike seen in palliative and intensive care studies, they are also remarkably similar to changes seen in healthy humans during dreaming and in seizure patients during visual hallucinations and OBEs [25]. These authors concluded that the dying brain can still be active in the near-death period and in a subsequent podcast they proposed that these near-death changes may be responsible for DBVs, OBEs, and TL as well as NDEs [26].

The thought of the dying brain becoming active at the edge of death may seem paradoxical, but according to one transpersonal psychologist, the template for transcendent experiences is hard wired into the human psyche as a normal constituent of the human personality and explains why dreams and visions occur with such clarity and frequency when someone is dying and seemingly midwife them into a deeper way of being [27, p. 25 & 154]. Christof Koch, a neuroscientist of some repute, is more 'cerebral' in his analysis and says that in life-threatening situations, neurons still capable of generating neural activity will construct images and stories that we have come to know as NDEs [28]. If this is true of NDEs, it's not unreasonable to propose the same may also be true of DBVs and ELDVs.

In studies involving ICU patients, it was the withdrawal of ventilator support and the resultant global hypoxia that led to the observed neurophysiological changes [24, 25]. In the palliative care situation, hypoxia at life's end may set up a similar dynamic, predisposing dying patients to a DBV. Whether a DBV actually ensues may not only depend on the rapidity and degree of hypoxia but also the person's innate propensity to dissociate. Bruce Greyson proposes that those who have an NDE are capable of dissociating or shifting their attention away from their physical body and the crisis that confronts it. This propensity to dissociate is what ultimately determines the likelihood of a NDE or an OBE [29] and could also explain why data from human studies show that some but not all dying patients have a surge in neurophysiological activity immediately before death [21, 25, 30, 31].

What remains unclear is why no patients in these palliative care studies exhibited any of the characteristic features of a DBV [6, p. 4] and why DBVs, once a common accompaniment of dying, are so rarely seen today. Both anomalies have been attributed to the sedating effect of end-of-life medication [32] even though the only reported study into the effect of palliative sedation on BIS scores indicates that opioid, benzodiazepine, and hyoscine preparations do not prevent the surge and may render DBVs covert [30]. Put more simply, DBVs are still experienced in the mind of the person dying, but as they are unaccompanied by any of the usual markers, they remain imperceptible to others unless the dream is powerful enough and/or the dose of medication small enough to favour manifestation. The effect of phenobarbitone is less clear. Based on four patients receiving cumulative doses of 4000, 1600, 2000, and 800 mg over 29, 24, 40, and 8 hours respectively, findings suggest phenobarbitone may prevent the BIS surge and that this effect is dependent on the total dose and duration of treatment [30].

Despite mounting evidence, neuroscientists are still reluctant to exclude yet unknown pathological changes unique to dying as a cause of the neurophysiological activity and cite reasons why the change in BIS scores could be spurious or artefact [33]. We are, however, reminded by others that the search for answers to this thorny question will always be limited by the absence of patient feedback and we must therefore rely on verifiable empirical evidence and anecdotal reports [17]. For many neuroscientists, accepting such circumstantial evidence would be considered overreaching, but for those who have witnessed a DBV, myself included, it's not difficult to associate that phenomenon with changes seen on the BIS and raw EEG.

2 Terminal Lucidity

Some of the most treasured recollections of grieving families are times when their previously unresponsive dying loved one had an unexpected episode of lucidity. Terminal lucidity (TL) [34], also known as lightening up [32] or pre-mortem surge [35], is extraordinary in its own right, but verges on the mysterious when it occurs in patients with a long history of dementia, schizophrenia, stroke, or other neurodegenerative disorders. This unexpected, spontaneous, and meaningful communication in patients assumed to have permanently lost the capacity for coherent verbal or behavioural interaction is referred to as paradoxical lucidity [36–38].

With TL, a previously unresponsive patient may utter a few words, deliver an important message, bid farewell or seek to set their house in order. Some ask for relief of pain or thirst while others are content to look, listen, and bask in the moment [35, 39]. A memorable example occurred when one of my patients who had been unresponsive for days, woke on her birthday and shared a glass of champagne with family at the kitchen table. After a short time, she returned to her bed and died the following day [4, p. 130].

Dying patients often resort to symbolism to explain their lived experience and for family as well as carers these lucid moments may seem anything but lucid [40]. This was the case with another of my patients who suddenly woke and said to her family, 'I'm climbing a steep mountain. When I get to the top, I have to do an appendix operation. I'm frightened because I've never done one before'. This woman was a doctor and, as is often the case, she resorted to metaphor to describe something that was beyond words—what dying was like for her. She shared little else before lapsing back into an unresponsive state and died some hours later.

Reporting on a series of six cases, Doctor Sandy MacLeod suggests the incidence of 'lightening up' or TL is much less now than previously recorded [32]. He attributes this to the increasing use of palliative sedation. As the vast majority of dying patients seek to be pain free in their last days, proportional doses of pain medication and sedation are prescribed to meet this request. In so doing, we ensure patient comfort, but we may also deprive them and those at the bedside of one final good-bye.

As with DBVs, terminal lucidity is thought to follow spontaneous surges in neurophysiological activity [26]. There is, however, some evidence to suggest that intimate communication and interpersonal connections made by close family in particular could precipitate the neurophysiological change that evokes the period of lucidity [41]. In the earlier anecdote of a patient waking on her birthday, it was her daughter's words, 'Mum, today is your birthday' that seemingly led to her brief period of lucidity.

3 The Lived Experience of Dying

In an article published in the early 1990s, Doctor Michael Kearney expressed concern about palliative care clinicians forsaking their role as healers by becoming what he called 'symptomatologists' [42]. Few would question the value of palliating symptoms in those who are dying, but the implication of Michael Kearney's words was unmistakably spelt out by one of my dying friends who stated, 'It does seem bitterly sad that my fate, the fate of me, will be decided, indirectly, through the functioning of a fleshly envelope. I see the soul, thus entrapped, as being the great and ultimate casualty of cancer's mortal war' [43, p. 105].

While we have learnt from those who are able to share their experiences, we know little about the lived experience of those who are unresponsive [18, 44]. We make assumptions about what they hear, feel, need, and understand, and decisions concerning care and medications are almost always based on objective measures that can be unreliable and misleading [18]. We have learnt that unresponsiveness does not equate to unawareness [45], but we cannot be certain if unresponsiveness equates to comfort nor do we know if and when covert experiences such as dreams, visions and OBEs occur and what these might mean for the patient. As ELDVs are known to be a source of peace and comfort to those who are conscious [9–15], it's quite possible the same is also true of DBVs.

For a specialty devoted to the care of the dying, palliative care has until now steered clear of research into the lived experience of unresponsive patients and the world they inhabit [2]. While research of this nature is ethically and methodologically challenging, its appropriateness cannot be based solely on the four prima facie ethical principles of beneficence, non-maleficence, respect for autonomy and justice. It must also take account of the patient's wishes and that of the immediate family. The belief that palliative care patients nearing the end of life are too sick to participate in research is often contrary to what they themselves feel and believe.

Indeed, the views expressed by palliative care patients towards research have been shown to be no different from that of other patient populations [46].

Symptom control is an essential step in the care of those with a life-limiting illness, but it must always be seen as the beginning of whole-person care. We are reminded of this by Richard Lamerton who is reputed to have said that palliative care seeks to make a person's body a comfortable enough place to live in for only then can they speak about the hidden and untold pain of dying or what he calls, 'the pain of the spirit' [47, p. 61]. While such discussions are not possible with those who are unresponsive or have lost the capacity to communicate, Blain-Moreas reminds us that these people maintain aspects of personhood—interpersonal connections and emotionally salient memories—even when moribund. She stresses that consciousness and personhood are independent constructs, and the absence of the former does not ipso facto deny the existence of the latter [41]. The way we engage, acknowledge, respect, and relate to unresponsive patients can be emotionally and spiritually therapeutic even for this vulnerable group of moribund patients. Dame Cicely Saunders constantly reminded us of this and the potential for healing wrought by the quality of one's presence.

4 Spiritual Care

The challenge in being a healing presence for someone who is unresponsive is dealt with at great length by Arnold Mindell in his seminal text, *Coma* [48], and by Rose and Ryan with their innovative teachings on end-of-life care [49]. In reference to altered states of consciousness, Mindell reveals how we attempt to interpret clinical changes without knowing if what we assume is right and whether the actions we take are appropriate to the situation that confronts us [48, p. 10]. For those nearing the end of life, a holistic, person-centred approach is advocated. In the context of end-of-life care, intuition and nuanced observations are found to be as valuable as any clinical assessment and care of the psyche and the soul is equally important and as necessary as care directed to the physical body.

Trisha Greenhalgh, Professor of Primary Health Care at University College Hospital, London, urges us to trust our intuition particularly in unfamiliar or challenging situations where we, more often than not, resort to the safety of protocols and reasoned-based practices. She does not suggest abandoning established practices, but that we remain sufficiently astute and aware to sense when evidence-based practice becomes evidence-burdened [50]. The skill, she says, is to respond to the subtle cues that signal a need to shift between the two approaches. Rose and Ryan also emphasise the need to be more fluid in our thinking when navigating challenges associated with the care of unresponsive patients. In so doing, we avoid getting stuck in a single paradigm of care, namely, the biomedical model [49].

Caring for someone at the edge of death asks more of clinicians and nurses than clinical expertise and deductive skills. It calls for a willingness to listen to one's intuition and to integrate this in a balanced way with the principles that underpin evidence-based medicine. The move to holistic care depends not only on what we know about our craft but also how much we know about ourselves. An authentic, open-minded approach to end-of-life care prepares us for patient experiences that are potentially transformative, but run the risk of going unseen, unheard, and of being misdiagnosed and mistreated. Hand in hand with this is a need to heed the comments and concerns expressed by family. These are nuanced and often more informed than observable behaviour and objective measures used by healthcare practitioners [51] and can only add to what we already know or don't know about the person.

5 Companioning the Unresponsive Patient

One of the most beneficial initiatives one can take when caring for an unresponsive patient is to create an ambience that respects their history, culture, beliefs, and wishes. The space should be as homely as circumstances allow and where an attitude of respect and reverence prevails. Music, prayers, readings, and rituals in keeping with the person's known preferences honour their personhood and contribute to the healing that can take place at a subliminal level. Times of silence may be as valuable as any other offering as they afford opportunities for dreaming and disembodied experiences both of which are believed to bring solace to the one dying. Family are encouraged to speak to and not about the dying person, to share emotionally salient memories and to validate them and the life they have lived. Tactile connections are also a valuable means of communication, particularly during times of silence and stillness. There are some, however, who are uncomfortable with touch, and if this is true of the person dying, this means of communication is best limited or avoided altogether.

All who visit, be they clinical staff, family, or friends, can show their respect by observing the same courtesies. This includes referring to the unresponsive person by name, informing them of their presence and by stating their intentions especially if this includes some form of intervention. Other courtesies shown to immediate family include respect, avoidance of trivial conversation, and keeping visits to an appropriate length of time.

In the early unresponsive phase, comatose and dying patients are constantly trying to make sense of their world, and it is the verbal and tactile connections made by family and carers that can have a profound settling effect. While we can never know how much is perceived or understood, research involving comatose patients gives us reason to believe the senses are, for the most part, doing what they are meant to do even though the person remains unresponsive. The therapeutic benefits of speaking to comatose patients was verified in a recent study that showed greater improvement in measures of arousal and awareness in patients who were spoken to regularly by those well known to them [52]. By way of illustration, the following comments were made by a man after he woke from a month-long coma, 'What made the big difference was my dear wife's presence. I could feel her hand in mine, our fingers intertwined. I knew it was her, though I could not figure out what she was doing in these strange worlds'. His message to clinical staff was equally clear, 'It was a bewildering, alien sensation of things being done to me by forces I could not see…if the nurses had not warned my apparently deaf ears of what they were going to do, I think I would have been scared indeed' [53].

It's presently unknown if the same degree of awareness is present in those who are dying, but anecdotal reports strongly suggest that covert awareness is present in the early unresponsive phase [18]. Further research is clearly required. Until then it's prudent and respectful to assume that unresponsive palliative care patients have some awareness of their outside world.

As Fig. 2 implies, awareness of the outer sensory world, also known as connected consciousness, gradually falls away, and the dying person is increasingly drawn to their inner world of dreams, visions, and disembodied experiences. In the neuroscientific world, this state is referred to as disconnected consciousness and is, in many ways, comparable to deep sleep. During this time, patients are unlikely to have any awareness of what is happening to them or around them. They are free of their tortured body, distressing thoughts and emotions that might otherwise engulf their mind. Just as we would not wake a person from a deep sleep, we honour this time with our silence and our reverence. We avoid drawing the person out of their peaceful state by limiting noise, maintaining relative silence, and refraining from non-essential interventions. For family, it is a good time for prayer and meditation, reading passages and poems softly or playing the person's favourite music at a volume that is just audible. As touch rather than sound is the last sense to go, holding hands or gentle stroking are good ways of maintaining a connection at this stage of the journey.

As a general rule, I prepare family for the possibility of a DBV and a lucid moment believing it is better for them to be forewarned rather than shocked by

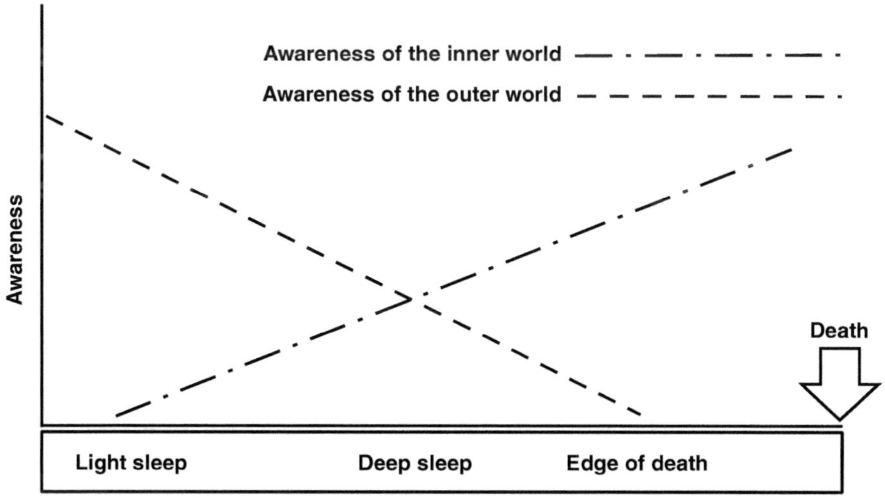

Fig. 2 A conceptual model illustrating the changing nature of awareness in dying patients as they journey from unresponsiveness to death

something they had not expected. I also explain why such experiences occur and reassure them that neither a DBV nor TL means their dying relative is delirious or distressed. I normalise both experiences by emphasising they are well recognised accompaniments of dying. As for the DBV, I recommended that family allow the experience to run its course and for them to not intervene in any way. Due to the enervating effect of medication, full-blown DBVs are now rare and those that do occur are often fragmentary and may manifest as hand movements, facial twitching, gesturing, eye opening or restlessness [49]. If these are part of a DBV, they will settle on their own accord within minutes. If not, a cause other than a DBV should be considered. With TL, greet the now lucid person as though they had just woken from a sleep. Allow them to orientate themselves and direct the conversation but take any opportunity to let them know how much they are loved.

The person is now nearing the end of their life's journey. They have disengaged from the manifest world and have melted into a progressively primal flow, which Buddhists call the clear light of death. One of our tasks is to ensure that they are not distracted from this process of letting go by anything we do or say. Rituals and some of the practices mentioned earlier may be adopted in softer tones. Knowing they are loved makes the dying person's journey easier to complete as it is an acknowledgement that they will not be forgotten. Such affirmations are best done earlier rather than later and repeated as often as one wishes.

Granting permission to 'let go' is tough love, but when done by a close family member, preferably the next-of-kin, anecdotal evidence suggests carefully chosen words may help the person surrender peacefully unto dying. If family ask what they could say, I recommend symbolic language rather than literal and to formulate their message around something their dying relative can readily relate to. 'Catch the next good wave and ride it all the way to shore' were the words a grieving mother whispered to her dying son who had been an avid surfboard rider. Others have said, 'Go to the light' or 'If you see (name) go to them. They are waiting to greet you'.

A protracted death is an extremely difficult time for family. The words, 'We would never allow an animal to die this way' is a reflection of their pain and suffering. Their grief needs to be heard rather than placated and their concerns addressed not only with answers but also in ways that exhibit authenticity and compassion. One counselling psychologist suggests, permission to visit troubling questions over and over may be as therapeutic as finding answers [54, p. 36].

Death is recognisable by the absence of respirations and a sense that the person is no longer there. It is a surreal moment. Clinicians may be asked to certify the death, but there is no immediate rush to do so. Confirmation of death, however, is something most families appreciate. It not only confirms what they already suspect, it also allows them to grieve openly. Family is encouraged to stay at the bedside for as long (or short) as they desire, to say goodbye and to partake of rituals they may have planned. This is time for the family. Depending on their wishes, clinicians, nurses, and carers can honour the occasion with their compassionate presence or by conferring privacy.

6 Summary

The dying person's connection to the outside slowly world diminishes in their final days. Apart from times of terminal lucidity, their awareness is increasingly directed inwards. During this stage of disconnected consciousness, dreams and visions become the dying person's reality. Provided the patient is pain free and comfortable, family and care providers can rest in the knowledge their loved one's inner world is probably rich with symbolism and that they are more at peace than at any other time in their illness. We are called to trust that the person dying is now following a trail that is foreign to the conscious mind, but unerringly familiar to the archetypal realm [27].

Unresponsiveness, often referred to as unconsciousness, is the next frontier waiting to be explored by those engaged in the care of the dying. The task in not so much one of understanding the mystery of death, but of learning more about the lived experience of those dying and how best to care for someone who no longer has a voice. While on this journey we can always take heart from the words of Janet Muff, a dream analyst who reminds us that the 'unconscious' will do its work even if we cannot [55, p. 81].

References

1. Taylor C. Dying: a memoir. Melbourne: The Text Publishing Company; 2016.
2. Kastenbaum R. The moment of death. Is hospice making a difference? Hosp J. 1999;14:253–70.
3. Betty LS. Are they hallucinations or are they real? The spirituality of deathbed and near-death experiences. Omega. 2006;53:37–49.
4. Barbato M. Caring for the living and the dying. Sydney: Self-published; 2010.
5. Blackmore S. Near-death experiences: in or out of the body? Skept Inq. 2006;16:34–45.
6. Barrett W. Deathbed visions. 2nd ed. Wellingborough: The Aquarian Press; 1986.
7. Osis K, Haraldsson E. At the hour of death. Norwalk: Hastings House; 1977.
8. Callanan M, Kelley P. Final gifts. New York: Bantam Dell; 1993.
9. Kerr CW, Donnelly JP, Wright ST, Kuszczak SM, et al. End-of-life dreams and visions: a longitudinal study of hospice patients' experience. J Palliat Med. 2014;17:296–303.
10. Brayne S, Lovelace H, Fenwick P. End-of-life experiences and the dying process in a Gloucestershire nursing home as reported by nurses and care assistants. Am J Hosp Palliat Med. 2008;25:195–206.
11. Fenwick P, Lovelace H, Brayne S. Comfort for the dying: five years retrospective and one year prospective studies of end-of-life experiences. Arch Gerontol Geriatr. 2010;51:173–9.
12. Ethier AM. Death-related sensory experiences. J Paediatr Oncol Nurs. 2005;22:104–11.
13. Depner R, Grant P, Byrwa D, et al. Expanding the understanding of content of end-of-life dreams and visions: a consensual qualitative research analysis. Palliat Med. 2020;1:103–10.
14. Nosek CL, Kerr CW, Woodworth J, et al. End-of-life dreams and visions: a qualitative perspective from hospice patients. Am J Hosp Palliat Care. 2015;32:269–74.
15. Devery K, Rawlings D, Tieman J, Damarell R. Deathbed phenomena reported by patients in palliative care: clinical opportunities and responses. Int J Palliat Nurs. 2015;21:117–25.

16. Borjigin J, Lee U, Liu T, et al. Surge of neurophysiological coherence and connectivity in the dying brain. PNAS. 2013;110:14432–7.
17. Shlobin NA, Aru J, Vincente R, Zemmar A. What happens in the brain when we die? Deciphering the neurophysiology of the final moments of life. Front Aging Neurosci. 2023;15:1143848. https://doi.org/10.3389/fnagi.2023.1143848.
18. Barbato M. Bispectral index monitoring in unconscious palliative care patients. J Palliat Care. 2001;17:102–8.
19. Roscow C, Manberg PJ. Bispectral index monitoring. Anaesthesiol Clin N Am. 2001;19:947–66.
20. Gambrell M. Using the BIS monitor in palliative care: a case study. J Neurosci Nurs. 2005;37:140–3.
21. Chawla LS, Akst S, Junker C, et al. Surges of electroencephalogram activity at the time of death: a case series. J Palliat Med. 2009;12:1095–100.
22. Chawla LS, Terek M, Junker C, et al. Characterization of end-of-life electroencephalographic surges in critically ill patients. Death Stud. 2017;14:385–92.
23. Auyong DB, Klein SM, Gan TJ, et al. Processed electroencephalogram during donation after cardiac death. Anaesth Analg. 2010;110:1428–32.
24. Vicente R, Rizzuto M, Sarica C, et al. Enhanced interplay of neuronal coherence and coupling in the dying brain. Front Aging Neurosci. 2022;14:813531.
25. Xu G, Mihaylova T, Li D, et al. Surge of neurophysiological coupling and connectivity of gamma oscillations in the dying human brain. PNAS. 2023;120:e2216268120.
26. ABC Health Report. Electrical activity observed in the dying brain. https://www.abc.net.au/radionational/programs/healthreport/electrical-activity-in-the-dying-brain/102449914. Accessed 20 June 2023.
27. Dowling SK. The grace in dying. San Francisco: HarperCollins; 1998.
28. Koch C. Tales of the dying brain. Sci Am. 2020;322:70–5.
29. Greyson B. Dissociation in people who have near-death experiences: out of their bodies or out of their minds? Lancet. 2000;355:460–3.
30. Barbato M, Barclay G, Potter J, Yeo W. The moment of death. J Pain Sym Manag. 2017;53:e1–3.
31. Masman AD, van Dijk M, van Rosmalen J, et al. Bispectral index monitoring in terminally ill patients. A validation study. J Pain Sym Manag. 2016;52:212–20.
32. MacLeod AD. Lightening up before death. Palliat Support Care. 2009;7:513–6.
33. Dahaba AA. Different conditions that could result in the bispectral index indicating an incorrect hypnotic state. Anaes Analg. 2005;101:765–3.
34. Nahm M, Greyson B, Kelley EW, Haraldsson E. Terminal lucidity: a review and case collection. Arch Gerontol Geriatr. 2011;55:138–42.
35. Schreiber T, Bennett MJ. Identification and validation of pre-mortem surge. J Hosp Palliat Nurs. 2014;16:430–5.
36. Mashour GA, Frank L, Batthyany A, Kolanowski AM, et al. Paradoxical lucidity: a potential paradigm shift for the neurobiology and treatment of severe dementias. Alzheimers Dement. 2019;15:1107–14.
37. Nahm M, Greyson B. Terminal lucidity in patients with chronic schizophrenia and dementia. J Nerv Ment Dis. 2009;197:942–4.
38. Nahm M, Greyson B, Kelly EW, Haraldsson E. Terminal lucidity: a review and a case collection. Arch Gerontol Geriatr. 2012;55:138–42.
39. Halford H. Essays and orations read and delivered at the Royal College of Physicians. 2nd ed. London: John Murray; 1833.
40. Dugan DO. Symbolic expressions of dying patients: communications, not hallucinations. Nurs Forum. 1989;24:18–27.
41. Blain-Moraes S, Racine E, Mashour GA. Consciousness and personhood in medical care. Front Hum Neurosci. 2018;12:306. https://doi.org/10.3389/fnhum.2018.00306.
42. Kearney M. Palliative medicine – just another specialty? Palliat Med. 1992;6:39–46.
43. Jones GC. Magnanimous despair. Mount Nebo: Boombana Publications; 1998.

44. O'Connor T, Paterson C, Gibson J, Strickland K. The conscious state of the dying patient: an integrative review. Palliat Support Care. 2021;20:731–43.
45. Sanders RD, Tononi G, Laureys S, Sleigh JW. Unresponsiveness ≠ Unconsciousness. Anaesthesiology. 2012;116:946–59.
46. White C, Hardy J. What do palliative care patients and their relatives think about research in palliative care? – a systematic review. Support Care Cancer. 2010;18:905–11.
47. Lamerton R. Care of the dying. Middlesex: Penguin Books; 1980.
48. Mindell A. Coma. Boston: Shambhala Publications; 1989.
49. Rose I, Ryan K. Doorways into dying. London: Austin Macauley Publishers; 2016.
50. Greenhalgh T. Intuition and evidence – uneasy bedfellows? Br J Gen Pract. 2002;52:395–400.
51. Bruera E. Perception of discomfort among relatives of unresponsive terminally ill patients. J Palliat Care. 2000;16:59–60.
52. Pape TL-B, Rosenow JM, Steiner M, Parrish T, et al. Placebo-controlled trial of familiar auditory sensory training for acute severe traumatic brain injury: a preliminary report. Neurorehabil Neural Repair. 2015;29:537–47.
53. Lean G. A matter of life and death. Sunday Mail, October 8, 2006.
54. Yoder G. Companioning the dying. Fort Collins: Companion Press; 2011.
55. Muff J. From the wings of night: dream work with people who have acquired immunodeficiency syndrome. Holist Nurs Pract. 1996;10:69–87.

Spiritual Care for the Bereaved

Bruce Rumbold and Samar Aoun

Abstract While understandings of the nature and scope of spirituality vary, it is nevertheless clear that spirituality, however understood, is not only disrupted by bereavement but can also be a resource for living with bereavement. The extent to which bereavement models take spiritual need and spiritual resources into account varies according to the assumptions and emphases of the disciplinary framework in which each model is based.

In this chapter, we discuss how the perspective provided by a spiritual care approach both complements and critiques current approaches to bereavement care; and how bereavement care might incorporate and contribute to spiritual care. We suggest that a spiritual perspective can hold together the insights offered by diverse bereavement theories, provide perspective on the importance and relevance of clinical interventions, and suggest further strategies to complement those currently recognised and funded (usually) through health services.

We also discuss the extent to which bereavement theories have been shaped by data from selected populations and show how paying attention to the ways bereavement is experienced in society in general shifts the focus of care away from professional interventions towards support provided in the community. Our contention in this chapter is that the social aspects of bereavement are the least developed in most

B. Rumbold (✉)
La Trobe University, Melbourne, VIC, Australia

Perron Institute for Neurological and Translational Science, Nedlands, WA, Australia
e-mail: b.rumbold@latrobe.edu.au

S. Aoun
La Trobe University, Melbourne, VIC, Australia

University of Western Australia, Perron Institute for Neurological and Translational Science, Nedlands, WA, Australia
e-mail: samar.aoun@perron.uwa.edu.au

M. C. Best (ed.), *Spiritual Care in Palliative Care*,
https://doi.org/10.1007/978-3-031-50864-6_41

bereavement theories and therapies, and that a public health approach can restore a more-nuanced social aspect that also accommodates spiritual aspects through their social expression. This public health approach needs to be grounded in the ecological perspective exemplified in compassionate communities' strategies. In such a framework, spiritual care can be provided implicitly as well as explicitly, so that spiritual care does not need to be initiated alongside debates about whether a spiritual care framework applies to all, or just some, people.

Keywords Bereavement · Spiritual care · Public health approach · Social networks · Compassionate communities · Palliative care

1 Spirituality in Human Life

As Chap. 2 of this collection shows, definitions of spirituality tend to vary from those narrowly constructed for researchers' purposes to those that attempt to encompass the range of activities, beliefs, and affiliations that people use to describe their spirituality. Debates around spirituality include whether it belongs to a distinct dimension of human existence—describable for example using a biopsychosocial-spiritual framework in which spiritual factors can be distinguished from psychological and social factors [1]—or a perspective that sees spirituality as expressed through physical, psychological, and social dimensions while nevertheless having the capacity to transcend them [2]. In this chapter, we align ourselves with an integrative understanding of spirituality, seeing it not as a separate variable distinguished by its unique content, but a distinctive perspective that connects aspects of human experience that are often in professional practice separated by each discipline's gaze. We also adopt a pragmatic stance, returning to the idea that what matters most is not what a practitioner thinks spirituality ought to be, but what it is for a person: that which lifts their spirits and gives them direction, hope, connection beyond their immediate circumstances.

Wright [3] mapped discussions of spirituality around the three key aspects of identity (who am I?), connection (who are we?), and meaning (why are we here?). He pointed out that at different stages of the life cycle our (largely implicit) answers to these questions can shift as we encounter different life challenges within changing settings. Our answers are seldom formed as direct responses to these key questions but tend to be embedded in narratives about our lives, our place in the world, and what matters to us. Spirituality develops across the life cycle, evolving through membership of different communities and experience of various life events. For some, faith communities may provide continuity, but for spirituality to remain lively, the shared beliefs and practices of those communities must continue to be grounded and tested in each person's experience.

As the definitions show us, many approaches to spirituality tend to favour one aspect or question over others, usually selected according to the disciplinary interests of the practitioner or researcher. Psychologists are thus often particularly interested in the question of identity, framing connection in terms of interpersonal engagement and meaning as self-understanding. Philosophers and theologians may be particularly engaged by questions of meaning and purpose, framing connection in terms of ideological alliances and identity through membership of faith communities or ideological affiliations. Sociologists, rather thinner on the ground in these discussions, may focus on connection and explore the other aspects through the tension between individual agency and social structure that constructs both a sense of self and knowledge of the world. At this point, it might be appropriate to declare that a social lens informs much of this chapter.

However, even if one of these three aspects is given priority, most understandings of spirituality continue to link them together. For example, Lartey [4] describes spirituality as involving relationships with places and things (spatial), with self (intra-personal), with others (inter-personal), among people (corporate) and with transcendence. This description makes it clear that spirituality is enacted: it is not just a matter of belief, but of practice. It's worth recalling that, traditionally at least, spirituality attends more to right practice than to right belief. Spiritual practices include individual and corporate disciplines of reflection, participation in rituals, and attention to breath, or to sacred text, or to nature. These practices usually contribute to experiential knowing and its communication through witness or testimony. Rather than being defined primarily by a set of propositional beliefs, spirituality often involves struggle with propositions and dogma: spiritual disciplines are intended to ground beliefs in everyday life—they facilitate the journey from head to heart. The core question of spirituality is how then shall we live, not what must we believe.

The way these three aspects engage with each other matters. Spirituality involves a good-enough coherence of a person's identity, significant connections and purpose (meaning) in life. Sense of coherence can thus be a measure of how belief connects with practice [5]. Spiritual distress arises from the loss of coherence or lack of coherence in the face of life's challenges. But as already noted, practice is embedded in—supported by and leading to—social narratives, stories that link an individual's experience with family and neighbourhood relationships and cultural stories. These stories best capture spirituality. The primary expertise required for spiritual care is understanding how stories are created and maintained and knowing how to listen to and work with stories.

2 Spirituality and Bereavement

Like spirituality, bereavement care in western societies has its roots in religious traditions and practices. At the end of the nineteenth century, bereavement was still managed principally through the funeral rituals provided by religious traditions, and bereavement practices that dictated social engagement and, for women in particular, signalled bereavement status through rules about clothing and personal adornment [6]. Many of these social rules that governed the period following bereavement were overwhelmed by the mass deaths of World War I and the influenza pandemic that followed immediately after. Overall, during the first half of the twentieth century there was a shift from traditional social organisation in which bereavement is an aspect of everyday life, managed through well-understood rituals based in shared frameworks of meaning, to social organisation where bereavement is an exceptional experience to be managed largely by the bereaved person [7].

In the mid-twentieth century, bereavement became the interest of some health-care professionals, particularly psychiatrists and psychologists [8]. The dominant ideas about bereavement today still have their roots in this pioneering psychiatric and psychological investigation and practice. While not dismissing the valuable insights provided by these disciplines, their work has placed bereavement care into clinical models that emphasise the contribution of professional practitioners working with individual clients, give priority to emotional expressive therapies, and thereby risk moving bereavement from everyday life into professionally managed settings. Therapy can thus be elevated, and social support downplayed: indeed, support can actually be reduced as family, friends, and neighbours give way to professionals because they see them as experts in this field. It has also led to continuing debate about links between bereavement and mental health, circumstances under which grief can be regarded as 'normal' and circumstances in which it can be diagnosed as a condition requiring clinical attention [9, 10]. A new discipline of grief counselling now operates at the interface between health system and community, strongly shaped by professional practice models, both in the theory underlying strategies and in fee-for-service provision even when located in community settings.

Adopting a spiritual perspective in this social context raises two major questions. First, to what extent can the scope of current bereavement care policies and models match the scope of a spiritual perspective? Second, how might current professional strategies be adopted and adapted to contribute to spiritual care?

In considering scope, it is interesting to recall a small empirical study that established a scope for loss that correlates with a spiritual perspective. Patricia Weenolsen [11] explored people's responses to a range of losses including, but not limited to, bereavement. She found that loss, or disruption, is experienced at a variety of levels, which she identified as:

- Primary (the loss itself)
- Secondary (associated losses)
- Holistic (future losses)
- Self-conceptual (loss of part of self)
- Metaphorical (loss of 'place' in the world).

For some people, even a major primary disruption such as bereavement can be handled with relative equanimity because their understanding of their place in life, their self, the relationships that hold them in place, and the meaning they ascribe to life events, can absorb the disruption. For others, what appears to be a minor disruption can have major consequences because it undermines their plans or aspirations for the future, or destabilises their sense of self, exposes their lack of social support or challenges their assumptions about the world and their place in it.

Weenolsen suggested that any loss must be transcended at each of these five levels, although she used '*transcendence*' in a rather utilitarian sense that includes living with or adjusting to loss at each level. That is, transcending in her sense begins with coping, although it may move towards the more usual sense of transcending as movement beyond the practical realities of loss to see the circumstances in a fresh and meaning-imbued way. As a framework, Weenolsen's work draws attention to the multiple levels at which life can be disrupted by loss and reminds us that coherence can be challenged even if a person's resources at several of these levels seem reasonably intact.

From a spiritual perspective, it is important that models for bereavement care have capacity to address all these levels of loss—or at least that providers of bereavement care use a range of models that encompass the potential scope of loss. Leget and Guldin in Chap. 25 of this volume review resources available for addressing loss at all of these levels and argue that adopting a spiritual perspective necessitates an integrative approach [12]. They demonstrate how various approaches address different elements of the bereavement experience, and by implication also expose limitations to the scope of many theories and practice models for bereavement care.

Some bereavement theories, developed for individual psychotherapy, focus largely on the inner world of the individual and adjustments that may need to be made. These theories often make assumptions about the need to reframe a person's life story, and particularly about the value of expressing emotion. The self becomes a rehabilitation project, undertaken by modifying or relinquishing attachment, involving activities which lead to the concept of grief work. But getting grief 'right' can put a lot of pressure on the grieving person if the focus is on 'grieving in your own unique way' or indeed relinquishing attachment in order to liberate emotional energy, as some of the earlier psychodynamic models proposed. Michael White [13] provided a classic example of the problem of assumptions embedded in such counselling models in describing his work with people who had been unable to grieve to the satisfaction of their grief counsellors—that is, had been unwilling to relinquish their emotional attachment to the deceased as the theory of the day required. He instead invited these people to 'say hullo again', to explore how their relationship with the deceased person had changed and what it was becoming. This finding was of course made in other places and in due course taken up in the continuing bonds model [14], an approach that has resonances with Eastern religious traditions and can provide space for explicit attention to spirituality [15].

Other bereavement models incorporate a focus on inner life but link this more explicitly with the process of re-engaging the world. Yet, others make re-engagement the focus, as in Attig's re-learning the world model [16]. In many of these approaches to bereavement, spirituality is mentioned as a factor that can contribute to the therapeutic task—that is, spirituality can be used to access a client's meaning system or ritual behaviours or sense of self. It is invoked functionally to achieve therapeutic goals, but the process of resolving grief—or learning to live with grief—may not teach us much about spirituality or attend to possibilities for spiritual growth.

Some approaches address spiritual aspects explicitly, most notably Neimeyer and colleagues making use of his meaning-making model [17, 18] but the very attempt to pay explicit attention to religion/spirituality can limit the approach to particular cultural contexts. Thus, the measure developed by Burke et al. [19] reflects the cognitive beliefs of evangelical Protestantism, a theological stance that does not capture even the diversity of Christian belief, let alone the ultimate concerns and questions of other faiths.

Overall, most bereavement theories work with issues that are of interest to a spiritual care perspective, but committing to any one of these theories without reference to others risks attending to only part of the spectrum of need and possibility identified by a spiritual care perspective. For example, a focus on an individual's inner work, or meaning-making, often sees social aspects reduced to interpersonal support. Similarly, as already noted, care has been drawn into professionalised spaces, and this has implications for our understanding, and practice, of spiritual care in bereavement. Bereavement studies, and hence theories, have not only tended to give priority to one of these three domains, but to do so predominantly through an individualistic lens. Connection is usually addressed through attachment theory, identity through a self-development lens, meaning-making as an individual's responsibility (or opportunity). An integrative approach reduces the risk of importing assumptions inherent to specific disciplinary interests.

The question then arises as to whether a spiritual care perspective can complement or challenge these strategies. A further question is whether a spiritual care perspective needs to be explicit. Our contention in this chapter is that the social aspects of bereavement are the least developed in most bereavement theory and therapy, and that a public health approach can restore a more-nuanced social aspect and accommodate spiritual aspects through their social expression, provided that a public health approach is informed by an ecological perspective [20]. Understanding social fabric is essential to a proper understanding of both spirituality and bereavement. Without it we have a psychological focus on identity independent of social networks or meaning as individual construction. Yet fundamentally, identity is constructed as self and others: hence the need to renegotiate a relationship with a person who has died. Our developmental communities nearly always include the living and the dead—and in old age the dead may vastly outnumber the living. Further, for many people, bereavement raises a series of acute questions about income, housing, parenting, etc. that may override 'inner work'. The dual process model of Stroebe and Schut [21] recognising that processing loss must go hand in hand with adjusting to changed circumstances is invaluable in this respect. The model attends to stories about loss and stories about continuity and recovery, respecting the oscillation between emotional pain and the socio-economic challenge of rebuilding life.

The inner work of bereavement cannot be divorced from the social world. Indeed, the pain of bereavement is strongly linked with social exclusion, or at least a sense of social exclusion. Here the period leading into bereavement can be crucial. Social networks enhanced during care for the dying person may be an asset brought into bereavement [22], and for some, their faith community may be at the heart of that support (Chap. 6–11). But for many others, protracted caregiving leads to a narrowing, or better a focusing, of the caregivers' purpose and a consequent shrinking of their social networks.

A spiritual care approach to bereavement thus needs to draw upon a range of theory and practice. But there is a practical problem inherent in explicitly framing an integrative approach as spiritual care—it can elicit a polarised response, particularly because of the continuing conflation of spirituality with religious belief and practice, more generally because an existential vocabulary is largely absent in secular societies. Offering a form of care that needs to begin with a discussion of core concepts [23] rather defeats the purpose. A reasonable response that has its origins in health (where bereavement care is largely located in policy) but capable of extending into social and cultural realms is a public health approach.

3 Public Health and Bereavement

Adopting a public health approach reminds us that most contemporary data concerning bereavement are selective. It is regularly noted that only a small proportion of any population avail themselves of bereavement services. Sometimes, this is interpreted as the result of insufficient availability of and access to these services. But in the decades during which bereavement theory was being built there was little or no testing of the implicit assumption that expressive therapies like counselling were best practice in bereavement care. Nor was there much investigation of how people who did not seek out bereavement counselling might manage their grief. Just as spirituality research often draws most upon those best able to articulate belief, so is bereavement research often focused upon those who ask for professional help in managing their bereavement. A public health approach however begins by asking about how bereavement occurs and is managed in extended communities or populations.

More than a decade ago we decided that, rather than assuming that professionals should decide the optimal ways of dealing with bereavement, we would explore where people actually found their support. The first empirical evidence that grief care has indeed been everyone's responsibility and that the community is shouldering this responsibility, came from a population based Australian Bereavement Survey [24]. An anonymous postal survey collected information from clients of six funeral providers in four Australian states (2014–15), 6 to 24 months after the death of their family member or friend, with 1139 responding. The questionnaire included a validated risk assessment screening measure (PG-13) for Prolonged Grief Disorder (PGD) [25] which enabled the categorisation of respondents' grief profiles into low, moderate, and high risk of PGD.

The findings were aligned to the *Public Health Model of Bereavement Support* [24], in its three-tiered approach to bereavement risk and need for support wherein the low-risk group (first tier) would need support principally from family and friends, the moderate risk group (second tier) would need support from the wider community through some general support from various professionals, and the high-risk group (third tier) would need support from mental health services (Fig. 1). Based on the literature, the model predicted that 60% of the sample would be low

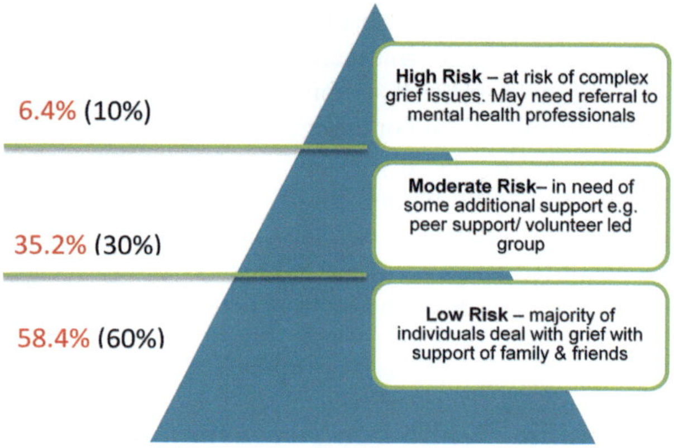

Fig. 1 The Public Health Model of Bereavement Support: predicted (in brackets) and actual proportions for the three at-risk groups of bereaved people. (Source: Aoun et al. [24])

risk, 30% moderate risk, and 10% high risk. Actual figures were very close at 58.4%, 35.2%, and 6.4%, respectively.

Low PG-13 scores typically arose from losses that were expected and less disruptive to daily routines (e.g. the death of an aged parent); moderate scores typically arose from deaths that were both expected and everyday-disruptive (e.g. the death of an ageing and ill partner); and deaths that are both unexpected or resisted and disruptive (such as a child or a younger spouse) led to high scores on the PG-13.

The sources of bereavement support were classified into three forms: Informal support, community support, and professional support. Informal support included support offered by family, friends, funeral directors, financial or legal advisors, religious or spiritual advisors, the Internet, or literature. Community support included support offered by general practitioners, nursing homes, hospitals, pharmacists, community groups, palliative care providers or school-based advisors. Professional support included support offered by trained counsellors, bereavement support groups, social workers, case coordinators, psychologists, and psychiatrists. The majority of the bereaved respondents in each of the three risk groups accessed support from family and friends (88–94%), followed by funeral directors (82%) and general practitioners (56%).

Access to mental health professional sources of support (counsellor, social worker, psychologist, and psychiatrist) was more frequently reported by the high-risk group (Fig. 2). The moderate risk group was particularly visible in the support accessed from community groups and palliative care services [24]. The supports that were deemed most helpful were in the informal category and those least helpful were in the professional category. It would appear that counsellors, or other professionals, need to remember that they are being consulted not to deal with bereavement as a singular event, but as one aspect of the tangible, multi-dimensional losses with which that bereaved person has to live.

In the informal sources of support, the findings revealed that attachment (emotional or affectionate bond, often provided by spouse/partner or close family) was the form of social support most frequently endorsed as helpful by respondents,

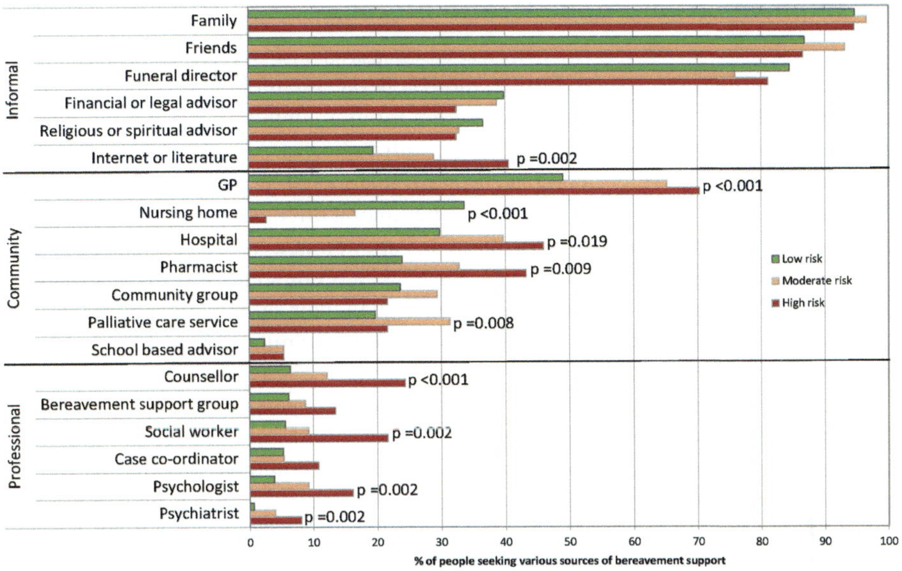

Fig. 2 Sources of bereavement support accessed by the three at-risk categories of bereaved people (low, moderate, high) grouped according to types of support (informal, community, professional). (Source: Aoun et al. [24])

suggesting that the majority of bereaved individuals value emotional support from those closest to them. This was followed in terms of frequency by reliable alliance (tangible assistance such as providing meals and transport often offered by family members) and social integration (perceived sense of belonging often provided by friends) [26].

The findings endorse social models of bereavement care that fit within a public health approach that can incorporate, but does not rely solely upon, professional care. As exemplified by Compassionate Communities policies and practices [27, 28], establishing collaboration between informal social networks, community organisations and professional services is vital for effective and sustainable bereavement care. A public health approach should be adopted to support the majority of bereaved people as much of this support is already provided in informal and other community settings by a range of people already involved in the everyday lives of those recently bereaved. Furthermore, a public health approach to bereavement care is needed to support these 'everyday assets' in the community who care for the majority of the bereaved, without the over-reach from professional services [29]. This study has provided empirical evidence for the need to strengthen the compassionate communities approach, not only for end-of-life care for dying patients but also along the continuum of bereavement support. Further population studies undertaken during the COVID-19 pandemic reinforce the significant contribution of the informal social networks which support—or fail to support—bereaved people [30, 31].

4 Implications of Public Health Findings

Some of these findings deserve further, more general, attention. One is the timeliness of support. It is notable that funeral directors rarely maintain ongoing relationships with their clients, yet their relatively brief contribution at the very start of bereavement is almost universally appreciated and remembered years later [32]. It seems that, in the initial chaos following a death, the funeral director provides structure and guidance that allows mourners to continue to function in a radically changed world. It is worth reflecting further on the extent to which clinicians too may be able to contribute in similar ways if they can foreshadow in their care the impending task of bereavement—affirm strengths, encourage connection, remind carers of the resources available to them (see Chap. 37).

Another is pointing beyond areas of professional expertise to other dimensions that can be explored. As Bury [33] puts it, 'Under conditions of adversity, individuals often feel a pressing need to re-examine and re-fashion their personal narratives in an attempt to maintain a sense of identity. Universal, cultural, and individual levels of human existence are tied together with narrative threads' (p. 264).

Bury identified three narrative forms through which people described their life with chronic illness, or more generally circumstances, such as bereavement, where change endures. They are:

- Contingent narratives
- *Origins, onset, symptoms, effects of illness*
- Moral narratives
- *Evaluating altered relationships with body, self, and society*
- Core narratives
- Changes *in identity and self-presentation*

Bury describes a process by which the focused story of a life-changing event develops and broadens to incorporate the ongoing effects of that event, the meaning that becomes attached to the changes, and the ways in which a person's understanding of themselves and the world changes. But for a complex and nuanced narrative like this to develop it needs an audience. Without someone who will hear and respond to the new narrative form emerging within the old, the teller is less likely to move beyond contingent stories to develop moral dimension to the story and in due course begin to reflect on implications for the core narratives that have previously held them in the world. People in informal networks can have a major role as consistent supportive listeners to a narrative that develops over months and years [34]. It is interesting to note that in our findings the constructive role of informal networks far out-weighs the somewhat-ambiguous contribution of professional caregivers. Perhaps in part this may be ascribed to the sort of listening professional helpers provide, some of whom may listen to a wider story, but others of whom may focus only on their own professional interests.

One strong implication of the findings is that the lens through which the professionals view loss, and hence the story they wish to elicit, is incompatible with what mourners are seeking at that stage of their bereavement. We were not able to explore this issue further, but we note that most in our sample appeared to be consulting professionals at a point where mobilising a restitution narrative (moral and core narratives in Bury's terms) was their issue, but professionals were wanting to focus on their contingent or loss narrative. It is understandable that a professional wants to understand the 'back story' in order to address a way forward. But this initial focus on loss narrative can disrupt the journey through grief. Hence, Walter's argument [35] that grief is best explored in the company of people who have known the deceased (and the mourner).

In comparison with studies of counselling clients who have sought a professionalised response, population studies show a real appetite for conversations to be held in everyday spaces, informally or using community for events such as a Grief Festival [36] or other public education programmes [37]. While it is vital that people can access professional support if they wish or are deemed to require it, conversations should begin where the loss is felt, in everyday experience. Contrast this with the standard institutional response of trying to separate everyday work and conversations about loss by bringing in the experts, the grief counsellors, to set up separate spaces rather than facilitate conversations in the classroom or office [38]. Nor does support need to take the form of facilitated conversation: various strategies for memorialisation can embed loss and celebration in everyday settings and everyday life [39].

5 Issues in Spiritual Care in Bereavement

We have already noted that a practical dilemma can arise from the way the different academic disciplines that inform different caring disciplines may be interested primarily in a particular aspect of the bereavement experience. That is, spirituality as an integrative quality can be fragmented by professionalised environments interested in particular parts of experience rather than the whole. A further dilemma of spiritual care provided by professionals at the end of life is that there is usually major discontinuity around the death. While a person is dying their professional caregivers may provide significant and vital support to the family, but this support becomes a memory once the person has died—most families are provided with bereavement resources, some are perhaps referred to a bereavement team with whom they may have had no, or only cursory, contact. The social network that sustained them through dying, if it included clinicians, is reduced.

Spiritual care in health settings is largely supportive: questions about any overarching goals of spiritual care are seldom addressed and are subsumed into person-centred approaches. Any goals mentioned are usually functional—reduction of distress, provision of comfort, capacity to endure illness and treatment. The focus is, due to its healthcare context, upon the individual. But spiritual care has a goal of transformation, expressed in a variety of ways in different belief systems. Transformation leads people to live creatively with their finitude and is shown in the coherence of belief and practice. Spiritual care assists people through their life cycle to find their gift, to develop it, and to give it away. That is, it impacts society, not just the inner life of the individual.

Spiritual care should not have to commence by trying to convince someone that they are a spiritual being (or for a religious person that spirituality is more about practice than orthodoxy). In a general sense, spiritual care is provided when connections are restored or renewed. More specifically, a spiritual approach pays attention to the multiple domains, captured in settings, stories, and systems of belief [40] that need to be addressed for coherence to be restored to a person's sense of self, of belonging, and contribution. Obviously, it is not only spiritual care practitioners who can support this sort of healing—but their contribution is to maintain steady attention to the whole spectrum of need and possibility, and not to assume that resolution in one aspect is 'closure', but a step towards achieving coherence elsewhere.

We have shown that spiritual care is implicit in a comprehensive public health approach, embedded in assumptions about individual, communal, and ecological health. Making this contribution explicit will enhance both public health and spiritual care. A public health approach restores the (currently marginalised) social aspects of connection by paying attention to the everyday situations in which bereavement is lived out (social networks, their capacities or their absence) and the structures that tend to frame bereavement as a healthcare problem.

What the public health model contributes to spiritual care includes insight into the ways the domains of identity, connection, and meaning are supported, maintained or re-developed in the informal social networks that are the bedrock of bereavement care and in the civic organisations that further equip and inform them. A bereavement care policy informed by this public health perspective should have its foundation in the strengthening and support of the principal resource for bereavement care, community social networks, linking these with formal funded bereavement care programmes that exist within community settings, primary care and some specialist palliative care programmes. Thus, while public health approaches to palliative care have been a major focus of public health end-of-life care, these must be accompanied by public health approaches to bereavement care if we are to develop relevant, coherent, and comprehensive end-of-life care policies and practices.

References

1. Sulmasy DP. A biopsychosocial–spiritual model for the care of patients at the end of life. Gerontologist. 2002;42:24–37.
2. Swinton J, Pattison S. Moving beyond clarity: towards a thin, vague, and useful understanding of spirituality in nursing care. Nurs Philos. 2010;11:226–37.
3. Wright M. Good for the soul?: the spiritual dimension of hospice and palliative care. In: Payne S, Seymour J, Ingleton C, editors. Palliative care nursing: principles and evidence for practice. Maidenhead: Open University Press; 2004. p. 218–40, 221.

4. Lartey E. In living colour: an intercultural approach to pastoral care and counselling. London: Cassell; 1997.
5. Jeserich F, Klein C, Brtinkhaus B, Teut M. Sense of coherence and religion/spirituality: a systematic review and meta-analysis based on a methodical classification of instruments measuring religion/spirituality. PLoS One. 2023;18:e0289203. https://doi.org/10.1371/journal.pone.0289203.
6. Jalland P. Death in the Victorian family. Oxford: Oxford University Press; 1996.
7. Walter T. On bereavement: the culture of grief. Maidenhead: Open University Press; 1999.
8. Small N. Theories of grief: a critical review. In: Hockey J, Katz J, Small N, editors. Grief, mourning, and death ritual. Buckingham: Open University Press; 2001. p. 19–48.
9. Horwitz A, Wakefield J. The loss of sadness: how psychiatry transformed normal sorrow into depressive disorder. New York: Oxford University Press; 2007.
10. Zisook S, Corruble E, Duan N, Iglewicz A, Karam E, Lanuaette N, Lebowitz B, Pies R, Reynolds C, Seay K, Shear M, Simon N, Young I. The bereavement exclusion and DSM-5. Depress Anxiety. 2012;29:425–43.
11. Weenolsen P. Transcendence of loss over the life span. New York: Hemisphere; 1988.
12. Guldin M, Leget C. The integrated process model of loss and grief – an interprofessional understanding. Death Stud. 2023;48:738. https://doi.org/10.1080/07481187.2023.2272960.
13. White M. Saying hullo again: the incorporation of the lost relationship in the resolution of grief. Adelaide: Dulwich Centre Newsletter; 1988. Re-printed in White C, Denborough D, editors. Introducing narrative therapy: a collection of practice-based writings. Adelaide: Dulwich Centre Publications.
14. Klass D, Silverman PR, Nickman S. Continuing bonds: new understandings of grief. Washington, DC: Taylor & Francis; 2014.
15. Klass D. The spiritual lives of bereaved parents. Philadelphia: Brunner-Mazel; 1999.
16. Attig T. How we grieve: re-learning the world. New York: Oxford University Press; 1996.
17. Burke L, Neimeyer R. Meaning making. In: Cobb M, Puchalski C, Rumbold B, editors. The Oxford textbook of spirituality in healthcare. Oxford: Oxford University Press; 2012. p. 127–33.
18. Neimeyer R, Sands DC. Meaning reconstruction in bereavement: from principles to practice. In: Neimeyer RA, Winokeur H, Harris D, Thornton G, editors. Grief and bereavement in contemporary society: bridging research and practice. New York: Routledge; 2011.
19. Burke L, Neimeyer R, Holland J, Dennard S, Oliver L, Shear M. Inventory of complicated spiritual grief: development and validation of a new measure. Death Stud. 2014;38:239–50.
20. Lang T, Rayner G. Ecological public health: the 21st century's big idea? BMJ. 2012;2012(345):e5466. https://doi.org/10.1136/bmj.e5466.
21. Stroebe M, Schut H. The dual process model of coping with bereavement: rationale and description. Death Stud. 1999;23(3):197–224.
22. Leonard R, Horsfall D. The evidence of the importance of informal care networks. In: Abel J, Kellehear A, editors. The Oxford textbook of public health palliative care. Oxford: Oxford University Press; 2022. p. 233–44.
23. Lepherd L. Spirituality: everyone has it, but what is it? Int J Nurs Pract. 2015;21:566–74.
24. Aoun SM, Breen LJ, Howting DA, Rumbold B, McNamara B, Hegney D. Who needs bereavement support? A population based survey of bereavement risk and support need. PLoS One. 2015;10(3):e0121101. https://doi.org/10.1371/journal.pone.0121101.
25. Prigerson HG, Horowitz MJ, Jacobs SC, et al. Prolonged grief disorder: psychometric validation of criteria proposed for DSM-V and ICD-11. PLoS Med. 2009;6(8):e1000121.
26. Aoun SM, Breen LJ, White I, et al. What sources of bereavement support are perceived helpful by bereaved people and why? Empirical evidence for the compassionate communities approach. Palliat Med. 2018;32(8):1378–88.
27. Patel M, Noonan K. Community development: compassionate communities. In: Abel J, Kellehear A, editors. The Oxford textbook of public health palliative care. Oxford: Oxford University Press; 2022. p. 107–16.

28. Wilson G, Malina EH, Flores SL, Kellehear A. Compassionate cities: a social ecology at the end of life. In: Abel J, Kellehear A, editors. The Oxford textbook of public health palliative care. Oxford: Oxford University Press; 2022. p. 117–25.
29. Rumbold B, Aoun S. An assets-based approach to bereavement care. Bereavement Care. 2015;34(3):99–102. https://doi.org/10.1080/02682621.2015.1115185.
30. Büssing A, Baumann K. Experience of loss and grief among people from Germany who have lost their relatives during the pandemic: the impact of healthcare professionals' support. Front Public Health. 2023;11:1230198. https://doi.org/10.3389/fpubh.2023.1230198.
31. Harrop E, Mirra RM, Goss S, Longo M, Byrne A, Farnell D, Seddon K, Penny A, Machin L, Sivell S, Selman L. Prolonged grief during and beyond the pandemic: factors associated with levels of grief in a four time-point longitudinal survey of people bereaved in the first year of the COVID-19 pandemic. Front Public Health. 2023;11:1215881. https://doi.org/10.3389/fpubh.2023.1215881.
32. Aoun SM, Lowe J, Christian K, Rumbold B. Is there a role for the funeral service provider in bereavement support within the context of compassionate communities? Death Stud. 2018;43:619. https://doi.org/10.1080/07481187.2018.1506835.
33. Bury M. Illness narratives: fact or fiction? Sociol Health Illn. 2001;23(3):263–85, 264.
34. Riches G, Dawson P. An intimate loneliness. Buckingham: Open University Press; 2000.
35. Walter T. A new model of grief: bereavement and biography. Mortality. 1996;1(1):7–25.
36. Selman L, Turner N, Dawson L, Chamberlain C, Mustan A, Rivett A, Fox F. Engaging and supporting the public on the topic of grief and bereavement: an evaluation of good grief festival. Palliat Care Soc Pract. 2023;17:1–17. https://doi.org/10.1177/26323524231189523.
37. Sallnow L. Prevention and harm reduction. In: Abel J, Kellehear A, editors. The Oxford textbook of public health palliative care. Oxford: Oxford University Press; 2022. p. 73–82.
38. Abel J, Kellehear A, Aoun S. Bereavement care reimagined. Ann Palliat Med. 2023;12:816. https://doi.org/10.21037/apm-23-24.
39. Rumbold B, Lowe J, Aoun S. The evolving landscape: funerals, cemeteries, memorialization, and bereavement support. Omega. 2020;84:596. https://doi.org/10.1177/0030222820904877.
40. Kellehear A. Spirituality and palliative care: a model of needs. Palliat Med. 2000;14:149–55.

Part VIII
Policy

The Ethics of Spiritual Care

Sandra Lynch

Abstract This chapter canvasses the broad set of ethical imperatives entailed in the provision of optimal spiritual and existential care. Beginning with consideration of the moral justification of the provision of spiritual care within the context of holistic person-centred care, it moves to explore the nature and quality of the education and training that healthcare professionals should receive to help ensure best practice, noting that lack of training, imprecision in the definition of terms and lack of institutional support combine to create particular ethical challenges in this field. The goal of the chapter is to assist healthcare professionals to develop a theoretically and practically informed framework that can guide them in competently responding to complex patient needs and in recognising the need for the development of organisational cultures and policies that facilitate best practice. Central to competence in this field is an understanding of the nature of spiritual and existential distress, how it is expressed and what barriers healthcare professionals might face in addressing it, both from personal and moral psychological perspectives and as institutional employees.

Keywords Spirituality · Religion · Holistic Care · Existential Distress · Spiritual Distress · Virtue · Death Anxiety · Self-awareness · Organisational Culture Spiritual care · Palliative care

S. Lynch (✉)
School of Philosophy & Theology, University of Notre Dame Australia, Broadway, NSW, Australia

IMPACCT Research Centre, Faculty of Health, University of Technology, Sydney, NSW, Australia
e-mail: sandra.lynch@nd.edu.au

M. C. Best (ed.), *Spiritual Care in Palliative Care*,
https://doi.org/10.1007/978-3-031-50864-6_42

1 Introduction

Eighty years ago, the medical historian Henry Sigerist published *Civilisation and Disease*, noting that to the individual patient disease 'is not only a biological process but an experience, and it may well be one that very directly affects his entire life' [1, p. 1]. Sigerist's comment encourages us to consider the ethical impact of the ways in which patients are viewed and the ways in which they view themselves. Concomitantly, the ways in which healthcare professionals (HCPs) are viewed and view themselves, and how these 'ways of seeing' might impact upon the structure and culture of healthcare institutions are matters for ethical consideration. Practising ethically in the context of spiritual care requires attention to dimensions of practice with which HCPs may or may not be familiar and which they may or may not regard as central to their own practice. Nonetheless, best practice implies an ethical responsibility both for healthcare institutions and for individual professionals to interrogate and evaluate these 'ways of seeing' to ensure that they impact positively on decision-making and action in the context of spiritual care.

The literature exploring the ethical issues and concerns arising in the context of the provision of spiritual care responds to a set of questions covering the philosophical and practical justification of its provision; the responsibilities of institutions in relation to its provision; and the professional training required for practitioners, which includes consideration of the nature of HCPs' attitudes towards, and engagement in, practice, all of which are explored below.

2 Justification of the Provision of Spiritual Care

Attempts have been made to defend the provision of spiritual care and ground its moral warrant in desire for, or consent to, its provision by patients, caregivers, and clinicians, or in purported correlations between spiritual care interventions and positive health outcomes. Sulmasy regards these attempts as unsuccessful in meeting empirical standards of proof [2]. Nonetheless, the literature does offer support for claims that spiritual care is an important component of holistic, person-centred care, arguing: that it contributes to improved health outcomes in a number of diseases [3]; that spiritual well-being in patients correlates with quality of life [4, 5]; and that spiritual well-being offers some protection against end-of-life despair in those for whom death is imminent [6]. The literature also suggests that spiritual care can contribute to improving relationships and increasing trust between patients and HCPs; to helping develop patients' coping mechanisms in the face of chronic illness and impending death; to giving patients confidence to ask difficult questions about prognosis; and to enhance patients' capacities to respond to distress [7]. A systematic review of the efficacy of religious and spiritual interventions in nursing care concluded that such interventions seem to effectively contribute to mental health, spirituality, and well-being outcomes, although the results were not unequivocal [8].

Sulmasy's approach to the moral justification of spiritual care is to ground it in the nature of healthcare and in the nature of spirituality [2], a view consistent with that of Kaldjian and Puchalski for whom best practice care includes responding to patients' ethical, spiritual, or religious beliefs and values [9, 10]. Sulmasy's argument is that healthcare demands caring for the whole person and as such it requires that spirituality is recognised as a valid focal point for professional concern in healthcare [2], a claim supported in the literature [11, 12]. Certainly, reluctance to recognise the spiritual dimension of life, or rejection and marginalisation of its place and significance in the context of healthcare are themselves issues of moral or ethical import if they impact negatively on the care of patients or undermine the capacity of others to provide spiritual care to patients. Indeed, failing to provide spiritual care has been found to increase the chance of depression and to adversely affect health conditions [13]. The strength of these ethical concerns is reflected in the International Council of Nurses' Code of Ethics, which recognises spiritual care as a human right [12]; in the World Health Organisation's quality of life assessment [14]; and in the work of Burkhart et al. [15].

Best practice in spiritual care requires that HCPs understand the force of arguments defending the moral warrant of spiritual care provision, and accept a set of interconnected, supporting propositions. The first of these propositions identifies the biopsychosocial-spiritual model of illness and health as the model which best supports holistic person-centred care. Exploration of the biopsychosocial, holistic, and whole person terminologies used in the literature reveals a multidimensional, integrated approach to care as a common theme, one in which spiritual care is a prominent additional factor [16]. Bozek et al. also report that a holistic view of health beyond biological and psychosocial well-being is frequently supplemented by the spiritual dimension of well-being, which they argue is a new construct [17]. However, like Puchalski, Ashley and O'Rourke in referring to medieval hospitals usually associated with religious monasteries, see the introduction of scientific and technological innovation as undermining past recognition of connections between spirituality and health [10, 18]. This innovation led to disassociation between spirituality and health, undermining spiritual care's potential therapeutic effects. Consequently, Puchalski argues that we are currently both re-engaging with the once accepted, but latterly neglected, spiritual dimensions of well-being in healthcare contexts and revising our understanding of the nature of healthcare [10].

The second proposition associated with defending the moral warrant of spiritual care stipulates that the training of HCPs must stimulate an appreciation of the broad nature of spirituality, its relevance in many people's lives, its relationship with religion and with existential concerns. Other associated propositions address imperatives crucial to the education of HCPs: firstly, that they understand the interaction between the different dimensions of the biopsychosocial-spiritual model and secondly, that they recognise and respond to existential and spiritual distress. While modern medicine does much to assuage physical suffering in dying patients, recognition of existential and spiritual distress is crucial if HCPs are to competently respond to the 'total' pain of the patient and to treat the dying patient holistically

[19]. Given the commitments these propositions imply, the third imperative is that HCPs develop an understanding of what it is that constitutes best practice within particular contexts and given particular patient needs [9, 13, 19, 20].

3 Educational Responsibilities of Institutions: Ethical

Including a spiritual dimension in the biopsychosocial model of health and illness logically implies that HCPs must have the capacity to recognise the spiritual dimension of life and to respond to spiritual need. These capacities require having some sensitivity to the role that spirituality and religion can play in the lives of patients and other stakeholders; and given that concepts mediate our experience of the world [21], HCPs' understandings of these concepts will frame and facilitate their engagement with patients needing spiritual care. Consequently, healthcare and educational institutions are responsible for ensuring: firstly, that HCPs have the conceptual knowledge and skills requisite to delivering spiritual care to patients facing chronic or terminal illness, as is appropriate to their role and ensures they do not undermine the provision of that care; and secondly, that HCPs have an opportunity to interrogate their own attitudes to death and the potential for moral suffering that HCPs face when unable to cure or help patients.

The importance of educating HCPs in spiritual care delivery is addressed in Chap. 27. However, Nissen et al. noting the time, attention, and training required to identify spiritual needs in daily, but patient-empowering, interactions with particular patients, address an ethically relevant point [22]. They warn that these kinds of interactions can be hindered in highly secularised contexts where spiritual needs may tend to be marginalised as irrelevant, unimportant or inappropriate. Thus, administrators must ensure HCPs are educated to provide spiritual care, while also addressing aspects of a secularised cultural context that can undermine its provision. The so-called 'privacy of religion argument' offers an example since it stipulates that patients must raise the topic of spirituality or religion, claiming that it is unethical for HCPs to ask directly about these matters or to engage in existential communication [13].

Certainly, it is unethical to force discussion or attempt to proselytise since this is inimical to patient-centred care [2, 23]. However, given claims that patients' existential distress is a clinical concern, responsiveness to that distress cannot justifiably be avoided. Leung and Esplen argue convincingly that the nature of clinicians' work determines that they are in relationship with patients and subject to the ethical responsibilities emerging from those relationships [24]. Consequently, where HCPs witness or suspect emotional or existential distress in patients and are not responsive to recognised need, their lack of response is an ethical concern. Open-minded inquiry about a patient's thoughts and feelings should be recognised as an exercise of genuine care, an attempt by HCPs to appreciate the potentially complex interplay of a patient's perceptions, fears, and desires in the face of illness, rather than an infringement of privacy. Whether or not the patient responds to such inquiry to open communication about fears or anxieties, the meaning and purpose of life, self-worth or identity, or about concerns of a specifically spiritual or religious nature, is a matter of patient choice.

In discussing how expectations and fears of overburdening others can discourage the initiation of end-of-life communication in informal settings (between patients and caregivers), von Blanckenburg et al. argue that it seems almost mandatory for professionals to initiate and foster end-of-life communication [25]. Best et al.'s research also supports professionalisation, given that palliative care patients whose doctors asked about their concerns were four times more likely to engage in spirituality discussions than others [26]. Professionalisation introduces a transparent process that invites exploration of unwarranted assumptions, facilitating spiritual and existential communication for those patients who desire or need it as they respond to what may be one of the greatest challenges of their lives.

At the same time, principles of justice and autonomy require that HCPs' rights be respected. Practising with integrity demands that HCPs cannot be expected to act against their own beliefs and understandings in relation to the delivery of spiritual care. Thus, the obligations of HCPs who are not personally appreciative of, or engaged in, the spiritual dimension of life extend only to respecting patients' wishes and ensuring their needs are met competently and appropriately. In fact, effective spiritual care may require specific carers who have an understanding and appreciation of the spiritual and religious beliefs of particular patients [13], since in some cases only a fellow believer might be able to comfort or pray with a patient. Joint acceptance of religious and spiritual truths may foster a depth of engagement that is impossible with a non-believer, even one approaching the patient with the best of intentions.

4 Terminology: Intersections and Disjunctions

Distinguishing between spiritual and existential care is complicated by imprecision inherent in the use of the terms, spirituality and religion. Spiritual and existential concerns often have much in common thematically, e.g. in terms of addressing meaning-making, fears, and anxieties, a sense of connectedness, and the nature and purpose of life. However, a definition of spirituality that includes a religious commitment, such as that of Koenig et al. discussed below, implies a clear differentiation [27]. The way in which patients and HCPs categorise this form of care may depend on their understandings of the terminology. Stereotypical and culturally entrenched ways of conceptualising and defining religion and spirituality increase the challenge of effectively providing spiritual care by undermining attempts to explore understandings of terms. Hence, HCPs need opportunities to critically reflect on those understandings, and to use their intellectual imagination to gain insight into the significance, or lack of significance, that spirituality and religion have in different people's lives.

Understanding varying definitions of spirituality, varying attitudes towards religion and its relationship to spirituality, and appreciating how these, and perhaps HCPs' own views, might impact care is integral to best practice. As Kaldjian argues, the way in which physicians respond to ethical challenges in medicine depends on what they believe and value and on their own capacity and willingness to interrogate the justifiability of their own beliefs, values, and actions [9]. This claim is no doubt relevant to the practice of all HCPs, and hence, healthcare and educational institutions must ensure that the education and training of HCPs serves as a catalyst to critical reflection on their own beliefs, values, and 'ways of seeing' as well as on patients' perspectives.

In considering beliefs about religion, Thuné-Boyle et al. note that while religion is often described in the literature as a form of escapism, denial, or avoidance, this view has been criticised as simplistic and stereotypical [28]. Nonetheless, it is not uncommon in current public debate, where dogmatic views are sometimes presented without substantiation and religion is associated with negative connotations of institutionalised thinking, moralism, and hypocrisy [27, 29]. Dismissive views of religion often imply that religious belief is unjustifiable or could only be justified via conclusive empirical evidence, but such views generally fail to grapple with either their own limitations or with more comprehensive definitions of religion and religious faith. Hence, HCPs may face personal ethical challenges in considering that calls for empirical evidence set standards that are inappropriate to debate on religion [30]. Dismissive views also fail to recognise and respect the diverse roles that religious and spiritual cognitions, practices and communities play in people's lives [28], regardless of whether these are static, orthodox views of religion or less orthodox views, which see religion as integral to an expansive spiritual horizon [31].

By comparison with religion, which is often defined as an institutionalised system of beliefs, rituals, and practices, spirituality is defined more broadly. It is a term that is difficult to standardise because it is not associated with a clearly defined worldview or ideology. Spirituality is sometimes referred to in non-religious, metaphysical or existential terms as a unique way of experiencing and exploring the essence of being, and finding hope, meaning, and purpose in life [32]. It is even used in anti-religious senses, when associated with negative or sceptical views of religion. Thus, it is unsurprising that research on caregivers' perspectives on existential and spiritual distress in palliative care identified the conceptualisation of spirituality as a concerning theme or that some authors use the terms spirituality and religiosity synonymously [8, 33].

Within the literature, the central feature of spirituality emerges as the beliefs and values that give a person a sense of meaning and purpose in life [34]. Koenig et al. accept broad definitions of spirituality in the clinical context but given spirituality's focus on a search for transcendent meaning, they argue that it must be defined more precisely in the research context and seen as intimately connected with organised religion and the supernatural [27]. It seems reasonable to postulate that an imprecise definition of spirituality may be problematic in the research context since as Koenig et al. argue, research must determine whether spiritual or secular sources of care generate positive outcomes or respond most effectively to distress in the face of life-threatening illness [27]. If spirituality is used as an umbrella term for both religion and secular humanism (i.e. non-religious forms of spirituality), then in the research context spiritual concerns may mistakenly be seen as synonymous with non-religiously related existential concerns; questions about religion may then be mistakenly downplayed [27].

The question of how HCPs are to understand spirituality and the role of the sacred or transcendent when meaning in life is experienced within a naturalistic or secular worldview remains unclear in the literature. Philosophical approaches to the topic that take a naturalistic stance see the impulse towards finding transcendent meaning in life as motivated by concern about our own mortality and the death anxiety that is to some extent natural to human beings [35]. Solomon argues that spirituality is akin to thoughtfulness, involving acceptance of death as the completion of life and providing closure that gives an individual life its narrative significance [36]. Thus, while engaging with the transcendent can be viewed as engaging with the supernatural and the divine, it can also reasonably be seen as getting beyond the particularities and travails of life to recognise—perhaps with gratitude, but not necessarily so—the broad trajectory of one's life, in terms of one's hopes, achievements, and participation in life.

Clearly, indefinite, intersecting, and competing notions of spirituality and religion present challenges for the education and training of HCPs. However, educators must ensure that HCPs develop a respectful understanding of divergent approaches to spirituality and religion so as to construct a coherent and workable framework within which: to reflect on the assumptions of patients and colleagues; and to engage in the clinical context with patients in the provision and planning of well-targeted spiritual and existential care interventions. HCPs must also be made aware that the specific nature of particular religious beliefs held by some patients may undermine spiritual well-being or at least make deterring end-of-life despair less effective [6]. Consequently, decisions about how best to care for such patients present ethical challenges requiring sensitive and respectful engagement.

Educators must also alert HCPs to debate among researchers as to how spirituality might best be defined to ensure that research investigating the impact of spiritual well-being and care on health is as robust as possible. However, a flexible, open-minded approach to the use of terms and concepts central to the provision of spiritual care is likely to best facilitate the delivery of care by providing a broad framework within which to relate to particular patients' concerns. In fact, Holyoke and Stephenson offer a challenge to HCPs to embrace a sweeping notion of spiritual care, noting that administering pain medication (and no doubt other forms of symptom management) can be seen as a spiritual act of compassion and sympathy, rather than simply as a biomedical act [37].

5 The Development of Best Practice: A Holistic Approach

While engagement with ways of conceptualising and defining religion and spirituality is requisite to the development of best practice, such engagement is not sufficient to acting on the ethical demands of practice within the spiritual care domain. Aristotelian ethics argues that it is through habituation or practice that we develop the complex rational, social, and emotional skills that allow us to appreciate the ethical dimensions of particular situations and to function well as human beings [38]. This implies that the development of ethical competence should be regarded by practitioners, healthcare and academic institutions as an educational process that has moral, practical, and psychological dimensions and occurs over time. Ideally, within processes of education and training, including in interactions with patients, colleagues, and other stakeholders, HCPs will come to understand the demands of responding to patient need in effective, ethical, and consistent ways. The fact that research has indicated that clinicians who participated in a spiritual care training programme were found within six months to have lost most of the competencies they initially developed suggests that regular professional development focused on best practice requirements is crucial for HCPs [39]. Tan et al. also identify ongoing staff education as an area of concern in the provision of spiritual care, along with evaluation of practice, accountability, and crisis management [20].

Kaldjian suggests that in the medical profession and in society generally, there is sufficient consensus about the beliefs, values, virtues, and goals that guide the work of HCPs to allow us to be relatively confident about the relevance of Aristotelian and other virtue-based approaches to ethics in guiding best practice in healthcare [9]. In the context of discussing skills that clinicians need to be able to guide patients during the course of illness, Kaldjian draws attention to an unusual set of communication skills [9]. He includes abilities to: initiate discussion, explain complex ideas plainly, respond to questions, listen to emotional responses, recognise subtle and non-verbal cues regarding patients' readiness to make decisions, and sustain hope despite disappointing and fearful realities. For Kaldjian adequately responding to patient need in the face of illness presumes that clinicians are also aware of the patient's biomedical state, capacity for social engagement, and psychological preparedness to engage in decision-making at the point of the particular interaction [9].

The list of skills Kaldjian enumerates provides a foundation for discerning the various aspects of existential and spiritual distress in healthcare settings. In the process of conceptualising and classifying existential distress, Kissane et al. provide a set of signposts to help HCPs recognise and respond to what might otherwise remain as unmet need, creating morbid distress and suffering [40]. The tasks of developing an understanding of these signposts, while also developing and refining the skills, capacities, and dispositions that Kaldjian identifies, are both practically important and ethically relevant aspects of spiritual care practice and training. They are relevant both to individual HCPs and institutions since they enable HCPs to respond competently to existential and spiritual distress in healthcare settings [9].

Kaldjian is clearly appealing to a set of virtues that are in interaction with particular skills in treating patients facing the progression of illness. Critical reflection on these virtues in the healthcare context is crucial to best practice [9]. Traditionally, virtues are seen as reliable, cross-situational dispositions or character traits, which appeal to a broad sense of value or human good [41, 42]. Sophisticated clinical and communication skills when combined with virtues, such as honesty, compassion, and sensitivity to the demands of best practice, are components of such a notion of value, not least for the sense of trust and security that they foster in patients. Kaldjian illustrates this when he discusses orchestrating transitions in goals of patient care with candour, compassion, and sensitivity to changing medical conditions and to emotional and spiritual needs in the face of progressive illness [9].

As noted above, facilitating HCPs' capacities to respond to patient need within a biopsychosocial-spiritual framework is partly an institutional responsibility, but it is also a matter of personal integrity, a matter of the individual HCP's commitment to virtuous practice and human reasonableness. Kaldjian's exhortation that ethical practice in medicine requires the integration of practical wisdom, conscience, and the goals of care implies practising with integrity so that professional commitments are consistent with, or at least not in conflict with, an individual's personal beliefs, values, and goals [9, 42]. Practical wisdom is seen as an overarching, intellectual virtue serving to guide the application of other virtues, facilitating consideration of the goals that are worth pursuing and preceding deliberation about the means that might most effectively achieve those goals.

The role of the virtue of compassion in healthcare contexts is emphasised by Crawford et al., who capture the force of philosophical treatments of compassion that see it as the basic social emotion or supreme ethical principle, given it engages us in attending to others and their suffering [43–45]. Compassion entails profound and active responsiveness to those in need and is like empathy or even mercy, which takes us beyond our own interests, needs, and values to lead us to invest time and effort in addressing the concerns of suffering patients [46]. Crawford et al. extend their focus on compassion beyond individual practice, to argue that it should also underpin the design of services and spaces and the development of supportive and nonthreatening organisational cultures, policies, and incentives [43]. They recognise the need to enhance HCPs' capacities to deliver competent and compassionate spiritual care to patients, as well as the need to minimise stress, and avoid compassion fatigue and burnout for HCPs involved in caring for dying and seriously ill patients [43].

Giddens provides us with an overarching concept that can help HCPs understand and respond compassionately to the experiences of patients as they face a diagnosis of chronic illness or impending death, regardless of whether they would engage with their experience in secular, religious, or spiritual terms [13, 47]. Giddens sees human beings as sustained in daily activity by *ontological security* or a sense of trust in others, the origin and need for which lies in a largely unconscious anxiety controlling mechanism. Like Erikson [48], Giddens argues that predictable routine maintains this security, but it is disrupted in critical situations, such as when we are faced with serious illness.

The foundational relationship between hope and the notion of trust in others relates to the provision of optimal spiritual and existential care, since trusting relationships may help remedy an unsettled mindset or a frail sense of life's meaning to sustain hope that possibilities of some kind remain [49]. Trusting relationships and the hope they engender can also mitigate against demoralisation or denial of terminal illness, a significant ethical concern given that patients in denial are three times more likely to be clinically depressed [50]. In addition, since clinicians in palliative care settings can spend up to 34% of their time guiding patients experiencing existential distress [51], HCPs ought also to be motivated to compassionately and competently respond to existential or spiritual distress for practical, as well as ethical reasons.

Symons focuses on a second overarching concept central to best practice: hospitality. Using Sontag's image of illness as a second but inferior 'citizenship' to that of wellness, he notes that illness can place a barrier between oneself and the world, such that patients feel alone and unsupported, despite receiving optimal medical care [52]. Sontag warns that during life most people will eventually be obliged to see themselves through the lens of illness [53]. Therefore, an attitude of hospitality, combined with honest, humble, and compassionate recognition that Sontag's warning applies not only to patients, but to HCPs and others, may well help address patients' feelings of isolation, by guiding them patiently through existential and spiritual distress towards hopefulness and reconciliation with the possibilities confronting them.

Yet as Leung and Esplen note, a synthesis of the literature reveals that many clinicians struggle with whether or not to engage with patients' distress and are unprepared to face the dilemmas and burdens of emotional involvement with patients [24]. This may be explained by lack of institutional support, but may also be explained by personal and moral psychological dimensions of practice such as caregivers' anguish or compassion fatigue, which will be discussed below.

6 Moral Psychological Dimensions of Practice

The literature generally emphasises the goodwill of HCPs committed to providing optimal patient care, but it also recognises the pressure under which HCPs often function and the impact this can have on the provision of care [50]. For example, the stress involved in the palliative care context can be debilitating given that demoralisation, distress, and depression are contagious in the absence of adequate self-care and debriefing sessions with a multidisciplinary team [19]. Knowledge gained within educational processes can enhance HCPs' capacities to function well in palliative care and other contexts, not least by allowing them to reflect on their own attitudes to death and the potential for moral suffering that HCPs face. Difficulty in relieving a patient's suffering can lead to anguish and feelings of helplessness and vulnerability to which caregivers can respond, consciously or even unconsciously, by employing defence mechanisms [54]; e.g. by rejecting the burden of emotional involvement with distressed patients, isolating themselves, hiding distress, disengaging from emotions, overworking, or alternatively losing interest in work [24, 54]. Pessin et al. argue that working with the dying and also the bereaved can encourage introspection about mortality among HCPs and elicit existential concerns that coexist with death anxiety [55].

Kohut and Wolf argue that healthy adult practitioners grow to recognise and straddle tension between empathetic concern for patients, awareness of their own mental and emotional capacities, and the demands of best practice [56]. Kohut describes an ethical project like that of Aristotelian habituation described above, where practitioners work towards becoming increasingly adept at sensitively establishing relationships of empathetic resonance with others, in which the interests and needs of those others, take precedence over practitioners' interests and needs [57]. Kohut sees introspection and empathy as informers of appropriate action in bringing practitioners in tune with the inner life of dying and seriously ill patients [57]. Introspection by HCPs, particularly when stimulated by participation in debriefing sessions with the team of interdisciplinary colleagues involved in provision of care, facilitates recognition of the impact of emotions on practice and reflection on differing perspectives and assumptions. Kissane provides an example of assumptions HCPs might interrogate when he warns clinicians that they should monitor their personal feelings about the value of a dying patient's continued life, given that clinicians tend to undervalue ratings of a patient's quality of life by comparison with the patient's own perceptions [19]. These reflective processes require honesty, courage, humility, and patience as HCPs critically explore their practice, acknowledging and normalising common challenges they face, increasing self-awareness, developing empathy, and generally coming to appreciate the complexity of providing optimal care. However, while personal awareness and the development of internal patterns of response to address behavioural tendencies, such as defensiveness due to fear or bias, are important in ensuring optimal care, mechanisms also need to be instituted by healthcare organisations to externalise the process of ensuring best practice, e.g. via incentives, deterrents, and debriefing opportunities.

The question of recognising and maintaining professional boundaries is also an ethical and moral psychological concern. Peeters warns that pastoral relationships are ethically complex due partly to the power imbalance that typically characterises them, but also to tension between interpersonal and professional aspects of these relationships [58]. To avoid the potential danger of undermining the professional character of such relationships, Peeters argues for a pastoral caregivers' code of ethics that provides explicit guidance about the nature of ethical conduct within these relationships [58]. Such guidance is crucial, but equally practical wisdom, honesty, humility, and self-awareness are requisite to appropriately managing relationships with patients. HCPs are closely engaged with patients dealing with personal and confidential information at highly stressful times in patients' lives. This may make patients emotionally vulnerable and lead HCPs to become more emotionally involved or take on more responsibility than is appropriate to such relationships.

7 The Delivery of Spiritual and Existential Care

There are broad administrative and prudential considerations of an ethical nature relevant to ensuring optimal practice in the delivery of spiritual and existential care, which are discussed below, but best practice firstly requires consideration of who is best equipped to deliver care. Tan et al. note rival approaches to delivery in the literature: from a single healthcare worker, often a nurse or a specific spiritual care worker, to members of a broad multidisciplinary team, the latter approach being regarded as optimal [20]. In a study of four hospices, Holyoke and Stephenson recommend recruitment, ongoing training and inclusion of volunteers in collaborative interdisciplinary healthcare teams [37]. Their research indicated that well-trained volunteers were essential given they have the time, inclination, and the capacities to help ensure the provision of optimal care in palliative care context.

Assigning the responsibility and privilege of delivering spiritual and existential care to patients in particular contexts or choosing which strategies to adopt (e.g. see Chap. 17 for consideration of meaning making and other strategies) are matters for investigation and discussion by HCPs aware of the capabilities, resources, and constraints inherent within those contexts. However, an underlying theme within the literature regarding the delivery of spiritual care is that it must be recognised as a domain of whole person care and integrated into the whole healthcare service, as wide recognition of and commitment to the biopsychosocial-spiritual model of health and illness imply it must. Additionally, the importance of the education of collaborative interdisciplinary teams to ensure best practice delivery is emphasised by the European Association for Palliative Care, in arguing for high quality, multidisciplinary, academically, and financially accessible spiritual care education for all palliative care staff [59]. These views reinforce the claim of this chapter that the provision of optimal spiritual and existential care is an ethical concern for the healthcare profession, one that is partly dependent on ensuring the quality of well-targeted professional education and training, but also dependent on the fulfilment of organisational responsibilities.

8 Organisational Culture

Organisational culture, policies, and incentives should serve as catalysts to skill development, professional and personal reflection and to the possibility of reform or refinement of practice, all of which help guarantee the currency of HCPs' skills. Gentile refers to this process in the context of business ethics as putting in place organisational enablers that help create alignment between an organisation's and an employee's sense of purpose to enhance the effectiveness of the overall enterprise [60].

As Tan et al. argue, best practice intervention does not happen in isolation [20]. It is part of a complex, collaborative system of care and is impacted by many factors within the organisational structure, including current inadequacy of professional training and support [20, 39]. For example, despite agreement among scholars that spirituality can be important in promoting health and well-being and therefore that responding to patients' needs for spiritual care is imperative, Hawthorne and Gordon report a lack of attention to spirituality in nursing training and practice, arguing that spiritual nursing care practices are invisible in many healthcare settings [7, 11]. These deficits persist even though educational bodies mandate the inclusion of spiritual care in nursing and medical education [12, 13].

Those in leadership positions in healthcare as administrators, clinicians, professional educators and researchers share a responsibility to take note of the growing literature in the field and to ensure that results of robust research are implemented within education, training and practice in the profession. Leaders must also ensure that further research addresses gaps in knowledge and equivocal results about the effectiveness of religious and spiritual care. For example, since healthcare costs require substantial public and private budgetary expenditure, there are practical and ethical imperatives to address the current inadequate supply of validated instruments capable of generating quantifiable evidence of the value of spiritual care services [61].

Apart from commitments to ongoing education, training, and engagement with research results in the spiritual care domain, administrators have a duty to establish systems of compliance, accountability, and evaluation that ensure all HCPs meet the obligations emerging from the values and goals their professions set as standards. Among specific recommendations for organisational best practice in the literature are the establishment of well-publicised, evidence-based assessment and referral processes in which compliance is monitored and supported. Appropriate levels of staffing, spiritual and existential care and support for staff (as needed) and mechanisms enabling staff to collaborate with management in developing its processes of accountability and evaluation are other expressions of best practice for which administrators are responsible [20]. Research also indicates the value of reminders of professional integrity; e.g. Ariely records an erosion of professional ethics within many professions, including medicine, and demonstrates the worth of employing 'moral reminders', oaths, and rules that are regularly and publicly recalled in support of best practice [62].

9 Conclusion

This chapter canvasses a broad set of ethical imperatives entailed in providing optimal spiritual and existential care, which is defended as an essential aspect of healthcare. The chapter's goal is to assist HCPs in developing a theoretically and practically informed framework that can guide them in competently responding to the complexity of patient need. Patients' needs for comfort, support, and understanding in the face of illness and death vary and are multidimensional [63]. This determines that responding to need is sometimes difficult and the chapter acknowledges that deficits in education, training, and organisational support combine to undermine the development of HCPs' competence in responding to patient need.

Failure to appreciate the ways in which spiritual and existential distress is expressed and the barriers HCPs might face in addressing it, personally and as institutional employees, are also identified as obstacles to best practice. Similarly, the chapter warns that bias and pervasive cultural criticism of religion can impact negatively on interaction between all stakeholders, a potential exacerbated by unappreciated power imbalances within relationships, which can also compromise the quality of patient care.

The role of organisations in developing and sustaining cultures that support HCPs in delivering optimal spiritual and existential care is addressed and the importance of shared purpose among individual HCPs and organisations is emphasised. Spiritual care practice is unique in respect to some of the challenges it presents for HCPs and administrators. Certainly, it shares many aspects of the provision of care in common with other healthcare fields, in that it entails care of people in times of stress and need, acknowledging physical, mental, and social dimensions of care [63]. However, spiritual care is unique in that significant responsibility for facilitating its provision falls on senior clinicians and administrators, some of whom will neither understand nor appreciate the significance of the spiritual realm for patients' lives. Consequently, while the duties of HCPs require that they show care and concern for patients, best practice requires that this be pursued with the intent of respecting and responding to spiritual need that may not resonate with the experience or understandings of particular HCPs.

References

1. Sigerist HE, Fee E. Civilization and disease. Ithaca, USA: Cornell University Press; 2018.
2. Sulmasy DP. Ethical principles for spiritual care. In: Cobb M, Puchalski CM, Rumbold B, editors. The Oxford textbook of spirituality in healthcare. Oxford: Oxford University Press; 2012. p. 465–70.
3. Best MC, Jones K, Merritt F, Casey M, Lynch S, Eisman J, et al. Australian patient preferences for the introduction of spirituality into their healthcare journey: a mixed methods study. J Relig Health. 2023;62(4):2323–40.
4. Goyarrola R, Lipsanen J, Saarelainen SM, Suviranta R, Rahko E, Lamminmäki A, et al. Spiritual well-being correlates with quality of life of both cancer and non-cancer patients in palliative care – further validation of EORTC QLQ-SWB32. BMC Palliat Care. 2023;22(1):33.
5. Kandasamy A, Chaturvedi SK, Desai G. Spirituality, distress, depression, anxiety, and quality of life in patients with advanced cancer. Indian J Cancer. 2011;48(1):55–9.
6. McClain CS, Rosenfeld B, Breitbart W. Effect of spiritual well-being on end-of-life despair in terminally ill cancer patients. Lancet. 2003;361(9369):1603–7.
7. Best M, Butow P, Olver I. Spiritual support of cancer patients and the role of the doctor. Support Care Cancer. 2014;22(5):1333–9.
8. de Diego-Cordero R, Suárez-Reina P, Badanta B, Lucchetti G, Vega-Escaño J. The efficacy of religious and spiritual interventions in nursing care to promote mental, physical and spiritual health: A systematic review and meta-analysis. Appl Nurs Res. 2022;67(October):151618.

9. Kaldjian LC. Practicing medicine and ethics: integrating wisdom, conscience, and goals of care. New York: Cambridge University Press; 2014.
10. Puchalski CM, Vitillo R, Hull S, Reller N. Improving the spiritual dimension of whole person care: reaching national and international consensus. J Palliat Med. 2014;17(6):642–56.
11. Hawthorne DM, Gordon SC. The invisibility of spiritual nursing care in clinical practice. J Holist Nurs. 2020;38(1):147–55.
12. International Council of Nurses. Code of ethics for nurses. Geneva: Switzerland; 2021. ISBN 978-92-95099-94-4
13. Nissen RD, Viftrup DT, Hvidt NC. The process of spiritual care. Front Psychol. 2021;12:674453.
14. Department of Mental Health and Substance Dependence WHO. World Health Organization Quality of Life (WHOQOL). WHO Document1 March 2012.
15. Burkhart L, Schmidt L, Hogan N. Development and psychometric testing of the spiritual care inventory instrument. J Adv Nurs. 2011;67(11):2463–72.
16. Thomas HMG, Rich J. Definition of whole person care in general practice in the english language literature: a systematic review. BMJ Open. 2018;8:e023758.
17. Bożek A, Nowak Paweł F, Blukacz M. The relationship between spirituality, health-related behavior, and psychological well-being. Front Psychol. 2020;11:1997.
18. Ashley BM, O'Rourke KD. Health care ethics: a theological analysis. 4th ed. Washington, D.C: Georgetown University Press; 1997.
19. Kissane DW. Psychospiritual and existential distress. The challenge for palliative care. Aust Fam Physician. 2000;29(11):1022–5.
20. Tan H, Arnison C, Venter N. Spiritual care in healthcare: elements of best practice – a scoping review 2022. Spiritual Health Association, Australia, and Spiritual Care in Aotearoa New Zealand Healthcare Co-design Rōpū; 2022.
21. McDowell J. Mind and world. Cambridge, MA: Harvard University Press; 1996.
22. Nissen RD, Gildberg FA, Hvidt NC. Approaching the religious psychiatric patient in a secular country: does "Subalternalizing" religious patients mean they do not exist? Arch Psychol Relig. 2019;41(2):123–40.
23. Sulmasy DP. A biopsychosocial-spiritual model for the care of patients at the end of life. The Gerontologist. 2002;42(suppl3):24–33.
24. Leung D, Esplen MJ. Alleviating existential distress of cancer patients: can relational ethics guide clinicians? Eur J Cancer Care. 2010;19:19 30–8.
25. von Blanckenburg P, Knorrenschild JR, Hofmann M, Fries H, Nestoriuc Y, Seifart U, Rief W, Seifart C. Expectations, end-of-life fears and end-of-life communication among palliative patients with cancer and caregivers: a cross-sectional study. BMJ Open. 2022;12(5):e058531.
26. Best M, McArdle MB, Huang Y, Clayton J, Butow P. How and how much is spirituality discussed in palliative care consultations for advanced cancer patients with and without a question prompt list? Patient Educ Couns. 2019;102(12):2208–13.
27. Koenig H, King D, Carson VB. Handbook of religion and health. 2nd ed. New York: Oxford University Press, Incorporated; 2012.
28. Thuné-Boyle IC, Stygall JA, Keshtgar MR, Newman SP. Do religious/spiritual coping strategies affect illness adjustment in patients with cancer? A systematic review of the literature. Soc Sci Med. 2006;63(1):151–64.
29. Death J. Governing child abuse voices and victimisation: the use of public inquiry into child sexual abuse in christian institutions. 1st ed. Milton: Taylor and Francis; 2017.
30. Forrest P. The epistemology of religion. In: Zalta EN, editor. The Stanford encyclopedia of philosophy. Fall 2021 ed.
31. Deignan K, Osgood L, editors. Teilhard de Chardin: a book of hours. Maryknoll, N: Orbis Books; 2023.
32. Gallacher R. Spirituality. Nurs Stand. 2015;30(26):61–2.

33. Boston PH, Mount BM. The caregiver's perspective on existential and spiritual distress in palliative care. J Pain Symptom Manag. 2006;32:13–26.
34. Puchalski C, Romer AL. Taking a spiritual history allows clinicians to understand patients more fully. J Palliat Med. 2005;3(1):129.
35. Bergo B. Emmanuel Levinas. In: Zalta EN, editor. The Stanford encyclopedia of philosophy. Fall 2019 ed.
36. Solomon RC. Spirituality for the skeptic: the thoughtful love of life. Oxford: Oxford University Press; 2002.
37. Holyoke P, Stephenson B. Organization-level principles and practices to support spiritual care at the end of life: a qualitative study. BMC Palliat Care. 2017;16(1):24.
38. Aristotle. The ethics of Aristotle: The Nichomachean ethics. Harmondsworth: Penguin; 335? BC; 1983.
39. van de Geer J, Veeger N, Groot M, Zock H, Leget C, Prins J. Multidisciplinary training on spiritual care for patients in palliative care trajectories improves the attitudes and competencies of hospital medical staff: results of a quasi-experimental study. Am J Hosp Palliat Care. 2018;35(2):218–28.
40. Kissane DW, Wein S, Love A, Lee XQ, Kee PL, Clarke DM. The demoralization scale: a report of its development and preliminary validation. J Palliat Care. 2004;20(4):269–76.
41. Sreenivasan G. In: Russell DC, editor. The situationist critique of virtue ethics. Cambridge, UK: Cambridge University Press; 2013.
42. Ramsay H. Beyond virtue: integrity and morality. London: Macmillan Press Ltd; 1997.
43. Crawford P, Brown B, Baker C, Tischler V, Abrams B. Health humanities. London, U.K.: Palgrave Macmillan; 2015.
44. Nussbaum M. Compassion: the basic social emotion. Soc Philos Policy. 1996;13(1):27–58.
45. Useless LE, Suffering. Entre nous: thinking-of-the-other. N.Y: Columbia University Press; 1998.
46. Oreopoulos DG. Compassion and mercy in the practice of medicine. Perit Dial Int. 2001;21(6):539–42.
47. Giddens A. The constitution of society: outline of the theory of structuration. Cambridge: Polity Press; 1986.
48. Erikson EH. Identity and the life cycle: selected papers. N.Y: International Press; 1959.
49. Ratcliffe M. The underlying unity of hope and trust. Monist. 2023;106(1):1–11.
50. Chochinov HM. Dignity in care: the human side of medicine. N.Y: Oxford University Press; 2022.
51. Kiely MT, Alison DL. Palliative care activity in a medical oncology unit: the implications for oncology training. Clin Oncol (R Coll Radiol). 2000;12(3):179–81.
52. Symons X. The hostility of illness and the therapeutic importance of hospitality. McGrath Institute for Church Life Church Life Journal; June 26, 2023.
53. Sontag S. Illness as metaphor. New York: Farrar, Straus and Giroux; 1978.
54. Sadler K. The price of compassion: letting go of your ideals to provide better care. Can Oncol Nurs J. 2016;26(3):233–7.
55. Pessin H, Fenn N, Hendriksen E, DeRosa AP, Applebaum A. Existential distress among healthcare providers caring for patients at the end of life. Curr Opin Support Palliat Care. 2015;9(1):77–86.
56. Kohut H, Wolf ES. The disorders of the self and their treatment: an outline. Int J Psychoanal. 1978;59(4):413–25.
57. Kohut H. In: Ornstein PH, editor. On empathy. Madison, CT: International Universities Press; 1981.
58. Peeters EJH. Quality pastoral relationships in healthcare settings: guidelines for codes of ethics. J Pastoral Care Counsel. 2020;74(1):42–52.
59. Best M, Leget C, Goodhead A, Paal P. An EAPC white paper on multi-disciplinary education for spiritual care in palliative care. BMC Palliat Care. 2020;19(1):9.

60. Gentile MC. Giving voice to values: how to speak your mind when you know what's right. New Haven, Conn: Yale University Press; 2010.
61. Hall EJ, Powell RA. Valuing the spiritual. J Relig Health. 2021;60(3):1430–5.
62. Ariely D. Predictably irrational: the hidden forces that shape our decisions. N.Y: HarperCollins; 2008.
63. Oben P. Understanding the patient experience: a conceptual framework. J Patient Exp. 2020;7(6):906–10.

Organisational and Leadership Factors for Spiritual Care Implementation

Csaba Szilagyi

Abstract Spiritual care (SC) plays a critical role in palliative care (PC). However, a substantial gap exists between our understanding of the role of religion/spirituality (R/S) in serious illness and the actual SC practices addressing R/S in PC. Spiritual care implementation addresses this knowledge–practice gap. In this chapter, we apply a blend of implementation, organisational, and leadership theories to help SC leaders close this gap by exploring how they might effectively influence organisational conditions and employ strategies for SC implementation at their institutions. Organisational and leadership factors critically impact SC implementation and integration. Therefore, the chapter presents frameworks and insights from implementation science, implementation climate, organisational readiness for change, implementation leadership, spiritual care leadership, and social entrepreneurship. These concepts offer opportunities for maximising leaders' capacity to lead, influence, and promote SC integration, producing consistent, widespread, and persistent SC implementation in PC. They help leaders develop comprehensive and strategic approaches to shape how their institutions understand, respond to, and incorporate SC, ultimately narrowing the knowledge–practice gap in SC and PC.

Keywords Implementation science · Organisational readiness for change
Implementation climate · Implementation leadership · Social entrepreneurship
Spiritual care · Palliative care

C. Szilagyi (✉)
Rush University Medical Center, Chicago, IL, USA
e-mail: Csaba_Szilagyi@rush.edu

M. C. Best (ed.), *Spiritual Care in Palliative Care*,
https://doi.org/10.1007/978-3-031-50864-6_43

1 Introduction

1.1 The Knowledge–Practice Gap in Spiritual Care in Palliative Care

A substantial gap exists between our understanding of the role of religion/spirituality (R/S) in serious illness and the actual practices addressing R/S in palliative care (PC). Implementation science refers to this as the knowledge–practice gap, illustrating the divide between evidence-based interventions and clinical models and their practical, everyday application [1–4]. A primary strategy to ensure high-quality healthcare and continuously improve patient outcomes is the implementation of evidence-based practices (EBPs).

A robust evidence base has been developed to support the importance of R/S and spiritual care (SC) in PC. In a recent systematic review, an appraisal of 371 research studies on spirituality in serious illness concluded with expert recommendations that advocate for the following actions: [1] 'routinely incorporate SC into the medical care of patients with serious illness'; [2] 'include SC education in the training of all members of the interdisciplinary medical team caring for seriously ill patients'; [3] 'include specialty practitioners of SC (e.g. chaplains) in the care of patients with serious illness' [5] (p. 188). Additionally, national PC clinical guidelines and quality frameworks have translated and applied the existing evidence for SC. The Clinical Practice Guidelines for Quality Palliative Care [6] in the United States (USA), the Netherlands Quality Framework for Palliative Care, [7] and the Existential and Spiritual Aspects of Palliative Care National Guidelines in the Netherlands [8] are all excellent examples. Compelling evidence and comprehensive clinical guidelines support the notion that addressing patients' R/S is indispensable for high-quality, holistic, and person-centred care. The scientific rationale and clinical consensus for incorporating SC into PC for improved patient outcomes is no longer a matter of serious debate. However, the question remains: How to effectively implement and strengthen the integration of SC in the daily care of people with serious illness?

A significant knowledge–practice gap persists between the evidence for SC and its practical integration as a routine and essential aspect of PC. Despite the proliferation of PC and national recommendations in the USA, only 38% of programmes have funded chaplain positions, [9] and just 48% of paediatric PC programmes employ chaplains [10]. Screening and addressing spiritual needs also lag behind. Research showed that only 55% of patients (n = 402) with serious illness and high PC needs were screened for SC in the last six months of life, with most of them expressing the desire to receive SC [11]. A study assessing hospices' organisational capacity and commitment to address spiritual concerns in New Zealand found that only 40% of staff conducted spiritual assessments regularly and 50% of surveyed hospices had SC policies [12]. Incorporating SC as a standard and integral part of care for all patients with serious illness remains a significant challenge and is considerably lacking in many settings. Therefore, implementation science is crucial to closing this knowledge–practice gap by identifying and applying strategies designed to accelerate the successful integration of EBPs, such as SC, into routine practice [2].

1.2 The Aim of the Chapter

Implementing SC is often a story of innovation adoption, leadership, and organisational change. Spiritual care leaders are poised to strategically affect organisational factors and hone their leadership capabilities, which is crucial for incorporating SC into PC. Therefore, the chapter applies a blend of implementation, organisational, and leadership theories to help SC leaders close the knowledge–practice gap by exploring how they might effectively influence organisational conditions and employ strategies for SC implementation and integration at their institutions.

1.3 Who Is a Spiritual Care Leader?

For our purposes, we understand SC leaders as persons who have the opportunity and capability to lead, influence, and promote the implementation and integration of SC in their setting, regardless of whether they have a formal leadership role within their organisation [13]. It can include chaplains in clinical or leadership positions and other clinicians and healthcare professionals who exhibit various leadership behaviours to influence SC delivery within their respective contexts.

1.4 Applying Implementation Science at the Organisational Level

The chapter uses an implementation language to refer to SC implementation and integration. The extent to which SC is implemented and integrated into PC as an essential and routine care domain moves across a broad spectrum and can vary from institution to institution. Whether leaders implement SC for the first time or expand existing services, assessing and addressing organisational and leadership factors affecting those efforts is vital and can determine outcomes. Moreover, the chapter focuses on leadership and organisational dynamics in the context of healthcare institutions rather than the national policy level. Still, the clinician, team, organisational, and national levels of implementation are interdependent and impact SC adoption.

2 Implementation Science for Spiritual Care

Spiritual care is an empirically and clinically supported care domain to implement in PC to achieve improved patient outcomes and comprehensive whole-person care. However, implementation science is a vital yet untapped resource to inform and support SC implementation and integration strategies.

Implementation science studies and informs the methods needed to translate research findings and enable the adoption of EBPs into routine healthcare in the clinical, organisational, health system, or policy contexts [2–4]. Livet et al. defined implementation science as 'the scientific study and application of strategies to promote the systematic uptake of research findings and other evidence-based practices into routine use, thereby improving the quality and effectiveness of health services. In other words, implementation science is about facilitating and understanding what it takes for healthcare settings to put an intervention or service into practice and do it well enough to maximise its desired clinical, humanistic, and economic outcomes' [2] (p. 491). Research on integrating SC consultation services into palliative home care groups in the Netherlands [11] is one of the few studies using an implementation science approach to examine the facilitators and barriers in adopting SC (see Chap. 44).

2.1 Phases and Levels of Implementation

Implementation Phases

Although systematic research on specific processes and strategies for SC implementation is limited, implementation science may inform, support, and accelerate the uptake and integration of SC in routine PC practice. Leaders can benefit from understanding the state of SC implementation in PC in relation to the three phases of implementation outlined by Tansella and Thornicroft [4]: adoption in principle, early implementation, and persistence of implementation.

Figure 1 depicts factors with a strong potential to influence SC implementation and move it through the implementation phases and multi-level changes. It outlines the implementation phases moving from left to right related to the levels at which relevant changes occur on the vertical axis. The organisational and leadership factors, highlighted on the left, influence and facilitate SC implementation and associated changes at each phase and each level. Understanding the dynamics of SC implementation and change efforts within this combined framework may guide implementation strategies to narrow the SC integration gap and move SC towards persistent implementation. Spiritual care leaders can identify and address facilitators and barriers at each phase and level. Yet, the particularities of SC implementation phases in PC may look different and vary depending on one's clinical, institutional, local, or national context.

Adoption in Principle

The adoption in principle phase is marked by the intention to implement EBP [4]. For instance, the endorsement of or commitment to the notion of addressing R/S in PC can be seen as adopting the general idea. National promotion of this concept

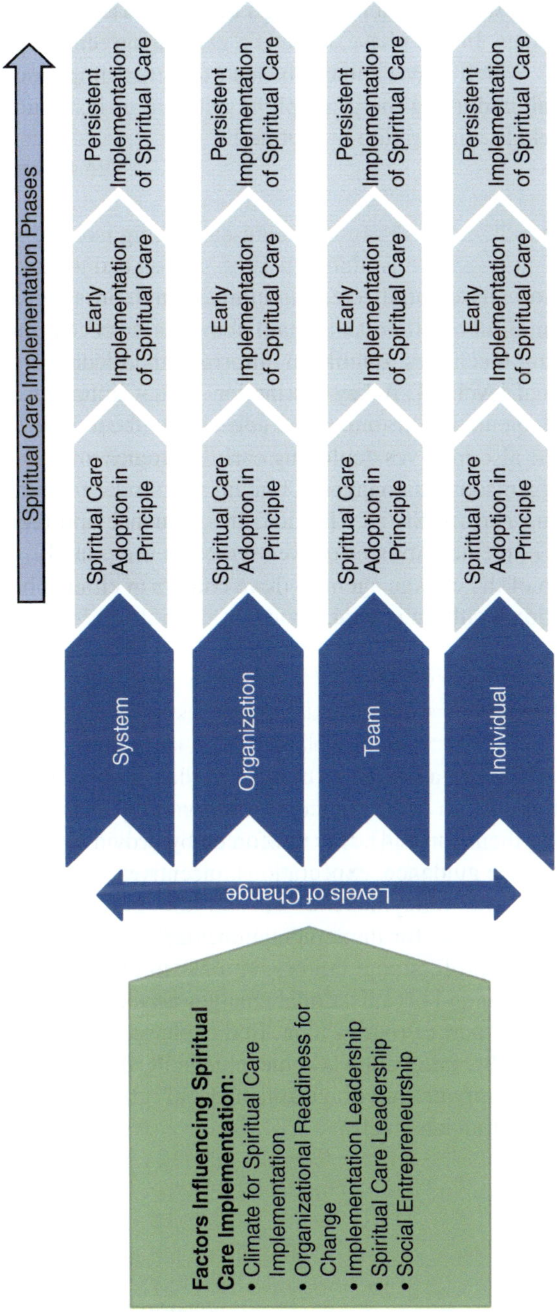

The figure depicts Organizational and leadership factors (on the left) with a strong potential to influence spiritual care Implementation to move through the implementation phases and multi-level changes (from left to right at each level). The levels of change and Implementation were adapted from Shortell, 2004 and Proctor et al., 2009. The phases of implementation were adapted from Tansella and Thornicroft, 2009.

Fig. 1 Organisational and leadership factors influencing spiritual care implementation may come from influential figures, experts, and advocacy groups in PC. Institutional leaders may also endorse the significance of SC in PC, while champions, opinion leaders, and early adopters within clinical teams go beyond the requirements set by policy or clinical guidelines. In this phase, there is a general agreement to incorporate R/S and SC in PC, which may or may not lead to actual implementation in practice. While essential, endorsing the principle at national or institutional levels does not necessarily yield SC integration in routine PC.

Early Implementation

The early implementation phase entails creating clinical guidelines viewed as feasible, flexible, and meaningful by clinicians, establishing a network of implementation sites, and developing incentives, quality monitoring, and feedback systems at the institution or national level [4]. A key distinction is that initial resources are made available for implementation, training, and adhering to local policy and practice guidance. This phase also involves deploying early strategies to induce the necessary behaviour and organisational changes. Clinicians' attitudes towards R/S and SC, bridging the training gap for SC as EBP, and the influence and reputation of advocates for SC affect implementation effectiveness. Most importantly, the persistence and determination of the change agent to drive change in clinical behaviours, practices, and organisational culture is vital.

Persistent Implementation

Consistently applying EBPs and adhering to clinical guidelines over the long term has a more substantial impact on health outcomes than merely endorsing them in theory and implementing them early [4]. It is reinforced by providing clear, consistent, and sustainable practice guidance, expectations, incentives, and feedback systems to teams, leaders, and policymakers. Beyond the initial resources, the availability of resources continues for implementation, staff training, and fostering the appropriate clinical and professional culture. It aims to coordinate, maintain, and consolidate the behaviour and organisational changes necessary for EBPs, such as SC, to become an integral part of routine care. In this phase, the sustained, comprehensive, and widespread SC integration is achievable in PC through the ongoing, consistent, and persistent application of established SC clinical guidelines at national, institutional, and clinician levels.

2.2 *Multi-Level Change and Implementation*

The success of implementation hinges on effectively addressing the multi-level changes inherent in the process. Proctor and colleagues [3] applied Shortell's [14] multi-level model of change for performance improvement to illuminate four distinct levels within the practice context where changes are essential for successful implementation: larger system/environment, organisation, group/team, and individual levels (Fig. 1). They emphasise the need for a systems perspective to align, navigate, and affect change at these interdependent levels to achieve significant and sustainable quality improvement and EBP implementation. Implementing SC in PC entails recognising and leveraging mechanisms to induce, manage, and maintain changes at each level.

System Level

Implementation-promoting changes in the larger healthcare system can be achieved through various policy, advocacy, regulatory, and economic activities at the national level, such as incentives, regulatory structures, and national guidelines to improve the quality of care, informed by empirical evidence [3, 14]. For instance, van de Geer and Leget describe the national programme and policy development for multidisciplinary SC as an integral part of PC in the Netherlands, [15] resulting in detailed practice guidelines for SC at the national level [7, 8].

Organisation Level

Organisational factors and context are pivotal in implementing empirically supported practices like SC. Institutional support for SC integration is crucial, as organisational culture significantly influences the acceptance of EBPs. Organisational efforts should target structural issues, including organisational redesign, learning, culture change, champion cultivation, professional and financial incentives, specialty recognition, and alignment with the institution's mission and strategy [3, 14]. SC leaders must assess and drive organisational-level changes for sustained implementation, not just focusing on teams and clinicians. Neglecting the organisational level can hinder SC implementation and lead to unsuccessful implementation or perpetual re-implementation efforts.

Team Level

Adopting and maintaining new practices requires change efforts to facilitate and improve effective coordination, collaboration, workflows, and knowledge sharing among health professionals [3, 14]. Moreover, understanding implementation barriers and facilitators in the interprofessional team context is instrumental for embedding SC in the team's culture, routine, and priorities. Organisational and team-based learning about the relationships between R/S, SC, and health not only enhances individual competencies but also has the potential to reshape team attitudes and the overall climate regarding SC [16, 17].

Individual Level

Individual behaviour among healthcare providers is crucial for implementing practice guidelines and EBPs. Efforts to drive change should address clinicians' and stakeholders' attitudes, barriers, and concerns related to these practices [3, 14]. Historically, healthcare quality improvement and implementation efforts have concentrated on individual factors, such as training, education, certification, and licensure, assuming that challenges primarily stem from a lack of individual knowledge and expertise [14].

Studies have revealed that many healthcare providers acknowledge the importance of R/S and SC but feel ill-equipped due to insufficient training, competencies, comfort, and time to address spiritual needs in patient care [18–22]. In response, clinician competencies [23, 24] and training programmes have been developed to address these individual barriers, generally leading to improved attitudes, comfort, and capabilities [17, 25–30] (see Chaps. 27, 30 and 31).

Achieving and sustaining practice changes depends on broader systems, organisational, and team environments. Individual change alone is insufficient. Research on serious illness programme implementation highlighted the need for multifaceted implementation strategies because training as a primary strategy had a limited impact on adoption since clinical culture-related barriers concerning clinicians' attitudes, motivations, and practice environment remained [31]. Despite significant progress in training clinicians, the SC integration into routine patient care varies widely across countries, institutions, and teams [9, 10, 32, 33]. A systems approach, planning and executing multi-level changes, can achieve lasting and consistent SC integration with persistent implementation across all interdependent levels: individual, team, organisation, and system (Fig. 1).

3 Leveraging Organisational and Leadership Factors for Spiritual Care Implementation

Organisational and leadership factors play a critical role in implementing and integrating SC in PC. A systematic review by Li et al. [34] distinguished six factors that interact to impact EBP implementation in organisations: (1) organisational culture; (2) leadership; (3) networks and communication; (4) resources; (5) evaluation, monitoring, and feedback; and (6) champions. Leadership emerged as a key influencer of the other five factors, creating an atmosphere instrumental for implementation. Thus, leaders' deliberate influence on organisational determinants can accelerate and sustain SC integration. It entails attention to implementation-specific leadership behaviours and organisational context for change [35–37].

3.1 Organisational Factors for Spiritual Care Implementation

Organisational culture, organisational climate, and implementation climate determine the adoption of EBPs and SC [38]. We explore the dynamics primarily at the organisational level of change and implementation (Fig. 1). These organisational-level changes interact with behavioural and practice changes at the team and individual levels. Additionally, larger socio-cultural, healthcare, regulatory, and economic environments shape organisations, including their cultures and change processes.

The Climate for Spiritual Care Implementation

Spiritual care leaders must carefully assess and shape their institution's climate for EBP and SC implementation. Implementation climate refers to individuals' shared perceptions and attitudes within an organisation regarding the importance of implementing EBPs, such as SC [38–40]. This climate strategically focuses on organisational elements responsible for achieving successful implementation outcomes. It consists of organisational members' collective views on the practices, processes, policies, and behavioural rewards, supports, and expectations regarding EBP implementation [39]. An institution's or a team's implementation climate reflects how much individuals 'perceive that the adoption, implementation, and use of an innovation such as EBP is expected, rewarded, and supported by the organisation' [39] (p. 2). These perceptions are formed by messages the organisation and its management communicate through their values, actions, processes, practices, and policies. Implementation climate positively correlates with effective implementation, requiring collective and coordinated behaviour change by many organisational members [40].

Leaders must appraise how much their organisation expects, rewards, and supports the uptake and use of EBPs like SC and how the existing climate aids or hinders SC implementation. Ehrhart and colleagues identified six implementation climate dimensions: Focus, Educational Support, Recognition, Rewards, and Selection for EBP, and Selection for Openness [39]. Using EBPs effectively is a main organisational goal and a top priority, and people think EBP implementation is important. Educational support for EBP comprises relevant conferences, workshops, in-services, and training resources. Evidence-based practitioners are respected clinical experts and are promoted and rewarded. Evidence-based practice use is rewarded with professional and financial incentives, including compensated time for EBP adoption. Selection for EBP favours team members who value and have utilised EBP and have formal EBP education. Selection for openness means recruiting team members who are flexible, adaptable, and open to new interventions. Moreover, leaders shape teams' implementation climate by disseminating EBP implementation information, synthesising it to team members' needs, mediating between high-level strategy and day-to-day activities, and selling and justifying implementation [41]. Improving the implementation climate for EBPs will also accelerate SC implementation, especially when framing SC as an empirically supported care domain.

Spiritual care leaders can also use this construct to evaluate and cultivate their institution's SC-specific implementation climate. *Spiritual care climate* is the extent to which the organisation expects, rewards, and supports SC adoption, integration, and interprofessional provision in routine patient care. Leaders may impact three major implementation climate domains: expectations, supports, and rewards for SC implementation and integration in their teams, organisational units, or institution. They may set evidence-based SC practices a top priority for their teams, tailor a range of educational supports to team members' SC training needs, recognise and reward the use of research-informed SC approaches, and build teams with flexibility, innovation, and skills to incorporate new interventions.

Organisational Readiness for Change

Integrating SC demands leaders' attention to the organisational readiness for change since implementing and improving SC bring about a cascade of changes across their organisational units and institutions. Success depends on skilfully managing organisational members' perceptions, motivation, and commitment regarding changes. Implementing complex SC practices and clinical models entails collective and coordinated action by interdependent individuals, teams, and departments, with each person or unit potentially contributing to or hampering implementation success. The theory of organisational readiness for change by Weiner [42] helps to ascertain and influence critical variables to create favourable organisational conditions regarding SC implementation at any institution. Weiner defines organisational readiness for change as the *shared* organisational *change commitment* and *change efficacy* to implement a specific organisational change [42]. Figure 2 shows the main factors influencing organisational readiness for change and the resulting initiation of persistent and cooperative change efforts, yielding effective implementation.

Change commitment means the collective motivation and determination to implement the change. When organisational members *want* the change (i.e. value the change), it yields the highest commitment to change, contrasting with situations when they have or ought to make a change. The SC leader's role is to guide the organisation towards a state where they genuinely desire SC integration and excellence rather than merely being told or feeling obligated to pursue it. Leaders can help organisational members see the value of SC more clearly and recognise values in SC that resonate with their own values.

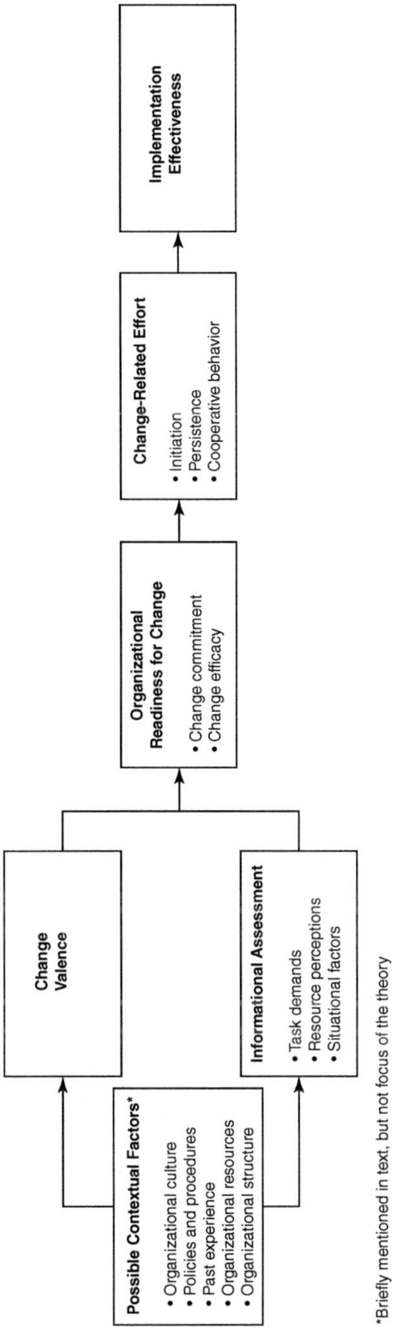

Fig. 2 Determinants and outcomes of organisational readiness for change. (Reproduced from Weiner, 2009 [42]. Originally published by Springer Nature and used with permission under the Creative Commons Attribution 2.0 International License)

Change efficacy entails 'organisational members' shared beliefs in their collective capabilities to organise and execute the courses of action involved in change implementation' [42] (p. 2). When individuals sense that their confidence and action capabilities are high regarding implementing a specific change or EBPs, like SC, they exhibit high change efficacy. Thus, SC leaders must increase the confidence and beliefs of the organisational members in their capabilities to provide, collaborate, and support SC as an essential and standard person-centred care domain.

Change commitment and efficacy are always context-specific and change-specific [42]. For example, an organisation may want and feel confident to adopt a new streamlined process to refer patients to the SC specialists, exhibiting high change commitment and efficacy. However, the same organisation may not see the value of the interprofessional SC model (i.e. lower change commitment) or have low confidence in their change efficacy to implement spiritual distress screening for all patients by healthcare providers.

This example also illustrates how to boost change valence and efficacy to prepare the organisation for practice change. Change commitment depends on the change valence. It shows how much people regard the change as important, essential, advantageous, or valuable [42]. Team members may appreciate SC deployment and integration at their institution for several reasons. Healthcare providers may respect SC's benefits for patients and their families. Spiritual care may resonate with their core beliefs or professional commitment to whole-person care acknowledging patients' spirituality. They may esteem it because organisational leaders, executives, informal opinion leaders, or peers endorse it. Others may value SC for its empirical support. Beyond individual motivations, organisational preparedness for change depends on whether members value the change enough to commit to its execution. Spiritual care leaders must communicate the value proposition of SC tailored to resonate with the values of various stakeholders.

Change efficacy depends on individuals' shared cognitive appraisals of key implementation capability determinants: task demands (e.g. clearly knowing what is asked of people), resource availability (e.g. the match or mismatch between task demands and available resources), and situational factors [42]. Leaders must explain how to implement SC practices or clinical models, what resources are available, and how the proposed change fits into stakeholders' current situation and context.

3.2 *Leadership Factors for Spiritual Care Implementation*

Adopting SC as a new aspect of PC or moving it to a higher degree of integration by implementing new initiatives requires a complex set of leadership capabilities. We discuss leadership behaviours and frameworks to help SC leaders strategically influence multi-level change and achieve persistent implementation.

Implementation Leadership

Implementation leadership refers to a specific and strategic approach to leadership that is instrumental for the successful implementation of EBPs in healthcare settings [43, 44]. It involves a set of influencing behaviours exhibited by leaders producing positive implementation outcomes. Aarons et al. characterised implementation leadership by four main dimensions: *knowledge* (i.e. being knowledgeable about the EBP being implemented), *proactivity* (i.e. proactive and anticipatory problem solving), *support* (i.e. supporting others in the implementation process), and *perseverance* (i.e. persevering through the ups and downs of the implementation process) [44]. Effective implementation leadership skills can be developed through training and significantly impact the implementation climate and readiness for change within an organisation [35, 45, 46].

To integrate SC into PC effectively, SC leaders should understand and cultivate domain-specific implementation leadership competencies, transcending their general leadership skills. General leadership theories provide frameworks for understanding different leadership styles and behaviours. Transformational leadership and Full Range Leadership [47] behaviours are associated with effective organisational change [35, 48–50] and innovative team behaviour [51, 52]. Therefore, leaders with these characteristics are likely to have the ability to support readiness for change, manage changes associated with implementation, and demonstrate expertise and persistence in implementing strategic initiatives.

However, it is unlikely that general leadership alone is effective for the successful and persistent implementation of EBPs and SC without considering implementation-specific behaviours and organisational context for change. Broad leadership theories may be insufficient to help us comprehend the connection between domain-specific leadership behaviours and specific aims and outcomes, such as implementation success [45]. Certain leadership activities and behaviours have been shown to influence implementation [36, 37, 53]. Thus, implementation leadership presents a subset or a specific application of leadership behaviours in the context of implementing EBPs and SC.

Gifford and colleagues [54] expanded the model and defined implementation leadership as 'a multidimensional process of influence' (p. 16) that enables the use and incorporation of EBPs in clinical practice and contains a set of activities and behaviours that influence team members, their setting, and organisational factors that facilitate implementation. Their comprehensive implementation leadership model includes *relations* behaviours, *change* behaviours, and *task* behaviours, in addition to having core leadership capabilities, expertise regarding the EBP and implementation methods, and developing a thorough implementation plan [54] (Fig. 3). Relations behaviours for implementation include recognising and supporting change efforts and facilitating interprofessional communication and consensus regarding the EBP. Change behaviours reflect the commitment to change, understanding and acting on challenges stemming from change, advocating for change, and reinforcing vision and goals for change. Finally, task behaviours seek to clarify roles and responsibilities, create and modify processes, policies, and workflows,

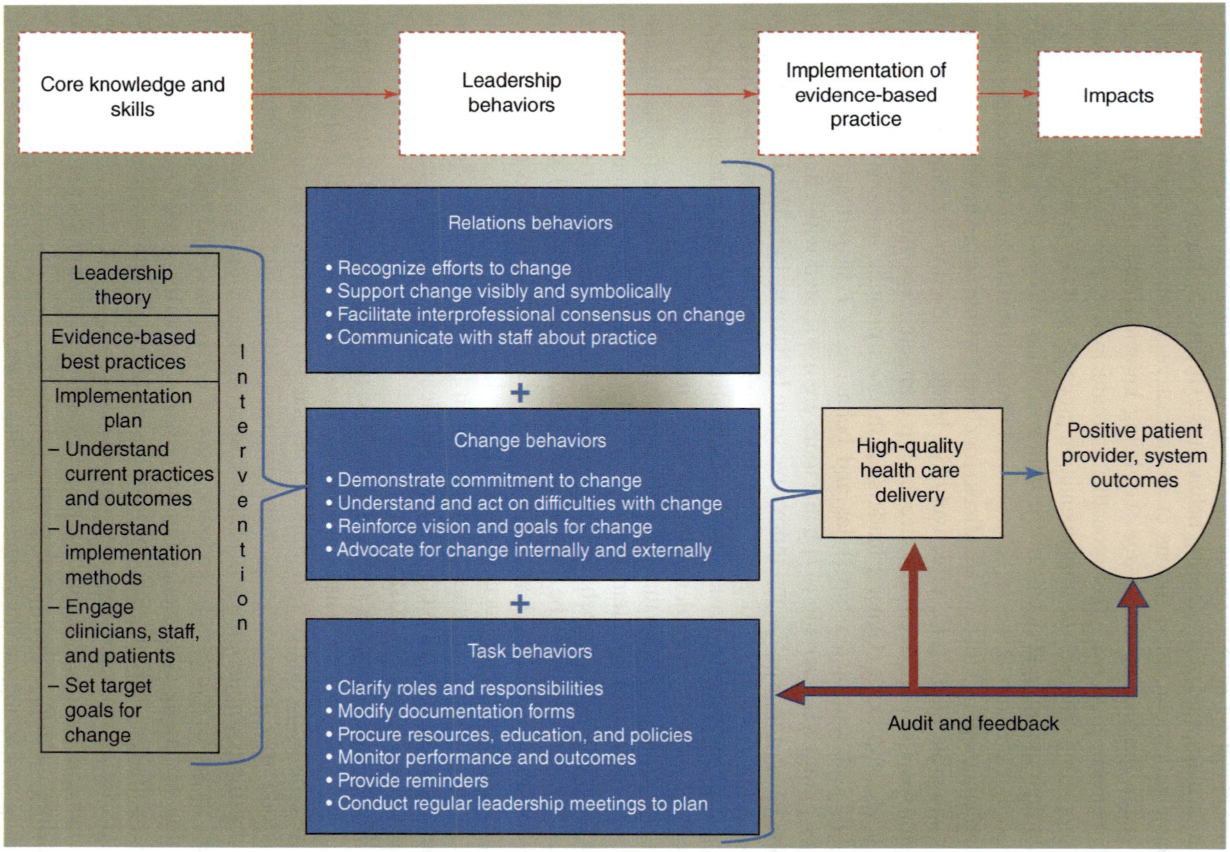

Fig. 3 O-MILe, Ottawa Model of Implementation Leadership. (Reproduced from Gifford et al. [54]. Originally published by and used with permission from Dove Medical Press Ltd.)

secure resources, ensure training, monitor performance and outcomes, provide reminders, and engage with leadership regularly.

Many SC leaders would likely have the general leadership capabilities to underpin these implementation-specific leadership behaviours [13, 55]. However, leading SC integration requires developing and using relevant implementation leadership skills to drive consistent and sustained implementation of SC as a routine and integral care domain in PC.

Spiritual Care Leadership

Research on SC leaders and SC leadership is scarce, with the most recent studies examining SC leadership in the context of the COVID-19 pandemic. An expert panel by Szilagyi et al. [13] focused on discovering leadership factors related to the integration, perceived value, and contributions of SC during the pandemic. They identified the importance of SC leaders' professional confidence, engagement and trust-building with executives, involvement with decision-making, innovation and creativity, building integrative and trusting connections with colleagues, and promoting cultural competencies, as impactful factors determining SC integration.

Muehlhausen and colleagues [56] explored the changing world of chaplaincy and the administrative role of SC leaders during the pandemic. Navigating the changing world of chaplaincy entailed themes relevant to our topic, such as managing shifting priorities, increasing interdisciplinary collaboration, improvisation, and innovation. In their administrative and leadership roles, SC leaders reported increasing assertiveness, creating policies to guide and implement new practices, making tough decisions, increasing assertiveness, allocating limited resources to ensure SC, and caring for and supporting team members. An analysis of SC leaders' responses to racial reckoning as a second pandemic during the COVID-19 pandemic in the USA [57] showed that some SC leaders exhibited leadership capabilities and felt empowered to act to create safety, confront issues of racism and discrimination, advocate for change, and educate and support team members. Kim et al. [55] applied the USA National Center for Healthcare Leadership (NCHL) [58] competency model to behavioural event interviews with spiritual care managers. Key qualitative themes reflected substantial use of achievement orientation, analytical thinking, and initiative leadership competencies in the Execution domain, collaboration and team leadership in the Relations domain, change leadership in the Transformation domain, and network/relationship development in the Boundary-spanning NCHL domain.

Overall, SC leaders demonstrated broad leadership capabilities in influencing and managing change, taking the initiative, innovating, executing, and supporting new SC delivery practices, and developing collaborations. Figure 4 highlights SC leadership attributes identified by research that are promising bases for developing implementation leadership's relations, change, and task behaviours [54]. Notably, fewer SC leadership qualities were related to the task behaviours indispensable for effective implementation. These SC leadership capacities suggest favourable precursors for gaining and using implementation leadership skills.

Implementation Leadership Behaviors by Gifford et al. 2017	Spiritual Care Leadership Attributes by Kim et al. 2020	Spiritual Care Leadership Attributes by Szilagyi et al. 2022	Spiritual Care Leadership Attributes by Muehlhausen et al. 2022	Spiritual Care Leadership Attributes by Muehlhausen et al. 2023
Relations Behaviors: • Recognize efforts to change • Support change visibly and symbolically • Facilitate interprofessional consensus on change • Communicate with staff about practice	• Collaboration • Team leadership • Network and relationship development	• Building integrative and trusting connections with colleagues • Engagement and trust-building with executives	• Increasing interdisciplinary collaboration • Caring for and supporting team members	• Supporting team members • Creating safety
Change Behaviors: • Demonstrate commitment to change • Understand and act on difficulties with change • Reinforce vision and goals for change • Advocate for change internally and externally	• Change leadership • Initiative • Achievement orientation • Analytical thinking	• Innovation and creativity • Professional confidence • Involvement with organizational decision-making • Promoting cultural competencies	• Managing shifting priorities • Improvisation and • innovation • Increasing assertiveness • Making tough decisions	• Advocating for change • Feeling empowered to act • Confronting issues of racism and discrimination
Task Behaviors: • Clarify roles and responsibilities • Modify documents and forms • Procure resources, education, and policies • Monitor performance and outcomes • Provide reminders • Conduct regular leadership meetings to plan			• Creating policies to guide and implement new practices • Allocating limited resources	• Educating team members

Fig. 4 Implementation leadership behaviours and key spiritual care leadership attributes

Kelly and Holmes [59] emphasise the shifts for chaplains to understand their roles and capabilities to initiate acts of leadership and for SC managers to embrace their leadership potential to envision and enact strategies to impact service delivery and policy in their organisations. They call for all SC providers to become strategically literate. It entails recognising their opportunities to strategically engage with, support, and transform priorities, policies, and systems to promote spiritual health and well-being and to collaborate with organisational and system-level leaders to advance this aim. Studies on SC leadership suggest that traits and abilities exist among SC leaders to practice strategic, transformative, and collaborative leadership.

Robust transformative and implementation leadership skills enable SC leaders to exert leadership influence horizontally (i.e. at individual and peer levels) and vertically throughout the multi-level model of change and implementation. Leaders must develop and leverage leadership behaviours specifically geared for moving SC from adoption only in principle towards persistent implementation and integration. Furthermore, SC implementation requires more than confidently navigating and leading organisational changes. It calls for strategic and sustained efforts aimed at systems transformation.

4 Social Entrepreneurship: Spiritual Care Leaders as Social Entrepreneurs

Social entrepreneurship (SE) offers a novel approach to expanding SC integration in PC. It helps leaders realise the full potential of SC by optimising and transforming systems to enhance the well-being and spiritual health of individuals with serious illness. Whether we use the term or not, advancing SC and PC in the healthcare ecosystem often requires an entrepreneurial spirit and approach.

Social entrepreneurship principles promote innovative and sustainable utilisation of human, organisational, clinical, economic, and technological resources, aiming to generate social value in response to complex human problems and to benefit the affected populations. Social entrepreneurship is broadly defined as an 'innovative, social value-creating activity' (p. 2) within or across organisations and sectors, which centres on the core social-value proposition as its integrating driver [60]. The social-value proposition ties together the main components of opportunity, people or human capital, financial resources, and context. The social entrepreneur innovatively combines and aligns resources to pursue opportunities to yield and sustain social value and benefits [60, 61]. Moreover, SE is not dominated by revenue production but prioritises generating multifaceted social value. It makes SE principles even more applicable since SC is considered a high-value yet non-revenue activity within the economic realities of healthcare systems.

Social entrepreneurship aims to create practices and systems that yield lasting positive change and innovative solutions to improve people's lives in the context of complex social problems. Spiritual care promises and delivers value in the context of serious and complex health, psychosocial, and spiritual problems. Evidence indicates that SC has a compelling social-value proposition for PC patients, their loved ones, and care teams, which can be readily contextualised and tailored to various clinical and sociocultural settings. Research and clinical experience illuminate the presence and prevalence of spiritual distress, spiritual pain, and spiritual needs in PC [62–64]. Spiritual care is clearly a service that produces social and health benefits by attending to patients' spiritual distress and concerns and supporting their well-being, quality of life, and coping with serious illness [5, 65, 66]. Social entrepreneurship helps SC deliver its value more fully by creatively combining and utilising opportunities, collaborations, and resources.

4.1 Integrating Service Provision and System Transformation

The integration of direct service provision and the aim to transform the existing system to a new, more optimal equilibrium are distinctive characteristics of SE. As such, SE occurs in the shared space of taking direct action to provide services and advocating for system change to address complex human issues [67].

Social entrepreneurship goes beyond direct service provision that addresses needs yet may leave the existing system unchanged or make incremental improvements while maintaining the current equilibrium. By directly engaging with the issue at hand, SE also differs from social activism that transforms systems indirectly by advocating policy and regulatory changes. Martin and Osberg [67] posit that SE centres on both forms of social engagement: direct action and seeking to transform the system. The goal is a transformed and sustained new equilibrium substantially different from the preceding system.

This understanding expands SC leaders' role in implementing SC in health systems. It encourages SC leaders to go beyond incremental improvements to existing processes and strive for a transformative shift where SC becomes integral and indispensable. Without this critical shift, SC implementation efforts may falter, linger in the incubation stage, or necessitate constant re-implementation rather than becoming a compelling, scalable, and sustainable social-value proposition. Whether the SC leader's ecosystem consists of a team, a department, a hospital, a healthcare system, or national healthcare delivery, they must envision and pursue a new optimal equilibrium of SC integration in their setting.

Transforming the system is especially difficult to imagine when the SC leader experiences a lack of organisational influence and control to induce system change. However, SE does not depend on the organisational hierarchy and power in a traditional sense. It leverages and combines the interconnected persons, resources, values, and priorities in a given system or organisation with ingenuity and strategic vision. Centring on empowerment rather than control, [68] SE cultivates and empowers partners—sometimes unexpected collaborators—to join and contribute to the vision and social-value proposition. Moreover, SE is often fuelled by social entrepreneurs' self-assurance, self-direction, willingness to take risks, persistence, and steadfast belief in the change and social-value proposition, in our case, SC promises to deliver. Thus, SE is accessible to any SC leader in any organisational position and role. Social entrepreneurship can empower SC leaders to influence system transformation, rather than view their organisations and systems as unchangeable or changing outside their control.

4.2 Stages of Transformation

Martin and Osberg outlined a four-stage process based on key patterns in successful social entrepreneurship: (1) understanding the world, (2) envisioning a new future, (3) building a model for change, and (4) scaling the solution [67]. The first two stages involve truly understanding and navigating the existing system dynamics as they are and envisioning a fundamental equilibrium change for targeted stakeholders to a new, stable, and sustainable system substantially healthier for that population. These efforts are followed by applying creativity and resourcefulness in building, testing, and refining a model for sustainable change. Subsequently, the focus shifts towards scaling the solution for sustainable equilibrium change, building a supportive ecosystem, and extending its benefits across populations and settings without needing to reapply effort and investment or re-implement constantly.

Cassel and colleagues [69] examined the adoption of palliative care in the USA using the SE framework. The percentage of hospitals with more than 50 beds implementing PC programmes tripled from 25% to 75% between 2000 and 2015. Social entrepreneurship principles and transformation stages explained the mechanisms of such rapid diffusion of PC as a high-value, low-revenue healthcare innovation. The initial step was to consider the dynamics of the broken healthcare delivery system for patients with serious illness characterised by insufficient training in communication, symptom management, and PC and the dominance of profit centres that incentivise overtreatment over whole-person care prioritising quality of life. The subsequent step was to envision the transformation of the care system for serious illness centred on the goals and needs of patients and their families and prioritising symptom relief and quality of life. The third step involved prototyping: building, testing, modifying, and improving care models. It led to the early implementation of PC programmes and generated research and education initiatives, published outcomes, and replication. It also contributed to developing evidence-based and consensus-based clinical guidelines and quality indicators over time. Widespread adoption was the focus of the final step through technical assistance, various training, train-the-trainer, and coaching approaches, and changes in regulatory and accreditation requirements and payment policy. Cassel et al. concluded, 'Dissemination of high-value, low-revenue innovations in healthcare takes dedicated expertise, persistence, and ingenuity' [69] (p. 238). This case study illustrates how PC moved towards persistent and widespread implementation through the multi-level change model. Parallels can be drawn with the implementation and diffusion of SC in PC. Spiritual care is a high-value, non-revenue innovation in healthcare that often faces comparable barriers.

Social entrepreneurship principles and stages of transformation offer valuable approaches for strategic and lasting transformation—whether that is the ecosystem of a team, organisation, or healthcare system —towards an equilibrium of persistent, consistent, widespread SC integration. Social entrepreneurship encourages SC leaders to view their setting as an ecosystem that can be skilfully and creatively influenced and transformed through its interdependent components, members, and resources. It enables SC leaders to deliver the compelling social value of SC to address the complex and pressing needs of the persons they serve by tapping their innovative and entrepreneurial mindset.

5 Conclusion

Evidence and clinical consensus support the vital role of R/S in serious illness. Nevertheless, the critical issue in SC implementation is the substantial knowledge–practice gap between what is known about R/S and SC and what is provided to patients in routine PC. Strategies informed by implementation science and relevant organisational and leadership theories will help SC leaders close the gap between SC as an empirically supported care domain and its availability in usual care.

Frameworks from implementation science, implementation climate, organisational readiness for change, implementation leadership, spiritual care leadership, and social entrepreneurship are highly applicable and expand our understanding of the dynamics inherent to implementation and organisational change. They empower leaders to develop comprehensive approaches and capabilities to make a difference in how their institutions understand, support, and incorporate SC. Concepts presented in this chapter will equip SC leaders to strive for consistent, widespread, and sustainable SC implementation and system transformation in the care of patients in palliative care.

References

1. Green LW, Ottoson JM, García C, Hiatt RA. Diffusion theory and knowledge dissemination, utilization, and integration in public health. Annu Rev Public Health. 2009;30:151–74. https://doi.org/10.1146/annurev.publhealth.031308.100049.
2. Livet M, Haines ST, Curran GM, et al. Implementation science to advance care delivery: a primer for pharmacists and other health professionals. Pharmacotherapy. 2018;38(5):490–502. https://doi.org/10.1002/phar.2114.
3. Proctor EK, Landsverk J, Aarons G, Chambers D, Glisson C, Mittman B. Implementation research in mental health services: an emerging science with conceptual, methodological, and training challenges. Admin Pol Ment Health. 2009;36(1):24–34. https://doi.org/10.1007/s10488-008-0197-4.

4. Tansella M, Thornicroft G. Implementation science: understanding the translation of evidence into practice. Br J Psychiatry. 2009;195(4):283–5. https://doi.org/10.1192/bjp.bp.109.065565.
5. Balboni TA, VanderWeele TJ, Doan-Soares S, et al. Spirituality in serious illness and health. JAMA. 2022;328(2):184–97. https://doi.org/10.1001/jama.2022.11086.
6. National Consensus Project for quality, palliative care. Clinical practice guidelines for quality palliative care. 4th ed. National Coalition for Hospice and Palliative Care; 2018. https://www.nationalcoalitionhpc.org/ncp
7. Boddaert M, Douma J, Dijxhoorn F, Bijkerk M. Netherlands quality framework for palliative care. IKNL/Palliactief; 2017. https://palliaweb.nl/getmedia/f553d851-c680-4782-aac2-2520632f2e8d/netherlands-quality-framework-for-palliative-care_2.pdf
8. IKNL. Existential and spiritual aspects of palliative care national guideline. IKNL; 2018. https://palliaweb.nl/getmedia/35a8c9d9-2fc8-4931-b2ed-1e7d8fa5bbd1/rl_Existential_and_spiritual_aspects_of_palliative_care.pdf
9. Spetz J, Dudley N, Trupin L, Rogers M, Meier DE, Dumanovsky T. Few hospital palliative care programs meet national staffing recommendations. Health Aff. 2016;35(9):1690–7. https://doi.org/10.1377/hlthaff.2016.0113.
10. Rogers MM, Friebert S, Williams CSP, Humphrey L, Thienprayoon R, Klick JC. Pediatric palliative care programs in US hospitals. Pediatrics 2021;148(1). https://doi.org/10.1542/peds.2020-021634.
11. Klop HT, Koper I, Schweitzer BPM, Jongen E, Onwuteaka-Philipsen B. Strengthening the spiritual domain in palliative care through a listening consultation service by spiritual caregivers in Dutch PaTz-groups: an evaluation study. BMC Palliat Care. 2020;19(1):92. https://doi.org/10.1186/s12904-020-00595-0.
12. Egan R, MacLeod R, Jaye C, McGee R, Baxter J, Herbison P. The spiritual environment in New Zealand hospice care: identifying organisational commitment to spiritual care. BMJ Support Palliat Care. 2014;4(3):299–302. https://doi.org/10.1136/bmjspcare-2013-000632.
13. Szilagyi C, Vandenhoeck A, Best MC, et al. Chaplain leadership during COVID-19: an international expert panel. J Pastoral Care Counsel. 2022;76(1):56–65. https://doi.org/10.1177/15423050211067724.
14. Shortell SM. Increasing value: a research agenda for addressing the managerial and organizational challenges facing health care delivery in the United States. Med Care Res Rev. 2004;61(3):12S–30S. https://doi.org/10.1177/1077558704266768.
15. van de Geer J, Leget C. How spirituality is integrated system-wide in The Netherlands palliative care national programme. Prog Palliat Care. 2012;20(2):98–105. https://doi.org/10.1179/1743291X12Y.0000000008.
16. Davis J, Oyedele O, Lion A, Szilagyi C, Puchalski C. Impacts of interprofessional spiritual care education within a healthcare team: a qualitative analysis. IMPRS 2022;5(1). https://doi.org/10.18060/26822.
17. Szilagyi C, Lion AH, Varner Perez SE, et al. Interprofessional spiritual care education in pediatric hematology-oncology: a pilot study. Pediatr Blood Cancer. 2022;69(3):e29515. https://doi.org/10.1002/pbc.29515.
18. Best M, Butow P, Olver I. Doctors discussing religion and spirituality: a systematic literature review. Palliat Med. 2016;30(4):327–37. https://doi.org/10.1177/0269216315600912.
19. Balboni MJ, Sullivan A, Enzinger AC, et al. Nurse and physician barriers to spiritual care provision at the end of life. J Pain Symptom Manag. 2014;48(3):400–10. https://doi.org/10.1016/j.jpainsymman.2013.09.020.
20. Bar-Sela G, Schultz MJ, Elshamy K, et al. Training for awareness of one's own spirituality: a key factor in overcoming barriers to the provision of spiritual care to advanced cancer patients by doctors and nurses. Palliat Support Care. 2019;17(3):345–52. https://doi.org/10.1017/S147895151800055X.
21. Palmer Kelly E, Paredes AZ, Hyer M, Tsilimigras DI, Pawlik TM. The beliefs of cancer care providers regarding the role of religion and spirituality within the clinical encounter. Support Care Cancer. 2021;29(2):909–15. https://doi.org/10.1007/s00520-020-05562-2.

22. Best M, Butow P, Olver I. Why do we find it so hard to discuss spirituality? A qualitative exploration of attitudinal barriers. J Clin Med Res 2016;5(9). https://doi.org/10.3390/jcm5090077.
23. Puchalski CM, Sbrana A, Ferrell B, et al. Interprofessional spiritual care in oncology: a literature review. ESMO Open. 2019;4(1):e000465. https://doi.org/10.1136/esmoopen-2018-000465.
24. Best M, Leget C, Goodhead A, Paal P. An EAPC white paper on multi-disciplinary education for spiritual care in palliative care. BMC Palliat Care. 2020;19(1):9. https://doi.org/10.1186/s12904-019-0508-4.
25. Jones KF, Paal P, Symons X, Best MC. The content, teaching methods and effectiveness of spiritual care training for healthcare professionals: a mixed-methods systematic review. J Pain Symptom Manag. 2021; https://doi.org/10.1016/j.jpainsymman.2021.03.013.
26. van de Geer J, Veeger N, Groot M, et al. Multidisciplinary training on spiritual care for patients in palliative care trajectories improves the attitudes and competencies of hospital medical staff: results of a quasi-experimental study. Am J Hosp Palliat Care. 2018;35(2):218–28. https://doi.org/10.1177/1049909117692959.
27. Best MC, Jones K, Washington J, Sullivan J, Kearney M, Puchalski C. Evaluation of the interprofessional spiritual care education curriculum in Australia: online. Palliat Support Care. 2022:1–9. https://doi.org/10.1017/S1478951522000244.
28. Wasner M, Longaker C, Fegg MJ, Borasio GD. Effects of spiritual care training for palliative care professionals. Palliat Med. 2005;19(2):99–104. https://doi.org/10.1191/0269216305pm995oa.
29. Dezorzi LW, Raymundo MM, Goldim JR, de Oliveira CAV. Spirituality in the continuing education of healthcare professionals: an approach to palliative care. Palliat Support Care. 2019;17(6):662–7. https://doi.org/10.1017/S1478951519000117.
30. van Meurs J, Wichmann AB, van Mierlo P, et al. Identifying, exploring, and integrating the spiritual dimension in proactive care planning: a mixed methods evaluation of a communication training intervention for multidisciplinary palliative care teams. Palliat Med. 2022;36(10):1493–503. https://doi.org/10.1177/02692163221122367.
31. Paladino J, Sanders J, Kilpatrick LB, et al. Serious illness care programme-contextual factors, and implementation strategies: a qualitative study. BMJ Support Palliat Care. 2022. https://doi.org/10.1136/bmjspcare-2021-003401.
32. Antoine A, Fitchett G, Marin D, et al. What organizational and business models underlie the provision of spiritual care in healthcare organizations? An initial description and analysis. J Health Care Chaplain. 2022;28(2):272–84. https://doi.org/10.1080/08854726.2020.1861535.
33. Tartaglia A, Corson T, White KB, et al. Chaplain staffing and scope of service: benchmarking spiritual care departments. J Health Care Chaplain. 2022:1–18. https://doi.org/10.1080/08854726.2022.2121579.
34. Li S, Jeffs L, Barwick M, Stevens B. Organizational contextual features that influence the implementation of evidence-based practices across healthcare settings: a systematic integrative review. Syst Rev. 2018;7(1):72. https://doi.org/10.1186/s13643-018-0734-5.
35. Aarons GA, Ehrhart MG, Farahnak LR, Hurlburt MS. Leadership and organizational change for implementation (LOCI): a randomized mixed method pilot study of a leadership and organization development intervention for evidence-based practice implementation. Implement Sci. 2015;10:11. https://doi.org/10.1186/s13012-014-0192-y.
36. Sandström B, Borglin G, Nilsson R, Willman A. Promoting the implementation of evidence-based practice: a literature review focusing on the role of nursing leadership. Worldviews Evid-Based Nurs. 2011;8(4):212–23. https://doi.org/10.1111/j.1741-6787.2011.00216.x.
37. Gifford W, Davies B, Edwards N, Griffin P, Lybanon V. Managerial leadership for nurses' use of research evidence: an integrative review of the literature. Worldviews Evid-Based Nurs. 2007;4(3):126–45. https://doi.org/10.1111/j.1741-6787.2007.00095.x.
38. Powell BJ, Mettert KD, Dorsey CN, et al. Measures of organizational culture, organizational climate, and implementation climate in behavioral health: a systematic review. Implement Res Pract. 2021;2:26334895211018862. https://doi.org/10.1177/26334895211018862.
39. Ehrhart MG, Aarons GA, Farahnak LR. Assessing the organizational context for EBP implementation: the development and validity testing of the implementation climate scale (ICS). Implement Sci. 2014;9:157. https://doi.org/10.1186/s13012-014-0157-1.

40. Weiner BJ, Belden CM, Bergmire DM, Johnston M. The meaning and measurement of implementation climate. Implement Sci. 2011;6:78. https://doi.org/10.1186/1748-5908-6-78.
41. Bunger AC, Birken SA, Hoffman JA, MacDowell H, Choy-Brown M, Magier E. Elucidating the influence of supervisors' roles on implementation climate. Implement Sci. 2019;14(1):93. https://doi.org/10.1186/s13012-019-0939-6.
42. Weiner BJ. A theory of organizational readiness for change. Implement Sci. 2009;4:67. https://doi.org/10.1186/1748-5908-4-67.
43. Castiglione SA. Implementation leadership: a concept analysis. J Nurs Manag. 2020;28(1):94–101. https://doi.org/10.1111/jonm.12899.
44. Aarons GA, Ehrhart MG, Farahnak LR. The implementation leadership scale (ILS): development of a brief measure of unit level implementation leadership. Implement Sci. 2014;9(1):45. https://doi.org/10.1186/1748-5908-9-45.
45. Richter A, von Thiele SU, Lornudd C, Lundmark R, Mosson R, Hasson H. iLead – a transformational leadership intervention to train healthcare managers' implementation leadership. Implement Sci. 2016;11(1):1–13. https://doi.org/10.1186/s13012-016-0475-6.
46. Richter A, Lornudd C, von Thiele SU, et al. Evaluation of iLead, a generic implementation leadership intervention: mixed-method preintervention-postintervention design. BMJ Open. 2020;10(1):e033227. https://doi.org/10.1136/bmjopen-2019-033227.
47. Avolio BJ. Full range leadership development. Sage Publications; 2011.
48. Bass BM. Two decades of research and development in transformational leadership. Eur J Work Org Psychol. 1999;8(1):9–32. https://doi.org/10.1080/135943299398410.
49. Eisenbach R, Watson K, Pillai R. Transformational leadership in the context of organizational change. J Organ Chang Manag. 1999;12(2):80–9. https://doi.org/10.1108/09534819910263631.
50. Avolio BJ, Reichard RJ, Hannah ST, Walumbwa FO, Chan A. A meta-analytic review of leadership impact research: experimental and quasi-experimental studies. Leadersh Q. 2009;20(5):764–84. https://doi.org/10.1016/j.leaqua.2009.06.006.
51. Masood M, Afsar B. Transformational leadership, and innovative work behavior among nursing staff. NursInq 2017;24(4). https://doi.org/10.1111/nin.12188.
52. Günzel-Jensen F, Hansen JR, Jakobsen MLF, Wulff J. A two-pronged approach? Combined leadership styles and innovative behavior. Int J Public Adm. 2018;41(12):957–70. https://doi.org/10.1080/01900692.2017.1303711.
53. Reichenpfader U, Carlfjord S, Nilsen P. Leadership in evidence-based practice: a systematic review. Leadersh Health Serv. 2015;28(4):298–316. https://doi.org/10.1108/LHS-08-2014-0061.
54. Gifford W, Graham ID, Ehrhart MG, Davies BL, Aarons GA. Ottawa model of implementation leadership and implementation leadership scale: mapping concepts for developing and evaluating theory-based leadership interventions. J Healthc Leadersh. 2017;9:15–23. https://doi.org/10.2147/JHL.S125558.
55. Kim DH, Fitchett G, Anderson JL, Garman AN. Management, and leadership competencies among spiritual care managers. J Health Care Chaplain. 2020:1–10. https://doi.org/10.1080/08854726.2020.1796076.
56. Muehlhausen BL, Desjardins CM, Chappelle C, Schwartzman G, Tata-Mbeng B, Fitchett G. Managing spiritual Care departments during the COVID-19 pandemic: a qualitative study. J Pastoral Care Counsel. 2022;76(4):294–303. https://doi.org/10.1177/15423050221122029.
57. Muehlhausen BL, Desjardins CM, Tata-Mbeng B, et al. Spiritual care department leaders' response to racial reckoning in 2020 and 2021. J Health Care Chaplain. 2023;29(3):292–306. https://doi.org/10.1080/08854726.2023.2167416.
58. National Center for healthcare leadership. Health leadership competency model 3.0. 2018. https://www.nchl.org/research/
59. Kelly E, Holmes C. Strategic leadership in healthcare chaplaincy. In: Kelly E, Swinton J, editors. Chaplaincy and the soul of health and social care: fostering spiritual wellbeing in emerging paradigms of care. Jessica Kingsley Publishers; 2019. p. 323–44.

60. Austin J, Stevenson H, Wei-Skillern J. Social and commercial entrepreneurship: same, different, or both? Entrep Theory Pract. 2006;30(1):1–22. https://doi.org/10.1111/j.1540-6520.2006.00107.x.
61. Mair J, Martí I. Social entrepreneurship research: a source of explanation, prediction, and delight. In: Blackburn RA, Brush CG, editors. Small business and entrepreneurship. Sage Publications; 2008. p. 256–67.
62. Damen A, Exline J, Pargament K, et al. Prevalence, predictors and correlates of religious and spiritual struggles in palliative cancer patients. J Pain Symptom Manag. 2021;62(3):e139–47. https://doi.org/10.1016/j.jpainsymman.2021.04.024.
63. Delgado-Guay M, Palma A, Duarte E, et al. Association between spirituality, religiosity, spiritual pain, symptom distress, and quality of life among Latin American patients with advanced cancer: a multicenter study. J Palliat Med. 2021;24(11):1606–15. https://doi.org/10.1089/jpm.2020.0776.
64. Delgado-Guay M, Hui D, Parsons HA, et al. Spirituality, religiosity, and spiritual pain in advanced cancer patients. J Pain Symptom Manag. 2011;41(6):986–94. https://doi.org/10.1016/j.jpainsymman.2010.09.017.
65. Balboni T, Balboni M, Paulk ME, et al. Support of cancer patients' spiritual needs and associations with medical care costs at the end of life. Cancer. 2011;117(23):5383–91. https://doi.org/10.1002/cncr.26221.
66. Balboni TA, Paulk ME, Balboni MJ, et al. Provision of spiritual care to patients with advanced cancer: associations with medical care and quality of life near death. J Clin Oncol. 2010;28(3):445–52. https://doi.org/10.1200/JCO.2009.24.8005.
67. Martin RL, Osberg S. Getting beyond better: how social entrepreneurship works. Boston: Harvard Business Review Press; 2015.
68. Santos FM. A positive theory of social entrepreneurship. J Bus Ethics. 2012;111(3):335–51. https://doi.org/10.1007/s10551-012-1413-4.
69. Cassel JB, Bowman B, Rogers M, Spragens LH, Meier DE, Palliative Care LC. Palliative care leadership centers are key to the diffusion of palliative care innovation. Health Aff. 2018;37(2):231–9. https://doi.org/10.1377/hlthaff.2017.1122.

Nation-Wide Guidelines for Multidisciplinary Spiritual Care: Implementation of the Netherlands' *Spiritual Care Guidelines* and *Grief Guidelines*

Marie-José H. E. Gijsberts and Erik Olsman

Abstract Spiritual care is the focus of the Netherlands' *Spiritual Care Guidelines* and is a central dimension in the Netherlands' *Grief Guidelines*. The objective of this chapter is to describe implementation of both evidence-based palliative care guidelines. In so doing, we draw from scientific evidence and from our experience taking several roles. We will highlight some content of both guidelines, after which we will describe what implementation minimally requires: (a) an early involvement of stakeholders, who represent relevant organisations, taking place from early development until authorisation of guidelines, (b) an emphasis on the guidelines' multidisciplinary nature, (c) education aimed at professionals developing spiritual care competency and multidisciplinary collaboration in spiritual care, and (d) investment in scientific research, with special attention paid to patient outcomes. We will finish the chapter with a description of a patient journey that highlights topics central to spiritual care, and contextual features that shape and are shaped by implementation. We conclude that more research on implementation of spiritual care guidelines is necessary and that in our country, sustaining ongoing implementation of spiritual care remains necessary. Our hope is that this chapter helps readers to contribute to a successful implementation of spiritual care into palliative care.

Marie-José H. E. Gijsberts and Erik Olsman contributed equally to this chapter.

M.-J. H. E. Gijsberts (✉)
End of Life Research Group, Vrije Universiteit Brussel & Universiteit Gent, Brussels, Belgium
e-mail: Marie-Jose.Gijsberts@vub.be

E. Olsman
Community & Care, Section of Spiritual Care & Chaplaincy Studies, Protestant Theological University, Utrecht, The Netherlands
e-mail: hjolsman@pthu.nl

M. C. Best (ed.), *Spiritual Care in Palliative Care*,
https://doi.org/10.1007/978-3-031-50864-6_44

Keywords Spiritual · Grief · Chaplaincy · Palliative · Guidelines · Implementation Multidisciplinary · Spiritual care · Palliative care

1 Introduction

In the Netherlands, spiritual care in palliative care is widely available, regardless of someone's religious or non-religious orientation. It takes place in all healthcare settings, and it is provided by many people as well: healthcare professionals and volunteers are expected to pay attention to the existential and spiritual needs of patients and their family members. This ideal implies that caregivers know what spirituality and spiritual care entail and how they can pay attention to spirituality, for example in times of grief. Also ideally, there is a role division between those seen as the experts in spiritual care, such as chaplains, and those seen as generalists in providing spiritual care, such as social workers, physicians, and nurses [1].

We focus on the implementation of guidelines that have spirituality and spiritual care as core topics. The objective is to describe implementation of two evidence-based palliative care guidelines in the Netherlands, in which spiritual care is a central topic. One is the *Spiritual Care Guidelines* (full title: Existential and Spiritual Aspects of Palliative Care) [1], which has spirituality and spiritual care at its heart, showing that spiritual care is a dimension that deserves attention in itself. The other is the *Grief Guidelines* (full title: Grief in the Palliative Phase) [2], in which spirituality is just one of the central dimensions next to, for example, psychological or social dimensions. We do so to make clear that, in order to successfully integrate spiritual care into palliative care, the different dimensions of palliative care should be seen in their mutual relationships [3, 4].

To put spiritual care in our country in context, it is necessary to understand that palliative care has started relatively recently in the Netherlands, as the discussion of euthanasia was settled first [5]. Once the government had funded a palliative care programme in the early 2000s, palliative care started to develop across the country [6], and the first manual that included an introduction on the characteristics of palliative care and guidelines on treatment of specific symptoms was launched [7]. By then, the only guideline referring to spiritual aspects of palliative care was the (psychological) guideline on existential crisis [7]. Some years later, however, the national policy plan for palliative care included the development of spiritual care [8]. The first guidelines on spiritual care and grief were published in 2010 [9, 10]. However, they needed revision because they were not evidence-based.

In this chapter, we will first sketch some content of the evidence-based *Spiritual Care Guidelines* and *Grief Guidelines*. Then, we will describe important elements or strategies that may facilitate or coalesce with implementation of these guidelines: early involvement of stakeholders, emphasising the guidelines' multidisciplinary nature, increasing professionalisation through education, and investing in scientific research. It should be noted that full implementation and integration of spiritual care (guidelines) into palliative care practice, research, and education has not been reached in our country, but we believe these elements or strategies to be paramount in this process. Before drawing some final conclusions, we will sketch a patient's journey. In this chapter, we draw from scientific evidence and from our experience taking several roles: developer of these guidelines, teacher of spiritual care, researcher, advisor of national policies, and respectively as physician and chaplain in palliative care.

1.1 Spiritual Care Guidelines

The *Spiritual Care Guidelines* utilise the consensus-based definition published by the European Association for Palliative Care (EAPC): 'Spirituality (or: a sense of meaning and purpose) is the dynamic dimension of human life that relates to the way persons (individual and community) experience, express and/or seek meaning, purpose and transcendence, and the way they connect to the moment, to self, to others, to nature, to the significant and/or the sacred' [11]. 'Existential' and 'spiritual' are used interchangeably throughout the guidelines and in this chapter. The spiritual dimension is considered to be multi-dimensional, containing [1] existential challenges, such as questions concerning identity, suffering, guilt and shame, hope and despair; [2] value-based considerations and attitudes, such as what is most important to the patient in relation to oneself, others and life; and [3] religious and spiritual considerations, such as beliefs and practices, and the relationship with the ultimate and/or God [1, 11].

The guidelines sketch a mutual influence between the spiritual and the physical, psychological, and social dimensions [3]. While the physical, psychological and social spheres, such as nausea, anxiety, or problems at work, are more directly visible, accessible, and addressed, the spiritual dimension, often the most intimate dimension, is not always directly visible, accessible, or addressed. As a consequence, the guidelines note that existential questions or spiritual needs may underlie problems that present as physical, emotional/psychological, or social symptoms. It refers to an ABC-model, which is a model that distinguishes between Attention (*Aandacht*), Spiritual Guidance (*Begeleiden*), and Crisis Intervention (*Crisisinterventie*), helping to propagate multidisciplinary spiritual care, which includes a division between professional roles.

Attention means that each caregiver is expected to listen, support, recognise, and screen for spiritual/existential issues. Recommendations include, for example, 'Create an atmosphere of calm, space and non-judgemental attentiveness to the patient's narrative' and 'Next to an open attitude of listening, a brief diagnostic exploration of the spiritual dimension could be performed (for several instruments, see the *Spiritual Care Guidelines*)'. Chaplains are additionally expected to *interpret* spiritual issues. Meanwhile, they represent other realities, such as a world in which, contrary to a medicalised world, humanity or a particular faith community and/or God reigns. Since spiritual care involves seeing each patient as a unique person, another feature of chaplains' work is that they try to connect to a person's unique life story with appropriate images, symbols, rituals, music, stories, poems, et cetera.

Although there is no clear demarcation between attention and spiritual guidance, the latter often is a longer process, consisting of several encounters. The guidelines indicate that chaplains in particular are specialists in spiritual guidance and other professionals are generalists. Spiritual guidance may start with the images or thoughts patients project onto different professional roles. Some patients, for example, project inaccurate, religious images onto the chaplain. Inaccurate projections require an 'evocative presence' of chaplains [12] and of each palliative caregiver, referring to bearing the thoughts and feelings evoked thanks (or due) to the professional role. These feelings and thoughts provide insight into how patients perceive (the relationship with) others, also marking the starting point for spiritual guidance. Another example is patients presuming that physicians and nurses can only provide physical care. Generalists becoming aware of these ideas and then correcting them may pave the way for spiritual care provision.

Crisis intervention may follow a spiritual crisis that may be precipitated by an acute situation, such as deep loss, terminal illness or the prospect of living longer than expected after having already said goodbye [13]. A spiritual crisis can threaten a person's self-understanding or result in a worsening in one of the following domains:

- Sense of purpose or meaning ('What is the point of suffering like this'?)
- Sense of inner peace ('How can I find peace within myself'?)
- Sense of connection, security, safety ('I feel so alone')
- Sense of faith in (or belonging to) God and the world ('Has God deserted me now'?)
- Need for forgiveness/feelings of guilt ('I'll no longer be able to make amends') [1].

Such crises may have negative outcomes, such as loss of energy, loss of control over emotions, suicidal ideation, withdrawal from others or existential loneliness. Positive outcomes frequently include a sense of renewal or spiritual awakening, like resilience or (renewal of) hope (post-traumatic) growth or renewal of relationships [14, 15]. The guidelines recommend referral to a spiritual care specialist, such as a chaplain, when a patient is facing a spiritual crisis.

1.2 Grief Guidelines

Based on other documents [10, 16], and its own expertise, the core authorship group for the *Grief Guidelines*, defined grief as follows (translation is ours):

> Grief is the set of physical, emotional, cognitive, social, behavioural and spiritual reactions that results from the loss of something or someone meaningful. Although grief in itself is not a reason for concern or a reason to provide professional care, being open and paying attention to the experience of the grieving person is experienced as supportive [2].

People with a life-threatening illness may mourn in response to a loss of, for example, meaningful roles, health, autonomy or meaning/spirituality. Family members, volunteers, and professional caregivers may grieve too. Grief may also consist of anticipatory grief, which is a response to a loss that will take place in the future [17, 18], and/or complicated grief referring to a clinically relevant condition that is central in the psychiatric diagnosis 'Prolonged Grief Disorder' [19, 20].

The core group took a critical stance towards normative grief models, like the stage-model of Kübler-Ross that saw grief processes as linear processes with sequential stages, starting with, for example, denial, and finishing with acceptance [21, 22]. Patients may rather hope for cure while preparing to die [23–25]. Bereaved family members and friends, when deviating from these stages, may furthermore feel unacknowledged in their grief [26].

The *Grief Guidelines* offer the following spiritual care related recommendations, in which each professional caregiver is expected to pay attention to spirituality (see also Sect. 1.1):

- Be aware that grief can manifest itself in patients and (bereaved) family members in several ways, such as physical, emotional, cognitive, behavioural, and spiritual
- In the case of complicated grief, consider consulting a chaplain, who—if required—can also refer to a colleague with a suitable spiritual and/or cultural background
- Consider offering chaplaincy care during the grief process, when existential/spiritual problems are at the fore
- Consider providing spiritual care, for example by a chaplain, and think about rituals that may offer support [2].

2 Involving Stakeholders

In the Netherlands, when the national guideline committee states that a guideline needs revision based on the available evidence, the Comprehensive Cancer Organisation (Dutch abbreviation: IKNL), a national organisation that supports the development of palliative care guidelines, approaches one professional association to appoint a chair, and several other ones to appoint representatives. Together, they constitute the core group that develops the guidelines, weighs their evidence and writes the modules. One author (Gijsberts) was a member of both core groups, acting on behalf of the Dutch Association of Elderly Care Physicians, and the other author (Olsman) acted on behalf of the Dutch Association of Chaplains, chairing the development of the *Grief Guidelines*. This demonstrates that implementation of spiritual care guidelines starts with involving stakeholders during the development of the guidelines.

Part of the development of guidelines is also to fine-tune the challenges healthcare professionals are facing when providing palliative care. Therefore, a survey among these professionals and other stakeholders is conducted. An invitation-only conference with experts is organised, where a priority of topics is discussed. Then, the core group makes the final prioritisation and determines which modules will (probably) be consensus or evidence based. With the help of a clinical librarian, the core group writes the evidence-based modules, based on systematic searches in several electronic databases. The other (consensus-based) modules are frequently based on review studies and on the expertise of the core group.

The drafts are shared with patient organisations, associations of professionals, and organisations with expertise in palliative care. They provide feedback on the guidelines, leading to a renewed version. Then, the renewed version is sent to the just-mentioned organisations again, with the request to accept it, meaning that the organisations' members agree to follow the recommendations. This process led to the acceptance of the Spiritual Care and Grief Guidelines by organisations such as the Alzheimer's Foundation in the Netherlands, the Collective Organisation for Palliative Care (Patients), and the Netherlands' associations for many professionals, including nurses and nursing aides, general practitioners, elderly care physicians, social workers, chaplains, and paramedics. Although guidelines are primarily written for professionals, patient input was incorporated during all phases of guideline development.

In summary, implementation of guidelines seems to be facilitated by or coalesces with an early involvement of several stakeholders representing relevant organisations, like patient organisations and associations for professionals. It is necessary to fine-tune to accommodate practitioners' challenges when trying to provide spiritual (and grief related) care. Also, organisations should be involved during revisions of the guidelines, and they should authorise or formally accept the guidelines, thereby recognising that it is a document to which they, and hence their members, want to adhere. This is an important step in ensuring that spiritual care guidelines are widely adopted.

3 Emphasising the Multidisciplinary Nature

Some people find it comforting or useful to receive support when they are struggling with spiritual or existential issues, while others prefer to be left alone. A minority requires the help of a specialised caregiver. When such care is provided, the guidelines propagate *multidisciplinary* spiritual care, which is in line with the idea that palliative care is best provided through a multidisciplinary team approach [27], which illustrates that implementation coalesces with an emphasis on the multidisciplinary nature of both guidelines.

In order for these guidelines to be genuinely multidisciplinary, spiritual care and spirituality should be visible. This means that spiritual care specialists, such as chaplains, need to be incorporated into organisations at the level of patient consultations, multidisciplinary team discussions, et cetera [28], which is in line with a survey study in our own country [29]. In a similar vein, Puchalski and colleagues emphasised the importance of interdisciplinary work in providing spiritual care [30], which may lead to an increase of the quality of and successful integration of spiritual care into healthcare in general.

Multidisciplinary spiritual care can only be provided when such care is properly organised, which includes facilitation of referral to specialist spiritual caregivers. This may be a chaplain or someone from the spiritual tradition of the patient and family—unless special expertise (for example, that of a psychologist or medical social worker) providing spiritual care on issues that have a strong social and/or psychological dimension is more suitable. The *Spiritual Care Guidelines* recommend making a referral, with the patient's permission, if the caregiver thinks (s)he cannot provide spiritual care that the patient and/or family is entitled to. This decision should be made on the following grounds:

- Content-based factors (spiritual crisis, need for rituals, etc.)
- Personal factors (lack of/insufficient expertise, subject matter that touches on one's own struggles)
- Practical factors (not enough time, professional boundaries)
- The availability of a specialised healthcare professional [1].

In a similar vein, the *Grief Guidelines* ask, 'When should a patient or family member be referred to a specialist healthcare professional?' and answers it as follows:

- Discuss the possibility of referral to a specialised healthcare professional if you are unable to provide that care yourself. Discuss this possibility:
  - When the patient/family member vocalises the need for care or guidance, or
  - When you notice this need
- When discussing this possibility, take into account whether the specialised care will be reimbursed financially [2].

To sum up, implementation seems to be facilitated by or associated with an emphasis on the multidisciplinary nature of the guidelines. This requires that, together with the other three dimensions of palliative care, the spiritual dimension should be made visible by specialists in spiritual care, such as chaplains. It also requires a proper organisation of spiritual care, which includes availability of referral options and financial reimbursement.

4 Increasing Professionalisation Through Education

For healthcare providers to optimally provide palliative care, education is important [31]. The same holds true for spiritual care, in which it is paramount to develop spiritual care competency, a process that includes reflection on the self and on one's own spirituality [28]. An intervention study in Brazil has provided some evidence for effects of educational interventions on spiritual care competency [32]. Interestingly, a South Korean mixed-methods study among 282 palliative care nurses found that the self-report on 'assessment and implementation of spiritual care' was, compared to other items, the lowest mean score [33], which adds to the urgency of good implementation of spiritual care guidelines into palliative care.

In our country, most curricula for physicians, nurses, psychologists, and social workers nowadays include a module on existential needs and spiritual care albeit sometimes as an elective course. Frequently, these modules refer to the *Spiritual Care Guidelines* and/or *Grief Guidelines*. Several chaplaincy curricula also include palliative care modules that help chaplain trainees to focus their spiritual care on a particular population, and within multidisciplinary settings. Also, various organisations in the Netherlands provide postgraduate training opportunities for spiritual care in palliative care. Among them are multidisciplinary masterclasses of one or more days, for physicians, chaplains, nurse specialists and nurses, sometimes organised as couples consisting of a chaplain and another professional, like a social worker, manager, nurse or physician. At a regional or local level, interdisciplinary spiritual care training is offered, often tailored to contextual needs, thus contributing to the implementation of spiritual care guidelines into palliative care as well.

In this section, we emphasised that education to develop spiritual care competency is paramount for the implementation of spiritual care guidelines into palliative care practices. In our own country, education on spiritual care frequently refers to spiritual care guidelines and, in many instances, it is part of curricula for nurses, social workers, physicians, psychologists, and several others. Most curricula for students in chaplaincy also include a module on palliative care that helps them to apply spiritual care to palliative care practices. Multidisciplinary postgraduate courses are also offered both to increase spiritual care competency and to stimulate multidisciplinary collaboration on spiritual care.

5 Investing in Scientific Research

A final element of implementation that we describe here is the investment in scientific research on spiritual care in palliative care. Both the evidence-based and consensus-based modules of the Grief and Spiritual Care Guidelines make clear that there is a lack of evidence in several areas. In particular, there is a lack of studies demonstrating spiritual care (in palliative care) patient outcomes [28, 34, 35], although we acknowledge that good spiritual care cannot be reduced to good outcomes [36].

A few years ago, the Netherlands Ministry of Health, Welfare and Sport assigned *ZonMw*, the Netherlands Institute for Health Care Innovation and Research [37], to develop a call for research in the field of spiritual care. This led to the ZonMw programme 'Spirituality and Chaplaincy at Home', [38] a programme that pays specific attention to implementation in home care situations, covering several action research studies. The programme has a broader focus than spiritual care in only *palliative* care at home. That broader focus is important because, while spiritual care in palliative care is available in our society, other clients and patients may need spiritual care as well.

A palliative care example of this programme is a study in which parents of a child with a life-threatening disease, caregivers, and researchers together explored the spiritual questions of parents and spiritual resources available to them. In another study, researchers tried to integrate tailor-made spiritual care from chaplains and volunteers for elderly people and people into palliative care settings [39]. The programme's projects have been successfully performed, and the outcomes are implemented into dissemination and implementation projects. Recently, the Ministry of Health Welfare and Sport (*VWS*) decided to follow up these implementation projects with funding for an overarching implementation project that will start in Autumn 2023.

Other already-existing ZonMw-research programmes on palliative care in our country, such as *Palliantie*, have funded the so-called *PLOEG-research*, which is a Dutch abbreviation for research on chaplaincy in palliative home care [40]. The projects resulted in the development of instruments to strengthen the embedding of spiritual care: a life story methodology that can be used by chaplains in palliative home care, and a referral tool for spirituality that may be used by all healthcare professionals.

In this section, we have elaborated on the importance of scientific research that explores the content of spiritual care in palliative care and that provides evidence in terms of patient outcomes. We have provided some examples of how spiritual care at home, and specifically chaplaincy in palliative care at home, have been studied, leading to implementation projects and simultaneously advancing the implementation of evidence-based guidelines into healthcare practices in several settings.

6 Spirituality in Various Healthcare Settings

In this section, we will describe a patient's journey (Mrs R). This example demonstrates how contextual features shape and are shaped by implementation. Meanwhile, some central topics in spiritual care in palliative care, like narrative, grief, hope, worries, and peace, are addressed.

6.1 Home

The General Practitioner (GP) of Mrs. R and her husband suggested that they should consider talking to a chaplain who could address their worries and possibly their anticipatory grief (see Box 1). Spiritual care may be provided in collaboration between chaplains, nurses, GPs, and others, like volunteers. For several years, chaplaincy at home has been reimbursed by the Netherlands Government of Healthcare, which illustrates that the implementation of spiritual care guidelines coincides with, or alternatively, may have affected, national healthcare policies. The centres for spiritual care at home match patients/family members and chaplains and offer training to improve spiritual care at home.

Box 1: Home

Mrs. R (82 years) lives in an assisted living facility, together with her husband. They have been married for 55 years and are very close. Over the past months, her health has been deteriorating, and she is increasingly suffering from fatigue and a lack of initiative after a bout of meningitis she contracted a year ago. During a meeting with the GP, Mr. R (84) asserts: 'Will the care provided by the nurses in the assisted living facility suffice? Or will, sooner or later, a nursing home be the only option'? It is difficult for Mrs. R to discuss her worries. She mostly falls silent when her husband mentions the topic. When the GP suggests that they talk to a healthcare chaplain, she declines the suggestion.

6.2 Hospital

The second night she is on a hospital ward, Mrs. R reveals her worries to a nurse, expressing the hope that rehabilitation would stimulate her recovery (see Box 2). Hope is a central topic in spiritual care [28], and this situation illustrates that, although hospitals recognise the importance of chaplains, for example during an existential crisis [41], nurses, because of their 24/7 presence, are frequently more likely to provide spiritual care, which is in line with other research [42]. This fact requires the training of hospital nurses in spiritual care provision [43], and chaplains remain necessary for referral or consultation. Hence, for palliative care guidelines to be adequately implemented into practices, contextual possibilities and restraints, like the presence or availability of caregivers, require attention.

Box 2: Hospital

A few weeks later, Mrs. R is admitted to the Intensive Care Unit, suffering from an urosepsis with high fever, low blood pressure and a very high pulse. After a few days, she improves and goes to a hospital ward, where the team tries to rehabilitate her. To alleviate her back pain, she is prescribed pain medication: paracetamol and NSAIDs and, if needed, oxycodone IR 5 mg. During the second night, she is in a lot of pain. The nurse gives oxycodone, and after half an hour, Mrs. R says, 'I have less pain', but she is crying silently. The nurse asks her if she would like to share anything about what is on her mind. Mrs. R replies, 'I'm worried that I can't go home anymore to spend the rest of my life with my husband'. When speaking with the night nurse, Mrs. R adds, 'All my hopes are set on rehabilitation', referring to a geriatric rehabilitation trajectory in a specialised nursing home ward. They sit together silently for a few minutes, until the nurse has to answer a call from another patient. When the nurse leaves, she asks for permission to report her worries and hope in the nursing chart. Mrs. R agrees and asserts, 'Thank you, for being here in such a supportive way'.

6.3 *Nursing Home*

During rehabilitation, Mrs. R and her caregivers try to realise her hope to improve (see Box 3). More than hospitals, nursing homes offer the opportunity to get to know patients and their life narrative, which could be seen as the start of spiritual care [28]. A narrative perspective on hope also helps to see the meaning that hope has to Mrs. R and her husband [14, 44]. When they receive the message that she cannot go home, however, the dynamics of hope take place, and the grief that comes with losing hope, requiring a compassionate attitude [14, 15]. Hence, for spiritual care to be implemented into palliative care, a focus on central themes, such as hope and grief, and narrative work is necessary, for which both guidelines offer several opportunities.

Box 3: Nursing Home
A few days later, Mrs. R is admitted to the Geriatric Rehabilitation Ward of a nursing home. She hopes rehabilitation will help her to walk independently with her walking frame, and make transfers independently from bed to chair, as well as going to the bathroom. These are the prerequisites to go back to the apartment in the assisted living facility. The physical therapist assesses her current abilities: Mrs. R needs help with transfers, and she walks under supervision with a walking frame. She turns out to be a very witty woman with a great ability for sharp observations of fellow patients and personnel. With passion, she talks about her former work as a social worker and how she combined this with caring for her family. During the first weeks of rehabilitation, the physician sees her often. During their conversations, she always returns to the wish to spend the last period of her life with her husband. Contact with the assisted living facility by the social worker shows that they cannot provide the help she needs. There is an interdisciplinary meeting with Mrs. R, her husband and daughter, physician, nurse, physical therapist, social worker, psychologist and chaplain. The social worker explains the limitations of the assisted living facility, and that, with the current results of Geriatric Rehabilitation, she will not be able to go back home. Her husband cries, and she comforts him silently.

6.4 *Hospice*

A process of grief may result in improved spiritual well-being, which may include, among many other elements, peace [45]. The link between hope, spiritual dimensions of dying, and peace has been described by others as well [46]. Typically, in a hospice setting, the implementation of guidelines with spiritual care as (one of) the central topic(s), is likely to include death and dying issues, like saying goodbye and searching or finding (final) peace. This seems to apply to Mrs. R as well, in expressing the wish to die at a hospice and having reviewed her life as a mother, and ultimately finding peace, also with the help of a psychologist. For her husband, the spiritual guidance by the chaplain was important, and helped him to stay and feel connected with his wife and other family members (see Box 4).

Box 4: Hospice
A few days later, Mrs. R tells her palliative care physician that she is trying to accept that she is not able to return home. She also seems to be preoccupied with the idea that she has not given her children the attention they needed when they were young. After an encounter with a psychologist, the latter states that Mrs. R is definitely not depressed, but actively looking back on her life, and taking stock. She is sad, the psychologist concludes, because she knows that she has to let go of her loved ones. For her husband, it is difficult to let her go: he is processing his own grief, and has four beneficial meetings with the chaplain. The following days, Mrs. R seems to be more peaceful. The last day the physician sees her alive is during the morning visit. Mrs. R states, 'I feel comfortable', and smiles, looking at her children. A little later that day, she passes away.

7 Conclusion

We conclude that implementation of the *Grief Guidelines* and *Spiritual Care Guidelines* seems to be facilitated by an early involvement of stakeholders, who represent relevant organisations, taking place from early development until authorisation. An emphasis on the guidelines' multidisciplinary nature also coalesces with or facilitates their implementation. Next to involvement of stakeholders and emphasis on their multidisciplinary nature, spiritual care guidelines can only be implemented when caregivers are trained in developing their spiritual care competency and multidisciplinary collaboration when it comes to spiritual care provision. All this, we conclude, should go along with scientific research, with a focus on the effects of spiritual care on patients and their family members.

While we drew from evidence, it should be said that no evidence is available for implementation of spiritual care guidelines in palliative care. Future studies should therefore explore what implementation of these guidelines actually looks like in various practices and determine what makes it successful. Another limitation is that we had to draw from our own experience when evidence was lacking. One of our biases is that we believe spiritual care to be important for good palliative care and have good reasons to do so (see Introduction). Nevertheless, implementation also requires that implementation is attuned to those who resist spiritual care.

Finally, this chapter does not describe everything necessary for successful implementation of spiritual care guidelines. Also, we have focused on nation-wide implementation, leaving aside local and regional implementation of spiritual care guidelines. It is worth mentioning the scoping review on strategies for implementation of palliative care organisational interventions and education in long-term care facilities by Collingridge Moore and colleagues [47]. Although they did not focus on spiritual care, there seem to be some overlap with our descriptions, as spiritual care is one of the four dimensions of palliative care, and their implementation strategies include multidisciplinary settings (nursing homes). Also, their study shows other factors that might be necessary for implementation, which we have not addressed in our chapter, such as sustaining ongoing change.

We do not believe that implementation of spiritual care guidelines in our country has been achieved entirely. Other elements and strategies than the ones described in this chapter may be necessary and starting to implement guidelines is not the same as permanent implementation. Nevertheless, we hope that this chapter helps healthcare providers, managers, policy makers and others to contribute to implementation of spiritual care (guidelines) into palliative care, with the ultimate goal to maintain or improve quality of life of patients with a life-threatening disease, their friends and family members.

Acknowledgement The authors thank Dr. Joep van de Geer, who was a member of the core group that developed the guideline Existential and Spiritual Aspects of Palliative care [1], for his helpful comments on several drafts of this chapter.

References

1. Integraal Kankercentrum Nederland. Guideline “Existential and spiritual aspects of palliative care”. Utrecht: IKNL; 2018.
2. Integraal Kankercentrum Nederland. Guideline “Grief in palliative care”. Utrecht: IKNL; 2022.
3. World Health Organization. Definition of palliative care [Internet]. 2002 [Updated 2020 Aug; cited 2023 Oct 28]. Available from: https://www.who.int/news-room/fact-sheets/detail/palliative-care
4. Liefbroer A, Ganzevoort RR, Olsman E. Addressing the spiritual domain in a plural society: what is the best mode of integrating spiritual care into healthcare? Ment Health Relig Cult. 2019;22(3):244–60. https://doi.org/10.1080/13674676.2019.1590806.
5. van de Geer J, Leget C. How spirituality is integrated system-wide in The Netherlands palliative care National Programme. Prog Palliat Care. 2012;20(2):98–105. https://doi.org/10.1179/1743291X12Y.0000000008.
6. Brinkman A, Gootjes J. NPTN: palliative care comes under the spotlight in The Netherlands. Eur J Palliat Care. 2009;16(3):151–3.
7. Integraal Kankercentrum Nederland. Richtlijnen palliatieve zorg altijd actueel online beschikbaar [Internet]. 2018 [cited 2023 Oct 28]. Available from: https://iknl.nl/nieuws/2018/richtlijnen-palliatieve-zorg-altijd-actueel-online

8. VWS (Ministry of Health, Welfare and Sport). VWS Plan van Aanpak Palliatieve Zorg 2008-2010 [Internet]. 2007? [cited 2023 Oct 28]. Available from: https://www.parlementairemonitor.nl/9353000/1/j4nvgs5kjg27kof_j9vvij5epmj1ey0/vi3ubexmomzt/f=/blg15483.pdf
9. Integraal Kankercentrum Nederland. Spirituele zorg. Landelijke richtlijn, versie 1.0 [Internet]. 2010 [cited 2023 Oct 28]. Available from: https://www.venvn.nl/media/qd5pzoi4/landelijke-richtlijn-spirituele-zorg-iknl-2010.pdf
10. Integraal Kankercentrum Nederland. Rouw. Landelijke richtlijn, versie 2.0 [Internet]. 2010 [cited 2023 Oct 28]. Available from: https://www.venvn.nl/media/m4chitge/richtlijn-rouw-pallialine-2010.pdf
11. Nolan S, Saltmarsh P, Leget C. Spiritual care in palliative care: working towards an EAPC task force. Eur J Palliat Care. 2011;18(2):86–9.
12. Nolan S. Hope beyond (redundant) hope: how chaplains work with dying patients. Palliat Med. 2011;25(1):21–5. https://doi.org/10.1177/0269216310380297.
13. Agrimson LB, Taft LB. Spiritual crisis: a concept analysis. J Adv Nurs. 2009;65(2):454–61. https://doi.org/10.1111/j.1365-2648.2008.04869.x.
14. Olsman E. Hope in palliative care: evidence, ethics, and aesthetics. In: van den Heuvel S, Scioli A, editors. The Oxford compendium of hope (in press). Oxford: Oxford University Press; 2024.
15. Olsman E, Willems D, Leget C. Solicitude: balancing compassion and empowerment in a relational ethics of hope-an empirical-ethical study in palliative care. Med Health Care Philos. 2016;19(1):11–20. https://doi.org/10.1007/s11019-015-9642-9.
16. Integraal Kankercentrum Nederland /Palliactief. Kwaliteitskader palliatieve zorg Nederland [Internet]. 2017 [cited 2023 Oct 28]. Available from: https://palliaweb.nl/zorgpraktijk/kwaliteitskader-palliatieve-zorg-nederland
17. Coelho A, de Brito M, Barbosa A. Caregiver anticipatory grief: phenomenology, assessment, and clinical interventions. Curr Opin Support Palliat Care. 2018;12(1):52–7. https://doi.org/10.1097/SPC.0000000000000321.
18. Patinadan PV, Tan-Ho G, Choo PY, Ho AHY. Resolving anticipatory grief and enhancing dignity at the end-of life: a systematic review of palliative interventions. Death Stud. 2022;46(2):337–50. https://doi.org/10.1080/07481187.2020.1728426.
19. Prigerson HG, Kakarala S, Gang J, Maciejewski PK. History and status of Prolonged Grief Disorder as a psychiatric diagnosis. Annu Rev Clin Psychol. 2021; May [cited 2023 Oct 30];17:109–26. Available from: https://www.annualreviews.org/doi/abs/10.1146/annurev-clinpsy-081219-093600
20. American Psychiatric Association. Grief: coping with the loss of your loved one [Internet]. 2020 [cited 2023 Oct 28]. Available from: https://www.apa.org/topics/families/grief
21. Corr CA. Coping with dying: lessons that we should and should not learn from the work of Elisabeth Kübler-Ross. Death Stud. 1993;17(1):69–83. https://doi.org/10.1080/07481189308252605.
22. Hagman G, editor. New models of bereavement theory and treatment: new mourning. New York, NY: Routledge; 2016.
23. Olsman E, Leget C, Duggleby W, Willems D. A singing choir: understanding the dynamics of hope, hopelessness, and despair in palliative care patients. A longitudinal qualitative study. Palliat Support Care. 2015;13(6):1643–50. https://doi.org/10.1017/S147895151500019X.
24. Robinson CA. "Our best hope is a cure." Hope in the context of advance care planning. Palliat Support Care. 2012;10(2):75–82. https://doi.org/10.1017/S147895151100068X.
25. Sachs E, Kolva E, Pessin H, Rosenfeld B, Breitbart W. On sinking and swimming: the dialectic of hope, hopelessness, and acceptance in terminal cancer. Am J Hosp Palliat Care. 2013;30(2):121–7. https://doi.org/10.1177/1049909112445371.
26. Stroebe M, Schut H, Boerner K. Cautioning health-care professionals. Omega. 2017;74(4):455–73. https://doi.org/10.1177/0030222817691870.
27. Fernando G, Hughes S. Team approaches in palliative care: a review of the literature. Int J Palliat Nurs. 2019 Sep;25(9):444–51. https://doi.org/10.12968/ijpn.2019.25.9.444.

28. Gijsberts MHE, Liefbroer AI, Otten R, Olsman E. Spiritual care in palliative care: a systematic review of the recent European literature. Med Sci. 2019;7(2):25. https://doi.org/10.3390/medsci7020025.
29. Ettema E, Wulp M, van Leeuwen R, Leget C. Embedding of the spiritual dimension in palliative consultation services in The Netherlands: inventory, evaluation, and recommendations. Prog Palliat Care. 2015;23(5):259–66. https://doi.org/10.1179/1743291X14Y.0000000113.
30. Puchalski C, Ferrell BR, Borneman T, DiFrances RC, Haythorn T, Jacobs C. Implementing quality improvement efforts in spiritual care: outcomes from the interprofessional spiritual care education curriculum. J Health Care Chaplain. 2022;28(3):431–42. https://doi.org/10.1080/08854726.2021.1917168.
31. World Health Organization. The role of education in palliative care [Internet]. 2021 [cited 2023 Oct 28], p. 15. Available from: https://iris.who.int/bitstream/handle/10665/345532/9789240033351-eng.pdf?sequence=1
32. Dezorzi LW, Raymundo MM, Goldim JR, de Oliveira CAV. Spirituality in the continuing education of healthcare professionals: an approach to palliative care. Palliat Support Care. 2019;17(6):662–7. https://doi.org/10.1017/S1478951519000117.
33. Kang KA, Chun J, Kim HY, Kim HY. Hospice palliative care nurses' perceptions of spiritual care and their spiritual care competence: a mixed-methods study. J Clin Nurs. 2021;30(7–8):961–74. https://doi.org/10.1111/jocn.15638.
34. Handzo GF, Cobb M, Holmes C, Kelly E, Sinclair S. Outcomes for professional health care chaplaincy: an international call to action. J Health Care Chaplain. 2014;20(2):43–53. https://doi.org/10.1080/08854726.2014.902713.
35. Liefbroer AI, Olsman E, Ganzevoort RR, van Etten-Jamaludin FS. Interfaith spiritual care: a systematic review. J Relig Health. 2017;56(5):1776–93. https://doi.org/10.1007/s10943-017-0369-1.
36. Olsman E. Resonance in a theopoetics of practice in practical theology. Int J Pract Theol. 2022;26(2):311–28. https://doi.org/10.1515/ijpt-2021-0031.
37. ZonMw. Working with knowledge to boost good health for all [Internet]. 2023 [cited 2023 Oct 28]. Available from: https://www.zonmw.nl/en
38. ZonMw. ZonMw-programma "Zingeving en geestelijke verzorging" [Internet]. 2020 [cited 2023 Oct 28]. Available from: https://www.zonmw.nl/nl/programma/zingeving-en-geestelijke-verzorging
39. ZonMw. CONNECT-studie: op weg naar passende geestelijke verzorging voor ouders van ernstig zieke kinderen in de thuissituatie [Internet]. 2020 [Updated 2023; cited 2023 Oct 28]. Available from: https://projecten.zonmw.nl/nl/project/connect-studie-op-weg-naar-passende-geestelijke-verzorging-voor-ouders-van-ernstig-zieke
40. ZonMw. PLOEG: Palliatief landelijk onderzoek eerstelijns geestelijke verzorging. Deelproject 2: in dialoog met je levensverhaal [Internet]. 2023 [cited 2023 Oct 28]. Available from: https://projecten.zonmw.nl/nl/project/ploeg-palliatief-landelijk-onderzoek-eerstelijns-geestelijke-verzorging-deelproject-2
41. van der Geer J. Learning spiritual care in Dutch hospitals: the impact on healthcare of patients in palliative trajectories [PhD thesis] Groningen: Rijksuniversiteit Groningen; 2017.
42. Taylor EJ. Client perspectives about nurse requisites for spiritual caregiving. Appl Nurs Res. 2007 Feb;20(1):44–6. https://doi.org/10.1016/j.apnr.2006.06.005.
43. Vlasblom JP, van der Steen JT, Jochemsen H. Spiritual care in a hospital setting: nurses' and patients' perspectives. Nurs Rep. 2012;2(1):e7. https://doi.org/10.4081/nursrep.2012.e7.
44. Olsman E, Leget C, Onwuteaka-Philipsen B, Willems D. Should palliative care patients' hope be truthful, helpful, or valuable? An interpretative synthesis of literature describing healthcare professionals' perspectives on hope of palliative care patients. Palliat Med. 2014;28(1):59–70. https://doi.org/10.1177/0269216313482172.
45. Gijsberts MJ, Echteld MA, van der Steen JT, Muller MT, Otten RH, Ribbe MW, Deliens L. Spirituality at the end of life: conceptualization of measurable aspects. A systematic review. J Palliat Med. 2011;14(7):852–63. https://doi.org/10.1089/jpm.2010.0356.

46. Swinton M, Giacomini M, Toledo F, Rose T, Hand-Breckenridge T, Boyle A, Woods A, Clarke F, Shears M, Sheppard R, Cook D. Experiences, and expressions of spirituality at the end of life in the intensive care unit. Am J Respir Crit Care Med. 2017;195(2):198–204. https://doi.org/10.1164/rccm.201606-1102OC.
47. Collingridge Moore D, Payne S, Van den Block L, Ling J, Froggatt K. Strategies for the implementation of palliative care education and organizational interventions in long-term care facilities: a scoping review. Palliat Med. 2020;34(5):558–70. https://doi.org/10.1177/0269216319893635.

GPSR Compliance

The European Union's (EU) General Product Safety Regulation (GPSR) is a set of rules that requires consumer products to be safe and our obligations to ensure this.

If you have any concerns about our products, you can contact us on ProductSafety@springernature.com

In case Publisher is established outside the EU, the EU authorized representative is:

Springer Nature Customer Service Center GmbH
Europaplatz 3
69115 Heidelberg, Germany

Batch number: 10732023

Printed by Printforce, the Netherlands